PRINCIPLES OF
# SOCIAL PSYCHIATRY

# PRINCIPLES OF
# SOCIAL PSYCHIATRY

EDITED BY

## DINESH BHUGRA
MSc MPhil MB BS MRCPsych
*Senior Lecturer*
*MRC Social & Community Psychiatry Unit*
*Institute of Psychiatry*
*De Crespigny Park, London*

AND

## JULIAN LEFF
BSc MD MRCP FRCPsych
*Director*
*MRC Social & Community Psychiatry Unit*
*Institute of Psychiatry*
*De Crespigny Park, London*

OXFORD

BLACKWELL SCIENTIFIC PUBLICATIONS

LONDON EDINBURGH BOSTON

MELBOURNE PARIS BERLIN VIENNA

First published 1993

Set by Excel Typesetters, Hong Kong
Printed and bound in Great Britain
at the University Press, Cambridge

DISTRIBUTORS

Marston Book Services Ltd
PO Box 87
Oxford OX2 ODT
(*Orders*: Tel:    0865 791155
        Fax:    0865 791927
        Telex: 837515)

USA
Blackwell Scientific Publications, Inc.
238 Main Street
Cambridge, MA 02142
(*Orders*: Tel:  800 759-6102
            617 876-7000)

Canada
Times Mirror Professional Publishing, Ltd.
130 Flaska Drive
Markham, Ontario L6G 1B8
(*Orders*: Tel: 800 268-4178
            416 470-6739)

Australia
Blackwell Scientific Publications Pty Ltd
54 University Street
Carlton, Victoria 3053
(*Orders*: Tel: 03 347-5552)

A catalogue record for this book is
available from the British Library

ISBN 0-632-03336-3

Library of Congress
Cataloging-in-Publication Data

Principles of social psychiatry/
    edited by Dinesh Bhugra and Julian Leff.
            p.        cm.
    Includes bibliographical references and index.
    ISBN 0-632-03336-3
    1. Social psychiatry.    2. Community psychiatry.
    I. Bhugra, Dinesh.    II. Leff, Julian P.
    [DNLM: 1. Community Psychiatry.    WM 31 P957]
    RC455.P72    1993
    616.89—dc20
    DNLM/DLC
    for Library of Congress

# Contents

# Contents

# List of Contributors

LEONA L.BACHRACH PhD, *Honorary Fellow, American Psychiatric Association, 19108 Annapolis Way, Gaithersburg, Maryland 20879, USA*

PAUL BEBBINGTON MA, PhD, MRCP, FRCPsych, *MRC Social and Community Psychiatry Unit, Institute of Psychiatry, De Crespigny Park, London SE5 8AF*

JENNIFER BEECHAM BA, *Research Fellow, Personal Social Services Research Unit, University of Kent at Canterbury, Canterbury, Kent CT2 7NF*

DINESH BHUGRA MSc, MPhil, MB, BS, MRCPsych, *Senior Lecturer, MRC Social and Community Psychiatry Unit, Institute of Psychiatry, De Crespigny Park, London SE5 8AF*

TRAOLACH S.BRUGHA MD, MRCPsych, *Department of Psychiatry, Clinical Sciences Building, Leicester Royal Infirmary, PO Box 65, Leicester LE2 7LX*

ALEC BUCHANAN MPhil, MB, ChB, MRCPsych, *The Maudsley Hospital, Denmark Hill, London SE5 8AZ*

ZAFRA COOPER DPhil, Dip. Clin. Psych., *Department of Psychiatry, University of Cambridge School of Medicine, Addenbrooke's Hospital, Cambridge CB2 2QQ*

ANTHONY D.COX MPhil, FRCP, FRCPsych, *Bloomfield Clinic, Guy's Hospital, St Thomas's Street, London SE1 9RT*

FRANCIS CREED MA, BChir, FRCP, FRCPsych, MD, *Professor of Community Psychiatry, University of Manchester, Department of Psychiatry, Rawnsley Building, Manchester Royal Infirmary, Oxford Road, Manchester M13 9WL*

MARTIN J.EALES MA, MB, PhD, MRCPsych, *The Maudsley Hospital, Denmark Hill, London SE5 8AZ*

MICHAEL GOSSOP BA, PhD, *Head of Research, Drug Unit, National Addiction Centre, The Maudsley Hospital, Denmark Hill, London SE5 8AZ*

ALAIN GREGOIRE MB, BS, MRCOG, MRCPsych, *Department of Psychological Medicine, King's College Hospital, Denmark Hill, London SE5 9RS*

TRUDY HARPHAM BA, PhD, *Urban Health Programme, Department of Public Health and Policy, London School of Hygiene and Tropical Medicine, Keppel Street, London WC1E 7HT*

PETER HILL MA, MB, BChir, MRCP, FRCPsych, *Professor of Child Mental Health, Department of Mental Health Sciences, St George's Hospital Medical School, Cranmer Terrace, Tooting, London SW17 0QT*

STEVEN HIRSCH BA, MD, MPhil, FRCPsych, *Professor of Psychiatry, Charing Cross and Westminster Medical School, Fulham Palace Road, London W6 8RF*

ANTHONY J.HOLLAND BSc, MPhil, MB, BS, MRCP, MRCPsych, *Institute of Psychiatry, De Crespigny Park, London SE5 8AF*

BRIAN JARMAN OBE, MA, PhD, FRCP, FRCGP, *Professor of Primary Health Care, St Mary's Hospital Medical School, Lisson Grove Health Centre, London NW8 8EG*

PHILIP JOSEPH BSc, MB, BS, MRCPsych, *Barrister at Law, Senior Research Fellow and Honorary Consultant in Forensic Psychiatry, Department of Forensic Psychiatry, Institute of Psychiatry, De Crespigny Park, London SE5 8AF*

STEVEN JOSEPH BSc, PhD, *Department of Psychology, University of Ulster, Coleraine, Co. Londonderry BT52 1SA, Northern Ireland*

MICHAEL B.KING MD, PhD, MRCP, MRCGP, MRCPsych, *Department of Academic Psychiatry, Royal Free Hospital, Pond Street, London NW3 2QQ*

MARTIN KNAPP BA, MSc, PhD, *Personal Social Services Research Unit, University of Kent at Canterbury, Canterbury, Kent CT2 7NF*

LIZ KUIPERS BSc, MSc, PhD, FBPS, *District Services Centre, Maudsley Hospital, Denmark Hill, London SE5 8AZ*

JULIAN P.LEFF BSc, MD, MRCP, FRCPsych, *Director, MRC Social and Community Psychiatry Unit, Institute of Psychiatry, De Crespigny Park, London SE5 8AF*

GLYN LEWIS MA, MSc, PhD, MRCPsych, *Institute of Psychiatry, De Crespigny Park, London SE5 8AF*

ANTHONY MANN MD, MPhil, FRCP, FRCPsych, *Institute of Psychiatry, De Crespigny Park, London SE5 8AF, and Royal Free Hospital School of Medicine, London NW3 2QQ*

PARIMALA MOODLEY MB, ChB, MRCPsych, *Senior Lecturer in Community Mental Health, Institute of Psychiatry, De Crespigny Park, London SE5 8AF*

EUGENE S.PAYKEL MD, FRCP, FRCPsych, *Department of Psychiatry, University of Cambridge School of Medicine, Addenbrooke's Hospital, Cambridge CB2 2QQ*

ANTHONY J.PELOSI MSc, MB, ChB, MRCP, MRCPsych, *Department of Psychiatry, Hairmyres Hospital, Glasgow G75 8RG*

BRICE PITT MD, FRCPsych, *Professor of Old Age Psychiatry, St Mary's Hospital Medical School, St Charles' Hospital, London W10 6DZ*

MICHAEL J.POWER BSc, MSc, DPhil, *MRC Social and Community Psychiatry Unit, and Department of Psychology, Royal Holloway and Bedford New College, University of London, Egham, Staines, London TW20 0EX*

GERALD F.M.RUSSELL MD (Ed), FRCP, FRCPEd, FRCPsych, *Institute of Psychiatry and The Maudsley Hospital, Denmark Hill, London SE5 8AZ*

JOHN STRANG MB, BS, MRCPsych, *Getty Senior Lecturer in the Addictions, National Addiction Centre, Institute of Psychiatry, London SE5 8AF*

GERALDINE STRATHDEE MB, BCh, BAO, MRCPsych, *Consultant Psychiatrist, The Maudsley Hospital, Denmark Hill, London SE5 8AZ*

BETSY THOM MA, BSc, CertEd, *Centre for Research on Drugs and Health Behaviour, 200 Seagrave Road, London SW6 1RQ*

GRAHAM THORNICROFT MB, BS, MA, MSc, MRCPsych, *The Maudsley Hospital, Denmark Hill, London SE5 8AZ*

PETER TYRER MD, MRCP, FRCPsych, *St Charles Hospital (St Mary's Hospital Medical School), London W10 6DZ*

JERRY WESTALL BA, *Research and Communications Officer, National Schizophrenia Fellowship National Office, 28 Castle Street, Kingston-on-Thames, Surrey KT1 1SS*

RUTH M.WILLIAMS MA, Dip. Psychol, CPsychol, *Department of Psychology, Institute of Psychiatry, De Crespigny Park, London SE5 8AF*

JOHN WING CBE, MD, PhD, FRCPsych, *Director, Research Unit, Royal College of Psychiatrists, 17 Belgrave Square, London SW1X 8PG*

LORNA WING MD, FRCPsych, *Centre for Social and Communication Disorders, Elliot House, 113 Masons Hill, Bromley, Kent BR2 9HT*

WILLIAM YULE MA, Dip. Psychol, PhD, FBPsS, CPsychol, *Institute of Psychiatry, De Crespigny Park, London SE5 8AF*

# Preface

This book is a celebration of the coming of age of social psychiatry. The interaction of brain and mind and the human being's social environment has been a topic of interest and debate for thousands of years. What is new, however, is the emphasis on the scientific study of the impact of social surroundings on mental health and illness. Urbanization, unemployment, poor housing, upbringing and culture are only some of the factors social psychiatry aims to look at. Relevant observations have been carried out by individuals in a variety of settings and from a diversity of backgrounds. For the first time authors from different disciplines, training and interest have come together to write what we hope will become a definitive text on social psychiatry.

The book should interest all those health care professionals who deal with human suffering and are looking for possible strategies to deal with various social factors. This book does not purport to cover psychiatry in its entirety, but encompasses major mental disorders and their inter-actions, as well as methodological and theoretical considerations. Clinicians of all levels in primary care and psychiatric care will find it useful, as will social workers, nurses and occupational therapists.

The problems involved in such a daunting task are many, but we have been fortunate in our authors who have delivered their manuscripts promptly. The authors, eminent experts in their chosen fields, have studied and written about the person – environment interactions as well as interpersonal relationships. The field is vast and ever expanding, but we hope we have provided a comprehensive view of the state of social psychiatry at the present time.

We would like to thank the staff of Blackwell Scientific Publications, and especially Dr Stuart Taylor and Mr Edward Wates for their help and patience in seeing this project through. We thank our authors for their contributions.

D.B., J.L.
*London, August* 1992

# List of Abbreviations

| | | | |
|---|---|---|---|
| ASQ | Attributional Style Questionnaire | GHQ | General Health Questionnaire |
| ATD | Aid to the Disabled | GMS | Geriatric Mental State |
| BAS | Brief Assessment Schedule | HIV | Human Immunodeficiency Virus |
| BDI | Beck Depression Inventory | HRSD | Hamilton Rating Scale for |
| CAMDEX | Cambridge Examination for | | Depression |
| | Mental Disorders of the Elderly | IES | Impact of Events Scale |
| CAP | Civil Addict Programmes | IMSR | Interview Measure of Social |
| CAPE | Clifton Assessment Procedures for | | Relationships |
| | the Elderly | IPDE | International Personality Disorder |
| CARE | Comprehensive Assessment and | | Examination |
| | Referral Examination | IPT | Interpersonal Psychotherapy of |
| CBA | Cost-Benefit Analysis | | depression |
| CBT | Cognitive Behavioural Therapy | IRU | Industrial Rehabilitation Unit |
| CEA | Cost-Effectiveness Analysis | LEDS | Life Events and Difficulties |
| CES-D | Centre for Epidemiologic Studies | | Schedule |
| | Depression Scale | MHA | Mental Health Act (1983) |
| CFI | Camberwell Family Interview | MHE | Mental Health Enquiry |
| CIS | Clinical Interview Schedule | MHF | Mental Health Foundation |
| CMHC | Community Mental Health Centre | MID | Multi-Infarct Dementia |
| CNS | Central Nervous System | MIND | National Association for Mental |
| COSTAR | Community Support Treatment | | Health |
| | and Rehabilitation programme | MMSE | Mini Mental State Examination |
| CPN | Community Psychiatric Nurse | NAMCS | National Ambulatory Care |
| CS | Conditioned Stimulus | | Survey |
| CSP | Community Support Programme | NETRHA | North East Thames Regional |
| CSR | Combat Stress Reaction | | Health Authority |
| CUA | Cost-Utility Analysis | NEWPIN | New Parents Infants Network |
| DIS | Diagnostic Interview Schedule | NSF | National Schizophrenic Fellowship |
| EAT | Eating Attitudes Test | PAQ | Patient Attitude Questionnaire |
| EE | Expressed Emotion | PAS | Personality Assessment Schedule |
| EI | Environmental Index | PDE | Personality Disorder Examination |
| EM | Explanatory Model | PHI | Physical Health Index |
| EMI | Elderly Mentally Infirm | PPV | Positive Predictive Value |
| EPDS | Edinburgh Postnatal Depression | PSE | Present State Examination |
| | Scale | PTSD | Post-Traumatic Stress Disorder |
| EPI | Eysenck Personality Index | QALY | Quality Adjusted Life Year |
| FACES | Family Adaptation and Cohesion | RAWP | Resource Allocation Working |
| | Scales | | Party |
| GDS | Geriatric Depression Scale | RDC | Research Diagnostic Criteria |

| | | | |
|---|---|---|---|
| RMPA | Royal Medico–Psychological Association | SID-P | Structured Interview for DSM-III Personality Disorders |
| RSU | Regional Secure Unit | SMR | Standardized Mortality Rate |
| SADS | Schedule for Affective Disorders and Schizophrenia | SNS | Social Network Schedule |
| | | SOS | Significant Other Scale |
| SANE | Schizophrenia: A National Emergency | SPAR | Standardized Psychiatric Admission Ratio |
| SAP | Standardized Assessment of Personality | SPS | Subsistence Production Society |
| | | SRE | Schedule of Recent Experience |
| SAS | Social Adjustment Scale | SRQ | Self Response Questionnaire |
| SBS | Social Behaviour Schedule | SSD | Social Service Department |
| SCAN | Schedule for Clinical Assessment in Neuropsychiatry | SSI | Supplemental Security Income |
| | | TAPS | Team for the Assessment of Psychiatric Services |
| SCANS | Sub-Clinical Anorexia Nervosa Scale | TOPS | Treatment Outcome Perspective Study |
| SCID-II | Structured Clinical Interview for DSM-III-R Personality Disorders | UPA | Underprivileged Area |
| SDAT | Senile Dementia of the Alzheimer Type | US | Unconditioned Stimulus |

# PART 1
# GENERAL PRINCIPLES
# AND RESEARCH METHODS

# Chapter 1
# Principles of Social Psychiatry

J.P. LEFF

## The historical development of social psychiatry in the UK

The simplest definition of social psychiatry is that it is what is done by social psychiatrists. This statement is not merely a tautology, since it allows individual practitioners the possibility of self-definition as social psychiatrists. This has indeed been part of the history of the subject since there is no universally accepted definition. The Royal Medico-Psychological Association (RMPA) had a Section of Psychotherapy and Social Psychiatry which was founded in 1946. The early meetings of the Section focused on social psychiatry, which, although never defined formally, was tacitly assumed to concern the study of social organizations. The group, large or small, was viewed as the entity on which social organizations were founded, and the term 'social' was used to mean 'appertaining to a group'. This conceptual framework arose from the experience during World War II of army psychiatrists, of whom the outstanding innovators were Maxwell Jones and Tom Main.

Jones was part of the Maudsley Hospital team at Mill Hill Emergency Hospital, and was in charge of the Effort Syndrome Unit with the remit to investigate the cause of chest pains experienced by soldiers under stress. He began to lecture to large groups of soldiers in the hospital on the origin of their symptoms and soon realized the therapeutic potential of the group itself (*The Guardian*, Obituary, 29 August 1990). At the same time Tom Main was working on a similar problem. He noted (personal communication, 1973) that the incidence of breakdown was higher in some army units than others, and these breakdowns could be legitimately viewed not only as throwing light on the problems of the sick indi-

vidual but on the organization to which he belonged (battalion, regiment, etc.). Main initiated studies of these social units in terms of disciplinary patterns, officer–man relations, welfare, social structure, roles, role-relations and culture. Main's research capitalized on a natural experiment. Assuming that the assignment of soldiers to units was relatively random and knowing that they were exposed to a similar level of combat stress, variations in psychiatric illness rates across units were very probably due to differences in the social organization of the units.

From the experiences of Jones and Main with group treatment and group structure emerged the concept of the 'therapeutic community', which Jones utilized first with returning prisoners of war and then established at Belmont Hospital, Sutton. It was therefore natural to associate social psychiatry with psychotherapy when the Section was founded in 1946. Incidentally, when Jones wrote about his innovatory establishment in 1952 his book was entitled 'Social Psychiatry'. In addition to an emphasis on therapy, the Section continued with studies of various organizations, especially hospitals.

The RMPA was superseded by the establishment of the Royal College of Psychiatrists in 1971, and two years later a Social and Community Psychiatry Group was set up within the College. Some continuity with the thematic concerns of the prior Section was maintained in that four members of the inaugural Executive Committee came from the Tavistock Institute of Human Relations and one other member was a therapist working with large groups. Furthermore, at the Annual General Meeting of the College in July 1974 the Group organized a session on 'Prospects in Social and Community Psychiatry', in which Tom Main was one of the three speakers. His topic was 'preventive psychiatry', which requires some explanation.

At the first meeting of the Executive Committee in November 1973, the concerns of the group were subsumed under three main headings:
1 Promotion of the best possible organization and disposition of community psychiatric services, both within the National Health Service (NHS) and outside it.
2 Development of a liaison with allied groups, such as general practitioners and social workers, and also with similarly relevant groups not directly involved with medical or social work functions such as teachers.
3 Fostering of educational and scientific interests, such as postgraduate training in social psychiatry, studies of social aspects of their treatment, and epidemiological, evaluative and operational inquiries.

It was anticipated that the Group would divide itself naturally into three working parties: the first area of concern would be dealt with under the heading of 'Services', the second under 'Prevention', and the third under 'Epidemiology'. In effect these divisions amounted to a recognition of major differences in interest, ideology and practice among the members of the newly established Group and its Executive Committee. The discipline of psychiatric epidemiology was well represented on the latter by eight members drawn largely from the three Medical Research Council Units dealing with that field and the General Practice Research Unit at the Institute of Psychiatry. The Committee also included a number of the pioneers in the development of community services for psychiatric patients. Although some of them had been involved in conducting research, their reputation had been established by their entrepreneurial activities in creating innovative services. They were obvious candidates for the Services working party. The third interest group on the Committee was mostly based at the Tavistock Institute of Human Relations. Its members can be viewed as providing the strongest link with the Section for Psychotherapy and Social Psychiatry in the RMPA. The Executive Committee of the Social and Community Psychiatry Group evidently considered that the most appropriate working

party for them to join was that on prevention, since Colin Murray Parkes was appointed as the convenor. Furthermore, at the AGM of the College in 1974 each of the three speakers in the session organized by the Group was clearly associated with one of the working parties. John Wing, Chairman of the Group, spoke on 'Epidemiology and research', and Jim Birley on 'Community services', while the topic addressed by Tom Main was 'Social and preventive psychiatry'.

To understand how the term 'preventive psychiatry' came to be associated with the therapeutic community movement, we turn to a paper by Hare (1969) in which he considered the relationship between social psychiatry and psychotherapy. He identified two growing points in preventive psychiatry, one of these being group methods of treatment. He viewed these as having close relations with psychotherapy, and in support of this cited a publication by David Clark (1965) on therapeutic communities. Clark was running a therapeutic community at Fulbourn Hospital, Cambridge, and later became a member of the Social and Community Psychiatry Group. Hare went on to argue that Maxwell Jones' view of the functions of a therapeutic community broadened from an initial focus on the treatment of established neurosis to include prevention. It is of interest that Hare considered the second growing point in preventive psychiatry to lie in the domain of public health and to be represented by facilities such as hostels and workshops. These were to become the remit of the Services working party of the College Group.

The claim that therapeutic communities, or indeed any other form of psychotherapy, constituted effective preventive psychiatry was viewed sceptically by the epidemiologists, since no research evidence was forthcoming. Considerable tension existed between the psychotherapists and the other members of the Psychotherapy and Social Psychiatry Section of the RMPA. Hare, himself an epidemiologist, argued forcefully 'that the epidemiological aspects of social psychiatry would develop more favourably in another soil, away from the immediate discussion and study of psychotherapy' (Hare 1969).

The uneasy association between psychotherapy

and social psychiatry within the RMPA was dissolved with the founding of the College, when Psychotherapy shared with Child Psychiatry the distinction of being the first Sections to be established. Interestingly, this was four years in advance of the official recognition of psychotherapy as a specialty by the Department of Health. Although psychotherapy achieved independence within the College south of the border, the Scottish branch retained a Section of Psychotherapy and Social Psychiatry. Correspondence from its chairman indicated continuing conflict in aims between the two arms of the Section. As we have recorded, within the Social and Community Psychiatry Group, continuity with one of the wellsprings of social psychiatry in therapeutic communities and group dynamics was maintained in the Prevention working party. In 1981 the Group was granted Section status, while under my chairmanship, and the existing working parties were discontinued, to be replaced by time-limited working parties constituted to deal with specific issues. In some respects this was a recognition that the initial ideological divisions had became less salient with the passage of time, and harmonious working relationships had become established. Nevertheless, there is a need to sustain a boundary between social psychiatry and psychotherapy, partly to limit the territory of the former to a manageable area, and partly to avoid acrimonious disputes over real or imagined imperialistic ambitions. Therefore we will propose a definition of social psychiatry and in its exposition will explore the possibility of establishing the boundary referred to above.

## A definition of social psychiatry

*Social psychiatry is concerned with the effects of the social environment on the mental health of the individual, and with the effects of the mentally ill person on his/her social environment.*

The phrase 'concerned with' is preferable to 'the study of' since, as we have noted, many people who regard themselves as social psychiatrists are primarily practitioners with little or no interest in research. The term 'mental health' is used in place of 'mental illness' since there is a tradition in this field of the promotion of health, beyond the prevention of illness and of the accumulation of handicaps.

In conceptualizing the social environment it may be helpful to invoke the image of a pebble thrown into water, surrounded by a set of concentric circles becoming ever fainter with increasing distance from the pebble. At the outer limit, culture exerts an effect, then moving progressively closer to the centre, workmates, friends and family are increasingly influential. What is the numerical lower limit of the social environment? Can two people be said to form an environment? The answer is clearly in the affirmative. Much of my own research has been concerned with the influence of the family on the course of psychiatric disorders. Depressed patients living with a spouse and schizophrenic patients living with a single elderly parent have been included in these studies (Vaughn & Leff 1976) and constitute legitimate subjects for research on social influences on psychiatric illness.

## Social psychiatry and psychotherapy

If dyadic relationships are fair game, then why not the relationship between a therapist and his/her client? It is not possible to find grounds on which this should be excluded. Indeed there are precedents for this topic being included in social psychiatric studies in the developing field of 'illness behaviour' and 'help-seeking behaviour'. This research has included investigation of the concepts of illness held by members of the public, their views as to appropriate treatments, and negotiation between clients and practitioners over their respective models of illness (Mechanic & Volkart 1960, Young 1981, Health Education Studies Unit 1982, Kleinman 1986). It would be logical to extend this work to encompass relationships between psychotherapists and their clients. Is the word 'relationships' the key for which we have been searching? Would it be tenable to argue that social psychiatry is legitimately concerned with client–therapist relationships but halts at the boundary to the psyche, ceding intrapsychic events to the psychotherapists and analysts? This would be tantamount to accepting B.F. Skinner's view of the individual psyche as a 'black box'. However, even within psychology, this approach has been superseded by the rapid development of cognitive theories incorporating the individual's concept of him/herself and the way he/she interprets external events (Brewin 1988). Within the extensive field of life events research, the notion of self-esteem has been invoked as a link between the lack of an intimate relationship and the depressing effect of events that represent a significant loss (Brown *et al.* 1986).

Life events research is one example of the longitudinal approach in social psychiatry (see also Chapter 10). Although the time-scale is relatively short, it entails the same assumptions as longer-term research, namely that experiences in the past are represented in the subject's memory and operate in the present to bring about pathological changes in the mental state. Past experiences include relationships as well as happenings (Brown *et al.* 1987). Whatever the theoretical construction proposed to represent past experiences, be it self-concept (George Brown) or latent schemata (cognitive theorists), it is difficult to maintain a clear distinction from psychodynamic theories concerning the self and its intrapsychic processes. Some psychoanalytical theories are easier to reconcile with a socioenvironmental view than others, for example, Freud's seduction theory rather than his later renunciation of it; the approach of the British Object Relations School rather than that of the Kleinian Group. However, the conclusion of this line of argument is that the topics that are of central concern to psychotherapy, in its broadest sense, also fall logically within the ambit of social psychiatry.

This conclusion is reinforced by the definition of psychotherapy proposed by Sutherland (1968): 'By psychotherapy I refer to a personal relationship with a professional person in which those in distress can share and explore the underlying nature of their troubles, and possibly change some of the determinants of these through experiencing unrecognized forces in themselves'.

Although psychotherapy and social psychiatry share a common interest in the origins of human distress, maybe they can be differentiated by their preferred methods of advancing understanding of its determinants. It is certainly true that social psychiatry has relied heavily on epidemiological techniques for its enquiries, involving large samples of subjects who are usually representative of a particular population. By contrast, research into psychotherapy and psychodynamics has tended to be hermeneutic, relying on the intensive study of individuals or small numbers of highly selected patients. However, current financial stringencies are placing increasing pressure on all practitioners to provide evidence for the effectiveness of their therapies. Partly in response to this pressure, psychotherapy is beginning to develop the academic arm of its discipline. Over the next few years it is predictable that psychotherapy will begin to utilize the research methods that are part of the stock in trade of social psychiatry, diminishing the differences in approach to which we have alluded.

This extended argument has not led to the erection of a solid barrier between social psychiatry and psychotherapy. The practitioners who belong to one or the other seem to have reduced the tensions that were evident in their joint Group in the RMPA by developing a gentleman's agreement on territorial demarcation. We shall respect this agreement and the reader will not find any chapters specifically dedicated to psychotherapy in this volume. However, many of the contributions deal with topics which lie in the area of overlapping interests between psychotherapy and social psychiatry.

## Cross-fertilization

Psychotherapy is not the only discipline which interdigitates with social psychiatry. Sociology, social psychology, social anthropology, and more recently cognitive psychology have all made valuable contributions to the development of social psychiatry. Durkheim's (1897) classical study of suicide provided central themes for two of the British MRC Units conducting research in social psychiatry (Norman Kreitman's and Peter Sainsbury's), while sociological critiques of institutions (e.g. Goffman 1968) stimulated Wing & Brown (1970) to initiate a line of research which continues to flourish to this day. The proposition that social support protects against mental ill health derived from both social psychology and social anthropology, and until recently was the major area of research in the Australian MRC Social Psychiatry Unit (Henderson *et al.* 1980).

Social psychologists have conducted numerous studies of group processes, which are of direct relevance to those roots of social psychiatry which emerged from group therapy. Medical sociologists have increased our understanding of the 'sick role' and of the relationship between doctors and their clients. Their work has illuminated the pathways traced by individuals as they undergo the transition into patients. The studies of migrants, which constitute a substantial corpus of research within the field of social psychiatry, would have been very ill-informed, if not fallacious, without the cooperation of social anthropologists. These related disciplines have provided a cornucopia of theories, concepts and techniques to enrich social psychiatry and stimulate its growth. Examples of this cross-fertilization will be encountered throughout this volume.

**The plan of the book**

In tracing the historical development of social psychiatry in the UK and in beating its bounds we have already encountered many of the important issues of principle and practice. The diversity of topics covered in this book are grouped into several sections, each of which we will introduce briefly here.

*Social causation*

The initial concern with groups rather than individuals has remained a dominant theme. Epidemiological studies have greatly enhanced our understanding of the links between factors in the social environment and the origin and course of psychiatric disorders. Inevitably, measurement has proved a major stumbling block, affecting both the delineation of psychiatric disorder and the quantification of social factors. In the absence of demonstrable pathological changes, classification of psychiatric illnesses remains contentious and subject to ideological fashion. Indeed in

recent years, the claim has been made by medical anthropologists that western psychiatric classification is a cultural construction that may be largely invalid when applied to non-western cultures (e.g. Littlewood 1990). This issue is addressed in Chapter 5. Despite these reservations, the standardization of psychiatric examination, for example by use of the Present State Examination (PSE) (Wing *et al.* 1974), and the setting-up of criteria for diagnostic classification, have revolutionized psychiatric epidemiology and made possible cross-cultural studies such as the International Pilot Study of Schizophrenia (World Health Organization 1973, 1979), and the Determinants of Outcome Project (Sartorius *et al.* 1986). The latter is a classical incidence study focused mainly on schizophrenia. Its value for social psychiatry hinges on the reliability and validity of measures of social factors. There is often a well-founded suspicion that qualities are being inappropriately treated as quantities. However, this area of measurement has been considerably strengthened by the development of non-parametric statistics, particularly modelling techniques.

While large-scale epidemiological studies have been informative, they can do no more than establish associations between social factors and the onset or course of psychiatric disorders. The gain from representative samples and large numbers of subjects is commonly offset by the lack of fine detail, making interpretation of the findings difficult. In an attempt to remedy this deficiency, in-depth interviewing has been combined with epidemiological survey techniques. This approach has characterized the work of George Brown (e.g. Brown & Harris 1978) and represents a significant advance in the technology of social psychiatry research. The contributions of epidemiology are the subject of a general review in Chapter 3, but are also referred to throughout Part 2, Social Causation. Research has focused on the effects on mental health of discrete happenings, such as life events (see Chapter 10) and disasters (see Chapter 27), and of large-scale social changes, including urbanization (see Chapter 20) and unemployment (see Chapter 21). Migration has been one of the outstanding social features of this century, with world wars and persecution providing the push, and the promise of economic betterment the pull. Migrants bring with them their own social and cultural values and afford opportunities for cross-cultural studies within a single country. These are considered in Chapters 5 and 29.

### Social consequences

The social consequences of psychiatric illness can be separated into those affecting the patient and those having an impact on the patient's social environment. The former may operate across the whole range of roles society expects the patient to perform: pair bonding, home making, parenting, working, and so on. Any psychiatric illness can impair one or all of these roles depending on its severity and chronicity, the premorbid level of social functioning attained by the sufferer, and the extent of social support available to cushion the impact of the illness. These issues are considered in Part 3, Social Consequences.

The effect of the psychiatrically ill patient on her/his immediate social environment is an area of increasing research activity almost exclusively focused on relatives, both within and outside the household. This upsurge is partly a response to relatives gaining enough confidence to voice their needs publicly and wield political power (e.g. in the National Schizophrenia Fellowship) and partly reflects the growth of consumerism in the NHS. These issues are taken up in Chapter 35.

The wider social environment, as represented by public attitudes to the mentally ill (see Chapter 22), has received sporadic attention over past decades. It has jumped into focus recently with the acceleration of programmes to move patients with learning difficulties and chronic psychiatric illnesses out of long-stay hospitals and into the community. There has undoubtedly been a reluctance to sample public attitudes, fuelled by the fear that asking questions would crystallize derogatory opinions. Furthermore, the results of attempts to educate the public on the subject of mental illness have been far from encouraging (e.g. Cumming & Cumming 1957). Nevertheless this field is beginning to open up with the dawning

awareness of the need to make positive efforts to integrate discharged long-stay patients into a more normal social milieu.

### Principles of management

A discussion of the setting-up of psychiatric services and their evaluation cannot proceed sensibly without an understanding of the local context. We will briefly describe the situation in the UK before highlighting specific chapters in this section of the book.

There is no doubt that the UK pioneered social psychiatry and remains at the forefront in this field. One reason for this pre-eminence lies in the activities of innovative individuals such as Maxwell Jones, who developed the concept of the therapeutic community, Tom Main, who became director of the Cassel Hospital in 1945, and Joshua Bierer, who opened the first psychiatric day hospital in the world. The novel services founded by these initiators stimulated similar developments in other countries, particularly North America, where Maxwell Jones eventually made his home. However, the NHS in the UK provided an ethos and a structure which was specially nurturant to such social methods of managing psychiatric illness. The ethos included a commitment to comprehensive care, which meant that every patient, however needy or lacking in resources, would find the services open to them. The NHS, even in its heyday, did not succeed in ironing out all inequalities of access to services, but the principle of equity led to the establishment of catchment areas in which there was at least an attempt to meet the needs of the whole population. There was also an advantage in the very small proportion of psychiatric services in the private sector, both from the standpoint of co-ordination of services and from that of the epidemiologist assessing service needs. One of the privileges bought with money is confidentiality, rendering data from private facilities virtually unobtainable. Another principle endorsed by the NHS is continuity of care. This was facilitated until 1983 by having health services and social services under the same management. Within the ambit of inpatient, outpatient and day patient services continuity can usually be guaranteed, and is certainly simpler to achieve than in the countries, like Germany, where the inpatient and outpatient facilities are staffed by different doctors belonging to separate institutions.

In the NHS, continuity between hospital services and general practitioners (GPs) has to be maintained by a positive effort on both sides, but there have always been professionals who were able to traverse any crevasses that opened up. In the past, social workers tended to fulfil this function. Recently, this role has increasingly become the remit of the relatively new cadre of community psychiatric nurses (CPNs). Whether based in hospital, community mental health centres, or in general practice, CPNs form a link between hospital services, GPs and patients in their own homes. Originally launched as an outreach service to bring depot neuroleptics to defaulting patients, CPNs soon came to undertake many therapeutic functions of a social nature. Another feature, which the NHS inherited, that facilitated the development of social psychiatry was the hallowed tradition of home visits by GPs. This made it acceptable for CPNs to come to patients' homes and enabled them to work with those families who could not or would not attend psychiatric clinics. This practice often evokes surprise in the USA, where doctors who are equivalent to GPs work in offices which patients are expected to visit.

The reader will have noticed the frequent use of the past tense in relation to the beneficial influence of the NHS on the development of social psychiatry. This should not be dismissed as nostalgia for a Golden Age. The NHS is facing radical reorganization, an increasing reliance on market forces to regulate the use of services, and a commensurate growth in the private sector. The future pattern is unpredictable, but both the ethos and the structure that were favourable to social psychiatry are almost certain to be eroded.

## EVALUATION OF SERVICES

One element in the new philosophy of the NHS is an emphasis on the responsibility of practitioners to ensure that they are providing an effective and efficient service. The notion of accountability has always been around, but has recently been accorded a high profile, the peak of which is cost-effectiveness. A critical attitude to health services characterized social psychiatry from its beginning. One of the principal aims of the therapeutic community movement was to flatten the hierarchy that psychiatry had inherited from medicine, in which the patient occupied the lowest stratum (Birley 1968). Furthermore one of the wellsprings of the early research in social psychiatry, such as Wing & Brown's (1970) three hospitals study, was the criticism levelled by sociologists at psychiatric institutions. It is now widely acknowledged that planning of services and evaluation must go hand in hand if planning is to have a rational basis. Ideally they constitute a cycle, in which new services are evaluated and then modified according to the results of the evaluation, and so on (Wing 1986).

Health services evaluation is generally looked down on in the research world as second class science. This is a consequence of the limited control the research worker can exert over the experiment. The first priority for any service developer is to get the service up and running and to convince the funders that it is doing a good job. The demands of scientific methods for randomized controlled trials and objective assessments often conflict with these aims, resulting in compromises over design issues. These problems need to be seen as challenges to the ingenuity of the best researchers rather than reasons for relegating this type of research to the bottom of the heap.

Evaluation of a service involves attention to all its components: the clients, the professional care-givers, the management and coordination of the service, and its impact on informal care-givers. The needs of the patients have often been considered, but rarely their views as to the adequacy of the service and their satisfaction or dissatisfaction with it. Given the current importance ascribed to consumerism, it is no longer acceptable to ignore the opinions of the clients, even when they happen to be long-stay residents in psychiatric institutions. The assessment of needs for services is no simple matter, even though it is the crux of rational planning. Epidemiological surveys have produced a plethora of data about the amount of psychiatric morbidity in specific populations, but it is by no means obvious what services should be provided to cope with it. The bulk of this morbidity is formed by depressive and anxiety neuroses, for which the most cost-effective services have yet to be identified.

Since establishing the effectiveness of treatments is an essential preliminary to recommending their incorporation in services, it is not surprising that trials of treatment have been undertaken by social psychiatrists. These have involved not only family interventions (e.g. Leff *et al.* 1982, 1989), but also drug trials, albeit of a preventive nature (e.g. Leff & Wing 1971). Studies of various types of intervention in families, including dyadic relationships, offer the added bonus of elucidating the direction of cause and effect between the patient's symptoms and her/his immediate social environment. This kind of research has become a very important adjunct to epidemiological studies.

At the other end of the scale are studies of policy, for instance that of replacing the traditional psychiatric hospital with district-based services. A study of this nature has been mounted by the Team for the Assessment of Psychiatric Services (TAPS) which was established by the North East Thames Regional Health Authority to evaluate reprovision for Friern and Claybury Hospitals (North East Thames Regional Health Authority 1990). The research has been proceeding for five years and will probably continue for another five. It includes assessment of all long-stay non-demented patients in both hospitals, numbering over 1000, evaluation of transfer of the services for dementia patients and the acute admission wards into the local health districts, a detailed comparison of the costs of hospital and community care for each service (Knapp *et al.* 1991) and a sociological study of the decision-making processes involved (Tomlinson 1990). Additional sub-studies are concerned with staff views about the appropriate training for community work, public attitudes towards the reprovision programme, and observation of patients' social interaction in informal settings (Dunn *et al.* 1990). The ramifications of a project with so broad a remit

are almost endless. If the research is of a high quality it affords the opportunity of influencing a policy which has already profoundly affected the lives of hundreds of thousands of people. In addition to the practical pay-off, there are important scientific issues that can be tackled, for instance whether the negative symptoms and the cognitive deficits of long-term schizophrenic patients improve when they live under less institutional conditions.

Many of the issues relevant to the evaluation of services are dealt with in Chapters 28–34. The book is rounded off with a look into the future (see Chapter 36).

## References

Birley J.L.T. (1968) The social psychiatrist's view of medical care. *Lancet* ii, 1181–1184.

Brewin C.R. (1988) *Cognitive Foundations of Clinical Psychology.* Lawrence Erlbaum, London.

Brown G.W., Andrews B., Harris T. *et al.* (1986) Social support, self-esteem and depression. *Psychological Medicine* 16, 813–831.

Brown G.W., Bifulco A. & Harris T. (1987) Life events, vulnerability, and onset of depression: some refinements. *British Journal of Psychiatry* 150, 30–42.

Brown G.W. & Harris T. (1978) *Social Origins of Depression: A Study of Psychiatric Disorders in Women.* Tavistock, London.

Clark D.H. (1965) *Administrative Therapy: The Role of the Doctor in the Therapeutic Community.* Tavistock, London.

Cumming E. & Cumming J. (1957) *Closed Ranks.* Harvard University Press, Cambridge.

Dunn M., O'Driscoll C., Dayson D., Wills W. & Leff J. (1990) The TAPS Project IV: an observational study of the social life of long-stay patients. *British Journal of Psychiatry* 157, 842–848.

Durkheim E. (1951) *Suicide: A Study in Sociology.* Free Press, Glencoe, Illinois. Originally published 1897, F. Alcan, Paris (translated by J.A. Spaulding & G. Simpson).

Goffman E. (1968) *Asylums: Essays on the Social Situation of Mental Patients and Other Inmates.* Penguin, Harmondsworth.

Hare E.A. (1969) The relation between social psychiatry and psychotherapy. In Foulkes S.H. & Stewart Prince G. (eds) *Psychiatry in a Changing Society.* Tavistock, London.

Health Education Studies Unit (1982) Final Report on the Patient Project. Health Education Council, London.

Henderson A.S., Byrne D.G., Duncan-Jones P., Scott R. & Adcock S. (1980) Social relationships, adversity and neurosis: a study of associations in a general population sample. *British Journal of Psychiatry* 136, 574–583.

Jones M. (1952) *Social Psychiatry: A Study of Therapeutic Communities.* Tavistock, London.

Kleinman A. (1986) *Social Origins of Distress and Disease: Depression, Neurasthenia and Pain in Modern China.* Yale University Press, New Haven.

Knapp M., Beecham J., Anderson J. *et al.* (1990) The TAPS Project, III: Predicting the community costs of closing psychiatric hospitals. *British Journal of Psychiatry* 157, 661–670.

Leff J., Berkowitz R., Shavit N., Strachan A., Glass I. & Vaughn C. (1989) Trial of family therapy vs a relatives group for schizophrenia. *British Journal of Psychiatry* 154, 58–66.

Leff J., Kuipers L., Berkowitz R., Eberlein-Fries R. & Sturgeon D. (1982) A controlled trial of social intervention in schizophrenic families. *British Journal of Psychiatry* 141, 121–134.

Leff J. & Wing J.K. (1971) Trial of maintenance therapy in schizophrenia. *British Medical Journal* 3, 599–604.

Littlewood R. (1990) From categories to contexts: a decade of the 'new cross-cultural psychiatry'. *British Journal of Psychiatry* 156, 308–327.

Mechanic D. & Volkart E.H. (1960) Illness behaviour and medical diagnosis. *Journal of Health and Human Behaviour* 1, 86–96.

North East Thames Regional Health Authority (1990) The Fifth Annual TAPS Conference Report.

Sartorius N., Jablensky A., Korten A. *et al.* (1986) Early manifestations and first-contact incidence of schizophrenia in different cultures. *Psychological Medicine* 16, 909–928.

Sutherland J.D. (1968) The consultant psychotherapist in the NHS: his role and training. *British Journal of Psychiatry* 114, 509–515.

Tomlinson D. (1990) Stick to the agenda. *Health Service Journal* 100, 392–394.

Vaughn C. & Leff J. (1976) The influence of family and social factors on the course of psychiatric illness: a comparison of schizophrenic and depressed neurotic patients. *British Journal of Psychiatry* 129, 125–137.

Wing J.K. (1986) The cycle of planning and evaluation. In Wilkinson G. & Freeman H. (eds) *The Provision of Mental Health Services in Britain: The Way Ahead.* Royal College of Psychiatrists Special Publication, London.

Wing J.K. & Brown G.W. (1970) *Institutionalism and Schizophrenia.* Cambridge University Press, London.

Wing J.K., Cooper J.E. & Sartorius N. (1974) *The Measurement and Classification of Psychiatry Symptoms.* Cambridge University Press, London.

World Health Organization (1973) *The International Pilot Study of Schizophrenia*, vol. 1. WHO, Geneva.

World Health Organization (1979) *Schizophrenia: An International Follow-up Study.* John Wiley, Chichester.

Young A. (1981) When rational men fall sick: an enquiry into some assumptions made by medical anthropologists. *Culture, Medicine and Psychiatry* 5, 317–335.

# Chapter 2
# Sociology and Social Psychiatry

M.J.EALES

## Introduction

There are many strands in the relationship between sociology and social psychiatry. Many areas of social psychiatry discussed in later chapters, such as social causes of psychiatric disorder, the implications of unemployment or urbanization, or the characterization of social networks, originated in the work of sociologists and utilize specific methods or concepts developed there. There is a particularly close relationship between sociology and psychiatric epidemiology. Studies into the distribution and causes of various types of problematical behaviour were a focus of social research from its beginnings, and much early work in what is now recognizable as psychiatric epidemiology was conducted by non-medical social researchers (Grob 1986). On one hand there are continuities between early fact-finding surveys of social problems such as Rowntree's studies of poverty in Victorian England or the national censuses originating in the same period in many countries, and modern epidemiological research directed at service planning. On the other hand, classic examples of sociological explanation focusing on the impact of wider social factors on individual behaviour (e.g. Durkheim's study of suicide) foreshadow modern epidemiological research into social causes of psychiatric disorders. Certainly much sociological research into causes of individual disorders has concentrated on macrosocial factors (e.g. social integration (Faris & Dunham 1939, Leighton et al. 1963) or economic factors (Brenner 1973, Catalano & Dooley 1977)), whereas modern epidemiological research has restricted attention closer to the individual level, largely for methodological reasons. But the interest in macrosocial factors continues in research into the mediation of wider social influences at the individual level, for example the relationship of social class or culturally based patterns of social attachment to factors predicting vulnerability to depression and anxiety (Brown & Harris 1978a, Prudo et al. 1981, 1984), or the interaction of social structures with individual lives to produce continuities in adversity across the life-span (Rutter & Madge 1976, Quinton et al. 1984, Harris et al. 1990). These important issues linking sociology with social psychiatry have now been largely incorporated within the discipline and are treated in detail in later chapters.

Sociology also has a role in providing a wider perspective on the lives of people with psychiatric disorders, and on the mental health services, by drawing attention to features and problems shared with other groups in society and other organizations. Examination of these common features highlights some wider social phenomena which may be highly relevant in explaining, for example, the social handicaps experienced by people with psychiatric disorders, or the development or maintenance of pathogenic social environments such as 'high Expressed Emotion' households, depleted social networks, or impoverished institutional conditions. Similarly, organizational processes of a more general nature have an important bearing on the functioning and effectiveness of the mental health services themselves. It is on this comparative approach that the present chapter focuses.

## Deviance and stigma

'Deviance' is an open-ended category which might include delinquency and criminality, vagrancy, drug or alcohol abuse, sexual deviance, and stigmatizing physical illness or disability, as well as psychiatric disorder. These groups are diverse and individuals falling within them are clearly not united by any common property of their behaviour or psychological make-up. The only justification for grouping them together is that they share certain aspects of their social situations and are exposed to common experiences in their dealings with members of the 'normal' community. 'Deviance' in this sense is closely linked with 'stigma', and the social processes to be discussed overlap with those affecting other groups subject to devaluation and discrimination by their fellow citizens, such as members of certain ethnic minorities, the poor or the unemployed. Some of the experiences faced by deviant individuals are also minor ingredients in the everyday lives of a much wider group of people who wish to conceal or neutralize disagreeable facts about themselves (Goffman 1968g). Although people with psychiatric disorders have to contend with the issues of deviance and stigma mostly in their contacts with the wider community, stigma may also be attached *within* the mental health services to particular groups of patients, such as those who are violent, socially unresponsive, or carry certain diagnoses (McGarry & West 1975, Mollica & Redlich 1980, Lewis & Appleby 1988). For such individuals the following discussion may be doubly relevant.

Deviant individuals occupy devalued statuses which carry practical and social disadvantages. They are liable to encounter disapproval or rejection and tend to be excluded from normal avenues of social participation, an exclusion that may range from mere awkwardness or distance in interaction with other members of society, through various informal sanctions and forms of discrimination, to enforced segregation. It is characteristic that a deviant status tends to dominate other aspects of a person's life, and influence all other statuses he might hold. This is mainly due to a range of denormalizing social phenomena which magnify the perceived difference between deviant individuals and other people, or cause them to acquire additional abnormal attributes.

### Social perception of deviant individuals

In the first place there is a tendency for deviant individuals to be perceived in a categorical way in which attention is focused on abnormal aspects of their behaviour or personality, and inferences are made about other personal attributes, often inaccurately, on the basis of widely held, over-generalized beliefs (*stereotypes*) about the characteristics of particular categories of person (Ashmore & Del Boca 1981, Tajfel 1981). These inferences may be triggered by an observable feature (e.g. a person talking to himself), or merely by the knowledge of an individual's deviant status. Some inferences, such as that of dangerousness in psychiatric patients, are relatively specific to the stereotypes of particular deviant groups, while others, such as incompetence, lack of cleanliness, moral blemish, are drawn from a common fund of undesirable attributes which is distributed across the stereotypes of various kinds of deviance. Beliefs embodied in stereotypes are not immune to change through experience, and those who have had social contact with people with psychiatric disorders are less likely to express unfavourable attitudes towards them (Jones *et al.* 1984a). Stereotypes which discourage such contact will therefore contribute to their own perpetuation.

Biased interpretation of observed characteristics is closely related to stereotyping. Examples from psychiatric settings are given by Goffman (1968b), where facts about patients' lives were highlighted by professional staff as evidence of abnormality which, in other persons, would have been regarded as innocuous and disregarded. While reflecting the self-validating property which stereotypes share with other cognitive schemata, this also illustrates the fact that the process of attending to and judging putatively deviant traits is context-dependent: 'allowances' or normalizing interpretations are less likely to be made where the person concerned is in an abnormal environment or is seen to be socially dissimilar in other ways to the person judging the behaviour (evidence relevant to mental illness is reviewed by Horwitz (1982)). This will usually tend to exaggerate the perceived abnormality of deviant individuals, but also accounts for the fact that early signs of mental illness tend to be discounted by close relatives of an affected individual, even when they are clearly apparent to outsiders (Clausen & Yarrow 1955, Schwartz 1957).

*Acquisition of additional deviant attributes*

At various times deviant individuals have been obliged to advertise their status, by such means as distinctive clothing or physical mutilation. Although the direct and deliberate creation of additional deviant attributes is no longer widespread, they continue to arise as consequences of social discrimination, or as unintended side-effects of official policies.

There is plentiful evidence that people with psychiatric disorders are discriminated against in areas such as employment and social relationships (see Chapter 22). Social contacts are inhibited by aversive stereotypes and by the propensity for stigma to spread to those who associate with a deviant individual (Davis 1961, Goffman 1968f), a phenomenon amply documented in relation to psychiatric disorder (Yarrow *et al.* 1955, Freeman & Simmons 1961, Birenbaum 1970, Jones *et al.* 1984b). At a later stage, discrimination and consequent social disadvantage tend to perpetuate themselves, through reduced opportunity and the stigma attached to disadvantage itself. A 'poor employment record' and lack of work skills and experience make it less likely that a person will be successful in getting a job; isolated individuals have fewer opportunities to meet people and form relationships, and are not widely sought as friends. Although not the only factors, phenomena of these kinds are probably important in the continuities in employment patterns and social contacts found in longitudinal studies of psychiatric patients (Monck 1963, Brown *et al.* 1966, Strauss & Carpenter 1974, 1977).

Official policies which unintentionally give rise to additional deviant attributes may do so gratuitously or with some degree of rational justification, although the balance between benefits and social costs in the latter case requires careful examination. Compare, for example, conspicuous side-effects caused by medication, and the practice (discontinued only relatively recently in some British institutions) of routinely shaving the heads of mentally handicapped individuals to prevent infestation with head lice. Gratuitously abnormal features of the physical and social environments in which people with mental illness or mental handicap may find themselves are discussed at length by Wolfensberger (1972).

*Restitutive processes*

Many of the processes described above are mutually reinforcing and tend to produce a widening penumbra of abnormality around an initial deviant trait. Over time there may be a partially orderly sequence of events making up a 'career', structured by the social institutions and subcultural groups which deviant individuals come into contact with, in the course of which an increasing range of abnormal attributes is collected and predictable changes in the individual's outlook occur (Goffman 1968c,e, Matza 1969). However, pressures in the opposite direction should not be overlooked. Official measures for the treatment or rehabilitation of various deviant groups are obvious examples, but informal restitutive processes are also widespread: for example, expectations about deviant behaviour may be 'self-defeating' where they lead to special provisions or allowances which assist the putative deviant individual in responding normally (Jones *et al.* 1984d). 'Normalization theory' (e.g. Wolfensberger 1970, 1972) has demonstrated the very wide scope for deliberate normalizing policies, both within and outside the official health and social services.

*Variability in social responses to deviance*

Although broad generalizations can be made, attitudes and responses to deviance are neither constant nor homogeneous. Individual differences in social attitudes towards deviant groups and ethnic minorities are related to personality attributes such as tolerance of ambiguity (Adorno *et al.* 1950, Allport 1954), but there are also shorter-term socioeconomic influences on the distribution of these attitudes. Authoritarianism and intolerance of deviant groups tend to increase in periods of economic recession, and subside during sustained economic expansion (Sales 1973, Scott & Scull 1980, Jones *et al.* 1984c). One reason for this is that in times of labour shortage there is a pressure for otherwise marginal members of society to enter normal roles in the work force. There may also be a general tendency for social norms to be defined more narrowly and inflexibly whenever social cohesion is disrupted, a relationship implicit in the much wider theory of social solidarity proposed by Durkheim (1893). Relevant evidence is scanty, but some data have been presented linking threats to social cohesion with escalations in such activities as the burning of 'witches' in New England, the lynching of black people in the southern USA, and attempts to eradicate homosexuality from the armed forces (Erikson 1966, Inveriarity 1976, Davies 1982).

There have also been obvious changes on a longer time-scale. Since the early twentieth century there have been substantial changes in orientation towards deviant and disadvantaged groups in western societies, and the stigma attached to some forms of behaviour has been considerably reduced. Discussion of the reasons for these secular changes, and of cross-cultural variation, is beyond the scope of this chapter.

## Individuals' management of stigma and disadvantage

Stigma and disadvantage have a predictable impact, although individuals' responses vary (e.g. Eales 1989). Feelings of shame are frequent where there is a pervasive sense of rejection or disapproval by other people, and studies among psychiatric patients and their relatives indicate that these consequences remain prominent (Yarrow *et al.* 1955, Freeman & Simmons 1961, Swanson & Spitzer 1970, Angermeyer *et al.* 1987). Nonspecific strategies adopted to deal with the resulting constraints on social interaction and relationships include the control or concealment of personal information, and selective avoidance of social contact (Davis 1961, Goffman 1968d, Jones *et al.* 1984e). Avoidant behaviour may lead to substantial social disability regardless of how other people actually behave.

Selective association with similarly placed individuals is often an important element in the management of stigma. Groups thus formed have a number of possible functions for their members: providing a protected milieu for interaction and

relationships, a source of information, and specific emotional support through the transmission or modelling of coping mechanisms, or through the availability of a set of ideas reinterpreting members' experiences, re-evaluating their status, or excusing their conduct (Bales 1944, Sykes & Matza 1957, Gussow & Tracy 1968). They may advocate their members' interests in a wider arena, as do some of the self-help organizations for people with psychiatric disorders and their relatives. Beside the possible benefits there may be 'membership costs', such as the public acceptance of a deviant identity, which may hinder integration with the 'normal' community (Birenbaum 1970). Support groups for patients or their relatives organized by public services share some of the same features (see Chapter 35).

### SECONDARY DEVIANCE

A more specific interaction between particular types of deviant behaviour and the social responses they elicit has been suggested by 'societal reaction' theory, first formulated systematically by Lemert (1951, 1967a; see also Becker 1963). The fundamental assertion of this approach was that by placing an individual in a deviant status, further deviant behaviour (*secondary deviance*) would occur as a result of his adjusting to, or reacting against, the expectations of others and the social constraints imposed on him (Lemert 1967b). It was suggested that this could initiate a cycle of interaction between the behaviour of the deviant individual and that of other people which would amplify or perpetuate a specific type of deviant behaviour. The official 'labelling' of deviance was regarded by some as critical in this process.

'Secondary deviance', and 'labelling' and its effects, each aggregate a number of distinct phenomena, and the concepts refer to areas of inquiry rather than specific causal processes (Plummer 1979, West 1985). However, particular emphasis was given to the motivation of deviant behaviour by the active adoption of an altered self-concept corresponding to the deviant status held, paralleling changes in motivation and conduct which occur with transformations of status in other, non-deviant, contexts: for example, the acceptance ('internalization') of expectations attached to an occupational role in the course of training or employment (Becker & Carper 1956, Becker & Strauss 1956, Strauss 1962). This type of explanation is most credible where novices undergo education into a deviant subculture: homosexuality, illicit drug use and delinquency provide examples (Becker 1953, Matza 1969). The explanations of psychotic symptoms offered using these concepts are generally unconvincing (Scheff 1966; see discussion by Gove 1970, Link 1982), although role expectations are relevant in explaining some aspects of illness-related behaviour in psychiatric disorders, discussed in the following section.

## Social implications of illness

A systematic approach to the social implications of illness was introduced by Parsons (1952), who identified a number of rights and obligations attached to being ill in modern western societies. He noted that individuals who were ill were not held responsible for their condition and enjoyed exemption from normal role obligations (depending on the seriousness of the illness, and its being recognized as legitimate by others); beside these rights were obligations to strive to regain health and to cooperate appropriately with medical advice in attaining this. Parsons' formulation of the 'sick role' has been criticized on a number of counts, and more elaborate frameworks have been proposed (e.g. Freidson 1970). In particular it assumes that expectations throughout society are uniform, and fails to distinguish between different types of illness, which may carry different social expectations. Chronic illnesses fit poorly into the scheme.

The related concept of 'illness behaviour' was introduced by Mechanic & Volkart (1961) to refer to individual differences in inclination to enter the sick role given a particular level of symptoms. Later it was given a more general meaning as it was recognized that individuals and social groups vary along multiple dimensions in their perception and appraisal of symptoms and the actions they take in response (Mechanic 1962, Helman 1990). Construed in this broad form,

illness behaviour depends partly on social norms and partly on a range of other factors. The social norms concerned – shared beliefs about the significance of and appropriate response to particular symptoms, social conventions about the seeking and providing of care – may be general throughout society, or more specific to smaller social groups such as ethnic groups, religious communities, or even families. The 'sick role', as formulated by Parsons, falls at one extreme of this continuum, covering those normative patterns of illness behaviour which are guided by the most widely held social expectations related to illness (and which therefore have the least scope for explaining individual variation). Hitherto the study of illness behaviour has tended to focus on the ill individual, but understanding the motivations and behaviour of *carers* is of increasing importance as the facilitation of family care becomes a central part of mental health practice (e.g. Gilleard 1984).

### *Implications in psychiatric disorder*

An obvious way in which illness-related role expectations are relevant to psychiatry is their potential for perpetuating disability. Families, doctors and institutions all play an active part in socializing people into roles in which they conceive of themselves as ill and in need of care or treatment, and behave accordingly. Usually this enables assistance to be rendered in an appropriate and coordinated manner. Disadvantages arise where the role expectations of the patient or those caring for him are discrepant with the degree or type of functional impairment which is actually present.

One reason for this is that role expectations have an inherent inertia, and may fail to keep up with changing needs for care or treatment as a patient's condition changes; this is particularly likely where a disorder has been prolonged, or there have been accommodating changes in other people's roles (Tarsh & Royston 1985). Another is that there may be an extrinsic pressure favouring such a discrepancy: where a carer derives satisfaction from caring for a dependant, where the self-conception of a doctor or other professional renders him unable to desist from 'therapeutic' activity, or where existing relationships of care and dependence are stabilized by organizational processes, for example where an institution exercises unnecessary constraint or supervision over its residents because avoidance of risk has become its foremost purpose, or routines of staff behaviour have been established which depend on patients behaving in a certain way. Finally there may be pressures arising from attributes of the *patient*, usually referred to by the term 'secondary gain'.

Normative patterns of illness behaviour are particularly suitable media in which to express distress, to communicate certain psychological needs to others and to solicit certain types of relationship with them (see Kreitman *et al.* 1970, Henderson 1974, Kleinman 1982). For these reasons, individuals who perceive their need for care or support as abnormally intense may find specific secondary gains in illness, and thus come into frequent or energetic contact with doctors or hospitals. In this and other instances, dysfunctional interaction between the patient and the doctor or institution, focused on the issues of care and dependence central to illness behaviour, may itself become the chief clinical problem (for examples of some typical forms this takes see Groves 1978).

## Social contingencies in psychiatric care

The nature and policies of mental health services (and other agencies) have an overriding influence on the careers of people with psychiatric disorders by defining the pathways which are open to them. Nosocomial factors were probably responsible for the apparent rise in the incidence of psychotic illnesses in the late nineteenth century, as patients previously more scattered became concentrated within mental hospitals (Tuke 1894, Scull 1979). Similarly, the presentation of many milder psychiatric disorders for medical treatment more recently reflects the availability of family doctor and outpatient psychiatric services catering for these conditions.

Ideally it is assumed that progress through the existing network of services is determined by individual needs for care and treatment, but in practice other social contingencies are also important. Service utilization is a complex topic and one example must suffice. Applying thresholds which would include most cases of depressive disorder treated by specialist services, it can be shown that substantial numbers of comparable cases remain undetected in the community (Brown & Harris 1978a, Dean *et al.* 1983, Brown *et al.* 1985). Those reaching psychiatrists are highly selected and knowledge of the factors governing selection through the series of 'filters' is incomplete (Goldberg & Huxley 1980). Symptom severity is an important influence at each stage (Wing *et al.* 1981), but others include the availability of alternative sources of social support, and constraints on access to medical services due to employment or child care responsibilities (Brown & Harris 1978b).

Some social factors influence what happens to patients *after* they come into contact with services because they are relevant to the social management of the disorder and its associated risks. Influences with a less rational basis have not been extensively studied. Research in the USA has shown the persisting influence of social class and ethnic group membership on the types of treatment and professional involvement offered to patients (Myers & Schaffer 1954, Hollingshead & Redlich 1958, Redlich & Kellert 1978, Mollica & Redlich 1980), and in Britain there is evidence suggesting that black patients are perceived by psychiatrists to be more dangerous than their white counterparts (Lewis *et al.* 1990). Inequitable practices may be especially important in psychiatry, through their potential to initiate interactive deviance-amplifying processes of the types described earlier.

## Psychiatric services and institutions

The nature and organization of psychiatric services have changed considerably in the last 150 years, with the rise of large, centralized, publicly regulated mental hospitals in the nineteenth century, and, more recently, the beginnings of their replacement by a range of dispersed community services. These have not been the result of isolated changes in social policy confined to the psychiatric services. In England, the introduction of the system of county asylums in the nineteenth century formed part of a more general establishment or transformation of segregated residential institutions for criminals, orphans, and a variety of dependent and destitute groups, which came to be organized in rather similar ways, residents experiencing a highly regimented and ordered existence governed by a centralized bureaucratic system of control. These institutions conformed to ideas of rational organization propagated elsewhere in Victorian society, notably in factories, and indeed in the absence of evidence of their efficacy the legitimacy of the asylums probably depended strongly on their conformity to existing institutional models (Rothman 1971, Meyer & Rowan 1977, Scull 1979).

The new institutions were none the less an improvement over what had preceded them. Some of the early asylums embraced rehabilitative principles ('moral treatment'), although these were probably not as widespread as is sometimes assumed, and were more readily available to middle-class patients (Bockoven 1956, Warner 1985). Moreover, some adverse features of the large mental hospitals arose not directly from their original design but from later institutional decline. In the late nineteenth and early twentieth centuries, mental hospitals in many areas showed a tendency to escalating size of resident populations, with increasing concentrations of chronically disabled patients, overcrowding, poorer staffing ratios and generally declining institutional conditions. At the same time, custodial goals replaced those of cure or rehabilitation. The precise reasons for these changes are uncertain. As mentioned earlier, social policy (including fiscal) pressures at the time favoured the accumulation of patients in this setting, and there may have been a process of mutual reinforcement between an increasing concentration of chronically disabled patients, on the one hand, and therapeutic nihilism, a custodial orientation and a progressively impoverished milieu, on the other.

As in their creation, the reform and dispersal of services based in mental hospitals has been one element in a wider process of social change, involving altered attitudes and practices concerning dependent groups in society. The poor and the physically disabled have been supported in the community for some time, and the care of children by public authorities in Britain has moved towards smaller institutions organized in family-type units, and increasingly to foster care in normal families. Indeed, the Curtis Report into child care institutions in 1946 identified broadly the same adverse features as did later studies of large mental hospitals – impersonal relationships between staff and residents, and lack of stimulation, variety and constructive activity. Changes in the mental health services have tended to lag behind those in other sectors, probably because of factors rendering hospitalization potentially long-lasting and difficult to reverse (age of onset, propensity for chronicity and secondary disability). Although the mental hospital population in England reached a peak in 1954 (Tooth & Brooke 1961), this does not necessarily indicate a decisive change in policy at or around that time, and there is evidence that hospital admissions began to shorten at least as early as the 1930s (Brown 1960). No doubt more specific factors, such as the introduction of effective physical and psychological treatments, have also contributed to changes in orientation in the psychiatric services, but probably to a lesser extent than is often assumed.

### Institutions and anti-institutions

Much debate accompanying the changes mentioned above focused on characteristics of institutions and their effects on people living in them, and the 1950s saw a series of case studies of the organization of mental hospitals, the interactional processes to which they gave rise, and the modes of adjustment within them by staff and patients (Stanton & Schwartz 1954, Belknap 1956, Caudill 1958). An influential description of a regime which prevailed in many of the older hospitals was given by Goffman (1968a), who emphasized parallels with other types of institution whose residents inhabited a self-contained social world segregated from the general community. He focused particularly on the pervasive limitation of residents' autonomy by depersonalizing procedures such as block treatment of groups of residents, lack of personal possessions or other opportunities to express choice, and deprivation of privacy and of the normal dignities of self-presentation. The impression was that this type of regime was likely to be damaging and the available evidence suggests that it was, both in terms of general social adaptation, and in its effects on specific impairments such as negative symptoms in schizophrenia (Wing & Brown 1970, King *et al.* 1971).

The work of Goffman and others tended to overstate the degree of uniformity among institutions, and to imply that adverse features identified in some were inherent and unavoidable characteristics of all. Two strands of thought undermined this assumption: First, advocates of 'therapeutic communities' had already proposed reforms involving new and different institutional models (Main 1946, Jones 1968, Manning 1989) (see also Chapter 1). These placed much emphasis on the dissolution of authority structures in favour of autonomy, personal responsibility, and democratic decision making. In fact the functioning of these organizations often depended on the unacknowledged retention of charismatic authority by senior staff members (Rapoport 1960, Punch 1974). None the less, the ideas they embodied overlap with the later philosophy of 'normalization', and some ingredients of the therapeutic community movement have been absorbed more diffusely into the mental health services.

Secondly, an increasing number of comparative studies have demonstrated that 'conventional' institutions themselves vary greatly in the type and quality of care they provide. Examples include studies of mental hospitals (Wing & Brown 1970), institutions for the mentally handicapped (King *et al.* 1971, Holland 1973, Raynes *et al.* 1979), residential schools for juvenile offenders (Street *et al.* 1966, Heal & Cawson 1975) and homes for the elderly (Townsend 1962). In the course of these studies, concepts and methods have been developed for assessing aspects of residential environments which have demonstrable effects on residents' social functioning. Important examples are measures of impoverished, unstimulating en-

vironments (Wing & Brown 1970), and of 'individual-oriented' versus 'institution-oriented' care practices (King *et al.* 1971).

## Organizational factors in psychiatric care

The recognition that institutions vary has naturally led to attempts to explain why they differ and to understand how good quality care may best be facilitated. Knowledge in this area remains fragmentary, and here it is only possible to mention a few of the issues involved (for further discussion see March & Simon 1958, Blau & Scott 1963, Scott 1966, Etzioni 1975, Hasenfeld 1983). It is important to recognize that the relevance of these organizational issues is not confined to large mental hospitals: many of the same issues are faced by community services, where there may be additional problems in coordinating dispersed activities (Redlich & Kellert 1978, Scott & Black 1986).

The official ideology or culture of an organization is an obvious and sometimes overlooked influence on the type and quality of care it is able to offer. Individualized care is unlikely to emerge unless staff are motivated to recognize and respond to the individual needs of clients, and this aim is incorporated into the attitudes and conceptions by which staff members understand and value their own activities. This has direct implications for staff training, but many studies of socialization into professional roles also demonstrate the importance of acquiring attitudes and styles of role performance through example and informal interaction with others, especially senior colleagues (e.g. Becker & Carper 1956). An organization's ability to educate its members in these ways may be impaired if there is marked role differentiation, senior staff being removed from interaction with clients to purely administrative duties (King *et al.* 1971).

Staff motivation is closely linked with the culture of the organization because criteria for success in role performance and in work with clients which arise from that culture largely define the intrinsic rewards staff draw from their jobs. But extrinsic rewards such as salary, prestige (both within and outside the organization), and other incentives such as opportunities for academic work are also important (Brown 1973). Low morale, whatever its cause, will make it difficult to deliver high quality care, and although a downward spiral in care quality and staff motivation may stabilize on the residual motivational base of a safe and undemanding routine, modest rewards and secure employment, in these situations an inability to attract or compete for resources may lead to further cycles of depletion and decline (see Leighton 1983).

Some sources of motivation are inherently unstable and their successes prone to be short lived. This is illustrated in organizations where gains initially achieved in the course of service reforms have been dissipated in a process of subsequent decline (see Wing & Brown 1970, Leighton 1983). It is especially likely to occur where the functioning of an organization or therapeutic regime depends critically on enthusiasm generated by a charismatic leader in the absence of (and perhaps in opposition to) other incentives inherent in the structure of the organization. In the first place the organization will be vulnerable to failure when the individual in question leaves. Secondly, enthusiasm has a limited natural life-span and unless other incentives are generally available, and are not monopolized by senior staff, it will need to be constantly replenished in the form of new staff (Manning 1976). The need for a high turnover of junior staff may have the advantage of malleability – for example in a context of reform, where vested interests and habit may produce resistance to change amongst longer-established staff (Raynes *et al.* 1979) – but it will give the organization a perverse interest in an unskilled or inexperienced work force.

Elements of an organization's structure may impede effective performance in spite of a high level of staff motivation. Poor communication procedures may lead to lack of coordination of activity, with duplication of effort, important tasks remaining undone, or inconsistency among staff which nullifies their efforts or creates new problems; conversely, measures to achieve good communication (e.g. staff meetings) can acquire an inappropriate priority over other, more fundamental organizational goals. Another important structural variable is the distribution within the organization of authority to make decisions. There is evidence that decentralization of some types of decision making to small semi-autonomous units facilitates individualized care (King *et al.* 1971, Holland 1973, Raynes *et al.* 1979). Discretion and autonomy on the part of front-line staff will be inhibited by a plethora of formalized rules and operating procedures which attempt to programme staff behaviour in detail, and the benefits of decentralization are probably due to the greater flexibility it allows in decisions about everday social care. But it needs to be recognized that if there are deficiencies in general staff quality or background training, a lack of programmed procedures may lead to aimless activity (or inactivity), or the adoption of dubious practices.

Decentralization also introduces problems in the monitoring and control of activities which are less obtrusive in centralized systems (Blau 1955, Scott 1966). If activities require particularly close control over staff behaviour for ethical, safety or other reasons, there may be overriding reasons for adopting or retaining standardized procedures. Where control is exercised more indirectly, the way in which performance is monitored may profoundly influence the priorities given by staff to various activities, and have unforeseen consequences for the goals being pursued (for examples see Scott 1966).

Effective performance by a service or organization may be hindered or distorted by pressures within it, the aims of which differ from those of the organization as a whole. These are ubiquitous and arise from the fact that individual members of staff have lives and motivations which originate and extend beyond the confines of the organization and which influence their attitudes and behaviour within it (Selznick 1948). A multitude of pressures can arise channelling activities and working relationships according to the convenience or enjoyment of staff, or the acquisition or maintenance of status or privileges for certain groups, irrespective of how they fit in with the supposed purpose of the organization. These are often conservative in effect ('vested interests'), but they can also be forces for the change or subversion of official policies. It should be remembered that the incentives associated with sectional interests may be congruent with the goals of the service, and enhance its overall performance; conversely, 'vested interests' in the pejorative sense often reflect a situation where incentives which *are* congruent with organizational goals are deficient.

Another pressure sometimes claimed to undermine organizational goals is the tendency for members' behaviour to become entrenched in habitual patterns. Routinization is, however, fundamental to social organization and its condemnation is usually misguided. Structure and inertia to change are indispensable in creating stability and continuity, and the predictability of behaviour which enables activities to be coordinated. Routinization of practices that lead to high quality care is not only possible, but strongly desirable. The clearest adverse consequence of routinization is its limiting of adaptability to changing external demands and opportunities to improve services. It is doubtful, however, whether even here it is ever really critical compared with other factors causing organizational inertia, such as vested interests, sinking of costs, and commitments to external constituencies. It is factors such as these, and the ultimate dependence of all organizations on their wider environment, that account for the finding (Hannan & Freeman 1984) that organizations are often capable of substantial change only in the sense that they are liable to disappear.

## Conclusion

Most attention in social psychiatry has been paid to the study of social factors at the individual level which influence the occurrence or course of psychiatric disorders and handicaps associated with them. This is an essential preliminary to any further development of the area, and sociology has played a part in it by providing specific concepts and methods which have been incorporated into a number of areas of social psychiatry discussed in detail in later chapters. However, a scientific basis for practice in social psychiatry will also require detailed knowledge of how pathogenic social environments and handicapping social processes develop and are maintained, and knowledge of factors fostering or militating against successful care in families or residential services. It is in these areas that an understanding of the more general social phenomena illustrated in the present chapter is likely to be especially important.

## References

Adorno T.W., Frenkel-Brunswik R., Levinson D.J. & Sanford R.N. (1950) *The Authoritarian Personality.* Harper, New York.

Allport G. (1954) *The Nature of Prejudice*, pp. 395–409. Addison-Wesley, Cambridge, Mass.

Angermeyer M.C., Link B.G. & Majcher-Angermeyer A. (1987) Stigma perceived by patients attending modern treatment settings. *Journal of Nervous and Mental Disease* 175, 4–11.

Ashmore R.D. & Del Boca F.K. (1981) Conceptual approaches to stereotypes and stereotyping. In Hamilton D.L. (ed.) *Cognitive Processes in Stereotyping and Intergroup Behaviour.* Lawrence Erlbaum, Hillsdale.

Bales R. (1944) The therapeutic role of Alcoholics Anonymous as seen by a sociologist. *Quarterly Journal of Studies on Alcohol* 5, 267–278.

Becker H.S. (1953) Becoming a marihuana user. *American Journal of Sociology* 59, 235–242.

Becker H.S. (1963) *Outsiders: Studies in the Sociology of Deviance.* Free Press, New York.

Becker H.S. & Carper J.W. (1956) The development of identification with an occupation. *American Journal of Sociology* 61, 289–298.

Becker H.S. & Strauss A. (1956) Careers, personality and adult socialization. *American Journal of Sociology* 62, 253–263.

Belknap I. (1956) *Human Problems of a State Mental Hospital.* McGraw Hill, New York.

Birenbaum A. (1970) On managing a courtesy stigma. *Journal of Health and Social Behaviour* 11, 196–206.

Blau P. (1955) *The Dynamics of Bureaucracy.* University of Chicago Press, Chicago.

Blau P. & Scott W.R. (1963) *Formal Organizations: A Comparative Approach.* Routledge Kegan Paul, London.

Bockoven J.S. (1956) Moral treatment in American psychiatry. *Journal of Nervous and Mental Disease* 124, 167–194, 292–321.

Brenner M.H. (1973) *Mental Illness and the Economy.* Harvard University Press, Cambridge, Mass.

Brown G.W. (1960) Length of hospital stay and schizophrenia: a review of statistical studies. *Acta Psychiatrica et Neurologica Scandinavica* 35, 414–430.

Brown G.W. (1973) The mental hospital as an institution. *Social Science and Medicine* 7, 407–424.

Brown G.W., Bone M., Dalison B. & Wing J.K. (1966)

*Schizophrenia and Social Care*, pp. 136ff. Oxford University Press, London.

Brown G.W., Craig T.K.J. & Harris T.O. (1985) Depression: disease or distress? Some epidemiological considerations. *British Journal of Psychiatry* 147, 612–622.

Brown G.W. & Harris T.O. (1978a) *Social Origins of Depression*. Tavistock, London.

Brown G.W. & Harris T.O. (1978b) *Social Origins of Depression*, p. 188. Tavistock, London.

Catalano R. & Dooley D. (1977) Economic predictors of depressed mood and stressful life events in a metropolitan community. *Journal of Health and Social Behaviour* 18, 292–307.

Caudill W. (1958) *The Psychiatric Hospital as a Small Society*. Harvard University Press, Cambridge, Mass.

Clausen J.A. & Yarrow M.R. (1955) Paths to the mental hospital. *Journal of Social Issues* 11, 25–32.

Curtis Report (1946) *Report of the Care of Children Committee*. Cmd 6923. HMSO, London.

Davies C. (1982) Sexual taboos and social boundaries. *American Journal of Sociology* 87, 1032–1063.

Davis F. (1961) Deviance disavowal: the management of strained interaction by the visibly handicapped. *Journal of Health and Social Behaviour* 7, 265–271.

Dean C., Surtees P.B. & Sashidharan S.P. (1983) Comparison of research diagnostic systems in an Edinburgh community sample. *British Journal of Psychiatry* 142, 247–256.

Durkheim E. (1893) *The Division of Labour in Society*. Free Press, New York. (Translated edition, 1933.)

Eales M.J. (1989) Shame among unemployed men. *Social Science and Medicine* 28, 783–789.

Erikson K. (1966) *Wayward Puritans: A Study in the Sociology of Deviance*. Wiley, New York.

Etzioni A. (1975) *A Comparative Analysis of Complex Organizations*, 2nd edn. Macmillan, London.

Faris R.E. & Dunham H.W. (1939) *Mental Disorders in Urban Areas*. University of Chicago Press, Chicago.

Freeman, H. & Simmons O. (1961) Stigma in the relatives of psychiatric patients. *Social Problems* 8, 312–321.

Freidson E. (1970) *Profession of Medicine*. Aldine, New York.

Gilleard C.J. (1984) *Living with Dementia: Community Care of the Elderly Mentally Infirm*. Croom Helm, London.

Goffman E. (1968a) *Asylums*. Penguin, Harmondsworth.

Goffman E. (1968b) *Asylums*, pp. 142ff. Penguin, Harmondsworth.

Goffman E. (1968c) *Asylums*, pp. 117–155. Penguin, Harmondsworth.

Goffman E. (1968d) *Stigma*. Penguin, Harmondsworth.

Goffman E. (1968e) *Stigma*, pp. 45–55. Penguin, Harmondsworth.

Goffman E. (1968f) *Stigma*, pp. 14, 41–45. Penguin, Harmondsworth.

Goffman E. (1968g) *Stigma*, pp. 151–165. Penguin, Harmondsworth.

Goldberg D. & Huxley P. (1980) *Mental Illness in the Community*. Tavistock, London.

Gove W.R. (1970) Societal reaction as an explanation of mental illness: an evaluation. *American Sociological Review* 35, 873–884.

Grob G. (1986) The origins of American psychiatric epidemiology. In Scott W.A. & Black B.L. (eds) *The Organization of Mental Health Services*. Sage, Beverley Hills.

Groves J.E. (1978) Taking care of the hateful patient. *New England Journal of Medicine* 298, 883–887.

Gussow Z. & Tracy G.S. (1968) Status ideology and adaptation to stigmatized illness: a study of leprosy. *Human Organization* 27, 316–325.

Hannan M.T. & Freeman J. (1984) Structural inertia and organizational change. *American Sociological Review* 49, 149–164.

Harris T., Brown G.W. & Bifulco A. (1990) Loss of parent in childhood and adult psychiatric disorder: a tentative overall model. *Development and Psychopathology* 2, 311–328.

Hasenfeld Y. (1983) *Human Service Organizations*. Prentice-Hall, Englewood Cliffs, New Jersey.

Heal K. & Cawson P. (1975) Organisation and change in children's institutions. In Tizard J., Sinclair I. & Clarke, R. (eds) *Varieties of Residential Experience*. Routledge Kegan Paul, London.

Helman C. (1990) *Culture, Health and Illness*. Wright, Oxford.

Henderson A.S. (1974) Care-eliciting behaviour in man. *Journal of Nervous and Mental Disease* 159, 172–181.

Holland T. (1973) Organizational structure and institutional care. *Journal of Health and Social Behaviour* 14, 241–251.

Hollingshead A.B. & Redlich F.C. (1958) *Social Class and Mental Illness*. Wiley, New York.

Horwitz A. (1982) *Social Control of Mental Illness*. Academic Press, New York.

Inveriarity J. (1976) Populism and lynchings in Louisiana. *American Sociological Review* 41, 262–279.

Jones E.E., Farina A., Hastorf A.H. *et al.* (1984a) *Social Stigma*, pp. 77–78. W.H. Freeman, New York.

Jones E.E., Farina A., Hastorf A.H. *et al.* (1984b) *Social Stigma*, pp. 72–76. W.H. Freeman, New York.

Jones E.E., Farina A., Hastorf A.H. *et al.* (1984c) *Social Stigma*, pp. 99–103. W.H. Freeman, New York.

Jones E.E., Farina A., Hastorf A.H. *et al.* (1984d) *Social Stigma*, p. 179. W.H. Freeman, New York.

Jones E.E., Farina A., Hastorf A.H. *et al.* (1984e) *Social Stigma*, pp. 185–294. W.H. Freeman, New York.

Jones M. (1968) *Social Psychiatry in Practice: The Idea of the Therapeutic Community*. Penguin, Harmondsworth.

King R.D., Raynes, N.V. & Tizard J. (1971) *Patterns of Residential Care*. Routledge Kegan Paul, London.

Kleinman A. (1982) Neurasthenia and depression. *Culture, Medicine and Psychiatry* 6, 174.

Kreitman N., Smith P. & Tan E. (1970) Attempted suicide as language: an empirical study. *British Journal of Psy-*

*chiatry* 116, 465−473.

Leighton A.H. (1983) *Caring for the Mentally Ill: Psychological and Social Barriers in Historical Context.* Cambridge University Press, Cambridge.

Leighton D.C., Harding J.S., Macklin D.B., Macmillan A.M. & Leighton A.H. (1963) *The Character of Danger.* Basic Books, New York.

Lemert E. (1951) *Social Pathology.* McGraw-Hill, New York.

Lemert E. (1967a) *Human Deviance, Social Problems and Social Control.* Prentice-Hall, Englewood Cliffs, New Jersey.

Lemert E. (1967b) *Human Deviance, Social Problems and Social Control*, p. 17. Prentice-Hall, Englewood Cliffs, New Jersey.

Lewis G. & Appleby L. (1988) Personality disorder: the patients psychiatrists dislike. *British Journal of Psychiatry* 153, 44−49.

Lewis G., Croft-Jeffreys, C. & David A. (1990) Are British psychiatrists racist? *British Journal of Psychiatry* 157, 410−415.

Link B. (1982) Mental patient status, work and income: an examination of the effects of a psychiatric label. *American Sociological Review* 47, 202−215.

McGarry M. & West S. (1975) Stigma among the stigmatized. *Journal of Abnormal Psychology* 84, 399−405.

Main T. (1946) The hospital as a therapeutic institution. *Bulletin of the Menninger Clinic* 10, 66−70.

Manning N. (1976) Values and practice in the therapeutic community. *Human Relations* 29, 125−138.

Manning N. (1989) *The Therapeutic Community Movement.* Routledge, London.

March J.G. & Simon H.A. (1958) *Organizations.* Wiley, New York.

Matza D. (1969) *Becoming Deviant.* Prentice-Hall, Englewood Cliffs, New Jersey.

Mechanic D. (1962) The concept of illness behaviour. *Journal of Chronic Diseases* 15, 189−194.

Mechanic D. & Volkart E.A. (1961) Stress, illness behaviour and the sick role. *American Sociological Review* 26, 51−58.

Meyer J. & Rowan P. (1977) Institutionalized organizations: formal structure as myth and ceremony. *American Journal of Sociology* 83, 340−363.

Mollica R.F. & Redlich F. (1980) Equity and changing patient characteristics 1950−1975. *Archives of General Psychiatry* 37, 1257−1263.

Monck E.M. (1963) Employment experiences of 127 discharged schizophrenic men in London. *British Journal of Preventive and Social Medicine* 17, 101−110.

Myers J. & Schaffer L. (1954) Social stratification and psychiatric practice. *American Sociological Review* 19, 307−310.

Parsons T. (1952) *The Social System*, pp. 437ff. Tavistock, London.

Plummer K. (1979) Misunderstanding labelling perspectives. In Downes P. & Rock P. (eds) *Deviant Interpretations.* Martin Robertson, Oxford.

Prudo R., Brown G.W., Harris T. & Dowland J. (1981) Psychiatric disorder in a rural and an urban population: sensitivity to loss. *Psychological Medicine* 11, 601−616.

Prudo R., Harris T. & Brown G.W. (1984) Social integration and the morphology of affective disorder. *Psychological Medicine* 14, 327−345.

Punch M. (1974) The sociology of the anti-institution. *British Journal of Sociology* 25, 312−325.

Quinton D., Rutter M. & Liddle C. (1984) Institutional rearing, parenting difficulties and marital support. *Psychological Medicine* 14, 107−124.

Rapoport R.N. (1960) *Community as Doctor.* Tavistock, London.

Raynes N.V., Pratt M.W. & Roses S. (1979) *Organizational Structure and the Care of the Mentally Retarded.* Croom Helm, London.

Redlich F. & Kellert S.R. (1978) Trends in American mental health. *American Journal of Psychiatry* 135, 22−28.

Rothman D. (1971) *The Discovery of the Asylum.* Little, Brown, Boston.

Rutter M.L. & Madge N. (1976) *Cycles of Disadvantage.* Heinemann, London.

Sales S. (1973) Threat as a factor in authoritarianism: an analysis of archival data. *Journal of Personality and Social Psychology* 28, 44−57.

Scheff T. (1966) *Being Mentally Ill.* Aldine, Chicago.

Schwartz C.G. (1957) Perspectives on deviance: wives' definitions of their husbands' mental illness. *Psychiatry* 20, 275−291.

Scott R.A. & Scull A. (1980) Penal reform and the surplus army of labour. In Bricky S. (ed.) *Law and Social Control.* Prentice-Hall, Toronto.

Scott W.R. (1966) Some implications of organization theory for research in health services. *Milbank Memorial Fund Quarterly* 44, Part 2, 4, 35−64.

Scott W.R. & Black B.L. (eds) (1986) *The Organization of Mental Health Services.* Sage, Beverly Hills.

Scull A. (1979) *Museums of Madness.* Penguin, Harmondsworth.

Selznick P. (1948) Foundations of the theory of organization. *American Sociological Review* 13, 25−35.

Stanton A. & Schwartz M. (1954) *The Mental Hospital.* Basic Books, New York.

Strauss A. (1962) Transformations of identity. In Rose A.M. (ed.) *Human Behaviour and Social Processes.* Routledge, London.

Strauss J.S. & Carpenter W.T. (1974) Prediction of outcome in schizophrenia. II. Relationships between predictor and outcome variables. *Archives of General Psychiatry* 31, 37−42.

Strauss J.S. & Carpenter W.T. (1977) Prediction of outcome in schizophrenia. III. Five-year outcome and its predictors. *Archives of General Psychiatry* 34, 159−163.

Street D., Vinter R.D. & Perrow C. (1966) *Organization for Treatment.* Free Press, New York.

Swanson R. & Spitzer S.P. (1970) Stigma and the psychiatric patient career. *Journal of Health and Social Behaviour* 11, 44–51.

Sykes G. & Matza D. (1957) Techniques of neutralization. *American Sociological Review* 22, 664–670.

Tajfel H. (1981) *Human Groups and Social Categories.* Cambridge University Press, Cambridge.

Tarsh M. & Royston C. (1985) A follow-up study of accident neurosis. *British Journal of Psychiatry* 146, 18–25.

Tooth G. & Brooke E. (1961) Trends in mental hospital population and their effect on future planning. *Lancet* i, 710–713.

Townsend P. (1962) *The Last Refuge.* Routledge Kegan Paul, London.

Tuke D.H. (1894) Alleged increase in insanity. *Journal of Mental Science* 40, 219–231.

Warner R. (1985) *Recovery from Schizophrenia: Psychiatry and Political Economy*, pp. 109ff. Routledge & Kegan Paul, London.

West P. (1985) Becoming disabled: perspectives on the labelling approach. In Gerhardt U.E. & Wadsworth M. (eds) *Stress and Stigma.* Macmillan, London.

Wing J.K., Bebbington P., Hurry J. & Tennant C. (1981) The prevalence in the general population of disorders familiar to psychiatrists in hospital practice. In Wing J.K., Bebbington P. & Robins L. (eds) *What is a Case?* Grant McIntyre, London.

Wing J.K. & Brown G.W. (1970) *Institutionalism and Schizophrenia.* Cambridge University Press, Cambridge.

Wolfensberger W. (1970) The principle of normalization and its implications for psychiatric services. *American Journal of Psychiatry* 127, 291–297.

Wolfensberger W. (1972) *The Principle of Normalization in Human Services.* National Institute for Mental Retardation, Toronto.

Yarrow M.R., Clausen, J.A. & Robbins P.R. (1955) The social meaning of mental illness. *Journal of Social Issues* 11, 30–41.

# Chapter 3
# Epidemiology

## A. MANN

### Epidemiology and clinical epidemiology

Epidemiology is concerned with the distribution of diseases in a population and the factors that influence that distribution (Lilienfield 1957). Its general aims are to describe disease in a population or groups within a population, explain the aetiology by discovering factors that put populations at risk and thus to predict occurrences and to prevent them. The descriptive function leads to a perspective against which a clinical population can be set, so-called 'completing the clinical picture'. The predictive function yields data for health service planning and a perspective against which treatment efficiency can be assessed. The definition of morbid risk is dependent upon a scientific method (to be detailed in the next chapter), which can be used for consideration of personal, demographic and environmental factors, as well as biological ones.

The development of epidemiology within psychiatry has largely been by research workers who would fit within the definition of a clinical epidemiologist. Clinical epidemiology has been defined as follows:

> the application by a physician who provides
> direct patient care of epidemiologic and
> biometric methods to the study of the
> diagnostic and therapeutic processes. I do not
> believe that clinical epidemiology constitutes
> a distinct or isolated discipline, but rather to
> reflect an orientation arising from both
> clinical medicine and epidemiology. (Sackett
> 1969)

The cross-fertilization between the clinician and the epidemiological method was also emphasized by Shepherd (1984):

> together these activities (categories of
> epidemiological study) make up nothing less

than the logical infrastructure of the clinical method, and the practising clinician who is aware of their significance may in turn stimulate epidemiological enquiry.

This research style – clinical epidemiology – has been attacked from the standpoint of community and social medicine on the grounds that epidemiology:

1 Is a science, not a technique in which a clinician can be trained. The roots of that science being ecological, demographic and political rather than clinical.

2 Concerns itself with the health of communities rather than individuals, its public face being community medicine.

3 Leads to solutions that may not have relevance for a clinician or even an individual patient; indeed the solutions may be sociopolitical rather than medical in their implementation (Smith 1980).

In subsequent discussions on this matter, Professor Smith recognized the contribution of the thoughtful doctor to the epidemiological method. In reality, virtually all epidemiological data in psychiatry have been generated by those from this category of 'thoughtful doctors'. The public health medicine sector in Britain has not taken a primary interest in the mental health of the population.

### Epidemiology and social psychiatry

The epidemiological method with its several functions must be one of the most important strands that make up social psychiatry, be this method mediated by the clinician who further explores ideas generated from his population of patients, or by a scientist whose starting point be population statistics. The social psychiatrist in the search for environmental causes for mental disorder will require data on non-clinic populations, a rapid method of detecting disease and of defining environmental risk factors, and a method of analysis that allows the relative contribution of the latter to the former to be determined – all part of the epidemiological research method. Outcome data are necessary for resource planning and service evaluation, another of social psychiatry's major themes. Secondary and tertiary prevention of disability from mental illness is in accord with the preventive function of epidemiological research. Finally, if the solutions for mental illness derived from epidemiological research do require governmental initiatives rather than clinical activity, then this too would be in keeping with some social theories of the nature of mental illnesses and the social psychiatrist's goal of greater public acceptance of the mentally ill.

However, while the epidemiological methods seem to meet the needs for research in social psychiatry, it is worth stressing the conceptual differences between a true epidemiological approach and a clinician's, even if the latter is very interested in social causation. Rose (1985) has described them, and they can be summarized as follows:

1 The clinician tends to focus on a case or near case, who is someone of high risk, and compares groups in terms of the numbers of affected individuals. With this approach, the remaining population, i.e. non-cases, is seen to be a homogeneous background against which these figures emerge. Such a model fits infectious diseases, or those with a dominant genetic aetiology. Yet most psychiatric conditions are multifactorial, with cases arising from those who are at an extreme end of a distribution of risk(s). In these circumstances the data on the whole population, in terms of risk, are of great interest. It may well be that greater demand for resources arises from the larger quantity of the population who are below the level of caseness, than from the smaller numbers of the severely affected. Rose (1989) has argued in the case of depression that the volume of social support required is larger for those who are mildly or moderately depressed, than severely depressed, as the former are more numerous in population.

2 Clinical research tends to focus on individuals or subgroups within a local population, rather than on a comparison of large populations. The problem here is that any one population may have a high or low level of key risk factor, meaning that important associations are missed or distorted. An association between smoking and lung cancer might have been missed if the studies had been carried out amongst a chest clinic population containing a high percentage of smokers.

3 The clinician, aiming to prevent disease, would target those at high risk, hoping that intervening with these would affect the number of cases likely to develop in a population. The creation of a high-risk register is the logical step. The public health doctor would tackle the level of risk factors in the population as a whole, by public education or by promoting social change, so that risk for every individual is lowered just a little. If the number of cases at the extreme of a distribution are determined by the mean level of risk in the whole population, then there will be fewer incident cases once the mean is lowered. This logic has been advanced as a basis for a population approach for reducing the number of alcohol-dependent individuals; the practical implications of such a policy are considerable (Harrison 1981). However, a case can also be made for reducing the numbers of individual patients with depression by this same strategy.

## Describing mental illness in a population: sources of data

The epidemiological approach, as a technique of research, is addressed in the next chapter. Its first aim, describing the distribution of mental illness in the population, will now be addressed. The results of many epidemiological studies show that most mental illnesses are in forms and in settings not in keeping with the day-to-day experience of practising clinical psychiatrists, whether community orientated or not. These results are a matter of major importance for the public health, need constant emphasis at times of resource planning, and during the education of professional workers.

The sources of data are three-fold: national or locally collected statistics on consultation and bed use, case registers and population survey. Each source has its advantages and disadvantages.

## Mental health statistics

Several sets of government statistics report data on the use of the health service by mentally ill patients. Formerly, psychiatric hospitals' statistics were presented separately in the Mental Health Enquiry, but they are now incorporated into the Hospital Inpatient Enquiry, which produces standard data on 10% of all discharges from hospital. The General Household Survey and Social Trends both provide data relevant to the mentally ill, for example, numbers of general practitioner consultations, uses of services by older people and the disabled, data on alcohol intake. The National Morbidity Statistics provide demographic and diagnostic details of consultations in general practice. At the moment, returns from the public health doctors on local morbidity and service use in their districts do not routinely record mental illnesses.

Brooke (1980) has criticized these health service statistics as a source of mental illness data and related health service activity on several grounds. First, these data are not complete. In the hospital sector, inpatient activity is emphasized, while the greater volume of day patient or outpatient activity is not detailed in the same way. Further, only institutions run by the health authorities are included, not those from the voluntary or private sector, nor data from the social services. Second, it is hard to be sure of the diagnoses shown in the statistics. Each return is dependent on a clinician's personal diagnosis, as it is later recorded on a summary sheet. Then from the point of view of research use of the statistics, it is important to add that the hospital returns report on admissions rather than on individual patients. Figures can be distorted by conditions that frequently relapse, as some patients will be counted several times. The returns, too, are by region, therefore losing variations between particular hospital services and districts.

Despite such limitations, national statistics have the considerable advantage of availability and thus have been used in monitoring mental illness in a population and its changes in prevalence. For instance, Lewis (1946) was able to predict the growing impact of the ageing of the population upon need for psychiatric services specifically for older people. The relative impact of deinstitutionalization programmes and the introduction of phenothiazine medication upon the proportion of long-term patients in mental hospital populations have also been analysed. Currently, a longitudinal view of hospital admissions is fuelling a controversy about 'disappearing' schizophrenia (Der *et al.* 1990, Prince & Phelan 1990). Broadly based statistics on hospital admissions have fostered international research. The first set of US/UK studies evolved from observations that admission rates for schizophrenia and affective disorder appeared to differ between New York and London (Cooper *et al.* 1972). The studies showed that these differences largely reflected diagnostic habits, American psychiatrists having broader criteria than the British for schizophrenia. The findings of their research seem to have been influential on the decision by the architects of DSM-III to narrow the diagnosis of schizophrenia considerably within the American context. A second set of US/UK studies concerned older people, where statistics have shown apparently higher rates of admission for organic psychoses among the over 65 year olds in New York and London. This time the research indicated some diagnostic discrepancies, but there was indeed a higher prevalence and incidence rate of dementia in New York (Gurland *et al.* 1983). This higher rate was not explained by greater admission of sufferers of dementia into residential care in New York (Mann *et al.* 1984). This institutional comparison, however, showed that the majority of residential care provision for dementia in London was provided within social service local authority homes, rather than by the health service. This finding is an illustration of how hospital statistics would grossly underestimate long-term care resources needed by patients with this condition.

Sharp & Morrell (1989) presented a cross-sectional view of consultations within the health service sector for mental illness, by drawing together statistics from general practice and from the Mental Health Enquiry in the year 1981.

These statistics showed that for disorders classifiable under ICD-9 sections 290–315, there were 22 980 consultations per 100 000 of the general population of all ages and sexes in general practice. This compared with 3532 outpatient attendances, 4943 day hospital attendances and 397 admissions in the same year. Thus, some two and a half times the number of 'psychiatric' consultations were taking place in general practice compared to the mental health sector. The conditions encountered in these surgeries met criteria for diagnosis, but they were largely for syndromes of depression and anxiety or for psychosomatic complaints rather than psychoses. These findings are paralleled by a similar analyses of statistics within the USA, where the majority of the psychiatric consultations are shown to occur in the general medical sector rather than the specific mental health sector (Regier *et al.* 1978).

## Case registers

The limitations of national statistics have led to the development of case registers: local systems that record contacts with designated medical and social services by psychiatric patients from a designated area (Wing 1989). A specific advantage of registers is that they obviate selection bias caused by the accumulation of certain types of patient at a particular inpatient unit, since only contacts from a particular area are counted. Secondly, individual patients can be identified as well as contacts with the services, avoiding double counting of relapsing patients. Thirdly, criteria for diagnoses can be standardized. Finally, all appropriate contact agencies in a locality can be asked to provide data, thus widening the net to include the likely points of contact for psychiatric patients. With all these features, a case register can provide prevalence rates for each diagnosis per unit of population for a district in a manner that allows comparison with other districts and other countries.

There are naturally problems with interpreting case register data. Some registers have been small and reflect only a segment of an inner city population, thus producing an unknown bias resulting from the setting of arbitrary boundaries. Further,

the register data can only reflect accurately community prevalence and incidence of diseases where symptoms make patients disturbed or visible, and thus likely to enter the psychiatric sector. Patients with depression and anxiety states who reach the psychiatric sector will be small, unrepresentative subsamples of a much larger group of sufferers. Third, registers do not deliver good data on recovery or outcome; patients no longer being recorded could have left the district, could be still symptomatic but out of touch, or could have recovered.

Case registers have provided valuable data over the last 20 years on trends for mental illnesses, particularly showing the interaction between specific diagnostic groups and services. They have also enabled specific patient groups to be identified for more detailed research. In the UK, registers have been successfully set up in Camberwell, Salford and Aberdeen. In Oxford, a linkage system enables contacts by patients with *all* branches of the health service, rather than just the psychosocial, to be traced. Central funding for registers, however, has been withdrawn, as each health district has now become obliged to provide data on patient contacts. The administrative need for specific detailed registers from certain districts to act as a planning base for the country as a whole, seems to have passed. In Europe, where successful registers have been instituted in Norway, Denmark and Germany, they have been under political attack from pressure groups, who see the storing of a patient's personal data in this way as an infringement of individual liberty. This attack has led to closure of the registers.

An example of a register is that set up in Salford by Fryers and colleagues in 1974, beginning with the inner city area of Salford East, and adding the suburban Salford West later (Fryers & Wooff 1989). Contacts with psychiatrists, psychiatric nurses in the community and mental health social workers are recorded. Census day was in January of each year, when current day patients and inpatients were enumerated and patients in contact with outpatients within a three-month band around census day. Analysis of prevalence figures between 1976 and 1987 showed a stable contact rate of approximately 7 per 1000 of the population for schizophrenia, but an increase from 2.4 to 8.2 per 1000 for depression and from 3.4 to 9.8 for other diagnoses which included alcoholism, personality disorder and anxiety. This increase was more marked among females. An analysis by age of patients contacting, showed the steepest rise to be in those over 75, in part explained by the establishing of a specialist psychogeriatric service during this period. Inception rates, new contacts to the register, showed the most marked increase during the same 11 years for the very old, inception contacts for those over 75 years old quadrupling in this period. Thus, if this register can be taken as illustrating a typical pattern over the last decade, it can be concluded that a continuing significant, but not increasing, demand is being made on services by patients with schizophrenia, whereas other groups, particularly the elderly, are making greater use of the local service.

### Surveying the population

Both health service statistics and case registers concern those patients in contact with some form of service, even if social service and general practice data are included in the latter. A population survey should yield the most comprehensive picture of the distribution of mental illness free from any quirk of self-selection into, or referral within, the care system. Such an exercise is not easy, requiring conceptual clarity and the surmounting of logistic difficulties. Nevertheless, they are successfully carried out.

CHOICE OF UNIT OF MEASUREMENT

The key conceptual decision is whether the survey will cover all forms of mental illness, or will focus on specific, clear-cut syndromes. For both, the survey planners will need to decide whether cases alone will be counted or whether the lesser levels of morbidity – a more dimensional approach – will also be recorded. The case/non-case approach is sympathetic to clinicians and health service planners. Diagnostic criteria can be determined in advance by the presence of certain symptoms, perhaps with subsidiary criteria for duration and disability; individuals meeting such criteria be-

coming the focus of the study. This approach fits most neatly for a survey of the psychoses. Examples of this style have been the Epidemiologic Catchment Area Study in the United States (Regier *et al.* 1984) and a survey in Camberwell, London (Bebbington *et al.* 1981). The disadvantage, however, as argued earlier, is that important information will be lost from not considering the whole range of morbidity. In practice, it often turns out that case definitions are called into question as many 'near misses' are discovered in the field. These subjects clearly possess symptoms, but don't meet precise caseness criteria. This problem appeared in surveys of eating disorders (Mann *et al.* 1983) and dementia (Livingston *et al.* 1990). Mild, subclinical or partial syndromes have to be described to identify this psychopathology. The need for many intermediate categories is more apparent when assessing depression or anxiety. Logic leads then to a dimensional approach to mental illness, allowing every respondent to be given a score on such a dimension. The classic Mid Town Manhattan Study (Srole *et al.* 1962) and Stirling County Study from Canada (Leighton *et al.* 1963) have adopted this strategy. They showed that, using this approach, the proportion of the population who suffer from psychiatric symptoms is much larger than arbitrary caseness criteria for these syndromes might suggest. The dimensional approach is criticized, as it is not possible to distinguish, for example, the 'unhappy' from the clinically depressed, or the 'worried' from those with an anxiety state.

In the UK, the Health and Lifestyle Survey (Stark 1987) reporting on a random sample of 9000 adults, followed a third approach. It documented individual symptoms without any preconceived arrangement into dimensions or diagnostic criteria. Respondents were asked about specific complaints such as fatigue, worry or impaired concentration. A caseness approach, however, was incorporated by use of the General Health Questionnaire.

CHOICE OF APPROACH

The major logistic step is the definition of the population and obtaining access to it, so that a satisfactory response rate is obtained from the survey. All population surveys will need a base from which to derive calculations. This base which becomes the denominator in a prevalence calculation will need geographical boundaries, but it will also need criteria for age at inclusion and definition by type of residence. The latter is particularly germane for psychiatric surveys, when patients being accommodated in hostel or residential homes are sometimes counted as living 'at home', sometimes not.

The procedure to obtain a base population will depend on the rarity of the condition being studied. It is inefficient to study rare conditions such as schizophrenia or anorexia nervosa by establishing a total population sample and interviewing all. For instance, less than 3 per 1000 of the population were shown to meet criteria for psychosis in the Camberwell Survey (Bebbington *et al.* 1981) and no case of anorexia nervosa meeting clinical criteria was detected amongst an unselected sample of 1000 schoolgirls in London (Johnson-Sabine *et al.* 1988). Such conditions with high visibility are better discovered by a survey of patients in contact with all health and social agencies in a locality (Campbell *et al.* 1990).

For conditions of greater frequency, however, a population survey is necessary and efficient. In the UK, most of the population registers with a general practitioner, so *practice lists* can be a ready base for a population sample. However, inaccuracies in these can occur as lists are not usually up to date and certain individuals perhaps of particular interest to psychiatrists, such as the paranoid, may avoid all doctors. In cities, patients may be registered with doctors away from their place of residence, consequently practice lists may not provide a comprehensive view of a local population. This is less of a difficulty in smaller towns, where administrative boundaries and practice lists may well be congruous. General practitioner lists have therefore proved useful (King 1986, Copeland *et al.* 1987). The *electoral roll* provides another source of names and addresses and is updated annually. It does not, however, provide the ages of the people listed, a handicap for surveyors interested only in those over or under

65 years. Certain individuals may choose not to register and these might well be the mentally ill, disabled or those suffering from dementia. Nevertheless, the electoral roll formed the basis of the Camberwell Survey (Bebbington *et al.* 1981) and a survey of the elderly in inner London (Lindesay *et al.* 1989). A final approach to obtaining a population list is *household enumeration*, necessary in the USA (Gurland *et al.* 1983, Regier *et al.* 1984), where there is no equivalent to general practice lists. This approach was also found to be necessary in another survey of the elderly in inner London, where practice list data seemed very inaccurate (Livingston *et al.* 1990). However, 'door knocking' to obtain names and addresses is time consuming, expensive in resources and needs prior public relations with the local police and community agencies.

Resources will determine whether the whole of the population identified by one such means is to be assessed, or only a sample. Sampling introduces its own error which needs to be estimated. Given any uncertainty of resource, it is usually wise to subdivide the chosen sample into a series of randomly determined subsamples. Assessment of each subsample is completed before the next is started. Should the study have to be curtailed, it is thus possible, after completing two out of three subsamples, to represent the total population. Were the sample to be treated as a whole, then those that are seen first will have been the easiest to access. Curtailment after two-thirds would provide an unrepresentative view of the total sample.

CHOICE OF ASSESSMENT MEASURES

The quickest means of determining the presence of mental illness will be by self-assessment questionnaires. These can be developed as a screen to predict disorder if validated against interview, or the questionnaire can be the actual dimensional measure of a disorder, such as anxiety or depression.

Unfortunately, for many important conditions, the mental state of the patient makes self-assessment impossible. Interviewer-administered schedules are thus necessary, particularly for psychotic patients and those suffering from dementia.

In these circumstances, a full diagnostic assessment by a psychiatrist would be ideal, this procedure now being made very reliable in research by the development of standardized schedules. However, such an exercise is time consuming, and thus expensive, for a large population survey. Brief interviews or interviewer-administered rating scales that can be used by other health professionals or even lay interviewers have, therefore, been developed. Such interviewers will need training and evidence of interrater reliability between the team of interviewers. Any such brief interview must have the specificity and sensitivity measured. Suffice it to say, specificity is the proportion of true non-cases below the cut-off value, i.e. correctly identified as non-cases, and sensitivity is the proportion of true cases correctly identified as such above the cut-off (see Wing *et al.* 1981 for details). Whichever method is chosen, a survey must be accomplished within a reasonable time. Cases may otherwise be admitted to hospital, and for some conditions, may die at a greater rate than those not affected. The results of such surveys are expressed as a prevalence rate, usually subdivided according to age, sex and social class. Groups may thus be identified with higher than average rates of disorder, observations that can generate hypotheses for more detailed research strategies (see Chapter 4). If a population is then rescreened, prevalence surveys become the basis of incidence studies. For many conditions within psychiatry, prevalence rates have been sufficiently and repeatedly determined for a new study not to be justified in its own right, unless it is to be the basis for intervention or for incidence studies (Sartorius 1977).

### Survey results

If the category of mental illness is extensive enough to include anxiety and depression, then the findings of UK population surveys show a broadly similar picture. Taking the Camberwell Survey as an example, a rate of 2 per 1000 for schizophrenia and 8 per 1000 for mania was found using Present State Examination (PSE) criteria (Bebbington *et al.* 1981). Depression, both reactive and endogenous, occurred at case level at 70 per 1000, while other neurotic disorders were found at a rate of 29 per 1000. The Camberwell Study was based upon an electoral roll, an approach that contrasted with that used in Camden, where two studies were specifically set up to determine the prevalence rate of schizophrenia in the borough (Campbell *et al.* 1990). Here, on two census days, all those over 18 who had a possible diagnosis of schizophrenia in contact with any branch of the health or social services were enumerated. A further detailed assessment provided an accurate diagnosis of those so identified and a rate of 5.6 per 1000 for schizophrenia in North Camden, and 9.8 per 1000 in the more economically deprived South Camden area, were discovered. The higher rate in Camden as a whole compared to Camberwell, another inner London area, probably reflects the difference in approach to case detection. The Epidemiological Catchment Area Study in the USA reported schizophrenia at a rate of about 10 per 1000 (Regier *et al.* 1984).

The ageing of the population and growing interest in dementia research has led to a burgeoning of surveys of older populations (also see Chapter 18). Some have adopted criteria applicable to younger age groups, thereby using instruments or screens validated for younger groups. A brief cognitive assessment scale is added to detect cognitive impairment (Regier *et al.* 1984). However, case definition may need modifying in old age. First, the nature of the symptoms that lead to the diagnosis of mental illness differ among older people and, secondly, physical disease plays a growing part as a covariant with mental state. For that reason, a second approach has been to begin again by devising specific instruments or scales for work with older people that take account of the changes in psychopathology and the role of physical illness and social factors in their manifestation (Gurland *et al.* 1983, Copeland *et al.* 1987). The disadvantage here is that change in case criteria and assessment make comparability of rates with those of younger ages difficult. Whichever approach has been used, rates of dementia seem to be fairly constant, affecting 40–50 per 1000 of the over 65 year olds in the population with a marked age-related increase in prevalence rate (Kay *et al.* 1985, Jorm *et al.* 1987). However, depression rates amongst older people differ widely. Depression affected 10–20 per 1000 according to the ECA (Epidemiologic Catchment Area) studies (Regier *et al.* 1984), contrasted to studies using the second method, which report rates of between 120 and 180 per 1000 of the older population (Gurland *et al.* 1983, Lindesay *et al.* 1989, Livingston *et al.* 1990).

Non-psychotic disorders always outnumber the psychoses in population surveys. This was emphasized again in the Health and Lifestyle Survey, a random survey of 9000 adults in the UK (Stark 1987). Approximately a third of the women and a quarter of the men respondents gave a positive response to the General Health Questionnaire (National Morbidity Statistics 1974), now the most widely used self-assessment screen for psychiatric morbidity of the non-psychotic type. In addition, specific complaints of fatigue, worry, nerves and insomnia were reported by between a quarter and a fifth of the population. Thus, while a definition of caseness for the non-psychotic disorders classified only 10% of the population as unwell, as in the Camberwell Study, the Health and Lifestyle Survey showed that the scale of the complaint in this area is very much larger. A major gap in knowledge at the moment is the degree of social handicap, health and social service use and economic wastage that arise from the large number of individuals with complaints of this type who would not be formally classified as cases. Thus, while prevalence surveys for specific case detection may no longer be justified, a 'public health' study that assessed symptoms of depression and anxiety throughout a population, and analysed their distribution in terms of the important determinants – personality abnormality and social disadvantage – would be interesting. Such a survey would then provide much needed data on the social and economic consequences of these symptoms, even when reported at low levels of severity.

The Health and Lifestyle Survey (Stark 1987) also showed disturbing trends in the relationship to alcohol consumption amongst the respondents. Each was asked to rate his/her level of drinking habit – light, moderate or heavy – and to keep a diary of alcohol intake in the past week. Whilst such data are imperfect, it seemed that moderate drinking was the most self-rated response amongst the men, at about 44% of those under 60. Even 27% of women rated themselves as moderate drinkers. However, it transpired that 'moderate' drinking among men meant a consumption of between 23 and 27 units per week, varying a little according to the age of the respondent. Such levels are well above the limit considered safe. The genesis of this drinking habit amongst people not in touch with services, who certainly wouldn't see themselves as more than moderate drinkers, must be determined. It would be particularly important to discover the nature of the link between this habit and widespread complaints, such as fatigue, worry and insomnia.

## Psychiatry in primary care settings

Epidemiological research suggests that neurotic disorders – syndromes of depression and anxiety or psychosomatic complaint – are the most common disorders at case level, but they arise from a very broad background of symptoms experienced by virtually everyone at sometime in life, such as fatigue, worry and low mood. Given that 98% of the population in the UK is registered with a GP and over 60% will consult in any one year, the primary care service is being faced with an enormous volume of psychiatric work. The numbers of consultations occurring in 1981 for psychiatric disorders have been quoted earlier; consultations with a definite psychiatric diagnosis make up 9.8% of all consultations (National Morbidity Statistics 1974), and this is the third most common category for consultation after respiratory and cardiovascular causes. While this is a burden for primary care, it is also an opportunity.

> The general practitioner, by nature of his provision of his primary care to a population, is well placed to monitor psychiatric disorder in the community as a whole and to identify those patients serious enough to warrant treatment. (Shepherd *et al.* 1966)

That quotation came from the first major study of psychiatric disorders in primary care. Since then, research into these disorders has been growing and is attracting increased interest. Although it has now been recognized that primary care has an integral part to play in the new strategies for community care of the mentally ill, it has been customary to refer to the psychiatric disorders managed in primary care as 'minor' when compared to the major or serious mental illnesses with which psychiatrists contend. The word 'minor' represents a value judgement, since 'minor' problems on a vast scale become major so far as resources are concerned. Croft-Jeffreys & Wilkinson (1989) recently estimated the direct costs of neurosis in primary care settings from consultation, prescription and certified sickness absence at over £300 million per year, equivalent to the cost of treating essential hypertension in primary care. However, by extrapolation from research studies, it is possible to estimate the hidden costs from neurosis resulting from uncertified sickness absence and permanent loss of employment at £5.6 billion per year. This figure can be contrasted with that recently quoted for schizophrenia as £310 million and £1.66 billion (Davies & Drummond 1990).

With a practice list of 2500, the GP would expect to see 300 cases annually of neurotic disorder, compared with 12 patients with severe depression and 55 with chronic mental illness (psychoses of all types). In addition, there would be 30 consultations from patients with recognized alcoholism and about 80 in which social problems were the main features (Royal College of General Practitioners 1973). These consultations for psychiatric disorder often occur concurrently with physical illness (Eastwood 1989). This association with physical morbidity makes another contrast, apart from the diagnostic distribution, with the type of clinical problems faced by psychiatrists. Only 5% of patients with neurosis are referred to psychiatric services from primary care settings, the remainder being managed entirely within primary care. Until recently, management in this setting has been overwhelmingly a pharmacological response (Williams 1979), although there is now a trend for use of other approaches involving community nurses, counsellors or psychologists in management.

Research in this field has led to the formulation of the Goldberg–Huxley model – to show the link between primary care and secondary services (Goldberg & Huxley 1980). This model based upon research evidence would suggest that, in the UK, the psychiatric services come at the end of selection processes that have occurred largely in primary care. The selection comes first from the patient with a psychiatric illness, who may or may not decide to consult a GP, and, second, from the GP, who may or may not recognize patients suffering from a psychiatric disorder and may or may not choose to refer them. It seems that the GP recognizes about two-thirds of those with psychiatric morbidity passing through the surgery. If this conspicuous morbidity, therefore, is combined with hidden morbidity, it can be estimated that there is a significant psychiatric component to a third of consultations (Johnstone & Goldberg 1976). Outcome for patients with neurosis in primary care settings is not uniformly good. Of a representative cohort of neurotic patients identified among primary care attenders, only a quarter remitted quickly. Fifty per cent showed intermittent symptoms throughout a year of follow-up, while 25% presented with persistent symptoms during the follow-up (Mann *et al.* 1981). This chronic group tends to be those that receive psychotropic medications, but without apparent benefit. A favourable outcome was shown to be associated with evidence of a supportive social network and good family relationships.

This brief review of primary care psychiatry is intended to expose the case for psychiatrists to become very much more aware of their GP colleagues, particularly for social psychiatrists whose interest is in the care of the mentally ill in the community. The GP is already at work in their field, dealing with many psychiatric problems – many of them chronic – at considerable cost to the Health Service. The new community care will, undoubtedly, add an unquantified further load to primary care. Strengthening the primary care team by better detection of psychiatric morbidity and by the introduction of broadly based management strategies involving multidisciplinary personnel who show sensitivity to social factors, will be an

34 *Chapter 3*

important part of developing community services. It must be a target of the social psychiatrist.

## References

Bebbington P., Hurry J., Tennant C., Sturt E. & Wing J.K. (1981) Epidemiology of mental disorders in Camberwell. *Psychological Medicine* 11, 561–579.

Brooke E.M. (1980) Information in mental health services: a tripartite system. In Stromgren E., Dupont A. & Nielsen J.A. (eds) *Epidemiological Research as Basis for the Organization of Extramural Psychiatry. Acta Psychiatrica Scandinavica Supplementum* 62, (suppl. 285), 291–297.

Campbell P.G., Taylor J., Pantelis C. & Harvey C. (1990) Studies of schizophrenia in a large mental hospital proposed for closure in the two halves of an inner London borough served by the hospital. In Weller M. (ed.) *International Perspectives in Schizophrenia Research: Biological, Social and Epidemiological Findings*, pp. 185–202. John Libbey, London.

Cooper J.E., Kendell R.E., Gurland B.J., Sharpe L., Copeland J.R.M. & Simon R. (1972) *Psychiatric Diagnosis in New York and London: A Comparative Study of Mental Hospital Admissions. Institute of Psychiatry Maudsley Monographs No. 20.* Oxford University Press, London.

Copeland J.R.M., Dewey M.E., Wood N., Searle R., Davidson I.A. & McWilliam C. (1987) Range of mental illness among the elderly in the community. Prevalence in Liverpool using the GMS-Agecat package. *British Journal of Psychiatry* 150, 815–823.

Croft-Jeffreys C. & Wilkinson G. (1989) Estimated costs of neurotic disorder in UK general practice 1985. *Psychological Medicine* 19, 549–558.

Davies L.M. & Drummond, M.F. (1990) The economic burden of schizophrenia. *British Journal of Psychiatry Bulletin* 14, 522–525.

Der G., Gupta S. & Murray R. (1990) Is schizophrenia disappearing? *Lancet* 335, 513–516.

Eastwood R. (1989) The relationship between physical and psychological morbidity. In Williams P., Wilkinson G. & Rawnsley K. (eds) *The Scope of Epidemiological Psychiatry*, pp. 210–221. Routledge, London.

Fryers T. & Wooff K. (1989) A decade of mental health care in an English urban community: patterns and trends in Salford 1976–87. In Wing J.K. (ed.) *Health Service Planning and Research*, pp. 31–52. Gaskell, London.

Goldberg D. & Huxley P. (1980) *Mental Illness in the Community: The Pathway to Care.* Tavistock, London.

Gurland B., Copeland J., Kuriansky J., Kelleher M., Sharpe L. & Dean L.L. (1983) *The Mind and Mood of Ageing. Mental Health Problems of the Community Elderly in New York and London.* The Haworth Press, New York.

Harrison L. (1981) Is a coordinated prevention policy really feasible? *Alcohol & Alcoholism* 21, 5–17.

Johnson-Sabine E., Wood K., Patton G. & Mann A.H. (1988) Abnormal eating attitudes in London schoolgirls – a prospective epidemiological study. *Psychological Medicine* 18, 615–622.

Johnstone A. & Goldberg D. (1976) Psychiatric screening in general practice: a controlled trial. *Lancet* i, 605–608.

Jorm A.F., Korten A.E. & Henderson A.S. (1987) The prevalence of dementia: a quantitative integration of the literature. *Acta Psychiatrica Scandinavica* 76, 465–479.

Kay D.W.K., Henderson A.S., Scott R., Wilson J., Rickwood D. & Grayson D.A. (1985) Dementia and depression among the elderly living in the Hobart community: the effect of the diagnostic criteria on the prevalence rates. *Psychological Medicine* 15, 771–778.

King M. (1986) Practice research: eating disorders in general practice. *British Medical Journal* 293, 1412–1414.

Leighton D.C., Harding J.S., Macklin D.B. et al. (1963) *The Character of Danger: Stirling County Study No. 3.* Basic Books, New York.

Lewis A. (1946) Ageing and senility. *Journal of Mental Science* 92, 150–170.

Lilienfield A.M. (1957) Epidemiological methods and influences in studies of non infectious diseases. *United States Health Services Science Reports* 2, 51–60.

Lindesay J., Briggs K. & Murphy E. (1989) The Guy's/Age Concern Survey – prevalence rates of cognitive impairment, depression and anxiety in an urban elderly community. *British Journal of Psychiatry* 155, 317–329.

Livingston G., Hawkins A., Graham N., Blizard R. & Mann A.H. (1990) The Gospel Oak Study: prevalence rates of dementia, depression and activity limitation among elderly residents in inner London. *Psychological Medicine* 20, 137–146.

Mann A.H., Jenkins R. & Belsey E. (1981) The twelve month outcome of patients with neurotic illness in general practice. *Psychological Medicine* 11, 535–550.

Mann A.H., Wakeling A., Wood K., Monck E., Dobbs R. & Szmuckler G. (1983) Screening for abnormal eating attitudes and psychiatric morbidity in an unselected population of 15 year old schoolgirls. *Psychological Medicine* 13, 573–580.

Mann A.H., Wood K., Cross P., Gurland B., Schieber P. & Haefner H. (1984) Institutional care of the elderly: a comparison of the cities of New York, London and Mannheim. *Social Psychiatry* 19, 9–102.

National Morbidity Statistics for General Practice 1971–72 (1974) HMSO, London.

Prince M. & Phelan M. (1990) Trends in schizophrenia. *Lancet* 335, 851–852.

Regier D.A., Goldberg I.D. & Taube C.A. (1978) The de facto US mental health services system: a public health perspective. *Archives of General Psychiatry* 35, 685–693.

Regier D.A., Myers J.K., Kramer M. et al. (1984) The NIMH epidemiologic catchment area (ECA) program: historical context, major objectives and study population characteristics. *Archives of General Psychiatry* 41, 934–941.

Rose G. (1985) Sick individuals and sick populations. *International Journal of Epidemiology* 14, 32–38.

Rose G. (1989) The mental health of populations. In Williams P., Wilkinson G. & Rawnsley K. (eds) *The Scope of Epidemiological Psychiatry*, pp. 77–85. Routledge, London.

Royal College of General Practitioners (1973) *National Morbidity Statistics*. HMSO, London.

Sackett D.L. (1969) Commentary: clinical epidemiology. *American Journal of Epidemiology* 89, 125–128.

Sartorius N. (1977) Priorities for research likely to contribute to better provision of mental health care. *Social Psychiatry* 12, 171–184.

Sharp D. & Morrell D. (1989) The psychiatry of general practice. In Williams P., Wilkinson G. & Rawnsley K. (eds) *The Scope of Epidemiological Psychiatry*, pp. 404–419. Routledge, London.

Shepherd M. (1984) The contribution of epidemiology to clinical psychiatry. *American Journal of Psychiatry* 141, 12.

Shepherd M., Cooper B., Brown A.C. & Kalton G. (1966) *Psychiatric Illness in General Practice*. Oxford University Press, Oxford.

Smith A. (1980) Epidemiology and the clinician. *Lancet* ii, 1987.

Srole L., Langer T.S. & Michael S.T. (1962) *Mental Health in the Metropolis: The Midtown Manhattan Study*, vol. 1. McGraw-Hill, New York.

Stark J. (1987) Health and social contacts. In *Health & Lifestyle Survey, Preliminary Report*, pp. 59–66. Health Promotion Research Trust, Cambridge.

Williams P. (1979) The extent of psychotropic drug prescription. In Williams P. & Clare A.W. (eds) *Psychological Disorders in General Practice*, pp. 151–160. Academic Press, London.

Wing J.K. (ed.) (1989) *Health Services Planning and Research: Contributions from Psychiatric Case Registers*. Gaskell, London.

Wing J.K., Bebbington P. & Robins L.N. (eds) (1981) *What is a Case? The Problem of Definition in Psychiatric Community Surveys*. Grant McIntyre, London.

# Chapter 4
# Epidemiological Methods in Psychiatry

ANTHONY J.PELOSI & GLYN LEWIS

## Introduction

Most medical research that involves human subjects will require a knowledge of epidemiological methods. Usually, even small-scale psychological or biological comparisons between groups of patients and controls are attempting to draw epidemiological conclusions. Epidemiology can thus be seen as the basic science of clinical and population-based study of disease.

Epidemiology has many uses (see Chapter 3), but amongst the most important is the study of aetiology (Morris 1975). Hypothesis-driven research on causes of disease is often called analytical epidemiology and will be the main focus of this chapter.

## Nomenclature

It is traditional within the epidemiological literature to write of 'disease' and 'exposure'. These will often seem rather inappropriate in psychiatry but the nomenclature will be retained as shorthand and to provide a link with general epidemiological texts. 'Disease' will be used to refer to any event, perhaps the onset of illness or even the decision to consult a GP. Likewise, the 'exposure' is any factor of interest that may be associated with the disease; from a real environmental exposure such as aluminium, through CT scan parameters to life events and social networks. They will not be restricted to a history of past contact with, for instance, a noxious chemical, infection or social adversity. A current physiological characteristic, such as enlarged ventricles on brain scanning, an abnormal dexamethasone suppression test, or a family history of mental illness will all be referred to as 'exposures'.

## Research strategies

When investigating the possible role of an aetiological agent, the first step must be to review the relevant published literature. A number of questions can be asked about the relationship between a study and existing published studies:

1 Is there epidemiological evidence for an association between the exposure and disease? This will be necessary both to persuade a funding agency and yourself of the value of performing the study.

2 Are there plausible psychological, biological or social mechanisms which can explain the association? Even in the absence of any epidemiological support for the hypothesis under test, a convincing case for a study can be made on the basis of such plausible mechanisms.

3 What is the probable strength of the association? This is necessary for estimation of the sample size needed for the study.

4 How does the proposed study add to the existing literature? There are many justifications for a new study, even if some evidence already exists for an aetiological association. Commonly previous studies have overlooked some important methodological points which will be addressed in your study design.

## Sources of data

It is wise to start with data that already exist in order to avoid the trouble and expense of collecting new information.

Government statistics and information collected by health service administrators (Wing 1989), by pharmaceutical companies and by other agencies have almost certainly been underutilized in psychiatry. It is more difficult to obtain population indicators for mental health than for physical health. However, the World Health Organization has suggested the following direct and indirect indicators: suicide and homicide rates, juvenile delinquency, alcohol consumption, drug addict notifications, and consumption of tranquillizers (World Health Organization 1981). Some useful data sources available to psychiatrists in various countries have been catalogued by Alderson (1988). With appropriate caution these data can be used to make comparisons of trends over time and of the mental health of various population groups in different areas. Investigations using routinely collected data can provide guidance to policy makers in planning health services. They are unlikely to provide convincing evidence on the aetiology of illnesses but may provide clues which can be tested in specifically designed epidemiological and laboratory studies.

Examples of this approach are the studies of Appleby (1991), who examined the 'Report on Confidential Enquiries into Maternal Deaths in England and Wales' and population data on deaths and births. He found that suicide was rare during pregnancy, with a standardized mortality ratio of 0.05. Der *et al.* (1990) have been able to suggest that there has been a decline in the incidence of schizophrenia on the basis of Mental Health Enquiry data.

It is important to emphazise that data collected by governments or information for audit of health services is often very poorly collected and subject to a variety of important biases. Such studies have to be interpreted with great care. Confounders, apart from age and sex, can only very rarely be taken into account. Time trends are particularly susceptible to changes in diagnostic habits, as such statistics use diagnoses which have not been standardized.

In addition to government and health service statistics there is a surprising amount of data already collected which may be able to answer research questions. These include publicly available data sets such as the Health and Lifestyle Survey (Cox *et al.* 1987), a survey of some 9000 individuals in Britain which contained extensive health assessments including the General Health

Questionnaire (Goldberg 1972) and alcohol intake. Furthermore, many researchers gather data for one purpose which can be used to address another hypothesis.

## The epidemiological approach

### Measures of disease frequency

The epidemiological method studies health problems in relation to specified populations. Raw numbers about clinical activity are of very limited value. To draw valid epidemiological conclusions the number of events – the numerator – must be related to the population at risk – the denominator – and to the specified time during which the events or phenomena occur. Failure to do this leads to the error that has been called a floating numerator. Examples are rarely difficult to find, particularly in newspaper articles. An example would be giving the number of murders in each region of Britain without the population of each region (*Observer Colour Magazine*, 17 February 1991).

Noble & Rodger (1989) is another example of using numerators without reference to population at risk. The authors were interested in violent incidents in the Maudsley Hospital. Unfortunately they presented graphs and tables of numbers of violent incidents, though they realized that these were not appropriate as the number of the beds in the hospital had changed over the years. Calculating the number of violent incidents per occupied bed would allow conclusions to be drawn.

The most frequently used measures of disease frequency are the prevalence and incidence. The *prevalence* is calculated using a cross-sectional survey and is the number of subjects with a given disease at a designated time divided by the population at risk, i.e. all the members of the survey. In one of the earliest community surveys in which mental disorders were investigated (see Lemkau 1986), a population of 55 129 people in Eastern Baltimore were assessed and those with serious mental disorders and mental handicap were identified. Three hundred and ninety-seven people with mental handicap were identified. The prevalence of mental handicap was 397/55 129; i.e. 0.0072, or, in a more manageable form, 7.2 cases of mental handicap per 1000.

The above example is the *point prevalence*. Other time periods can be used for prevalence figures depending on the purposes of the investigator. It may be valuable to know how many people have been ill at any time during the past year. This would include those currently ill but also those who have been sick in the past year and have become well. This is the *annual prevalence*. For example, Brown & Harris (1978) interviewed a random sample of 458 women in Camberwell. Of these, 76 met their criteria as cases of current psychiatric disorder, or had been psychiatrically disturbed at some time in the year prior to interview but had recovered. The annual prevalence was 76/458 or 0.17 (17%).

The *incidence rate*, on the other hand, is usually calculated from a cohort study, or occasionally from government statistics. It is the rate of *new* events or new cases of disease occurring within a defined time period. The denominator is the population at risk of experiencing the event during this period. If someone dies or is lost to follow-up, subjects can still be included in the study but only for the period during which the subject was 'at risk' of developing the disorder. This adjustment is only necessary for common conditions, or in cohorts where a substantial proportion of people are lost to follow-up. The incidence rate can be generally expressed as follows:

$$\text{Incidence rate} = \frac{\text{No. of new events}}{\text{No. of person-years at risk}}$$

Further details can be found in Breslow & Day (1987).

Incidence and prevalence are interrelated; it will be apparent that prevalence of a disease will depend on its incidence and its duration. Prevalence measures are of value in assessing the public health impact of illnesses, especially chronic conditions, and are vital in guiding health care provision. Chronic illnesses could have a low incidence rate but a relatively high prevalence. Incidence figures are of greater value in aetiological studies. The use of prevalence measures in exploring aetiology must be done with caution as an association between an exposure and prevalent cases may be due to the exposure increasing the risk of disease, or leading to a prolonged illness.

There are also differences in the statistical methods used in the analysis of these measures. Most commonly used statistics are estimating sampling variation, for example in the analysis of a cross-sectional prevalence survey in which a random sample of a much larger population is taken. In contrast, in incidence studies variation derives from the variability of rates and is statistically estimated using Poisson statistics (see Armitage & Berry 1987). For example, the suicide rate in Britain uses the whole population, all 55 000 000, as the denominator and all suicide deaths as the numerator. Sampling variation therefore does not arise but variation between years arising due to chance is estimated using Poisson statistics.

### Measures of association

The contribution of epidemiology to elucidating the causes of illnesses has essentially involved comparing rates of disease. These can involve comparisons over time or can be of different geographical areas, or of different types of people. On some occasions this work has provided sufficient evidence for policy makers to consider that a factor shown to be associated with an illness is causal, and therefore preventive action is taken.

In medical epidemiology it is fairly easy to choose from a range of examples where research on human subjects has produced universally or generally accepted evidence of an important causal factor in disease leading to preventive measures. For example, in Victorian times it was noted that there was an association between cancer of the scrotum, a very rare condition, and working as a chimney sweep. This cancer is almost unheard of in young men in the general population and the association was accepted as evidence for a causal link. This brought about appropriate changes in work practices. More recently, epidemiological evidence has led to the conclusion that smoking is a causal factor in the development of lung cancer, leading to campaigns to discourage smoking and changes in the fiscal policies of some governments.

Clear-cut examples are less readily available from the mental health field. A number of associations with emotional and psychiatric disorders have been firmly established. Examples include the tendency for schizophrenic illnesses to run in families (Kendler 1988) and the association between adverse life events and depressive disorders (Brown & Harris 1978) (also see Chapters 7 and 10). However, debate continues on the causal relationships in these associations. Even when there is general agreement on aetiological factors, preventive interventions involve complex and controversial political decisions or may not be possible for ethical reasons.

The associations demonstrated by epidemiological research are, in effect, statistical associations. In other words evidence is sought that those who have been in contact with a hypothesized causal factor have a greater likelihood of developing the illness than those not in contact. There are naturally a number of problems in attempting to move on to infer causation, and these are discussed below.

RELATIVE RISK

The most useful measure of association between a possible risk factor and an illness is the relative incidence. This can be defined as the incidence rate in those exposed to the risk factor divided by the incidence rate in those not so exposed (Table 4.6):

$$\frac{\text{Relative}}{\text{incidence}} = \frac{\text{Incidence in exposed}}{\text{Incidence in those not exposed}}.$$

Relative risk is a shorthand term that will be used here, though strictly 'risk' refers to probability rather than an incidence 'rate'. A relative risk of 1 indicates no association between that particular exposure and the disease of interest.

Relative risks are also estimated from prevalence data by dividing the prevalence in those exposed with the prevalence in those not exposed to the hypothesized risk factor. Odds ratios (or relative odds) are also increasingly being used in cross-sectional surveys (see Appendix to this chapter).

**Table 4.1** Some associations in medicine and psychiatry

| Association | Approximate relative risk |
| --- | --- |
| Employment in asbestos industry and lung cancer | 14 |
| Cigarette smoking and lung cancer | 10 |
| Heavy cigarette smoking and lung cancer | 30 |
| Schizophrenia in one parent and development of schizophrenia | 12 |
| Schizophrenia in two parents and development of schizophrenia | 35 |
| Low socioeconomic status and schizophrenia | 3 |
| Adverse life events and depressive illness | 2–9 |
| Life events and onset of schizophrenia | 3–6 |
| Life events and suicide attempt | 10 |
| Birth in winter and schizophrenia | 1.1 |

Adapted from Doll (1955), Doll & Hill (1964), Paykel (1978), Eaton (1985), Eaton *et al.* (1988).

In case-control studies, subjects have been chosen for study specifically because they either do or do not have the illness of interest. Therefore, neither prevalence nor incidence of illness in the groups can be calculated. However, the observed odds ratio in a case-control study provides an estimate of the relative risk in the population from which the cases and controls have been drawn.

Table 4.1 outlines some *approximate* relative risks of association which have been identified using epidemiological research methods. The advantages of this summary measure should be clear from the table. When associations are presented only in terms of statistical significance of differences within particular investigations (i.e. by providing a *P* value), the strength of the association is not immediately apparent. However, the relative risk (with appropriate confidence intervals in individual studies) provides a useful summary measure, with implications for the interpretation of the finding and its importance.

There are other advantages of using relative risks as measures of association. First, they are easy to understand. Second, a large relative risk cannot be explained by a smaller relative risk. For instance, the large association between being of Afro-Caribbean descent in Britain and being diagnosed as suffering from schizophrenia (relative risk around 10; Harrison *et al.* 1988) cannot be explained by, for example, the season of birth effect (around 1.1). Third, it seems that relative risks are relatively constant between cultures and countries, even when the prevalence of a condition varies. Under those circumstances the attributable risk (see below) varies. Relative risk is usually taken to be a measure of aetiological 'force'.

ATTRIBUTABLE RISK

The attributable risk (AR) provides information on the absolute effect of an exposure, i.e. the excess risk (rather than the relative risk) of disease in those exposed compared with those not exposed.

It can be defined as the difference between the incidence rates in the exposed and non-exposed:

AR = Incidence rate in exposed
       − incidence rate in unexposed.

It therefore gives the increase in risk associated with the exposure. For an individual, the attributable risk is more useful than the relative risk in deciding upon which exposures need to be avoided. For example, smoking cigarettes increases the risk of heart disease two times and lung cancer ten times. These relative risks might suggest to an individual that lung cancer is the main risk for cigarette smokers. However, this ignores the prevalence of heart disease (very common) and lung cancer (rare) in the non-smokers. Ten times a very small risk is less attributable risk than two times a large risk. Smokers are much more likely to die of heart disease.

A similar point can be made in assessing suicide risk. For instance there is epidemiological evidence that divorced people have an increased risk of suicide. However, because suicide is so rare, this information is of little use to a psychiatrist attempting to predict suicides because the attributable risk for a rare event will be very low. Attributable risks are therefore valuable in assessing individual risks and the effectiveness of preventive measures.

POPULATION ATTRIBUTABLE RISK

One further measure of the importance of an exposure can be made. The population attributable risk is the proportion of the condition in the population of interest that can be explained by a risk factor. It is a measure of the public health importance of an exposure and it gives an assessment of how many cases of the disease can be explained by the exposure, assuming it is causal in nature.

The data of Mullen *et al.* (1988) on sexual abuse and the prevalence of depression can be used to illustrate its utility. Population attributable risk can be calculated knowing the relative risk, the proportion of the population with the exposure and the prevalence of the disease in the unexposed group (for details see Last 1988). If one applies the rate from the unexposed group to the exposed group, any excess cases of disease are assumed to be due to the exposure. The excess proportion is the population attributable risk. The data of Mullen *et al.* suggest that about 25% of the cases of depression in the survey could be explained by previous sexual abuse. Though this is a considerable proportion, such a difference could not explain, as the authors suggested, the sex difference in depression, particularly considering that men are also subject to sexual abuse.

## Study designs in psychiatric research

### Clinical description – case reports and series

Some of the most influential research papers in clinical psychiatry have been single case reports, especially the famous patients described by Freud. These are not epidemiological studies but they can provide clues to associations and causes of illnesses.

Single case reports can be used within epidemiological research to illustrate important points. A fine example is found in Robertson's cohort study of the manner of death in convicted male offenders who had been given compulsory hospital orders in

1963 (Robertson 1987). The most striking finding was relative risk of around three for suicide and other violent death. Robertson illustrated his data with a vignette on one of his seriously disturbed subjects which underlined the importance of the study and the reasons for undertaking it: 'Statistics tell one side of the story but cannot reflect the misery wrought by these illnesses on the patients and their families...' (Robertson 1987).

Reporting clinical case series remains an important and useful research activity, especially in psychiatry in view of the rudimentary nature of so much of our knowledge. These series usually do not refer to a specified population, and cannot therefore be described as epidemiological in nature. This method often provides pointers to associations with psychiatric conditions, although it is unusual that these are so strong as to give evidence for an association; further investigations with appropriate comparison groups are required.

Examples of influential case series can be found in the eating disorders literature. Many of the hypotheses tested in epidemiological research were stimulated by such work, for example Bruch's descriptions of anorexic patients (Bruch 1973). Russell's series of patients with bulimia nervosa (Russell 1979) spawned extensive and productive investigation of this illness which had previously not been adequately delineated.

### Case-control studies

*In a case-control study, individuals with a particular condition or disease (the* cases) *are selected for comparison with a series of individuals in whom the condition or disease is absent (the* controls). *Cases and controls are compared with respect to existing or past attributes or exposures thought to be relevant to the development of the condition or disease under study.* (Schlesselman 1982a)

Case-control studies thus estimate the relative risk of association between a disease and a factor of interest and are widely used as a quick, efficient, and relatively inexpensive means of exploring possible aetiological factors. Mantel & Haenszel (1959) observed that the method is 'adapted to

the limited resources of an individual investigator and places a premium on the formulation of hypotheses for testing, rather than on facilities for data collection'.

The refinement of this methodology has been one of the major advances in epidemiological research over the past three decades. Many of the technical developments have been by epidemiologists interested in the aetiology of cancer who have done much to remove the disreputable image of the 'quick and dirty' case-control study that provided unreliable results requiring confirmation with other study designs. Case-control studies now have a central and respected place in epidemiology.

This design is also extensively used in clinical research; for example, it has been used to study the association between schizophrenia and CT scan parameters (e.g. Smith *et al.* 1988) and obstetric complications (e.g. Lewis & Murray 1987), risk factors for tardive dyskinesia (e.g. Mukherjee *et al.* 1986) and depression and corticosteroid metabolism (e.g. Carroll *et al.* 1981). Geneticists who study the association of a disorder with an increased familial risk are also using a case-control design (e.g. Coryell & Tsuang 1982).

The case-control study can be considered an extension of the traditional clinical description of a series of cases. The prevalence of exposure in the cases can be compared with that in a comparison group, the controls. The control group gives an estimate of the prevalence of exposure in the population from which the cases were drawn. The researcher therefore starts by selecting a source of cases and then chooses an appropriate control group. This is often the most difficult step in the design which we will discuss in the section on selection bias. It can be seen that 'control' is not very appropriate to describe members of the comparison group but alternatives have not gained widespread acceptance.

Since case-control studies start with identified cases, they have a particular advantage in investigating uncommon illnesses. As illustrated in Chapter 3, screening of a general population sample of perhaps 10 000 subjects could be required to identify 100 people with schizophrenia. A specific cohort study of schizophrenia would be even less feasible (but see Andreasson *et al.* 1987, as described below, for an example of a retrospective cohort study of schizophrenia).

Case-control studies can be designed to test a single hypothesis or can be used to explore numerous possible associations. The exploratory approach is the strategy of choice in several situations:

1 When studying a rare disease in which it is difficult and expensive to obtain a sufficient number of cases, making it desirable to maximize the information obtained from each project.

2 When the state of knowledge of a disease is such that no single hypothesis can be convincingly formulated to make a focused study worthwhile – this is sometimes the case with psychiatric conditions. The 'fishing expedition' approach of the exploratory study may provide aetiological clues which justify further testing in specifically designed case-control or cohort studies and in laboratory research.

A fine example of an exploratory investigation has been reported by Amaducci and his colleagues (1986), who assessed possible risk factors for Alzheimer's disease. Information was obtained on over 70 possible causes or pointers to aetiology and clear statistical associations were found with several different factors. The authors are rightly cautious in interpreting their findings, but they provide important clues worthy of further research.

## AN EXAMPLE OF A CASE-CONTROL STUDY – CRAIG & BROWN (1984)

Craig & Brown (1984) used the case-control method to study the possible importance of life events in the aetiology of painful gastrointestinal conditions. They identified patients suffering from 'functional' illness in a gastrointestinal clinic and compared them with patients from the same clinic with organic gastrointestinal disorder and with another group of healthy people from the local community. Table 4.2 has been constructed from just some of their results; an environmental stress is defined as a severe life event or major difficulty in a 38-week period preceding the interview.

The efficiency and relative cheapness of the

**Table 4.2** Life events and painful gastrointestinal (GI) disorder

|  | Functional GI disorder | Organic GI disorder |
| --- | --- | --- |
| Environmental stress | 53 | 26 |
| No environmental stress | 14 | 42 |

Odds ratio = $53 \times 42/14 \times 26 = 6.1$ (95% CI 2.8–13.1).

design is clear. If Craig & Brown had designed a cross-sectional community survey to test their hypothesis they would have had to interview many thousands of people before a sufficient number with gastrointestinal disorders would be identified.

Are these life events of causal significance in functional bowel symptoms? The difference in the cases and controls may have arisen by *chance* but this is most unlikely, as indicated by the usual tests of statistical significance. The 95% confidence limits for the odds ratio are from 2.8 to 13.1 (for method of calculation see Schlesselman 1982a). Functional bowel illness could conceivably lead to a greater number of life events, perhaps mediated by its effects on work performance, relationships, etc. However, the assessment plays close attention to timing and independence of life events and reduces the likelihood that the association can be explained by *reverse causality*. Sex and social class, for example, are possible *confounders* and a number of possible biases have to be considered. A selection or referral *bias* appears to be the most important. For example, are those with functional bowel symptoms more likely to be referred for hospital treatment if they have recently had life stresses and does this apply to the same extent to the hospital controls?

### Cross-sectional surveys

In this design a sample is selected, usually in a random fashion, from a population. The subjects are then assessed in regard to the presence of one or more illnesses and also for current and past exposure to possible risk factors. Findings can be expressed in terms of the prevalences of the

**Table 4.3** Schematic representation of a cross-sectional survey

| | |
|---|---|
| I | Selection of a random sample of population of interest |
| II | Participants assessed in regard to presence of disease and past and present exposures |
| III | Prevalence of disease compared in those with and without exposures and relative risks estimated |

**Table 4.4** General results of a community survey

| | Ill subjects | Well subjects | Total |
|---|---|---|---|
| Risk factor positive | $a$ | $b$ | $a + b$ |
| Risk factor negative | $c$ | $d$ | $c + d$ |

illnesses under study. Also risk factors will be explored by comparing the prevalence rates of illness in exposed subjects with those in the unexposed. A simplified outline of the design is shown in Table 4.3.

For risk factors which are continuous measures, such as weight and height, the appropriate statistical comparison will be used. For categorical risk factors (e.g. whether there have been recent life events, whether subjects are smokers or non-smokers) the results can be expressed as shown in Table 4.4.

The relative risk will be obtained by dividing the proportion of ill subjects exposed to the risk factor by the proportion of those without the disease who are so exposed. Using the above notation this is:

$$\text{Relative risk} = \frac{a/(a + b)}{c/(c + d)}.$$

Commonly, odds ratios are also calculated for cross-sectional surveys for various reasons (see Appendix). In most circumstances this will approximate to the relative risk:

$$\text{Odds ratio} = \frac{a/b}{c/d}.$$

This scheme is of course the simplest illustration of the presentation of results. At times there will be several different levels of severity of illness and exposure and these will be analysed in similar ways.

There have been many important and highly influential studies of this type in the field of psychiatry. The most ambitious was the Epidemiological Catchment Area study (ECA; Regier *et al.* 1984, Eaton & Kessler 1985) in which surveys were conducted in five different areas of the USA

to obtain basic prevalence data, to assess health service needs, and to explore risk factors with many operationally defined psychiatric illnesses.

Cross-sectional surveys usually draw on representative samples of the population and therefore avoid most of the problems of selection bias encountered in case-control studies. It is, of course, important that participation rates are as high as possible and, where possible, details are obtained on non-participants. Information biases (arising from both subject and observer) can occur in the assessment of presence of disease and exposure status. Some workers have used tape-recordings of interviews to address the problem of observer bias (e.g. Surtees *et al.* 1983).

The major problem with cross-sectional surveys arises from their inefficiency in studying uncommon conditions as it is necessary to assess large numbers of subjects to identify enough cases to permit meaningful statistical analysis. Out of nearly 9500 subjects assessed as part of the ECA, only 144 were diagnosed as suffering from schizophrenia (Myers *et al.* 1984). Clearly it would be difficult to justify setting up an investigation of this scale to study only this one uncommon condition.

It should also be borne in mind that these surveys identify prevalent cases; therefore relative risks for having the disease (rather than developing the disease) are calculated. The identified cases may mainly be those with longstanding illness. Associations identified may thus relate to the causes of chronicity rather than causes of the illness.

AN EXAMPLE OF A CROSS-SECTIONAL SURVEY – MULLEN *ET AL.* (1988)

Mullen and his colleagues used a cross-sectional survey to examine the association between current psychiatric disorder and past and recent sexual and physical abuse. To maximize the efficiency of their design they used questionnaires to obtain data on a first sweep of a random sample of adult women and then followed this up with a more detailed interview; a two-stage design. The following results are a simplified version of their overall findings on childhood sexual abuse.

Approximately 10% of adult women reported childhood sexual abuse. Those abused in childhood had higher mean scores on the General Health Questionnaire. The subjects were categorized as 'cases' or 'non-cases' of psychiatric disorder (predominantly depressive illness) using the Present State Examination, and some adapted results are presented in Table 4.5. The study shows a statistically significant association between childhood sex abuse and the presence of depression in adulthood, with an odds ratio of 3.6.

Mullen and colleagues examined their data for some potential confounding variables, for example they showed that the association could not be explained by social class or educational background. Biases could arise in the reporting of current mental state and past abuse. Also, interviewers may have been influenced by their views on the hypothesis under test causing them to overestimate systematically levels of depression in abused women. Additionally, euthymic subjects may underreport their past experience of emotional and physical trauma. Mullen and colleagues considered these various possibilities and dealt with them in the design and analysis of the study wherever possible. They drew cautious conclusions that sexual abuse in childhood is likely to be an important causal factor for subsequent depression in adult women.

### Cohort studies

The cohort study is the most scientifically satisfactory of the non-experimental designs in medical research; it is also usually the most difficult and expensive type of investigation to conduct.

It starts with subjects who are free of the illness of interest. A group of subjects who are exposed to a putative risk factor and a group not so exposed are identified and followed over the

**Table 4.5** Results from a cross-sectional survey: child sexual abuse and depression (Mullen *et al.* 1988)

|  | Case | Non-case | Total |
|---|---|---|---|
| Sexual abuse in childhood | 8 | 33 | 41 |
| No sexual abuse in childhood | 17 | 256 | 273 |

Odds ratio = 8 × 256/17 × 33 = 3.6 (95% CI 1.4–9).

**Table 4.6** Schematic representation of cohort study

| | |
|---|---|
| I | Study subjects identified and exposure status determined |
| II | Subjects followed up over the years and outcome of interest measured in the participants |
| III | Incidence rates of illness in the exposed group and in the unexposed group compared and relative risks estimated |

years. The incidence rates in the two groups are calculated and the relative rates of developing the illness when exposed to the risk factor can then be calculated. The simplified general scheme for conducting a longitudinal study is shown in Table 4.6.

The disadvantages of these studies mainly relate to their scale. For conditions that are at all uncommon the cohort design requires very large samples of exposed and unexposed subjects. A cross-sectional survey of a large number of subjects is difficult and expensive, but in cohort studies there is the additional problem of follow-up, often over many years.

For example, assume that in a study of schizophrenia the annual incidence rate in a group of young adults under study is around 1 per 1000. If 1000 people were followed up for ten years only around ten people in this large group will have developed the illness. This may be barely adequate for statistical analysis, making it difficult to justify the effort and expense put into the project. This design is clearly more feasible with commonly occurring non-psychotic psychiatric disorders.

Cohort designs have the important advantage that subjects' exposure to the hypothesized risk factor is assessed while they are all healthy; therefore, unlike cross-sectional surveys and case-control studies, there will be no scope for observer bias in the assessment of exposure status, nor for recall bias by the subjects. Other biases can occur however. There may be so-called migration bias in which those who were unexposed at the beginning of the study become exposed to the risk factor of interest during the course of a prolonged follow-up period. This bias should be considered in the design as it can be measured and allowed for in the analysis. There can also be important selection biases affecting exposure status (see below).

A clear-cut advantage of cohort studies in most of medical epidemiology is that reverse causality is not a plausible explanation for the finding of an association between exposure and disease; subjects do not have the disease at the beginning of the study. However, with the more subtle and ill-defined disorders studied in psychiatry this may not be the case. In the example below in which cannabis consumption by healthy people is seen to be statistically associated with the subsequent development of schizophrenia, the possibility of reverse causality still has to be considered – could the mental experiences of an incipient schizophrenic illness lead some subjects to find solace in the use of illegal psychotropic substances?

There is an additional advantage of this study design in mental health research. In, for example, cancer epidemiology the investigators are interested simply in whether or not the subjects develop the illness of interest. However, in the mental health field changes in outcome over time in different individuals can be of interest and cohort studies with several assessments of outcome over the years permit this (see Rutter 1988).

The time and resources involved in a cohort

study are obviously considerable and any serious investigation of this type is a major undertaking. It is possible however to conduct a retrospective cohort study. This makes use of data collected in a large group of subjects some years before, in which one or several possible exposures of interest have been measured. If it is possible to identify which subjects have become ill over the years then the incidence rates of illness in the exposed and in the unexposed can be established.

## AN EXAMPLE OF A RETROSPECTIVE COHORT STUDY – ANDREASSON *ET AL.* (1987)

Andreasson and his colleagues had access to the results of a survey conducted in all the men in Sweden conscripted into the army in 1969/70 – a total of 50 465. Data had been obtained on social background, psychiatric history and drug habits. Members of this cohort could be identified in the national register of psychiatric care up until 1983, which contains all psychiatric inpatient admissions in Sweden. Rates of schizophrenia could therefore be calculated.

Table 4.7 presents some of their findings. A dose–response relationship between the level of cannabis consumption and the subsequent development of schizophrenia can be seen.

A study such as this has to be interpreted with caution, as is pointed out by the authors of the report. Is it reasonable to draw the conclusion from this study that the intake of cannabis has been a causal factor in the development of schizophrenia? The association is fairly strong, with a relative risk of 2.4 overall, and there is clear evidence of a dose–response relationship ranging from a relative risk of 1.3 at low levels of consumption to as much as 6 with high consumption. However, there is a possibility that personality traits act as a confounder, having an association both with the tendency to consume illicit psychotropic substances and later development of schizophrenia. Nevertheless, this remains an impressive study and provides good evidence of an association which requires further investigation.

The authors calculated odds ratios rather than incidence ratios because schizophrenia is so

**Table 4.7** Results from retrospective cohort study: cannabis and development of schizophrenia

| Consumption (no. of times) | Total subjects (no.) | Cases of schizophrenia (no). | Odds ratios |
|---|---|---|---|
| 0 | 41 280 | 197 | 1 |
| 1–10 | 2 836 | 18 | 1.3 |
| 11–50 | 702 | 10 | 3.0 |
| >50 | 752 | 21 | 6.0 |

**Table 4.8** Diagram of the design of a randomized
controlled trial

| | |
|---|---|
| I | Identification of group of patients with an illness and consent to participate obtained |
| II | Subjects *randomly* allocated to treatment type |
| III | Mean level of improvement after treatment measured in each group and compared |

uncommon, and follow-up was virtually complete, so that a person-years correction was unimportant.

### Randomized controlled trials

This study design is frequently encountered and will be well known to readers as it is extensively used to evaluate the efficacy of medical treatments, especially new drugs (Pocock 1983).

The controlled trial essentially involves the *random* allocation of study subjects to receive or not to receive a treatment under investigation (Table 4.8). Those allocated not to receive the treatment constitute the controls who should be treated in exactly the same manner as the experimental group except for the intervention under test. When a new drug is being tested the control group receives a dummy medication. Both the patients and the investigating doctors are kept unaware of which subjects have been allocated to each group.

The outcome of the experiment is evaluated after a defined time period and the rates of recovery or improvement in health in the study groups are compared. Because the investigators and the patients are blind as to treatment there should not be bias in assessing or reporting outcome. It should be remembered, of course, that certain side-effects may reveal the treatment allocation either to the patient or the investigator. This potential source of bias can be measured by asking the doctors and patients to make a guess about whether active drug or placebo is being taken.

In controlled trials the random allocation means that problems due to confounding only arise by chance. Usually the first table in the results of a trial gives details of the comparability of the two groups (e.g. mean ages, weights, severity of illness, etc.) to allow the reader to assess the possibility of confounding. This procedure is usually known as checking the randomization. The purpose of randomization is therefore to ensure that confounders are unsystematically allocated between the different treatment groups. Even confounders of which the researcher is unaware are randomly allocated, and should not affect the conclusions (except by chance).

In many instances an effective treatment for the illness may be available and it will therefore not be ethical to give a placebo medication; in this circumstance the comparison will usually be between the standard therapy and the new treatment under investigation.

Important problems arise when the treatment is not a medicine but, for example, a form of psychotherapy. In these circumstances it is not possible to keep the patient or the therapist blind to treatment allocations. It may however be possible to keep the investigator responsible for measuring outcome blind to the treatment received by each subject.

Another problem may arise because of the complexity of some psychiatric treatments, which can demand considerable commitment from the patients. Dropout may be a major problem. In a recent study by Leff *et al.* (1989) the effect on relapse prevention of family therapy was compared with that of attendance at a relatives' group. Unfortunately only 6 of the 11 families continued attendance at the relatives' group. There are various strategies for dealing with this situation; the main recommendation is to maintain the advantages of the randomization procedure by presenting results according to 'intention to treat' rather than the completion of treatment. Both sets of results can, of course, be presented, allowing the reader to judge the possible effects of treatment dropout.

One useful distinction is that between explanatory and pragmatic trials (Schwartz & Lellouch 1967). Most clinical trials are conducted to address a pragmatic clinical problem; which of the treatments should be used? On other occasions, a trial is designed to address a theoretical issue. It is important to keep the aims of a trial clear, as confusion about this issue will lead to a badly conducted study which may address neither theoretical nor practical issues.

The above scheme has not included the steps prior to the random allocation of participants. Details must also be provided of the type of patients who are being approached to enter the study, which subjects were unsuitable because of concerns about compliance, and who chose not to participate. It is useful here to consider the notion of internal and external validity. A randomized controlled trial may have very high internal validity – each stage of the study from randomization may be conducted entirely satisfactorily and provide good evidence of efficacy of the therapy under study. However, a study conducted in a highly specialized clinic in which subjects were rigorously screened for likely compliance may lead to excessive claims for the value of a treatment that do not apply in standard clinical practice (see Elwood 1988). Again, the explanatory/pragmatic distinction is relevant here; some researchers advocate using case-control studies to assess immunization programmes in less developed countries because these give a much more realistic measure of actual clinical effectiveness, rather than the more idealized picture obtained from rigorously conducted clinical trials with highly motivated subjects (Smith *et al.* 1984).

EXAMPLE OF A CLINICAL TRIAL –
FREEMAN *ET AL.* (1988)

Freeman and his colleagues compared the efficacy of three different types of treatment in bulimia nervosa: cognitive behaviour therapy, behaviour therapy and group therapy. In addition they had a further group of subjects who remained on the waiting list. Patients were randomly allocated to the treatments but because group psychotherapy was one of their treatments a stratified randomization procedure was used.

Numerous outcome measures were used which tended to demonstrate the efficacy of each of the psychological treatments. Recommendations could be made from the study on the type of treatments that are likely to be most cost-effective in this disorder.

Their study provides important examples of the difficulties in conducting trials of this complexity. There were a number of safeguards against biased results and there is discussion of the misleading effects of conducting analysis only on those completing treatment, rather than according to the intention to treat. Although one of the best studies of its type in psychiatry the trial had to stop one year earlier than planned due to the high rates of dropout. Of the 92 patients randomized to a psychological treatment, 55 were available for assessment of outcome at three months, 38 at six months, 28 at nine months, and only 24 at one year.

## Conclusions

This section has presented brief details of the methods of investigating groups of human subjects. The randomized controlled trial has an established place in testing pharmacological treatments in psychiatry; despite difficulties it could be more widely used to guide clinicians in their use of non-pharmacological methods and in the planning of their services. However, observational research designs (case-control, cross-sectional and cohort) are the only available means for investigating aetiological factors in human disease. Although there are problems in applying these methods in psychiatry, these are mostly shared with our medical colleagues and well-conducted studies should continue to identify associations with psychiatric disorder.

## Interpreting associations

It is extremely difficult to infer cause of disease from an association with an exposure. There are, however, only a limited number of possible explanations for an association, apart from the possibility that it reflects a causal relationship. These explanations are chance, reverse causality, confounding and bias, and they will be discussed in turn.

## Chance

An association can arise by chance. The standard tests of statistical significance give an estimate of the probability that the data could have arisen by chance – the *P* value. This means that a result which is significant at the 5% level will, on average, be found once in every 20 studies, even if no true association exists. When this occurs it is known as a type 1 error. It is a particular problem if many possible associations are examined within one study and repeated significance tests are performed. It is therefore important to distinguish hypotheses for which the study was designed and findings gleaned after 'data-dredging' to discover a few 'significant' results.

Less commonly recognized is the opposite error. A research project may find no association; but a real association may have been missed because the study is too small and the variation correspondingly large. The study therefore lacks statistical power. Such type 2 errors are a particular problem in biological studies in psychiatry (see Bearn *et al.* (1988) and Evans (1988) for an example and discussion of this problem), and they are also common in social psychiatry and psychology research, because the investigations or other assessments are complex and expensive and sample sizes are inevitably small.

Sartorius *et al.* (1986) conducted a large study to ascertain the incidence of schizophrenia in a number of countries. They concluded that the incidence of (narrowly defined) schizophrenia did not show any difference amongst the countries. However, there was about a twofold difference in incidence between countries with the highest and lowest rates and though this failed to reach statistical significance the authors did not give sufficient weight to the possibility there was a real difference but the study was not statistically powerful enough to detect it. If an investigator wishes to conclude that there is *no* association between disease and exposure it is important to conduct a statistically powerful study.

The routine use of confidence intervals would help resolve this problem. Confidence intervals provide more information than the *P* value (Gardner & Altman 1986), as they indicate the statistical precision of an estimate as well as the probability of its having occurred by chance. Thus confidence intervals indicate whether an association is statistically significant but also whether

a non-significant result is compatible with a clinically important association.

The statistical power of a study gives the probability that a type 2 error will *not* occur. It depends on four factors:
1 The strength of the expected association.
2 The prevalence of exposure.
3 The significance level, usually taken as 5%.
4 The sample size.
For example, a case-control study looking for a relative risk of 2 at the 5% level where the prevalence of exposure is 15% has a power of 80% when there are 200 cases and 200 controls (see Schlesselman (1982a) for tables of required sample sizes in case-control studies). Unless the researcher is expecting a very strong association between the disease and exposure, a case-control study needs to be quite large to have sufficient statistical power. Though the case-control approach usually needs less resources than cohort studies or surveys, by current standards within psychiatry, statistically powerful case-control studies would still be considered large investigations.

This point should be noted by those doing detailed and expensive biological 'exposures' such as scanning and neuroendocrine studies or conducting social investigations with lengthy assessments. The usual sizes of reported psychiatric studies imply that investigators are pursuing massive differences which are unlikely to emerge in view of the multifactorial nature and likely heterogeneity of mental disorders. This means that many important group differences could be under study but remain undetected due to small sample sizes.

### Reverse causality

An association can result if the disease causes the exposure. This is often a particular problem in case-control studies and cross-sectional surveys because data on exposure are usually collected retrospectively. For instance, severe marital discord may be a causal factor for depression. Alternatively depression could lead to marital problems. Likewise, the observation that low social class is associated with schizophrenia is widely held to result from the illness rather than be a cause (Goldberg & Morrison 1963). There-fore, the timing of exposure and onset of disease is important. Similarly, in life events research much attention is paid to 'independent' life events as opposed to those which may be influenced by the illness under study (Brown & Harris 1978). In scanning investigations, ventricular enlargement may be on the causal pathway to schizophrenia, but on the other hand it could be a result of the effects of a schizophrenic illness or its treatment. Recent case-control studies exploring the asso-ciation between CT scan appearances and schizo-phrenia have attempted to address this possibility (Andreasen *et al.* 1990).

Reverse causality is less of a problem in cohort studies, as they start by identifying exposed sub-jects who do not, at that stage, have the disease.

Reverse causality can be an explanation of interest. Some authors have suggested that the association between the abnormal dexamethasone suppression test in depressive illness has aetio-logical significance, in that the hormonal findings are markers of hypothalamic disorder underlying severe depressive illness. In contrast, Mullen *et al.* (1986) have suggested that changes in corti-costeroid metabolism are a result of the anorexia and insomnia of depression.

## Confounding

Confounding is the most important of the possible interpretations of an association and is the main problem in making the leap from association to aetiology. Adjusting for confounding in design and analysis is one of the major preoccupations of medical research, and one of the main difficulties facing psychiatrists in their attempts to explore the causation of mental disorders. A confounder is an independent risk factor, or a protective factor, for the disease which is causally related to the study disease and which varies systematically with the exposure of interest; it is not, however, on the causal pathway between exposure and disease. A confounding factor can lead to a spurious asso-ciation or can eliminate a real association.

A simple illustration is provided by the ob-servation that more women have Alzheimer's dementia than men. Could this indicate that, for

example, hormonal factors could be related to the development of Alzheimer's disease? In fact, this arises from two other associations. First, between age and Alzheimer's disease, which becomes commoner with age; secondly women are more likely to live longer than men. Thus age is said to confound the relationship between sex and Alzheimer's disease. Age is a common confounder and needs to be taken into account in almost any study.

Another example from medical epidemiology helps explain confounding. A study designed to test the hypothesis that high alcohol consumption is causally related to lung cancer would probably demonstrate a statistical association. However, people who drink heavily are more likely to smoke than non-drinkers or moderate drinkers; smoking is therefore a confounding factor. The association between alcohol consumption and lung cancer would disappear if re-examined with separate consideration of smokers and non-smokers.

This example from cancer research highlights one of the problems faced by psychiatrists. There is general agreement that any aetiological study of lung cancer would have to take smoking habits into consideration. However, in psychiatry there are relatively few risk factors known to be im-portant. Thus our research may be exploring aetiological associations that are being distorted (either overestimated or obscured) by the presence of confounding factors of which we are unaware. Professor Geoffrey Rose uses the aphorism that 'one cannot account for the confounding factor one does not know about' and this is a useful reminder both to think about confounders when designing studies, and also that definite conclu-sions about aetiology are difficult to make.

In experimental scientific studies, such as clinical treatment trials, random allocation of individuals to experimental groups reduces the problem of confounding. But people are not randomly allo-cated to possible causes of disease. Observational studies (cross-sectional, case-control and cohort) remain the only way to investigate environmental causes of illness in humans, and so the problem of confounding is introduced. In attempting to interpret an association it is often helpful to ask 'what are the determinants of exposure in this group, why were some exposed others not?'. In other words 'How does this study situation differ from a randomised trial?' (G. Rose 1987, personal communication).

The scheme used by Schlesselman (1982a) to illustrate the nature of confounding factors is shown in Fig. 4.1 to help orientate the reader. A single-headed arrow indicates a causal association and a double-headed arrow indicates non-causal association.

When the factor is causally related to the disease of interest and the hypothesized exposure

is associated with this factor then an investigation which fails to take it into account will reveal a statistical association. The alcohol (exposure), smoking (confounding factor) and lung cancer (disease) relationship is an example of this. Similarly, when the study exposure does increase the risk of disease and is independently related to another risk factor an investigation which fails to take this second risk factor into account will over-estimate the relative risk.

Two separate risk factors do not confound each others' relationship with disease; a confounder has to be associated with both the disease and the exposure. A factor that is related to disease because it is on the causal pathway between exposure and disease does not confound the association (Fig. 4.1(b)). If you statistically adjust for the factor on the causal pathway, however, you will appear to eliminate the association between the exposure and the disease.

A further hypothetical numerical example is shown in Tables 4.9–4.12. It has been deliberately designed with unrealistically large associations. Suppose a case-control study is attempting to measure the association (if any) between life events and schizophrenia. The raw data, illustrated in Table 4.9, finds no association, with an odds ratio of 1. However, schizophrenics are less likely to have children at home, and if we further suppose that life events are commoner in households that have children, the presence of children in the home confounds the relationship between schizophrenia and life events. When the results are stratified by the presence or absence of children (Table 4.10), there now appears to be a strong association, previously masked by the confounder with an overall odds ratio of around 5.

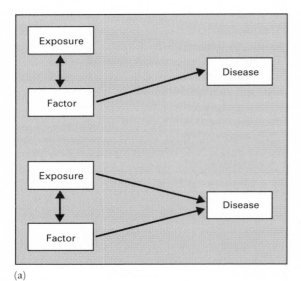

(a)

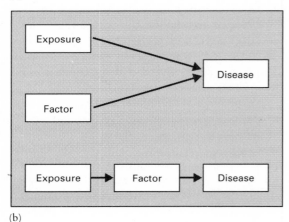

(b)

**Fig. 4.1** (a) Situations in which there is confounding. (b) Situations in which there is no confounding.

**Table 4.9** A hypothetical example of confounding: the relationship between schizophrenia and life events

|                | Cases | Controls |
|----------------|-------|----------|
| Life event     | 100   | 100      |
| No life event  | 100   | 100      |
| Total          | 200   | 200      |

Odds ratio = 1.0

**Table 4.10** Stratifying by the confounder: the presence of children at home

|  | Children | | No children | |
|---|---|---|---|---|
|  | Cases | Controls | Cases | Controls |
| Life event | 45 | 95 | 55 | 5 |
| No life event | 5 | 50 | 95 | 50 |
| Total | 50 | 145 | 150 | 55 |
|  | Odds ratio = 4.7 | | Odds ratio = 5.8 | |

**Table 4.11** Stratifying by the exposure: life events

|  | Life events | | No life events | |
|---|---|---|---|---|
|  | Cases | Controls | Cases | Controls |
| Children | 45 | 95 | 5 | 50 |
| No children | 55 | 5 | 95 | 50 |
| Total | 100 | 100 | 100 | 100 |
|  | Odds ratio = 0.04 | | Odds ratio = 0.05 | |

**Table 4.12** Stratifying by the disease: cases or controls

|  | Cases | | Controls | |
|---|---|---|---|---|
|  | LE+ | LE− | LE+ | LE− |
| Children | 45 | 5 | 95 | 50 |
| No children | 55 | 95 | 5 | 50 |
| Total | 100 | 100 | 100 | 100 |
|  | Odds ratio = 15.5 | | Odds ratio = 19 | |

LE+, life events; LE−, no life events.

A confounder is associated with the disease at each level of the exposure. This is illustrated in Table 4.11, as the data are now stratified by the exposure, life events. The odds ratios now illustrate the association between the confounder (the presence of children) and the disease. The odds ratio of 0.05 in this hypothetical example indicates that schizophrenics are about 20 times *less* likely to have children at home than the controls. For a factor to confound a relationship it must also be associated with the exposure, both within the cases and within the controls.

Stratifying the results by the case/control distinction (Table 4.12) illustrates a strong association between life events (the exposure) and the presence of children (the confounder) in this imaginary example.

ADJUSTING FOR CONFOUNDERS

Adjusting for confounders can occur in the design (restriction and matching) and/or in the analysis (stratified analysis and multivariate methods) but is only effective if they are measured accurately. Inaccurate measurement can result in a false sense of security, since residual confounding may occur despite the presence of a design or analysis that has apparently taken account of the confounder. This can also occur if what is actually measured is an imperfect proxy for the true underlying confounder, for instance if social class is used as a proxy for differences in lifestyle.

Often many (or even all) of the four main methods of adjusting for confounding will be used in the same study.

*Restriction*

Subjects are only selected if they have the same value of the confounding variable. For instance, if sex is a potential confounder then only women may be selected for study (Brown & Harris 1978). Jenkins (1985) investigated the sex difference in minor psychiatric morbidity by restricting her sample to one grade of the civil service, thus reducing the confounding effects of occupational status and education. Controlling for confounding by restriction makes it impossible to look for interactions (see below).

*Matching*

Matching can be carried out in case-control studies and less commonly in cohort studies. Thus the unexposed subjects in a cohort study or the controls in a case-control study can be deliberately selected so as to be similar to the subjects of the index group in regard to any number of potential confounders, but commonly age and sex.

This technique has different consequences in the

analysis of cohort studies and case-control studies. In both, however, its main advantage is to increase power. There is a common misapprehension that matching, by itself, improves the validity of studies. This is not so, and in case-control studies it can sometimes actually lead to a biased estimate unless the matching is retained in the analysis. In a matched cohort study, if matching is not retained in the analysis there will have been no gain in statistical power, and the effort involved in the matching procedure will have been wasted.

Matching is most often used in case-control studies. Matching of cases and controls is, at first sight, a straightforward technique. If controls are chosen to be similar to each case in regard to confounding factors then their effects will be removed. Also balance will be created in numbers of cases and controls according to the presence or absence of the confounder; a matched study, therefore, is usually statistically more efficient than an unmatched one as long as the matched variable *is* a confounder. However, the association between the matched variable and the disease cannot be studied.

Individual matching is most frequently used – and misused. Here, the presence or absence of possible confounding variables is noted for each case, and a control subject (or subjects), similar in regard to these features, is grouped with each individual case. For example, it may be decided that matching on neighbourhood (in an attempt to control for social class and also social adversity/advantage, poor housing, etc.) could best be done by taking the next-door neighbour of the same sex as each case. Individual pairing will be appropriate here. Amaducci *et al.* (1986), in their Alzheimer's disease study, used a friend or acquaintance of the same sex and neighbourhood and to within three years of age of each individual case (see below).

Individual matching should not be used when there are many subjects in each matching category. Cases may be categorized on the basis of confounders and then controls, similar in regard to these confounders, are chosen such that numbers of cases and controls are equal, or in a fixed ratio, within each stratum. Thus, age may be considered an important confounding variable. If there are 10

cases between 21 and 30 years, and 20 between 31 and 40 years, frequency matching would involve the deliberate inclusion of twice as many controls who are in the older age range no matter what is the age distribution in the sampling frame for the controls. In this situation, it would be pointless to pair control subjects with individual cases, i.e. to match individuals according to age alone.

*Matched design-matched analysis.* The most important principle is that matching must be retained in the analysis. This is not always adhered to in clinical research. If it is ignored at this stage then a confounding structure, different from that present in the population from which subjects were drawn, may actually be built into the studies by the investigators. This can lead to a biased relative risk estimate, usually biased towards unity. A detailed explanation of how this arises is given by Rothman (1986).

The methods of analysis of individually and frequency matched studies are explained in detail by Breslow & Day (1980) and Schlesselman (1982a).

*Advantages and disadvantages of matching.* The advantages of matching seem clear. Each subject in the study contributes to the results and therefore a more precise estimate of relative risk will be obtained than with stratified analysis of an unmatched study. In a small-scale study in which several confounding variables have to be taken into consideration there may be no alternative but to individually match. Such a design is recommended when the exposure under study involves an elaborate investigation; in this case the extra time and effort spent on matching will be compensated for in the increase in statistical precision of the study result.

The major disadvantage involves administrative difficulty. It may not be possible to match some controls to cases, therefore time and money spent in these assessments will have been wasted (see McKinlay (1977) for discussion of this point and examples). Frequency matching has similar practical disadvantages but these are less extreme. Another problem is that the analysis of matched studies is more complex and it is impossible to conduct stratified analyses.

Therefore there is a balance between putting resources into a careful matching of subjects or alternatively increasing the sample size of an unmatched study. The researcher has to decide which strategy will lead to the most efficient investigation.

### An example of an individually matched study: risk factors for Alzheimer's disease (Amaducci et al. 1986)

Amaducci *et al.* (1986) individually matched 116 cases of Alzheimer's disease to two different control groups – hospital patients and healthy neighbours. Information had to be obtained from a relative of the cases because of their dementia, and to minimize a recall bias relatives also provided information on the controls. Table 4.13 gives just one comparison of the cases and their hospital controls; the exposure here is the history of dementia in any first-degree relative.

The association may have arisen by chance, although this is highly unlikely as indicated by the *P* value of 0.005. However, it should be borne in mind that almost 200 statistical comparisons were made in this study and so there is a real possibility that some positive findings arose by chance. Reverse causality is not a possibility with this

exposure. However, the authors weigh up the possibilities of selection and information biases. In particular they consider whether families with multiply affected members would have been more likely to have an Alzheimer's disease patient referred to a study hospital. Also, the informants for the cases may have been more aware of a family history of dementia than informants for the control subjects.

### STRATIFICATION

The principle of a stratified analysis is straightforward. The relative risk is calculated within each level of the confounding variable and a summary statistic, a weighted average of some sort, is calculated (Breslow & Day 1980). The details of analysis will not be described here, but the principle is illustrated in the hypothetical example given above (Tables 4.9 and 4.10). With stratification the relative risk of disease at each level of the confounding variable cannot be affected by the confounder.

### Standardization

Age and sex standardized rates are a common way to present data on mortality, particularly when using government statistics when age and sex are the only potential confounders on which information is usually available. Standardization is merely a specific way of carrying out a stratified analysis in order to adjust for differences in (usually) the age and sex structure of the population (see Kahn 1983).

As in the examples given above, comparing raw rates can be misleading in certain comparisons. For example, the prevalence of dementia in a seaside town could be found to be much higher than in an inner city area. However, different age structures in these areas will have to be taken into account if there are more elderly people in the seaside town – rates will have to be *standardized* for age. This is a further example of age acting as a *confounder* accounting for an apparent association between, in this example, dementia and area of residence.

In planning health services in the area the actual experience of the local population may be all the

**Table 4.13** An individually matched study

| | | Controls | |
| --- | --- | --- | --- |
| | | No. of case-control pairs | |
| | | Dementia in first-degree relative | No dementia in first-degree relative |
| *Cases* | Dementia in first-degree relative | 2 | 25 |
| | No dementia in first-degree relative | 5 | 82 |

$$\text{Odds ratio} = \frac{\text{no. of pairs with case exposed and control unexposed}}{\text{no. of pairs with control exposed and case unexposed}} = \frac{25}{5} = 5$$

Adapted from Amaducci *et al.* (1986).

information required and standardization may not be necessary. If a hypothesis on aetiology were being investigated comparisons of unstandardized rates could be misleading.

Unfortunately, the confounding effects of age have been relatively ignored in some published studies in psychiatry. For example, Der *et al.* (1990) failed to adjust for age in their study of time trends in schizophrenia, while Sartorius *et al.* (1986) compared the incidence of schizophrenia in developed and developing countries without explaining how they took account of the differing age structures of the populations involved (Jablensky *et al.* 1992).

MULTIVARIATE TECHNIQUES

It is often difficult to control for more than one or two confounders by stratification because the number of subjects in each stratum becomes very small or non-existent. For example, stratifying by sex, age (in six age groups), and social class (six groups) would yield $2 \times 6 \times 6 = 72$ strata. Even with a large study there may be few or no cases or controls in certain strata, which will therefore not be of value in estimating relative risk. Multivariate analysis is conceptually similar to stratification but makes a simplifying assumption which increases the apparent power of the study (Dunn 1981). Epidemiological studies are often analysed using logistic regression, which assumes a linear relationship between the logarithm of the odds (logit) of being a case and the exposures. This model can take account of a large number of variables simultaneously, including continuous measures. Detailed accounts are given in Breslow & Day (1980, 1987).

However, there are problems with this method. It assumes a linear (or logistic) relationship (Warr (1987) discusses non-linear relationships in mental health) and distances the investigator (and the reader) from the data being analysed. It is wise then to use multivariate techniques in conjunction with simpler stratified analysis.

*Interactions or effect modification*

It is convenient at this point to outline the meaning of interactions in medical research. Some

**Table 4.14** An example of an interaction

| | Working class | | Middle class | |
|---|---|---|---|---|
| | Cases | Controls | Cases | Controls |
| Life events | 15 | 18 | 4 | 15 |
| No life events | 8 | 40 | 8 | 33 |
| | Odds ratio = 4.17 | | Odds ratio = 1.10 | |

Adapted from Bebbington *et al.* (1984).

factors may influence the size of an effect in a different way from that produced by a confounder. Interaction or effect modification occurs when the value of an exposure alters the size of the association between the disease and another risk factor. This is illustrated in Table 4.14 with results from a cross-sectional survey (Bebbington *et al.* 1984). The study was examining the relationship between life events and the onset of depression. The table shows the results stratified by social class. The association between depression and life events is only apparent in the working class group. Social class is therefore described as an effect modifier, or alternatively that there is an interaction between life events and low social class in increasing the likelihood of developing depression.

It is useful to compare Table 4.14 with the hypothetical example given in Table 4.10. In the latter, when results are stratified by the presence of children, the odds ratios between life events and the disease are quite similar in the strata – there is no interaction.

*Bias*

The other important explanation for the finding of an association between an illness and exposure is bias, generally defined as 'any process at any stage of inference which tends to produce results or conclusions that differ systematically from the truth' (Sackett 1979).

The numerous possible sources of bias in clinical and epidemiological research have been listed and described by Sackett (1979) and Last (1988), and they have identified six different stages where bias can occur: in reading the published literature; in specifying and selecting the study sample; in measuring exposures and outcomes; in analysing the data; in interpreting results; in publishing results.

This section will introduce some of the most important biases, concentrating on those arising from the selection of study samples (selection bias) and those related to the measurement of information on both illness and exposure (information bias).

Bias is least likely to arise in the experimental situation of the randomized clinical trial as subjects are randomly chosen for inclusion in a particular group and because patients and observers are kept blind, wherever possible, to the allocations. In observational studies, the scope for bias is greater the more the study differs from the ideal clinical trial situation.

It is important to stress that error must be systematic for bias to arise during the collection of data. Random errors in, for example, the measurement of subjects' exposure or disease status, should not lead to the finding of a spurious association (although they will bring about an underestimate of the relative risk or a reduction in the statistical precision of an estimate). However, the more random error, the more a sceptical researcher will fear that there are also systematic errors.

### BIASES DUE TO THE SELECTION OF STUDY SAMPLES

Selection biases are most problematic in case-control studies. Epidemiology is the population-based study of disease and the case-control study is no exception to this rule. The rationale of the design is that the control group should give an estimate of the prevalence of the *exposure in the population from which the cases have been drawn*. Simple algebra illustrates that only under these circumstances will the odds ratio derived from a case-control study conform with the 'true' odds ratio in the study population (Schlesselman 1982b). For this reason choosing the control group becomes one of the major problems. Selection bias occurs when the controls give a biased estimate of the prevalence of exposure in the study population.

Recently, it has been suggested that selection bias may be important in explaining different results obtained in investigations of the association between the size of the cerebral ventricles and schizophrenia (Smith *et al.* 1988). These authors consider that the variation between studies could be explained by differences in the control groups rather than differences amongst the samples of schizophrenic patients.

Another example is found in the study of illnesses in which psychosomatic factors may be relevant. A case-control study, comparing emotional factors in clinic attenders with asthma and that in patients with more serious structural lung disease, may demonstrate an association between psychiatric disorder and asthma. This may be of aetiological importance. However, most asthmatics are managed at primary care level and emotional distress may partially determine hospital referral. Such a process is less likely to occur with more serious lung disease. Dealing with this important problem in case-control studies often hinges on the choice of the control group (or control groups).

There are a few simple guidelines which are worth considering when deciding on the best possible control group:

1 If possible, cases should relate to a study population. For instance, in a specialized hospital, restricting cases to those of the catchment area may make it easier to choose appropriate controls.

2 In some circumstances, researchers choose more than one control group in the hope that if a consistent association is found in both comparisons, selection bias is unlikely to be a reasonable explanation.

3 A control subject would become part of the sampling frame for the cases if he/she were to develop the disease. For instance, if the cases are all first-contact schizophrenics from a defined catchment area, it would be reasonable to choose a population-based sample from the catchment area as controls. This assumes that everyone with schizophrenia in the catchment area eventually contacts the psychiatric services. The situation with affective disorder is quite different. There is a considerable literature illustrating that most of those with affective disorder never contact the

psychiatric services (Goldberg & Huxley 1980, Shepherd *et al.* 1981). Therefore, general population controls for hospital cases of depression could lead to an important selection bias (see 'Examples of selection bias' below).

**4** Patients attending the same facility but who are suffering from a psychiatric disorder different from that under study can provide an unbiased estimate of the exposure in the study population, so long as the exposure is not associated with the control illness and the probability that controls are selected is not influenced by exposure. It may be desirable to avoid using control subjects all of whom have the same condition. Thus, if there is an association between one of the illnesses suffered by controls and the exposure, a large discrepancy in the relative risk estimate will be avoided.

**5** Healthy volunteers are most commonly used in studies where a blood, imaging or other test is being investigated. In this situation, it is difficult to assess potential biases. If volunteers are used, the investigators must make every attempt to describe who they were, why they volunteered and their response rate. For example, a recent study exploring positron emission tomography scan abnormalities in obsessive-compulsive disorder used volunteer controls but no details were given on who they were. There was no way of knowing whether they differed markedly from the study population (Baxter *et al.* 1987). The general point made above, that controls would be included in the sampling frame for cases if they become diseased, tends to outlaw the use of volunteer controls in most psychiatric centres.

**6** In studying common minor psychiatric disorders, one approach may be to screen a population and study a smaller sample of likely cases and controls in more depth. This has been called a two-stage screening procedure (Williams *et al.* 1980, Bebbington *et al.* 1981).

Selection biases also arise in cohort studies. In general and occupational epidemiology, investigators are well aware of the problems of the healthy worker effect. Thus, there may be an association between an occupational exposure and development of an illness. However, the job in question may demand especially good health; a comparison of subsequent illness with the general population may give a misleading impression of the health-damaging effects of the occupation. For example, most cohort studies of the nuclear industry find that the death rate of the employees is around 80% of the general population. However, nuclear industry employees are selected for good health and given a health check before starting work. Presumably, similar factors are acting on the mental health of occupational cohorts. The damaging effects of, for example, a mentally stressful job may be obscured by self-selection or selection by the employers of psychologically very stable workers.

Biases may also arise due to self-selection by those approached to participate in a cohort study. Thus non-participants may differ in important ways from the eventual study sample in regard to exposure and their likelihood of developing disease. For this reason it is important that information is obtained on a sample of non-participants to examine any systematic differences. Also, those who become lost to follow-up during a prolonged cohort study may be systematically different in regard to exposure and illness experience from those who complete the study. In population-based surveys there is data to suggest that non-responders are more likely to be psychiatrically ill (Clark *et al.* 1983, Williams *et al.* 1986). However, the physically ill and disabled are more likely to respond to health surveys (Sheikh & Mattingly 1981).

Selection biases do not arise with randomized controlled trials as subjects are allocated to treatment groups in a random manner. In a recent

**Table 4.15** An example of selection into treatment

|  | 3 + Children | | % with 3+ children |
|---|---|---|---|
|  | Yes | No |  |
| Patient cases | 9 | 105 | 8 |
| Community cases | 9 | 28 | 24 |
| Community controls | 30 | 352 | 8 |

Odds ratio for patients = 1.01 (95% CI: 0.47–2.19)
Odds ratio for community cases = 3.77 (95% CI: 1.63–8.72)

Adapted from Brown & Harris (1978).

evaluation of the use of 'alternative' treatments in cancer care, which include psychosocial interventions, the participating centre did not allow their patients to be randomized. An attempt was made to study efficacy of the treatments by comparing outcome in attenders at different clinics (Bagenal *et al.* 1990). The subsequent debate about the results of the study has been dominated by the possibility of selection biases, whereby those with more severe illness were referred to or selected themselves for attendance at the alternative treatment clinic.

## Examples of selection bias

Brown & Harris (1978) interviewed a sample of inpatients and outpatients in addition to their population sample. It is therefore possible to compare the presence of risk factors for depression in patients and community cases. The results are shown in Table 4.15.

They illustrate that the association between having three or more children under 14 years old at home and the onset of depression was only apparent when the cases ascertained by community survey were compared with the community controls (odds ratio = 3.77). In contrast there was no apparent association between the presence of three or more children and depression if patients were the source of cases and the controls were chosen from the general population. It is possible to speculate that the presence of young children increases the risk of depression, and also reduces the risk of receiving psychiatric care.

The study by McGuffin *et al.* (1988) may be subject to selection bias. They noted an increase in the incidence of life events in the relatives of depressed hospital patients compared with the results of a population survey. Their results suggest however that the relatives were not very representative, because there was a marked preponderance of women (145:99). In addition, many relatives were not living in the Camberwell area when the study was conducted and so their comparison with Camberwell community data is less than ideal. Furthermore, they began by choosing relatives of depressed hospital patients who are

unrepresentative of depressed people in the community. A case-control study could try to minimize the possible selection bias by choosing an appropriate control group.

### INFORMATION BIASES

Once again problems due to information biases are most problematical in case-control studies. It is convenient to divide information bias into that derived from the subject and that from the observer, though more exhaustive classifications exist (see Sackett 1979).

## Subject-derived bias

When ill subjects are asked about past exposure to a possible risk factor, which is the situation in most case-control studies and cross-sectional surveys, recall of exposure may be influenced by disease status. This is often termed 'recall bias'.

One of the best-known examples is the study of Stott (1958), which found that mothers of babies with Down's syndrome more frequently reported an emotional stressor during pregnancy than women who delivered a healthy baby. This finding is now thought to be due to the mothers' attempt to explain bearing a handicapped child, an 'effort after meaning'.

Recall bias is important in life events research. A depressed subject may remember aversive life events more readily than someone without depression (Lloyd & Lishman 1976). This would increase the apparent association between life events and depression.

There are a number of overlapping strategies for minimizing and evaluating recall bias. Their use should be considered at the design stage of a case-control study.

1 Using a structured questionnaire and standardizing the criteria for exposure is an essential prerequisite for reducing information bias, including recall bias. Relying upon recognition rather than recall by supplying the subject with a comprehensive series of prompts, should also minimize this bias. This method is now routinely adopted in life events research.

2 Recall bias is less likely if the illness is of recent

onset, another reason for favouring the study of incident rather than prevalent cases.

**3** Control subjects who are themselves suffering from an illness may be as motivated as the cases to search their memories in regard to exposure. A more appropriate comparison in the Down's syndrome study mentioned above would have been with the mothers of babies with a different handicap of known cause rather than the mothers of healthy babies.

**4** The validity of self-reported exposure data can be tested, for example by interviewing a close relative or consulting medical records.

**5** Raphael (1987) suggests that if other intuitively plausible exposures, which are known not to be risk factors, are not differentially recalled by the study groups this lends weight to a finding of association with the hypothesized exposure. In addition subjects could be asked about their own causal hypothesis, to see if this corresponds with that of the experimenter.

**6** Social network (Henderson *et al.* 1981), personality measures (Katz & McGuffin 1987), early aversive experiences (Wolkind & Coleman 1983) and marital discord, are all probably influenced by current mental state. Therefore case-control methodology and cross-sectional surveys may lead to misleading results. One potential approach is to design a case-control study within a cohort. For instance, Brown *et al.* (1987) followed a group of women at increased risk of becoming depressed. At the start of the follow-up period they collected data liable to be influenced by mental state. They then compared those who became depressed with those who did not using a case-control design. A similar design is often adopted in attempting to study risk factors for postnatal depression (e.g. Kumar & Robson 1984).

*Observer bias*

An interviewer may introduce bias when aware of which subjects have the illness of interest. Similarly, in cohort studies and in community surveys, knowledge of past or current exposure may influence diagnosis in doubtful cases. For example, in an investigation of the aetiology of depression carried out in subjects' homes, obvious

bad housing may lead to an overestimation of levels of depression.

Once again it is useful to assess the standards of an observational study by comparing it to the design of the ideal clinical trial. 'Blind' assessment in clinical trials arose from the observation that knowledge of the treatment condition can seriously bias the results of a clinical assessment (Hill 1962). Similar standards must also pertain to observational research and so assessments should be 'blind' to exposure, disease status or both whenever possible.

A number of strategies can be used to avoid observer bias. Epidemiologists who investigate the aetiology of physical diseases prefer to use non-medically trained interviewers as they are more likely to follow questionnaires exactly and not to use their own judgement in deciding on exposure and occasionally disease status. Another possibility is to tape-record interviews which can then be co-rated (see Surtees *et al.* 1983), preferably keeping the co-rater unaware of each subject's disease status (in case-control and community studies) or exposure status (in cohort studies). In research using imaging or laboratory techniques it is relatively easy for assessments to be performed by a 'blind' rater.

Observer bias is eliminated by self-administered questionnaires and computerized assessments (Lewis *et al.* 1988). On the other hand there is concern that subjects may not fully understand self-administered questionnaires, and that those who read poorly or are illiterate may be unable to respond. Other sources of bias, for instance when the subject's responses are influenced by disease status, will remain when self-administered measures are used.

It is also possible to try to keep interviewers unaware of the purpose of the study. In practice this may be impossible, especially in small-scale research as the author of the research proposal also acts as interviewer. Also it is hard to sustain the interest and morale of a research team if they are unaware of the study purpose.

*Measuring bias*

If it is possible to measure a bias then it can be treated as a confounder and adjusted for in the analysis of results. Unquantifiable biases are a major problem because it becomes difficult to interpret the results of a study. A bias may have a trivial effect or alternatively lead to a major distortion. The only solution to this difficulty is to attempt to measure bias. Thus, in a randomized controlled trial patients may experience a distinctive and unusual side-effect when on the active agent. At the end of the trial both they and the investigators can be asked to say whether they think they were on the active drug or the placebo; the results can be taken into account in the analysis. However, 'Efforts to compensate for it [bias] in the analysis must be viewed with suspicion' (Rose & Barker 1978).

## AN EXAMPLE OF POSSIBLE INFORMATION BIAS

Goldberg & Morrison (1963) compared the social class of the parents of schizophrenic patients with that of the general population. The general population is probably an appropriate sample to compare with schizophrenic first admissions since almost all people with schizophrenia in a community will eventually come to the attention of the local psychiatric services. However, Goldberg & Morrison ascertained parental social class from the birth certificates of the schizophrenics and compared this with census data on the general population. Social class was therefore collected in different ways in cases and 'controls'. This can result in a well-documented bias as social class tends to be 'higher' when recorded on birth certificates than when recorded by census (Leete & Fox 1977). This suggests that a traditional case-control design would be more appropriate and would enable the social class of both cases and controls to be ascertained in the same way.

### Inferring a cause from an association

The last explanation for a statistical association identified in an epidemiological study is that the exposure does increase the risk of disease; that it is a cause or is on the causal pathway.

The final conclusion regarding causality depends on judgement, argument and the uses to which

the conclusion will be put. In studies which bear directly upon important areas of social policy, one would expect more convincing evidence to be produced by the researcher. Laboratory work provides plausible final pathways for causes, thus supplementing epidemiological studies that indicate the importance of aetiological factors in the population at risk.

Hill (1965) and others have published guidelines to help in the judgement of whether an association is a causal one. These include the following:

1 *Strength of an association.* The stronger the association between a hypothesized risk factor and a disease, the likelier it is that the association is causal.

2 *Consistency with existing knowledge.* Evidence from other sources, such as laboratory and animal research and clinical description, may help support evidence for a causal association arising from epidemiological studies.

3 *Time sequence.* The putative causal mechanism has to have taken effect before the onset of illness and efforts should be made to determine this in studies of ill subjects. This may not always be possible with some chronic conditions. For example, the overall evidence suggests that there is a modest increase in the size of the ventricular system in patients with schizophrenic illness (Andreasen *et al.* 1990). This may be a marker for the neuropathological mechanisms leading to this illness but such studies have to depend on the case-control method and therefore the possibility of reverse causality remains. It is impossible to address this issue with a cohort study as this would involve obtaining large groups of healthy people with enlarged and non-enlarged ventricles and then following them over the years.

4 *Dose–response relationship.* The finding of a dose–response relationship, i.e. a relationship in which a change in amount, intensity, or duration of exposure is associated with an increase or decrease in risk of illness (Last 1988), is usually considered as further evidence that an association is a causal one. This dose–response relationship is, for example, very clear in the relation between smoking and lung cancer – those who smoke 40 cigarettes a day are more likely to develop lung cancer than those who smoke 20 a day.

## Conclusion

This chapter describes a number of the methodological problems in the design and interpretation of psychiatric research. Of particular importance for readers of this text is the use of case-control studies. Since they are relatively small-scale studies they are commonly used, but on many occasions the problems associated with them are poorly understood. As Breslow & Day (1980) have pointed out:

> As a form of research the case-control study continues to offer a paradox: compared with other designs it is a rapid and efficient way to evaluate a hypothesis. On the other hand, despite its practicality, the case-control study is not simplistic and it cannot be done well without considerable planning. Indeed, the case-control study is perhaps the most challenging to design and conduct in such a way that bias is avoided. Our limited understanding of this difficult study design and its many subtleties should serve as a warning – these studies must be designed and analysed carefully with a thorough appreciation of their difficulties.

In research of all types the main intellectual challenge comes before the data are collected; in choosing the design, deciding on potential confounders and their appropriate measurement, and assessing the importance of biases. Almost all the problems can (or should) be foreseen and, wherever possible, dealt with in the design. This chapter has tried to demonstrate how an epidemiological approach is relevant in the design of all quantitative psychiatric research projects involving human subjects, whether the hypothesis to be examined is social, psychological or biological in nature.

## Appendix: odds and odds ratios

There are a number of advantages to using odds rather than using probability in assessing the risk of disease. There are two main reasons for this. First, the mathematics associated with manipulating odds ratios is easier. Second, the regression coefficients in a logistic regression model can be exponentiated and expressed as odds ratios. Therefore it is possible to present results before and after multivariate adjustment in terms of odds ratios. Finally, odds ratios are the only valid method of analysing case-control studies when the data are categorical (as shown in Schlesselman 1982a).

To illustrate calculating odds and odds ratios, the following table can be thought of as the results of either a cross-sectional survey, cohort study or case-control study.

|            | Cases | Controls | Total |
|------------|-------|----------|-------|
| Exposed    | $a$   | $b$      | $a + b$ |
| Not exposed| $c$   | $d$      | $c + d$ |

The probability of being a case in the group of exposed subjects is $a/(a + b)$. The odds of being a case in the exposed group is $a/b$. Similarly in the unexposed group, the probability of being a case is $c/(c + d)$ while the odds is $c/d$. The odds ratio is therefore $(a/b)/(c/d)$, and after manipulating algebraically this is $(a \times d)/(b \times c)$. The odds ratio is therefore a 'relative odds'. The odds in the exposed group is usually divided by the odds in the unexposed group, as in calculating relative rates.

Probability and odds are related to each other.

$$\text{Probability} = \frac{\text{odds}}{1 + \text{odds}}$$

Likewise:

$$\text{Odds} = \frac{\text{probability}}{1 - \text{probability}}$$

The following table will give an idea of the relationship between odds and probability.

| Probability | Odds     |
|-------------|----------|
| 0.001       | 0.001    |
| 0.01        | 0.01     |
| 0.1         | 0.11     |
| 0.25        | 0.33     |
| 0.5         | 1.00     |
| 0.75        | 3.0      |
| 0.9         | 9.0      |
| 1.0         | infinity |

A few points are worthy of note. First, a probability of 0.5 corresponds to an odds of 1.0 and probabilities greater than 0.5 therefore have odds larger than 1. Also, odds can go up to infinity and so are unlike probability, which only varies between 0 and 1. Odds, however, do not meaningfully exist below 0.

## References

Alderson M.R. (1988) *Mortality, Morbidity and Health Statistics*. MacMillan Press, Basingstoke.

Amaducci L.A., Fratiglioni L., Rocca W. *et al.* (1986) Risk factors for clinically diagnosed Alzheimer's disease: a case-control study of an Italian population. *Neurology* 36, 922–931.

Andreasen N.C., Swayze V.W., Flaum M., Yates W.R., Arndt S. & McChesney C. (1990) Ventricular enlargement in schizophrenia evaluated with computed tomographic scanning. Effects of gender, age and stage of illness. *Archives of General Psychiatry* 47, 1008–1015.

Andreasson S., Allbeck P., Engstrom A. & Rydberg U. (1987) Cannabis and schizophrenia: a longitudinal study of Swedish conscripts. *Lancet* ii, 1483–1486.

Appleby L. (1991) Suicide during pregnancy and in the first postnatal year. *British Medical Journal* 302, 137–140.

Armitage P. & Berry G. (1987) *Statistical Methods in Medical Research*. Blackwell, Oxford.

Bagenal F.S., Easton D.F., Harris E., Chilvers C.E.D. & McElwain T.J. (1990) Survival of patients with breast cancer attending Bristol Cancer Help Centre. *Lancet* ii, 606–610.

Baxter L.R., Phelps M.E., Mazziota J.C., Guze B.H., Schwartz J.M. & Selin C.E. (1987) Local cerebral glucose metabolic rates in obsessive-compulsive disorder. *Archives of General Psychiatry* 44, 211–218.

Bearn J., Treasure J., Murphy M. *et al.* (1988) A study of sulphatoxymelatonin excretion and gonadotrophin status during weight gain in anorexia nervosa. *British Journal of Psychiatry* 152, 272–276.

Bebbington P., Hurry J., Tennant C., Sturt E. & Wing J.K. (1981) Epidemiology of mental disorders in Camberwell. *Psychological Medicine* 11, 561–579.

Bebbington P., Sturt E., Tennant C. & Hurry J. (1984) Misfortune and resilience: a community study of women. *Psychological Medicine* 14, 347–363.

Breslow N.E. & Day N.E. (1980) *Statistical Methods in Cancer Research*: vol. I. *The Analysis of Case Control Studies*. Oxford University Press, Oxford.

Breslow N.E. & Day N.E. (1987) *Statistical Methods in Cancer Research*: vol. II. *The Design and Analysis of Cohort Studies*. Oxford University Press, Oxford.

Brown G.W., Bifulco A. & Harris T.O. (1987) Life events, vulnerability and the onset of depression: some refinements. *British Journal of Psychiatry* 150, 30–42.

Brown G.W. & Harris T. (1978) *Social Origins of Depression*. Tavistock, London.

Bruch H. (1973) *Eating Disorders: Obesity, Anorexia Nervosa and the Person Within*. Basic Books, New York.

Carroll B.J., Feinberg M., Greden J.F. *et al.* (1981) A specific laboratory test for the diagnosis of melancholia. *Archives of General Psychiatry* 38, 15–22.

Clark V.A., Aneshensel C.S., Frerichs R.R. & Morgan T.M. (1983) Analysis of non-response in a prospective study of depression in Los Angeles County. *International Journal of Epidemiology* 12, 193–198.

Coryell W. & Tsuang M.T. (1982) DSM-III schizophreniform disorder. *Archives of General Psychiatry* 39, 66–69.

Cox B.D., Blaxter M., Buckle A.L.J. *et al.* (1987) *The Health and Lifestyle Survey*. Health Promotion Research Trust, Cambridge.

Craig T.K. & Brown G.W. (1984) Goal frustrating aspects of life events, stress and aetiology of gastro-intestinal disorder. *Journal of Psychosomatic Research* 28, 411–421.

Der G., Gupta S. & Murray R.M. (1990) Is schizophrenia disappearing? *Lancet* 335, 513–516.

Doll R. (1955) Mortality from lung cancer in asbestos workers. *British Journal of Industrial Medicine* 12, 81–86.

Doll R. & Hill A.B. (1964) Mortality in relation to smoking: ten years' observations of British doctors. *British Medical Journal* 1, 1399–1410.

Dunn G. (1981) The role of linear models in psychiatric epidemiology. *Psychological Medicine* 11, 179–184.

Eaton W.W. (1985) Epidemiology of schizophrenia. *Epidemiologic Reviews* 7, 105–126.

Eaton W.W., Day R. & Kramer M. (1988) The use of epidemiology for risk factor research in schizophrenia: an overview and methodologic critique. In Tsuang M.T. & Simpson J.C. (eds) *Handbook of Schizophrenia* vol. 3. *Nosology, Epidemiology and Genetics of Schizophrenia*. Elsevier, Amsterdam.

Eaton W.W. & Kessler L.G. (eds) (1985) *Epidemiologic Field Methods in Psychiatry: The NIMH Epidemiologic Catchment Area Program*. Academic Press, Orlando.

Elwood J.M. (1988) *Causal Relationships in Medicine. A Practical System for Critical Appraisal*. Oxford University Press, Oxford.

Evans C. (1988) Melatonin secretion and anorexia nervosa – a serious type II error. *British Journal of Psychiatry* 153, 121.

Freeman C.P.L., Barry F., Dunkeld-Turnbull J. & Henderson A. (1988) Controlled trial of psychotherapy for bulimia nervosa. *British Medical Journal* 296, 521–525.

Gardner M.J. & Altman D.G. (1986) Confidence intervals rather than *P* values: estimation rather than hypothesis testing. *British Medical Journal* 292, 746–750.

Goldberg D. (1972) *The Detection of Psychiatric Illness by Questionnaire. Maudsley Monograph No. 21*. Oxford University Press, Oxford.

Goldberg D. & Huxley P. (1980) *Mental Illness in the Community*. Tavistock, London.

Goldberg E.M. & Morrison S.L. (1963) Schizophrenia and social class. *British Journal of Psychiatry* 109, 785–802.

Harrison G., Owens D., Holton A., Neilson D. & Boot D. (1988) A prospective study of severe mental disorder in Afro-Caribbean patients. *Psychological Medicine* 18, 643–657.

Henderson A.S., Byrne D.G. & Duncan-Jones P. (1981) *Neurosis and the Social Environment*. Academic Press, Sydney.

Hill A.B. (1962) *Statistical Methods in Clinical and Preventive Medicine*. Livingstone, Edinburgh.

Hill A.B. (1965) The environment and disease: association or causation? *Journal of the Royal Society of Medicine* 58, 295–300.

Jablensky A., Sartorius N., Ernberg G. *et al.* (1992) Schizophrenia: manifestations, incidence and course in different cultures. A World Health Organization ten country study. *Psychological Medicine* Monograph Suppl. 20. Cambridge University Press, Cambridge.

Jenkins R. (1985) Sex differences in minor psychiatric disorder. *Psychological Medicine Monograph No. 7*. Cambridge University Press, Cambridge.

Kahn H.A. (1983) *An Introduction to Epidemiologic Methods*. Oxford University Press, New York.

Katz R. & McGuffin P. (1987) Neuroticism in familial depression. *Psychological Medicine* 17, 155–161.

Kendler K.S. (1988) The genetics of schizophrenia: an overview. In: Tsuang M.T. & Simpson J.C. (eds) *Handbook of Schizophrenia* vol. 3. *Nosology, Epidemiology and Genetics of Schizophrenia*. Elsevier, Amsterdam.

Kumar R. & Robson K.M. (1984) A prospective study of emotional disorders in childbearing women. *British Journal of Psychiatry* 144, 35–47.

Last J.M. (1988) *A Dictionary of Epidemiology*, 2nd edn. Oxford University Press, New York.

Leete R. & Fox J. (1977) Registrar General's social classes: origins and uses. *Population Trends* 8, 1–7.

Leff J., Berkowitz R., Shavit N., Strachan A., Glass I. & Vaughn C. (1989) A trial of family therapy v. relatives group for schizophrenia. *British Journal of Psychiatry* 154, 58–66.

Lemkau P.V. (1986) The 1933 and 1936 studies on the prevalence of mental illnesses and symptoms in the Eastern Health District of Baltimore, Maryland. In: Weissman M.M., Myers J.K. & Ross C.E. (eds) *Community Surveys of Psychiatric Disorders*. Rutgers University Press, New Brunswick.

Lewis G., Pelosi A.J., Glover E. *et al.* (1988) The development of a computerized assessment for minor psychiatric disorder. *Psychological Medicine* 18, 737–745.

Lewis S.W. & Murray R.M. (1987) Obstetric complications, neurodevelopmental deviance and risk of schizophrenia. *Journal of Psychiatric Research* 21, 413–421.

Lloyd G. & Lishman A. (1976) The effect of depression on speed of recall of pleasant and unpleasant experiences. *Psychological Medicine* 5, 173–180.

McGuffin P., Katz R., Aldrich J. *et al.* (1988) The Camberwell collaborative depression study. II: Investigation of family members. *British Journal of Psychiatry* 152, 766–774.

McKinlay S.M. (1977) Pair matching – a reappraisal of a popular technique. *Biometrics* 31, 731–735.

Mantel N. & Haenszel W. (1959) Statistical aspects of the analysis of data from retrospective studies of disease. *Journal of the National Cancer Institute* 22, 719–748.

Morris J.N. (1975) *Uses of Epidemiology*, 3rd edn. Churchill Livingstone, London.

Mukherjee S., Rosen A.M., Caracci G. *et al.* (1986) Persistent tardive dyskinesia in bipolar patients. *Archives of General Psychiatry* 43, 342–346.

Mullen P.E., Linsell C.R. & Parker D. (1986) Influence of sleep disruption and calorie restriction on biological markers for depression. *Lancet* ii, 1051–1054.

Mullen P.E., Romans-Clarkson S.E., Walton V.A. & Herbison G.P. (1988) Impact of sexual and physical abuse on women's mental health. *Lancet* i, 841–845.

Myers J.K., Weissman M., Tischler G. *et al.* (1984) Six-month prevalence of psychiatric disorder in three communities. *Archives of General Psychiatry* 41, 959–967.

Noble P. & Rodger S. (1989) Violence by psychiatric inpatients. *British Journal of Psychiatry* 155, 384–390.

Paykel E.S. (1978) Contribution of life events to causation of psychiatric illness. *Psychological Medicine* 8, 245–253.

Pocock S.J. (1983) *Clinical Trials. A Practical Approach*. John Wiley & Sons, Chichester.

Raphael K. (1987) Recall bias: a proposal for assessment for control. *International Journal of Epidemiology* 16, 167–170.

Regier D.A., Myers J.K., Kramer M. *et al.* (1984) The NIMH Epidemiologic Catchment Area Program. Historical context, major objectives, and study population characteristics. *Archives of General Psychiatry* 41, 934–941.

Robertson G. (1987) Mentally abnormal offenders: manner of death. *British Medical Journal* 295, 632–634.

Rose G. & Barker D.J.P. (1978) Observer variation *British Medical Journal* 2, 1006–1007.

Rothman K. (1986) *Modern Epidemiology*. Little Brown, Boston.

Russell G.F.M. (1979) Bulimia nervosa: an ominous variant of anorexia nervosa. *Psychological Medicine* 9, 429–438.

Rutter M. (1988) *Studies of Psychosocial Risk. The Power of Longitudinal Data*. Cambridge University Press, Cambridge.

Sackett D.L. (1979) Bias in analytic research. *Journal of Chronic Disease* 32, 51–63.

Sartorius N., Jablensky A., Korten A. *et al.* (1986) Early manifestation and first contact incidence of schizophrenia in different cultures. *Psychological Medicine* 16, 909–928.

Schlesselman J.J. (1982a) *Case Control Studies*. Oxford University Press, New York.

Schlesselman J.J. (1982b) *Case Control Studies*, p. 36. Oxford University Press, New York.

Schwartz D. & Lellouch J. (1967) Explanatory and pragmatic attitudes in therapeutic trials. *Journal of Chronic Disease* 20, 637–648.

Sheikh K. & Mattingly S. (1981) Investigating non-response bias in mail surveys. *Journal of Epidemiology and Community Health* 35, 293–296.

Shepherd M., Cooper B., Brown A.C. & Kalton G. (1981) *Psychiatric Illness in General Practice*, 2nd edn. Oxford University Press, Oxford.

Smith G.N., Iacono W.G., Moreau M., Tallman K., Beiser M. & Flak B. (1988) Choice of comparison group and findings of computerised tomography in schizophrenia. *British Journal of Psychiatry* 153, 667–674.

Smith P., Rodriguez L. & Fine P.G. (1984) Assessment of the protective efficacy of vaccines against common diseases using case-control and cohort studies. *American Journal of Epidemiology* 113, 87–93.

Stott D.H. (1958) Some psychosomatic aspects of causality in reproduction. *Journal of Psychosomatic Research* 3, 42–55.

Surtees P.G., Dean C., Ingham J.G., Kreitman N.B., Miller P.Mc.C. & Sashidaran S.P. (1983) Psychiatric disorder in women from an Edinburgh community: associations with demographic factors. *British Journal of Psychiatry* 142, 238–246.

Warr P. (1987) *Work, Unemployment and Mental Health*. Oxford University Press, Oxford.

Williams P., Tarnopolsky A. & Hand D. (1980) Case definition and case identification in psychiatric epidemiology: review and assessment. *Psychological Medicine* 10, 101–114.

Williams P., Tarnopolsky A., Hand D. & Shepherd M. (1986) Minor psychiatric morbidity and general practice consultations: the West London Survey. *Psychological Medicine. Monograph Supplement* 9.

Wing J.K. (1989) *Health Services Planning and Research. Contributions from Case Registers*. Gaskell, London.

Wolkind S. & Coleman E.Z. (1983) Adult psychiatric disorder and childhood experiences: the validity of retrospective data. *British Journal of Psychiatry* 143, 188–191.

World Health Organization (1981) *Development of Indicators for Monitoring Progress Towards Health For All by the Year 2000*. WHO, Geneva.

# PART 2
# SOCIAL CAUSATION

# Chapter 5
## Influence of Culture on Presentation and Management of Patients

DINESH BHUGRA

## Introduction

Any meaningful study of mental illness across cultures, and therapy when the therapists and their clients come from different cultures, requires an understanding of the diverse premises used within each culture in constructing and defining the concepts of mental health and illness. Such concepts underlie help-seeking behaviours, as well as acceptance or rejection of help offered. This chapter aims to outline some of the issues that therapists must be aware of when dealing with patients from other cultures. The practical issues vital for setting up services are dealt with in Chapter 29.

As social psychiatry deals with forces in the social environment that affect the ability of groups or individuals to adapt, adjust or to change the self or the environment, a framework is essential to understand the effects of migration and acculturation. Not only does it attempt to clarify, identify and increase understanding of how groups of people adapt but also to define the processes and social structures that damage or enhance adaptive capacity (De Vos 1982). Cohen (1987) postulates that the processes of adaptation to a new culture are gradual. The migrant's coping abilities are founded on a scale of personal values, including responsibility, dependence–independence, loyalty and perceived control of the environment. These coping abilities are likely to be put into use once a set of experiences are seen to be distressing, be these experiences social, physical or psychological.

In this chapter we will not look at the epidemiological data of psychiatric diagnosis across cultures and nations, nor do we propose to review the possible hypotheses for varying rates of psychiatric illness across different communities. The aim here is to discuss issues that affect doctors and patients who come from different cultures and the patients' help-seeking behaviour, and to offer some general guidelines for therapist–patient interactions.

Culture comprises values, explicit and implicit behaviour patterns and historically derived and selected ideas; the entire conglomerate thus being observed, mediated, acquired, absorbed and then transacted through the use of distinctive, sometimes almost unique symbols. The conceptualization and definition of culture has often led to it being seen as consisting of everything that is human made (Herskovits 1955) or involving shared meanings (Geertz 1973). Al-Issa (1982) suggests that most definitions regard culture as those aspects of the environment that are man-made. These obviously include the subjective environment which consists of beliefs, norms, myths and valves that are shared by the group and symbolically transmitted to its members. Under this rubric are included the physical environment, such as buildings, bridges and roads, handed down through generations. Culture can be perceived as a system which may be symbolic, personal cognitive or structural (for further discussion see Gudykunst *et al.* 1988). Gudykunst *et al.* (1988) recommend that culture be distinguished from the social system and society. They perceive culture as a shared phenomenon which influences interpersonal communications. We shall follow a broader perspective of culture rather than simply race here. Wilkinson & King (1987) offer a valuable insight into the use of race as a variable. As Tiwari *et al.* (1986) argue:

> Various cultures are not chance products . . .
> culture is the ground substance, the matrix
> within which the psychological, sociological
> and biological forces operate, imparting

meaningfulness and affecting not only the experiences of mental illness but also the biological theories, diagnostic procedures and therapeutic approaches to mental illness. Culture includes categories, plans and rules that people use to interpret their world and act purposefully within it and is learnt as the child grows up in society (Spradley & McCurdy 1974). Thus it is 'acquired' as a 'member of the society' (Rack 1982). Not surprisingly cultures are modified in response to changes in the environment and these alterations may be accepted by its members with reluctance. Culture may exercise powerful pathogenic and pathoplastic as well as health-sustaining influences (Varma 1986). Communication and culture reciprocally influence each other. The culture from which individuals come can affect their mode of communication and this pattern of communication in turn can change the culture they share (Gudykunst *et al.* 1988). Patterns of communication are particularly important in diagnosing mental illness where objective tests are few and not easily available to all clinicians. Therefore, any comparative studies undertaken across cultures often create a collage of distorted pictures. The interface of anthropology and psychiatry has produced an interesting debate. As Skultans (1991) points out, the differences between new cross-cultural psychiatry and 'old' cross-cultural psychiatry exist in the placement of disease categories. In the former a contextual analysis of the indigenous disease categories is recommended ignoring the importation of western categories, whereas the latter proposes that hidden within the 'illness' is a core which is common to all people. The debate continues (see Leff 1990, Littlewood 1990, Skultans 1991). In order to understand the patterns of interpersonal communication, it is important that we begin by looking at some historical facts concerning migration.

## Migration and types of migrants

People have migrated from one place to another, from one country to another and from one culture to another for centuries. Various systems of classifications of migration have been offered (see Anwar 1979). Patterson (1963) has argued for a simple push–pull distinction in migrants – whether the migrant moved to the new country as a result of positive attraction or simply to escape from the old. Rack (1982) proposes a classification of *Gastarbeiters*, exiles and settlers. In addition, in the ever-shrinking global village, students and businessmen often move around regularly and at short intervals. There are a number of people who maintain more than one residence across continents and the stresses experienced by such individuals may be qualitatively and even quantitatively different from other more geographically stable groups.

*Gastarbeiter* is a German word which means migrant worker, but has a specific legal implication. *Gastarbeiter* migration is a result of industrialization, which in developing countries leads to movement from rural to urban areas. This itself exposes the individual to certain stresses which have been discussed in Chapter 29. Typically though, a young man sets out for a developed country in which he never intends to remain permanently. His family is left behind and regular remittances home mean that his own current financial status may be less than comfortable. Since the primary aim is to save as much as possible and also to send as much home as possible, he often has to live in poor housing conditions. He works long hours and may have more than one job, allowing him no spare time to mix with the 'host' community. He may share his living quarters with others in a similar situation and may prefer to spend most of his working and non-working time with his countrymen. There may not be any incentive to mix with his 'hosts' since he perceives his roots still to be in his country of origin. In the 1950s and 1960s migrants from the Indian subcontinent often lived in cramped conditions sharing bedrooms. Subsequently when their families joined them they became 'settlers'.

Settlers on the other hand arrive in a new country with the specific intention of settling down there permanently. This group often consists of young families or young married couples who may have innovative and adventurous ideas and who may feel creatively suffocated at home (Rack

1982). Two types of settlers can be identified: first those who took an active decision, for example, the workers from Ireland leaving for the USA after the potato famine; and secondly those who were made to leave against their will, for example, 'criminals' sent to the colonies. This type of migration is limited nowadays, largely because of stringent migration laws in most countries.

The decision, specially if taken actively, may lead to premigration preparation – learning about the new country and its customs, learning new languages, etc. This in turn will help the new migrants to settle down quicker with less stress. However, each individual's experience has to be understood at his/her particular level, taking into account his/her background and upbringing. The adoption *of* the new country as well as *by* the new country may be entirely successful or it may be superficial. It is also hypothetically possible that the individual and his family may take to the new country but prevalent attitudes and prejudices there may result in their being rejected. On the other hand they may not take to the country either because of geography, climate, social or political factors, even though the country may be perfectly willing to assimilate them. The stresses in the two situations are likely to be dissimilar. Furthermore, variations in social support and personal resources between individuals may lead to different outcomes. Reactions may vary from alienation to paranoid projection. As Rack (1982) has argued, it is possible that by the simple act of emigration, the individual gives one clue that he might be the kind of person who looks for the causes of his problems in his environment rather than in himself. Apart from this explanation, it is also possible that the individual's self-concept and self-esteem were strong enough initially for him to emigrate, and his/her genuine expectations or 'what he was led to believe' may not be fulfilled. This is bound to add to a feeling of let-down and loss – not only of family left behind but also of self-esteem and expectations – creating a discrepancy between achievement and expectation and therefore adding to stresses experienced.

Exiles or refugees face a different set of problems. In due course the exile may become a 'settler' and adapt rapidly to the new country. On the other hand a persistent feeling of nostalgia and loss may continue to haunt the individual. In addition to groups of exiles, for example, massive migration after World War II in Europe and migration across India and Pakistan at the time of partition, there are, of course, individual political refugees. The latter group may include those who come to the country for a particular reason, for example, as students, and then discover that it is unsafe for them to go back. The two broad types of exiles again face different kinds of stresses. Mass displacement may lead to being settled in refugee camps with associated problems of diet, documentation, stretched medical services, etc. The individual refugee may have to cope with often incredulous officialdom, rapidly shrinking financial resources, etc. The stresses of leaving families, property and a feeling of belonging behind produce alienation, anger and despair – an extended bereavement reaction. Tyhurst (1977) has delineated an acute condition called a 'Social Displacement Syndrome', characterized by paranoid behaviour, generalized hypochondriasis, anxiety and depression, disorientation and confusion and desocialization. Gross behavioural disturbances (Rahe *et al.* 1978), emotional outbursts of anger and crying (Stein 1980) and alcoholism (Rack 1982) have been reported. This general personal disequilibrium is said to reach its peak at about six months after entry into a new country. These are complex problems and once again the reader is reminded that only general principles are being applied to here. Migration from one sociocultural system to another implies a radical change in the environment of the migrant, thereby adding to the bewilderment, shock and stress.

Migration is not a unitary experience but rather a continuous one: the stresses and processes continue to change. Rogler *et al.* (1987) argue that the migration experience encompasses three potential sources of primary strain:

1 Insertion into the host society's socioeconomic system.
2 Acculturative processes in reaction to the host society's culture.
3 Change in the interpersonal bonds entangling the migrant's role.

They define primary strains as deeper, more en-veloping, more persistent parameters of external stress which condition broader segments of a migrant's life than do role strains as described by Pearlin *et al.* (1981). Thus it becomes obvious that the process of acculturation is dynamic and con-tinuous, and it may never be complete. The stresses vary in influences, and difficulties, though chronic, may affect the psychological status of the individual. The impact of racism and issues of cross-cultural adaptation are discussed further by Cashmore (1987) and Kim & Gudykunst (1988).

### Doctor–patient interactions

The patients bring to the doctor a series of com-plaints that are their formulations in their own words of 'experiences of dissolved changes in states of being and in social functions' (Eisenberg 1977). Thus social function gets included in the definition of complaints. These social functions encompass not only failures to meet social obligations, for example, inability to cope with housework, concentrate on studies, but also dis-satisfaction with interpersonal relationships (Leff 1988). In some cultures complaints about rela-tionships are never presented *explicitly* to doctors or traditional healers, though this may occur using different idioms of distress (see Nichter 1981a,b). As Leff (1988) points out, 'In selecting from his uncomfortable or painful experiences what to complain about, the patient is influenced by his expectation concerning what the doctor is qualified to deal with'. Patients want to get better quicker. A discrepancy in the time schedules for getting better between what they think is right and what the doctor thinks is possible only adds to their confusion and negative attitudes about the health care system. In addition, it has been reported that differential perceptions of illnesses as well as reporting biases exist between blacks and whites in the USA (Anderson *et al.* 1987). Being black skinned is not detrimental to one's mental health, though stressful social conditions which come about as a result of being black, for example, experiences of loss or failure, denial of respect, are (Cannon & Locke 1977). However, not all immigrants are black. Neff (1984) urges

researchers to take into account other factors like urbanicity as well. Bochner (1982) offers a detailed account for readers interested in the field of cross-cultural interactions.

A knowledge of symptoms is not sufficient to make sense of the 'use' of physicians. Help seeking may reflect a need for social support or secondary gain reflected in release from various obligations and other social processes which may or may not be directly related to the illness or symptoms (Mechanic 1975). Thus presentation of somatic symptoms (reflecting psychological distress) to the doctor has been interpreted by some patients as what doctors are there for. However, the role of the doctor is perceived differently across cultures. Recent studies from the East End of London have suggested that among the Bangladeshi community the doctor is often approached as much for non-health problems as for health problems, taking on a similar role in helping solve family problems as a village elder would do back home (MacCarthy & Craissati 1989). Neighbors *et al.* (1983) reported that among blacks in their sample older and female respondents were more likely to seek formal assistance, and that too through hospital emergency rooms, private physicians and minis-ters. They explain this on the grounds of social conditions and recommend that these be changed. The patient's expectations of the doctor are also moulded by the concepts of illness they hold, which in turn are affected by their culture and experiences (Fig. 5.1).

Helman (1978) reported that among his general practice attenders the commonest model used among the white patients was that of folk medi-cine. The folk classification used by older patients was of two basic polarities: hot and cold and wet and dry. Some areas of the body were seen as more vulnerable to environmental influences than others. This distinction can also be applied to concepts of mental illness. Kleinman (1980) argues that in order to understand patients and their healers, they must be studied in their par-ticular cultural environments and cross-cultural comparisons made only then to seek generaliza-tion about these fundamental human experiences. Since health care systems are socially and culturally constructed, he further argues that medicine

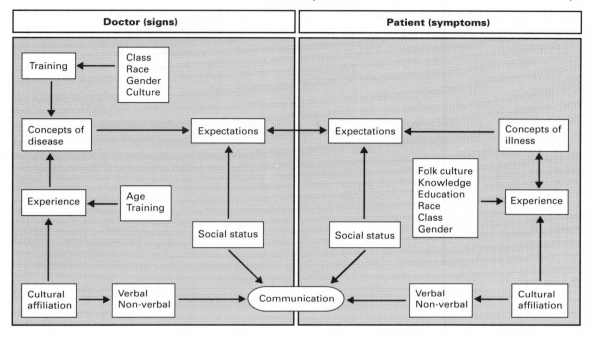

**Fig. 5.1** Therapist—client interaction and influencing factors. (Modified from Leff 1988).

itself is a cultural system of symbolic meanings anchored in particular arrangements of social institutions and patterns of interpersonal interactions. Such a system therefore is influenced by internal and external structures. The former include popular, professional and folk sectors of care. Kleinman (1980) observes that 70–90% of all illness episodes in the USA are managed within the popular sector – within the individual–family–social networks.

Kleinman's emphasis on the dichotomy between two aspects of sickness, disease and illness, is well worth noting (Kleinman 1980). In his view, disease refers to a malfunctioning of biological and/or psychological processes, while the term illness refers to the psychosocial experience and meaning of perceived diseases. As he states:

> Illness includes secondary personal and social responses to a primary malfunctioning (disease) in the individual's physiological or psychological status (or both). Illness involves processes of attention, perception, affective responses, cognition and valuation

directed at the disease and its malfunctions (i.e. symptoms, role impairment etc.).

Though disease affects single individuals, illness experience will often affect others as well (e.g. family, friends, colleagues). Eisenberg (1977) on the other hand argues that patients suffer 'illnesses' whereas physicians diagnose and treat diseases, though he goes on to acknowledge that diseases are abnormalities in the structure and function of body organs and systems whereas illnesses are experiences of devalued changes in states of being and in social function.

Illness is thus the shaping of disease into behaviour and experience, which, needless to emphasize, are modified by personal, social, and cultural influences. Most cultures maintain a wide range of social norms which are considered appropriate for different age groups, genders, occupations, social ranks and cultural minorities within the society (Helman 1990). Every society has the notion of a spectrum extending between what is regarded as normal and abnormal social behaviours. Helman (1990) goes on to argue that different culture-bound mental illnesses can be located at various points along the spectrum of abnormal social behaviours. Even though their timing and setting may be unpredictable, their clinical presentations and behaviour changes are patterned by culture. Simons (1980) has argued that culture-bound syndromes can be seen as universal phenomena. He takes the example of language learning to argue that the basic neuro-developmental template remains within a certain range no matter where one is born. However, depending upon the location of one's birth one may learn to speak German, English, Spanish or Japanese fluently. However, Kenny (1985) takes Simons to task for taking a universal approach at the expense of specific social and cultural contexts (for fuller discussion see Simons & Hughes 1985).

In the past there had been a tendency in the psychiatric literature, especially when describing 'culture-bound syndromes', to focus on exotic and dramatic non-western patterns of behaviour (e.g. Latah, Koro, Amok) while ignoring the cultural embedding of western psychopathology (Gaines 1982). As Lipsedge (1989) observes, 'Although the physical symptoms associated with menstruation appear to be experienced universally, the mood changes associated with the pre menstrual syndrome in the U.K. and the U.S.A. do not seem to occur cross-culturally'. Littlewood & Lipsedge (1987) consider that overdoses, agoraphobia, some forms of shoplifting and baby snatching are western culture-bound syndromes. Pfeiffer (1982) points out the difficulties in integrating culture-bound syndromes with psychiatric nosological systems. A major difference in these two approaches is the way in which symptoms are perceived and ordered in qualitatively different ways. Cultural influences contribute differentially to the causation, formation and interpretation of psychopathological syndromes on four dimensions: culture-specific areas of stress; culture-specific shaping of conduct; culture-specific interpretations, and culture-specific interventions. Pfeiffer goes on to discuss these further. This chapter does not propose to enter into the debate about nosology of culture-bound syndromes (see Simons & Hughes 1985).

Explanatory Model (EM) attempts to explain

**Table 5.1** Suggested questions to elicit Explanatory Models (modified from Kleinman 1980)

| | |
|---|---|
| Q1 | What do you call your problem? What name does it have? |
| Q2 | What do you think has caused your problem? |
| Q3 | Why do you think it started when it did? |
| Q4 | What do your symptoms do to you? How do the symptoms affect you? |
| Q5 | How severe is your problem? Do you think it will have a long course or a short one? |
| Q6 | What do you fear most about your symptoms? |
| Q7 | What are the chief problems your symptoms have caused you? |
| Q8 | Do you think you need treatment for this? What kind of treatment do you think will help? What kind of results do you expect to receive from the treatment? |

aetiology, time and mode of onset of symptoms, pathophysiology, course of sickness and treatment. Explanatory Models differ from general beliefs about sickness and are marshalled in response to a particular illness (for details see Kleinman 1980). Various questions that need to be asked in order to elicit EM are listed in Table 5.1.

The conversion of disease experience to illness leads on to interpretation of symptoms and help-seeking behaviour. These stages are shown in Table 5.2.

It becomes apparent that the doctor–patient interaction would depend very much on the stage at which help is being sought. The interaction will also be affected by the nature of consultation, quality of pre-existing relationship with the doctor and attitudes of both participants. Idioms of distress can be utilized in different modes, for example, psychological, mechanistic, somatic, spiritual. The indigenous practitioners have had greater success in dealing with non-life-threatening chronic diseases and somatization (Kleinman 1980). Bakx (1991) argues that cultural practices in the west have changed in parallel with the changes in economy, whereas in some cultures folk healers are used either because of a cultural

**Table 5.2** Conversion of disease into illness and help seeking

Perceiving and experiencing symptoms
↓
Recognizing the symptoms
↓
Labelling and evaluating the symptoms
↓
Developing a disease
↓
Recognizing an individual's 'sick role'
↓
Deciding what to do
↓
Engaging in specific health care-seeking behaviour
↓
Applying treatment in popular/professional or folk sector
↓
Evaluating the effects of treatment
↓
Altering modes of help seeking

distance between the biomedical fraternity and the local population (Sharpston 1976) or because of a lack of infrastructure (Workneh and Giel 1975, Nchinda 1976). In the west, however, folk medicine is becoming more popular, perhaps due to increased consumer awareness of the failing of modern medicine. Chen (1975) points out from studies in Malaysia that though traditional medicine is giving way to modern scientific medicine, the latter is not replacing traditional medicine but is rather being added on to largely vigorous and continuous systems of traditional beliefs and practices. Dunn (1974) observes that Malaysian Chinese medicine although firmly rooted in tradition is also a modern innovative and changing system which he calls 'modern and traditional'. In an interesting study in Malaysia, Strange (1973) found that illnesses perceived to be due to natural causes were initially self-treated but would be presented to a leader or a cupper if the condition persisted or worsened, and that if the cause was believed to be due to a malign spirit a *bomah* (traditional medicine man) will be called. If there was no improvement or further deterioration occurred even after several *bomahs* had been consulted, only then a doctor would be called for. Orley & Leff (1972) reported that among the Ganda, diseases are classified not only according

to the part of the body affected but also on the basis of other criteria which include the idea of whether the disease was thought to have been caused by supernatural means or to have come by itself, and whether it is Ganda or European in origin. In an earlier participant observation study one of the authors noted that the diseases were seen as weak or strong, the former having a natural causation and the latter attributed to witchcraft or the action of spirits. Thus the diseases were Ganda (caused by witchcraft) or European – the former including epilepsy or madness, not treatable by European methods (Orley 1970a,b). Hartog (1972) observed a similar pathway to that of Strange's (1973) in cases of 'mental deviance'. Unlike other systems of medicine, modern scientific medicine has its basis in biological and experimental thinking. This has produced an emphasis on disease processes rather than the whole person. With the development of subspecialization within medicine the sick person becomes even more 'fragmented'. People from other cultures who have often had exposure to other systems of medicine may be looking for a holistic approach. Beliefs evolve of person's cultural heritage and are also affected constantly by concurrent social conditions (Lin 1980).

### Interrelationship of culture and mental illness

Culture can influence mental illness through its definitions of 'normality' and 'abnormality' in a particular society, through forming the aetiology of certain illnesses, and by influencing the clinical presentation and help-seeking behaviours.

Cultural mechanisms can have a beneficial effect on mental health through: provision of emotional outlets and cathartic strategies; synchronization of individual differences which make a meaningful universal and consistent world view available to its members. It can also affect mental health by provisions of mechanisms to lessen the stresses created by ecological adaptation and social rules; through methods of dealing with its sick members through isolation, marginalization or treatment, and by creating a gratifying environment by socioeconomic organization, political control and leadership.

Culture may predispose, precipitate or perpetuate mental disorders by: creating basic vulnerable personality types; stressful roles; pathological family interactions; acculturation; fostering sanctions against certain behaviours and rewarding certain maladjusted behaviours, as well as establishing unhealthy practices and rigid patterns, e.g. mating.

In making a clinical diagnosis of mental illness in a patient from a different culture, the clinician must bear in mind the following points:

1 Whether the specific cluster of symptoms and signs as well as behavioural changes demonstrated by the patient are interpreted by them and by their community as evidence of a 'culture-bound psychological disorder'.

2 The extent to which cultural factors affect some of the diagnostic categories and techniques of western psychiatry.

3 The role of the patient's culture in helping them to communicate and understand their own psychological distress.

4 The perception of the patient's abnormal behaviour and complaints by the patient's personal, family and social networks.

5 Whether the patient's experience can be understood in terms of social, economic and political pressures on them (Burke 1974).

6 The experiences of patients in a different culture may not only affect their presentation but also their symptomatology (Littlewood & Lipsedge 1989).

The process of acculturation has been defined as a complex process whereby the behaviours and attitudes of a migrant group change toward those of the host society as a result of exposure to a cultural system that is substantially different (Rogler 1989). As noted earlier, this is a continuous process and the stage of acculturation will also determine the style of communication of distress.

### Non-verbal communication in doctor–patient interaction

In the doctor–patient relationship non-verbal communication is as important as verbal forms in understanding the patient's distress, particularly in psychiatric assessment. Silence in conversation, for example, tends to be construed differently in different cultures. The English and the Arabs may use it to denote private thoughts, Indians may use silence as a sign of respect for their elders, whereas the French and Spaniards may read it as agreement among the parties. The Chinese and Japanese use it as a floor-yielding signal but emphasizing the point just made. Americans on the other hand may feel the need to fill the silence with more talk. Patterns of speech are as susceptible to the influence of other cultures as are those of behaviour. It is quite possible that an Indian who has lived in the USA for a considerable length of time may adopt similar usage of silence.

Non-verbal communication is affected by personal expectations as well as usage of a language that is not understandable by the patient. Feelings of surliness, anger, desperation or frustration are often kept in check in order not to alienate the doctor, but these may surface in non-verbal behaviour. There exist unspoken rules about interpersonal distance across cultures. In western societies, for example, these zones can be intimate (contact to 45 cm), personal (45 cm to 1.20 m), social (1.20 m to 3.6 m) and public. In other cultures these will be different. In India, for example, the intimate and personal zones are very similar. Among Africans, Indonesians and Mediterraneans the conversational distances are much closer. Thus the location of the furniture and seating arrangements might imply totally different messages to a patient from another culture than those intended. Sex roles, gender expectations and power structures within a culture will all affect communication – verbal or non-verbal. Eye contact is another important aspect of non-verbal communication. White middle class people when speaking to others look away approximately half the time. However, when whites listen they make eye contact with the speaker four-fifths of the time. Blacks, on the other hand, when speaking make greater eye contact and when listening only infrequent contact. In some cultures being in the same room and close proximity themselves indicate attentiveness. Some of these factors need to be borne in mind while assessing the patient's responses. The patient may be expecting some form of understanding from the doctor and may therefore respond in a manner when it is not forthcoming and this manner may be perceived by the unwary as docile or aggressive.

## Verbal communication in doctor–patient interaction

Doctors trained in the western system of medicine learn to ask what is wrong before asking the reason why, whereas the patient often believes he knows what is wrong but wants to know why it has happened. Unless the clinician is sensitive in the line of questioning there is plenty of scope for friction. An additional problem which is often undervalued, especially in the mental health field, is that of stigma. There has been some work done to understand stigma, to determine public attitudes to mental illness and help seeking, or to study social distancing of the self from someone who is perceived as mentally ill (see Chapter 22) but very little in cross-cultural psychiatry.

Whilst the practitioners of biomedicine are satisfied when a child's bronchopneumonia or gastroenteritis can be traced to a microbial infection, practitioners of traditional medicine tend to pursue the question a step further and ask 'but why this child; is there not an underlying supernatural or predisposing cause?' In other words, as Chen (1975) goes on to argue, the traditional medicine-man and his system deal with the real causes of diseases while modern scientific medicine appears to him to deal only with the palliation of the manifestations of disease. As noted earlier, in countries around the world quite often the two systems have come to function in a harmony which at the surface appears incomprehensible and even contradictory. This feeling is often carried over to the new cultures. The expectations from the health system do not change even though the 'new' health system may prove to be alien. Thus a discrepancy between expectations and delivery of services creates a feeling of being let down.

Awareness of the cultural norms and taboos can certainly help engage a patient in treatment. Among Punjabis, for example, the concepts of hot and cold and Vai-badi are extremely common. As Bhopal (1986) notes, these concepts, akin to those noted by Helman (1978), are not necessarily alien to western medicine. The patients may use various indigenous or folk remedies. These in turn may interact with western medicines if the patient's explanatory model has been ignored.

A sympathetic understanding of cultural values as well as religious beliefs is important in obtaining patient compliance. The needs of people from ethnic minorities of different generations are often assumed to be the same, which is as inappropriate as making the same assumption across generations of white patients. Another problem is that of the role and the position of the doctor. The doctors are likely to be of a higher social status than their patients, but even when the two are of equal social standing the doctors still carry an advantage by virtue of the power their professional skills and knowledge offer them. Their expectations, therefore, will influence not only the nature of the complaints that are presented to them but also the acceptance of treatment.

A thorough knowledge of the relevant culture is essential in decoding and then treating some of the complaints presented. In addition, as we know, not all migrants have the same experiences, stresses or responses. The upward or downward mobility of the migrants also adds to the variables. Higher rates of psychopathology among lower classes especially among black Americans (Neighbors 1986), moving up the social ladder (Kessler & Cleary 1980), and moving down the social ladder (Parker & Kleiner 1966) have major implications not only for research but also for social policy. Neighbors (1987, 1990) recommends that social engineering through environmental change (i.e. to reduce racism or eliminate poverty) would lead to mental health improvements. Miller (1987) suggests that both universality and targeting (of services) have to be employed. The programmes on offer are almost always utilized more effectively by those with more education and resources. Thus at a macropolitical level several issues, for example, unemployment and poor education, need to be tackled as a matter of some urgency before the health care system becomes acceptable to all.

In a study of Havik Brahmin females in South

India, taking the commonest presenting examples of 'head turning' as dizziness, Nichter (1981b) studied 22 clients of a traditional healer and reported that the common theme among the problems presented was that these induced uncertainty and disorientation. These were expressed symbolically by the somatic symptom of dizziness. Traditional healers are adept at back-translating from bodily complaints to psychosocial problems (Leff 1988). This is further emphasized by Chen (1975) who states, 'when modern medicine is exported to traditional societies, it fails to provide the necessary ritual and philosophic basis which is considered necessary for such societies'. Traditional medicine may be perceived as supportive, personal and holistic in its approach, in contrast with modern scientific medicine which may be seen as mechanistic, impersonal, organ-oriented and individualistic. Leff (1988) further observes that if the doctor is perceptive enough to appreciate that the somatic symptoms presented signify emotional distress but is unable to make the link with the patient's life circumstances, he/she may provide reassurance and/or psychotropic medication. This may result in temporary relief but is almost certain to lead to the patient returning later or seeking help elsewhere. Parsons & Wakeley (1991) reported similar findings from Australia. They found that their sample presented distress in emotional, somatic as well as sociocultural dimensions. The severity of duties was organized in the minds of the sample after the event. Taking pain as an example, Pugh (1991) found that the appeal of eclectic practitioners lay in their ability to tap virtually the whole course of pain's semantic associations even if only superficially.

Kleinman (1986) illustrates some of the issues discussed above. This study needs to be discussed in some detail. One hundred consecutive patients given a local diagnosis of neurasthenia in an outpatient department in Hunan (Taiwan), were interviewed for several hours about symptoms, course, illness behaviour, help-seeking behaviour and ethnomedical beliefs associated with the current illness. A DSM-III diagnosis was made. Using a western classificatory system 93 patients were diagnosed as suffering from clinical depression and 87 of these met the criteria for major

depressive disorders. One-third of the latter gave evidence of melancholia – a particularly severe form of the disorder – and in 60% depression had lasted for more than two years. One-quarter of the sample was diagnosed as suffering from hysteria – the term covering both conversion and somatic disorders. However, there was some overlap between hysteria and depression. Forty-four of the neurasthenic patients met the criteria for chronic pain syndrome – pain in a single site or several sites lasting for more than two years and causing disability with social impairment in family or work settings.

Of the 100 patients, each volunteered a mean of seven complaints of which five were somatic. Of 93 depressives only nine complained of depression and of the 87 with major depressive disorder nearly one-third complained entirely of somatic symptoms. The great majority (78%) maintained that their disorder was wholly or partly organic, but most ascribed it to work problems (61%) and a quarter to political problems. In 43% of cases the significance of the illness was judged to be the communication of personal or interpersonal distress or unhappiness. When Kleinman treated all 87 patients of major depressive disorder with tricyclic antidepressant medication, a six-week follow-up showed that 65% reported substantial improvement and another 17% slight improvement. However, 30% considered their social impairment to be worse and more than one-third (37%) sought further help from traditional health practitioners. A three-year follow-up of 21 patients with both chronic pain syndromes and major depressive disorder revealed that possible explanations of the illness had changed along with altered patterns of help seeking. Thus patients with a good response to antidepressants may have perceived their social impairment to be worse, possibly because they did not get social support from their therapist or because their 'cognitive schemata' had only partially changed. The perceived lack of support from the therapist may be another factor which may have led the patients to the traditional healers' doors.

The use of narrowly defined categories by a cross-cultural researcher is likely to suppress cultural variability (Rogler 1989), a problem to

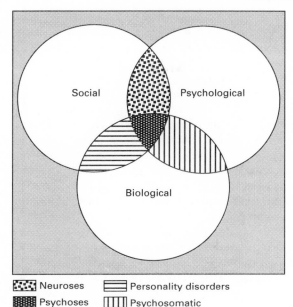

Neuroses

Psychoses

Personality disorders

Psychosomatic

**Fig. 5.2** Interactions of phenomenological realities.

**Table 5.3** Possible questions for migrant's migration experiences

| | |
|---|---|
| Q1 | How long ago did the subject migrate? |
| Q2 | At what age did the subject migrate? |
| Q3 | Motives for migration? |
| Q4 | Difficulties in migration and its perceived reversibility? |
| Q5 | Preparedness? |
| Q6 | How great was the difference? |
| Q7 | Experience before and during the journey? |
| Q8 | Migrated alone or in a group? |
| Q9 | Intentions at the beginning about duration of stay |
| Q10 | Attitude to the culture of new country? |
| Q11 | The role of the new society in helping the subject to adjust? |
| Q12 | Previous life experiences? |

which Kleinman's research calls attention. Rogler (1989) advocates research that departs from the prevailing, almost routinized, a priori commitment to standing measures of mental health. The issues related to cross-cultural research are not being discussed in this chapter (see Flaherty *et al.* 1988, Rogler 1989).

Kleinman & Lin (1980) argue that psychocultural interactions relate core symbolic meanings and behavioural norms to universal psychophysiological processes in such a way as to constitute a biosocial bridge between different phenomenological levels of reality (i.e. biological, psychological and social). These three levels then interact to produce different types of distress, as shown in Fig. 5.2.

Hamburg *et al.* (1970) also specify these three levels as influencing the development of serious disorders of behaviour but caution that the relative importance of each influence is not always clear. There is no doubt that sociocultural factors and sociopsychological factors are important in the genesis of functional psychiatric disorders (see Dohrenwend (1975) for a detailed discussion).

An accurate assessment of these phenomenological levels of reality is of paramount importance in managing individual patients, specially if they come from a different background from that of the therapist. Rack (1982) proposes a list of questions to be asked of migrants which may offer some help in assessment. These are shown in Table 5.3.

### Principles of treatment

The principles of treatment across cultures do not vary much. It is the mode of treatment which does. Both the doctor trained in western methods and the traditional healer provide their patients with a fundamental therapeutic tool, namely a set of codes for ordering disrupted perceptions and for restoring the discontinuity between physical and social state which is implied by illness (Comaroff 1978). The manner in which these tools are compared varies across cultures. Among the indigenous populace in India, western medicine is often preferred; however, this, as noted earlier, depends upon the type of disorder. On the Indian subcontinent quite often indigenous and folk healers use western methods of treatment including drugs and injections. The general expectation among some groups is that the doctor should be able to work out the diagnosis because 'after all he is the doctor'. This reflects not only on the doctor's special skills in diagnosis and management but also a degree of respect for somebody who is perceived as knowledgable and wise. Under these expectations, the therapist has to alter the questions being asked and only gradually home in on specific complaints. By contrast with a western patient the approach may be direct and to the point.

It has been argued that the traditional healer can be seen as a ritual specialist and a focus of social and emotional support for the patient (Nichter 1981a) – a role complementary to that of a western physician – a point also made by Chen (1975). Thus there is no reason why the two approaches may not be combined.

The issues of gender and class within various groups are often ignored. It has been noted by Heller *et al.* (1980) that perceptions of mental illness are class related. They were able to support Hollingshead & Redlich's (1958) and Langner & Michael's (1963) observations that lower classes are more prone than their middle class counterparts to focus on concrete problems rather than mental states in determining the state of an individual's mental health. The position of women in the Indian subcontinent is subject to a considerable amount of stress and the joint family system may offer some protection. However, studies in the west have shown that the recognition by a spouse is likely to occur more quickly when symptoms are persistent (rather than intermittent), communication of feelings is free and when there are opportunities for checking the spouse's observations with the observation of others, especially those who are relatively sophisticated in the evaluation of behaviour (Clausen & Huffine 1975). These authors go on to argue that higher educational status and high mutual respect in the couples are conducive to early recognition of symptoms. However, early recognition does not always mean early help seeking. Help seeking will depend upon the nature of symptomatology, resources available for keeping the patient at home or taking him/her to the nearest source of

help, and the reluctance of the spouse to seek help. Hammer (1963–64) argued that the central status of pre-patient was more important in early help seeking. However Clausen & Huffine (1975) modify the observation by stating '... to the extent that a husband or wife performs the most salient roles effectively, many symptoms will be tolerated, but when crucial role functions are not performed, hospitalization tends to occur quickly'. Post migration or in an alien society the role of the woman undergoes a change. Thus she may leave to be an earner yet still be expected to carry out all household chores with little support from men folk.

Psychiatric distress among ethnic minorities may be complicated by the effect of migration as well as perceived and real racism. Counselling and managing patients under these conditions can be difficult. The use of a counsellor who is from the same cultural background and preferably bilingual can alleviate some of the problems. The use of interpreters and associated difficulties are discussed elsewhere in this volume (see Chapter 29). A culturally sensitive counsellor can often achieve a greater rate of success in engaging the patient. Sometimes it may be difficult because the treatment paradigms being offered may not fit in with the individual's expectations. In a study of Asian couples with sexual dysfunction, Bhugra & Cordle (1986) reported low rates of success due to an inability to engage such couples in behavioural paradigms. d'Ardenne (1987) overcame this problem by involving elders in the extended family. Thus therapy needs to be tailored according to the individual's perceptions of the problems and expectations of treatment and management. With increasing emphasis on the community mental health movement, the needs of minority communities and their expectations of treatment are bound to affect help-seeking behaviour (Bhugra 1992).

Leff (1990) suggests that ascription of equal values to folk beliefs about mental illness and its categorization as to the western biomedical system of psychiatry is an essential first step. He urges the study of people who are considered to be mentally ill by the local population, most of whom may be treated by traditional healers in the first instance. To this end the healers themselves must be interviewed to ascertain their diagnostic systems. Anthropologists, sociologists, psychiatrists and other mental health professionals need to work together to develop a better understanding of psychosocial factors in the genesis of mental disorders across cultures and the service needs of each group. MacCarthy (1988) offers some sensible practical advice for psychologists working with ethnic minorities. The basic preventive strategies have to look at person-centred approaches (Neighbors 1990).

In summary the therapists need to be flexible, sensitive and aware of cultural factors affecting their clientele. A different perspective offered by the patients in terms of their preferences and choices does not mean that they do not need help or are likely to reject it when offered. What it means is that any successful therapeutic interaction has to strike the right balance between the patient's cultural and preferred treatment norms and those of the health care systems and health care providers.

## References

Al-Issa I. (1982) Does culture make a difference in psychopathology? In Al-Issa I. (ed.) *Culture and Psychopathology*. University Park Press, Baltimore.

Anderson R.M., Mullner R.M. & Cornelius L.J. (1987) Black-White differences in health status: methods or substance? *Millbank Quarterly* 65, suppl. 1, 72–99.

Anwar M. (1979) *The Myth of Return*. Heinemann, London.

Bakx K. (1991) The eclipse of folk medicine. *Sociology of Health and Illness* 13, 20–38.

Bhopal R.S. (1986) Bhye–Bhaddi: a food and health concept of Punjabi Asian. *Social Science Medicine* 23, 687–688.

Bhugra D. (1992) Setting up services for ethnic minorities. In Weller M. & Muijen M. (eds) *Dimensions of Community Psychiatry Setting Up Services for Ethnic Minorities*. Baillière–Tindall, London (in press).

Bhugra D. & Cordle C. (1986) Sexual dysfunction in Asian couples. *British Medical Journal* 292, 111–112.

Bochner S. (ed.) (1982) *Cultures in Contact: Studies in Cross-cultural Interaction*. Pergamon, Oxford.

Burke A. (1974) Is racism a causatory factor in mental illness. *International Journal of Social Psychiatry* 30, 1–3.

Cannon M.S. & Locke B.Z. (1977) Being black is detri-

mental to one's mental health: myth or reality? *Phylon* 38, 408–428.

Cashmore E.E. (1987) *The Logic of Racism*. Unwin Hyman, London.

Chen P.C.Y. (1975) Medical systems in Malaysia: cultural bases and differential use. *Social Science and Medicine* 9, 171–180.

Clausen J.A. & Huffine C.L. (1975) Sociocultural and social-psychological factors affecting social responses to mental disorder. *Journal of Health and Social Behaviour* 16, 405–420.

Cohen R.E. (1987) Stressors: migration and acculturation to American society. In Gaviria M. & Arana J. (eds) *Health and Behaviour: Research Agenda for Hispanics*. Simon Bolivar Research Monograph No. 1, pp. 59–71. University of Illinois, Chicago.

Comaroff J. (1978) Medicine and culture: some anthropological perspectives. *Social Science and Medicine* 12B, 247–254.

d'Ardenne P. (1987) Sexual dysfunction in a cross-cultural setting: assessment, treatment and research. *Sexual and Marital Therapy* 1, 23–34.

De Vos G.A. (1982) Adaptive strategies in US minorities. In Jones E.E. & Korchin S.J. (eds) *Minority Mental Health*. Praegar, New York.

Dohrenwend B.P. (1975) Social cultural and social psychological factors in the genesis of mental disorders. *Journal of Health and Social Behaviour* 16, 365–392.

Dunn F.L. (1974) Medical care in the Chinese communities of Peninsular Malaysia. Cited in Chen (1975) Medical systems in Malaysia. *Social Science and Medicine* 9, 171–180.

Eisenberg L. (1977) Disease and illness: distinctions between professional and popular ideas of sickness. *Culture, Medicine and Psychiatry* 1, 9–23.

Flaherty J., Gaviria F.M., Pathak D. et al. (1988) Developing instruments for cross-cultural psychiatric research. *Journal of Nervous and Mental Disease* 176, 257–262.

Gaines A.T. (1982) Cultural definitions, behaviour and the person in American psychiatry. In Marsella A.J. & White G.M. (eds) *Cultural Conceptions of Mental Health and Therapy*, pp. 167–192. Reidel, Dordrecht.

Geertz C. (1973) *The Interpretation of Culture*. Basic Books, New York.

Gudykunst W.B., Ting-Toomey S. & Chua E. (1988) *Culture and Interpersonal Communication*. Sage, Newbury Park, California.

Hamburg D.A., Bond D., Eisenberg L., Grinker S. et al. (1970) *Psychiatry as a Behavioral Science*. Prentice-Hall, Englewood Cliffs, New Jersey.

Hammer M. (1963–64) Influence of small networks as factors in mental hospital admissions. *Human Organisation* 22, 243–251.

Hartog J. (1972) The intervention system for mental and social deviants in Malaysia. *Social Science and Medicine* 6, 211.

Heller P.L., Chalfant H.P., Worley M., Quesada G.M. &

Bradfield C.D. (1980) Socio-economic class, classification of 'abnormal' behaviour and perceptions of mental health: a cross-cultural comparison. *British Journal of Medical Psychology* 53, 343–348.

Helman C.G. (1978) 'Feed a cold, starve a fever': folk models of infection in an English community, and their relation to medical treatment. *Culture, Medicine and Psychiatry* 2, 107–137.

Helman C.G. (1990) *Culture, Health and Illness*. Wright, London.

Herskovits M. (1955) *Cultural Anthropology*. Knopf, New York.

Hollingshead A.B. & Redlich C. (1958) *Social Class and Mental Illness: A Community Study*. John Wiley, New York.

Kenny M.G. (1985) Paradox lost: the latah problem revisited. In Simons R.C. & Hughes C.C. (eds) *The Culture Bound Syndromes*, pp. 63–76. Reidel, Dordrecht.

Kessler R.C. & Cleary P.D (1980) Social class and psychological distress. *American Sociological Review* 45, 463–478.

Kim Y.Y. & Gudykunst W.B. (1988) *Cross-cultural Adaptation: Current Approaches*. Sage, Newbury Park, California.

Kleinman A. (1980) *Patients and Healers in the Context of Culture*. University of California Press, Berkeley.

Kleinman A. (1986) *Social Origins of Distress and Disease: Depression, Neurasthenia and Pain in Modern China*. New Haven, Yale University Press.

Kleinman A. & Lin T.-Y. (1980) *Normal and Abnormal Behaviour in Chinese Culture*. Reidel, Dordrecht.

Langner T. & Michael S. (1963) *Life Stress and Mental Health*. Crescent Press, New York.

Leff J. (1988) *Psychiatry Around the Globe*. Gaskell, London.

Leff J. (1990) The new cross-cultural psychiatry: a case of the baby and the bathwater. *British Journal of Psychiatry* 156, 305–307.

Lin K.-M. (1980) Traditional Chinese medical beliefs and their relevance for mental illness and psychiatry. In Kleinman A. & Lin T.-Y. (eds) *Normal and Abnormal Behaviour in Chinese Culture*, pp. 95–111. Reidel, Dordrecht.

Lipsedge M. (1989) Cultural influences on psychiatry. *Current Opinion in Psychiatry* 2, 267–272.

Littlewood R. (1990) From categories to contexts: a decade of the new cross-cultural psychiatry. *British Journal of Psychiatry* 156, 308–327.

Littlewood R. & Lipsedge M. (1987) The butterfly and the serpent: culture, psychopathology and biomedicine. *Culture, Medicine and Psychiatry* 11, 289–336.

Littlewood R. & Lipsedge M. (1989) *Aliens and Alienists*. Unwin and Hyman, London.

MacCarthy B. (1988) Clinical work with ethnic minorities. In Watts F.N. (ed.) *New Developments in Clinical Psychology*, pp. 122–139. John Wiley, Chichester.

MacCarthy B. & Craissati (1989) Ethnic differences in response to adversity. A community sample of Bangladeshis and their indigenous neighbours. *Social Psychiatry and Psychiatric Epidemiology* 24, 196–201.

Mechanic D. (1975) Sociocultural and social-psychological factor affecting personal response to psychological disorder. *Journal of Health and Social Behaviour* 16, 393–404.

Miller J.M. (1987) Race in the health of America. *Millbank Quarterly* 65, suppl. 2, 500–531.

Nchinda T.C. (1976) Traditional and Western medicine in Africa: collaboration or confrontation. *Tropical Doctor* July.

Neff J.A. (1984) Race differences in psychological distress: the effects of SES, urbanicity and measurement strategy. *American Journal of Community Psychology* 12, 337–351.

Neighbors H. (1986) Socio economic status and psychological distress in black Americans. *American Journal of Epidemiology* 124, 779–793.

Neighbors H.W. (1987) Improving the mental health of Black Americans: lessons from the community Mental Health Movement. *Millbank Quarterly* 65, suppl. 2, 348–380.

Neighbors H. (1990) The prevention of psychopathology in African Americans: an epidemiologic perspective. *Community Mental Health Journal* 26, 167–179.

Neighbors H.W., Jackson J.S., Bowman P.J. & Gurin G. (1983) Stress, coping and black mental health: preliminary finding from a national study. *Prevention in Human Services* 2, 4–29.

Nichter M. (1981a) Negotiation of the illness experience: Ayurvedic therapy and the psychosocial dimension of illness. *Culture, Medicine and Psychiatry* 5, 5–24.

Nichter M. (1981b) Idioms of distress: alternatives in the expression of psychosocial distress: a case study from South India. *Culture, Medicine and Psychiatry* 5, 379–408.

Orley J.H. (1970a) *Culture and Mental Illness*. East African Pub House, Nairobi.

Orley J.H. (1970b) African medical taxonomy. *Journal of the Anthropological Society of Oxford* 1, 137–150.

Orley J.H. & Leff J.P. (1972) The effect of psychiatric education on attitudes to illness among the Ganda. *British Journal of Psychiatry* 121, 137–141.

Parker S. & Kleiner R. (1966) *Mental Illness in the Urban Negro Community*. Free Press, New York.

Parsons C.D.F. & Wakeley P. (1991) Idioms of distress: somatic responses to distress in everyday life. *Culture, Medicine and Psychiatry* 15, 111–132.

Patterson S. (1963) *Dark Strangers*. Tavistock, London.

Pearlin L.I., Lieberman M.A., Menaghan E.G. *et al.* (1981) The stress process. *Journal of Health and Social Behaviour* 22, 337–356.

Pfeiffer W.M. (1982) Culture bound syndromes. In Al-Issa I. (ed.) *Culture and Psychopathology*, pp. 201–218. University Park Press, Baltimore.

Pugh J. (1991) The semantics of pain in Indian culture and medicine. *Culture, Medicine and Psychiatry* 15, 19–43.

Rack P. (1982) *Race, Culture and Mental Disorder.* Tavistock, London.

Rahe R.H., Looney J.G.M., Ward H.W., Tung T.M. & Liv W.T. (1978) Psychiatric consultations in a Vietnamese refuge camp. *American Journal of Psychiatry* 135, 185–190.

Rogler L.H. (1989) The meaning of culturally sensitive research in mental health. *American Journal of Psychiatry* 146, 296–303.

Rogler L.H., Gurak D.T. & Cooney R.S. (1987) The migration experience and mental health: formulations relevant to Hispanics and other immigrants. In Gaviria M. & Arana J. (eds) *Health and Behaviour: Research Agenda for Hispanics*, pp. 72–84. Simon Bolivar Research Monograph No. 1. University of Illinois, Chicago.

Sharpston M.J. (1976) Health and human environment. *Finance and Development* 13, 1.

Simons R.C. (1980) The resolution of latah paradox. In Simons R.C. & Hughes C.C. (eds) *The Culture Bound Syndromes*, pp. 43–62. Reidel, Dordrecht.

Simons R.C. & Hughes C.C. (eds) (1985) *The Culture Bound Syndromes.* Reidel, Dordrecht.

Skultans V. (1991) Anthropology and psychiatry: the uneasy alliance. *Transcultural Psychiatric Research Review* 28, 5–24.

Spradley J.P. & McCurdy D.W. (1974) *Conformity and Conflict: Readings in Cultural Anthropology.* Little, Brown, Boston.

Stein B. (1980) The refugee experience. Cited in Rack P. (1982) *Race, Culture and Mental Disorder.* Tavistock, London.

Strange H. (1973) Illness and treatment in a Malay village. *Asian Journal of Medicine* 9, 362.

Tiwari S.C., Katiyar M. & Sethi B.B. (1986) Culture and mental disorder: an overview. *Indian Journal of Social Psychiatry* 2, 403–425.

Tyhurst L. (1977) Psychosocial first aid for refugees: an essay in social psychiatry. *Mental Health and Society* 4, 319–343.

Varma V.K. (1986) Cultural psychodynamics in health and illness. *Indian Journal of Psychiatry* 28, 13–34.

Wilkinson D.Y. & King G. (1987) The case of race as a variable: conceptual and methodological issues in policy implications: *Millbank Quarterly* 65, suppl. 1, 56–71.

Workneh F. & Giel R. (1975) Medical dilemma: a survey of the healing practice of a coptic priest and an Ethiopian sheik. *Tropical and Geographical Medicine* 27, 431–439.

# Chapter 6
# Social Causation of Schizophrenia

PAUL BEBBINGTON & LIZ KUIPERS

Schizophrenia is pre-eminently a condition which responds to changes in social circumstances. Both the positive and the negative symptoms which characterize it are affected by the level of stimulation. This chapter will review the scientific evidence for what good clinicians already know and work with from their own experience.

## Early social theories of schizophrenia

The early theories linking parental behaviour with the onset of schizophrenia have been reviewed elsewhere (Kuipers & Bebbington 1988, 1990). These attempted to provide a virtually complete explanation of the emergence of the disease in essentially cognitive terms: early experience was held to result in ways of perceiving (and therefore of interacting with) the social world that correspond to the observed symptoms of schizophrenia. Examples include 'double bind' communication (Bateson *et al.* 1956), 'fragmented' or 'amorphous' parental styles of communication (Wynne & Singer 1963, 1965), and 'schism' or 'skew' in parental marriages (Lidz *et al.* 1957). Finally, Laing & Esterson (1964) held that schizophrenia was an understandable response to pressures in the family and in society at large.

These theories linger on in the consciousness of many psychiatric professionals, but probably should not. The experimental evidence for them is really very thin indeed (Hirsch & Leff 1975). The oddities of the parents do not appear marked, and are certainly not the cause of the condition. Moreover, Hirsch & Leff (1975) were themselves unable to replicate the findings of Wynne & Singer (1963, 1965) in the only independent attempt to test out these parental-style theories of the origins of schizophrenia.

These studies are now to be seen mainly as interesting failures. Although it should not be forgotten that they did at least have the effect of obtaining acceptance for a social dimension to the disorder, opening the door for more refined hypotheses, they also seem to have been responsible for the tendency of some professionals to blame families for the state of the patient. This is inappropriate: apart from any other consideration, the evidence for major genetic and physical environmental components cannot sustain a belief that relatives by their behaviour actually 'cause' schizophrenia.

The bugbear of these early investigations is the impossibility of establishing causal direction from retrospective studies. True prospective studies of whole populations would be prohibitively expensive, as most of the people laboriously followed up will never develop schizophrenia. It is less costly to follow up families with children who may be at 'high risk' of developing schizophrenia (e.g. Venables 1977, Goldstein 1985), although attendant difficulties remain, such as the length of time required to complete the study, high dropout rates, and the ethics of not intervening (Shakow 1973).

The study of Doane and her colleagues (Doane *et al.* 1981, Goldstein 1987) chose to equate attendance at a psychiatric outpatient department for disturbed adolescents with an increased risk of schizophrenia. They have now reported results available after a 15-year interval. Only four adolescents developed definite schizophrenia in this time, although several more met criteria for schizophrenic spectrum disorder. If these groups are conjoined to give a 'broad' definition of schizophrenia, it appears that this diagnosis is associated with parental abnormalities of communication and affective style, together with a measure of family atmosphere, all rated at induction.

However, it is not clear what these findings actually say about the causes of schizophrenia defined in a narrower and more usual sense. Moreover, it is possible that the more disturbed adolescents drew extreme reactions from their parents, and happened also to be those who went on to develop the disease. In other words, although the study is nominally prospective, it cannot resolve the ambiguity of causal direction.

## Social influences on the timing and course of schizophrenia

Modern social theories of schizophrenia start from the sensible proposition that social influences act together with factors at other levels to determine at least the timing, and perhaps the fact, of schizophrenic breakdown. They fall mainly into two groups, those relying on measures of 'life events' and those relying on the concept of 'Expressed Emotion'.

### Life events

Several sources of evidence suggest that *changes* in the social environment may lead to the emergence of schizophrenic symptoms in susceptible individuals. So, for instance, acute florid symptoms may reappear in patients subjected to too much pressure in rehabilitation programmes, or discharged before they are ready (Wing *et al.* 1964, Stevens 1973, Goldberg *et al.* 1977, Drake & Sederer 1986).

The evidence from specific life event studies that stress has some part in precipitating episodes of schizophrenia is still not beyond doubt. Most have been of retrospective case-control design, although where events are dated accurately over a sufficient period, within-case comparisons can be suggestive of an effect. In other words, significant peaking of events before onset in the individual case can be taken as prima facie evidence of an association.

Case-control comparisons do carry the assumption that people with schizophrenia are influenced by life events that would have an impact on anyone, although their response is obviously idiosyncratic in that it leads to the emergence of schizophrenic symptoms. Consider, however, the real possibility that schizophrenic subjects are hypersensitive to the social environment and that this leads to a social withdrawal that cuts down their exposure to events. The schizophrenic patients might then have less events than the normal controls, and the events that precipitated their onset might be so trivial that they are normally excluded from analysis. We would then have to fall back on the less powerful technique of using subjects as their own controls in order to reveal a relative excess of pre-onset events, possibly of a minor significance. There is in fact some evidence that people with schizophrenia view events in ways that might make them more susceptible to their impact (J. Ventura 1991, personal communication). Hirsch and his colleagues (1973) obtained findings suggesting that patients without the protection of medication may be particularly likely to break down in the face of stressful events.

The first study of life events and schizophrenia was that of Brown & Birley (1968). They used fairly sophisticated methods for the time, and found an increase in events of various degrees of impact, limited to the three-week period before onset. The main objection to this study is that only in 29 of the 50 cases was onset from a state of normality to the emergence of schizophrenic symptoms. Jacobs & Myers (1976) also used sophisticated methods. Their findings were inconclusive and cannot be interpreted easily as they chose to examine events in the six-month antecedent interval. They may have thereby obscured a real increase in frequency limited to the weeks immediately before onset. The same might be said of the negative results in the study of Malzacher and his colleagues (1981), although they did give results for a three-month period before onset. Al Khani and his co-workers (1986) used reasonably adequate methods in a Saudi Arabian study, but with complicated results, showing an effect of life events restricted to certain groups. Canton & Fraccon (1985) included events that could have occurred after onset, thus disqualifying them from consideration as causal agents. The study of Chung and his colleagues (1986) was based on a small number of patients with mixed diagnoses and adds little to the literature.

However, we have recently seen the publication of a large World Health Organization (WHO) collaborative study conducted in nine catchment areas from around the world (Day *et al.* 1987). Although limited by the lack of control groups, it is important. The selection of cases was deliberately broad, and included an appreciable minority of doubtful diagnosis. All told, the study included 386 cases out of the 435 screened and in scope. 'Onset' could be from a state without symptoms, from one with only minor neurotic symptoms, or from one with minor psychotic symptoms. Cases were only included when onset had occurred within six months of screening and was capable of being dated to within a one-week period. Events were recorded for the three-month period preceding onset.

In the absence of control groups, the value of the findings comes from the patterning of life events before onset. Although this could be artefactual, for instance, due to recall effects, or the 'search after meaning' (Brown 1974), the results are suggestive. In all the centres, events tended to cluster in the three weeks before onset, and perhaps, to a lesser extent, in the three-week period before that. When all events were considered together, these findings were significant in six of the nine centres, and similar trends in the remaining three centres probably fail of significance because of small numbers of cases or a low event rate.

An alternative design involves the assessment of life events over a period in patients who have recovered from a known episode of schizophrenia. Michaux and his colleagues (1967) published an early and unsophisticated study in which they gave a life events scale monthly to schizophrenic patients, and were able to show an increase in stress in the month preceding that in which hospitalization occurred.

Ventura and his colleagues (1989) have carried out a prospective study in which life events were recorded at monthly intervals for 12 months in a group of schizophrenic patients. They found that the frequency of events in the month preceding onsets was significantly greater than in analogous months not followed by onset in the same patient. It was also greater than the mean monthly rate in non-relapsing patients.

Malla and his colleagues (1990) have published results of another study of this type, in which they followed 21 patients over one year in an aftercare programme. The PERI life event schedule (Dohrenwend *et al.* 1978) was administered. In addition, daily hassles were recorded ('minor events'). Events were rated by a blind rater for whether they arose independently of the patient's symptoms at weekly or fortnightly intervals. Relapse was essentially defined as the re-emergence of positive psychotic symptoms. There tended to be more events, both major and minor, in the three-month period before relapse compared with any *other* three-month periods in relapsing patients, or with *any* three-month periods in those who did not relapse. However, only in the latter comparison was the trend significant, and then only when events and hassles were taken together. This study is greatly hampered by small numbers, but is at least consistent with the possibility that events tend to peak before onset.

Jolley, Cramer and Hirsch (personal communication 1990) have set up another study with this design. Fifty-six patients have been analysed so far; life events were rated at two-monthly intervals, and there was a significant increase in event frequency in the four-week period immediately preceding onset compared with the three preceding four-week periods, and also with any of the four-week periods in the non-relapsed patients. In addition, it appeared that the risk of relapse following an event was increased tenfold in those not receiving medication.

These studies thus add to the evidence for a causal role of life events, although the subjects are inevitably restricted to those who have had at least one previous episode of schizophrenia.

It has been argued that life events play a 'formative' role in depression but a merely 'triggering' one in schizophrenia (Brown *et al.* 1973, Brown & Harris 1978). This really just means that dispositional factors are more important in the latter.

Paykel (1979) has calculated that in the six months following the occurrence of a major event, the risk of developing schizophrenia is increased three- or fourfold over the general population rate, while that of developing depression is increased sixfold.

Recently, the author and his colleagues (Bebbington *et al.* 1992) have conducted a study of episodes of psychosis of recent and definable onset. This included 52 subjects with schizophrenia. Life events were identified in the six-month period before onset using the Life Events and Difficulties Schedule (LEDS) of Brown & Harris (1978). There was a highly significant increase in events of all degrees of severity in the three-month period before onset. However, there was also an increase in the three-month period before that. This study used good methods and obtained a very significant effect of life events. The results differ from other studies in showing a much more prolonged influence of events. They are presented graphically in Fig. 6.1.

It is plain from reviewing these studies that there is still some debate about the role of life events in schizophrenia. The proposition that the condition is significantly affected by social circumstances is, however, considerably strengthened by the literature on Expressed Emotion.

### Expressed Emotion

Expressed Emotion (EE) is now a long-established concept, which has been reviewed at length elsewhere (Kuipers 1979, Hooley 1985, Leff & Vaughn 1985, Koenigsberg & Handley 1986, Kuipers & Bebbington 1988, 1990, Vaughn 1989). The story is a nice one: it began in an unexpected finding, which was then seized upon, leading first to a series of increasingly sophisticated corroborative studies, and ultimately to planned interventions with families and prescriptions for routine clinical practice.

The original finding was reported in a study by Brown and his colleagues of the prognosis of male mental patients with a variety of discharge arrangements (Brown 1959, Brown *et al.* 1958). Against expectation, patients who went back to live with parents or spouses did surprisingly

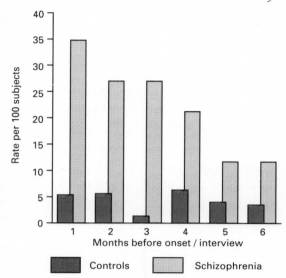

**Fig. 6.1** Camberwell Psychosis Study (Marked and Moderate Life Events).

badly; moreover, this effect seemed to be dose related: it depended on the amount of contact between relative and patient. The authors tentatively concluded that certain intense relationships might increase the risk of relapse.

Brown and his colleagues (1962) subsequently developed a semi-structured interview to assess the emotional atmosphere in the home. They thought that from this they would be able to identify specific qualities of the relationship that might be important in relation to relapse. The modern rating of EE is based on the Camberwell Family Interview (CFI – Brown & Rutter 1966, Rutter & Brown 1966). Relatives are assessed in terms of the number of *critical comments* they made, and their overall *hostility* and *emotional overinvolvement*. EE is a composite derived from these components. It has been found to predict relapse rates during follow-up in studies from around the world (Table 6.1).

The early studies (Brown *et al.* 1972, Vaughn & Leff 1976) suggested that reduced levels of face-to-face contact and medication both offered protection against the adverse effects of a high EE family environment. There are a number of implications from this work: first, it does indeed appear that relapse in schizophrenia is influenced

*Chapter 6*

**Table 6.1** Results of prospective studies of EE

| Author | Location | Subjects (no.) | Episode | Follow-up | Relapse rate (%) High EE | Low EE |
|---|---|---|---|---|---|---|
| Brown et al. 1962* | S London | 97 (male) | All | 1 year | 56 | 21 |
| Brown et al. 1972 | S London | 101 | All | 9 months | 58 | 16 |
| Vaughn & Leff 1976 | S London | 37 | All | 9 months | 50 | 12 |
| Leff & Vaughn 1981[†] | S London | 36 | All | 2 years | 62 | 20 |
| Vaughn et al. 1984 | Los Angeles | 54 | All | 9 months | 56 | 28 |
| Moline et al. 1985[‡] | Chicago | 24 | All | 1 year | 91 | 31 |
| Dulz & Hand 1986[§] | Hamburg | 46 | All | 9 months | 58 | 65 |
| MacMillan et al. 1986 | N London | 67 | First | 2 years | 63 | 39 |
| Nuechterlein et al. 1986[‖] | Los Angeles | 26 | All | 1 year | 37 | 0 |
| Karno et al. 1987 | S California | 44 | All | 9 months | 59 | 26 |
| Leff et al. 1987 | Chandigarh, India | 76 | First | 1 year | 33 | 14 |
| Tarrier et al. 1988b[¶] | Salford, UK | 48 | All | 9 months | 48 | 21 |
| Parker et al. 1988** | Sydney, Australia | 57 | All | 9 months | 48 | 60 |
| McCreadie & Phillips 1988 | Nithsdale, Scotland | 59 | NA | 6 months 12 months | 13 17 | 11 20 |
| Budzyna-Dawidowski et al. 1989 | Cracow, Poland | 36 | All | 1 year 2 years | 32 72 | 9 18 |
| Ivanovic & Vuletic 1989 | Belgrade, Yugoslavia | 60 | All | 9 months | 64 | 7 |
| Mozny 1989 | Rural Czechoslovkia | 68 | All | 1 year | 60 | 29 |
| Cazzullo et al. 1989 | Milan, Italy | 45 | All | 9 months | 58 | 21 |
| Stricker et al. 1989 | Munster, W Germany | 99 | All | 9 months | 'Significantly higher' | – |
| Ferrera & Vizarro 1989 | Madrid, Spain | 31 | All | 9 months | 44 | 38 |
| Barrelet et al. 1990 | Geneva, Switzerland | 41 | First | 9 months | 32 | 0 |
| Vaughn et al. 1992a | Sydney, Australia | 87 | All | 9 months | 52 | 23 |

* Their measure of 'emotional overinvolvement' was the prototype of EE.
† Follow-up of same patients as Vaughn & Leff (1976).
‡ Non-standard criteria for high EE.
§ An unknown number of subjects were not living with their EE-rated relatives.
‖ All patients on fixed dose fluphenazine.
¶ Patients receiving standard care with or without education in the authors' intervention.
** All relatives were parents. An unknown number of subjects were not living with parents at the time of readmission or reassessment.

by social circumstances; secondly, patients with a high risk of relapse can be identified; and thirdly, since factors associated with relapse were pinpointed, so too were the targets of a possible intervention programme. These targets comprise the effective provision of medication, a reduction of face-to-face contact, and a lowering of EE in the family.

Only three studies definitely show no predictive value of EE (Köttgen *et al.* 1984, McCreadie & Phillips 1988, Parker *et al.* 1988). The first of these has major methodological flaws that vitiate its findings (Vaughn 1986). The most crucial defects are that not all the patients were actually living at home and an unknown number of patients counted as relapsing had not recovered in the first place. Idiosyncrasies and flaws are also apparent in the other two studies, but it seems inappropriate to make too much of these – after all, none of the studies reporting positive findings are without blemish. Although there are several failings in the Australian study of Parker and his colleagues (1988), they anticipate criticism by providing analyses that take account of most of them. They did have very high rates of relapse in their low EE patients, and it is just possible that they were an unusual and chaotic group – they often changed residence and their very inconsistency may have taken them out of close contact with their relatives.

The study by McCreadie & Phillips (1988) is the first in which assessments of EE have been made on patients *in remission living in the community*. It is thus a study of *prevalence*, rather than of index episodes of acute symptoms. Several comments may be made. First, the overall relapse rate was extremely low at 17%. This is not surprising in a prevalence study, as it would be expected to pick up more of the good prognosis cases. The inclusion of good prognosis cases makes it harder to demonstrate the effect of factors influencing course, and the effect itself may be less, relative to unknown intrinsic factors. Indeed, the generally accepted beneficial effects of medication were also absent in this study. As McCreadie & Phillips suggest, this might be due to selective use by the prescribing psychiatrists, but on the other hand it might not.

The predictive studies of EE should be evaluated overall: the specific finding of an effect of the time relatives spend together has only shown up in studies carried out by the original group of British workers, but, that apart, the literature provides an impressive consensus for the value of EE.

Hogarty (1985) has raised the possibility that EE predicts relapse only in men, not women: this seems to have some support from the available evidence (e.g. Vaughn *et al.* 1984). Brown and his colleagues (1972) did claim that EE was equally predictive for male and female sufferers, but, even so, EE may be of less clinical significance in women because the prognosis is relatively better for other reasons (Salokangas 1983). The question of the role of EE in female patients therefore remains open.

If EE is a robust predictor of relapse, the relapse rate of schizophrenia should be affected by anything that affects EE. One example is the different organization of family life in many Third World countries in comparison with the industrialized west. In particular, extended families are the norm in the former. It is clear from Table 6.2 that the proportion of families rated high in EE is at its greatest in western industrialized societies.

The better course and outcome of schizophrenia in developing countries is well established (World Health Organization 1979): could it be the result of different family characteristics as reflected by the EE measure? Wig and his colleagues (1987a) carried out an EE study in the area around the Indian city of Chandigarh. As expected, relapse rates were low, particularly in the rural areas. Nevertheless, an association remained between hostility expressed by relatives and subsequent relapse a year later. This suggests that the good outcome of schizophrenia in this culture might indeed be the result of beneficial family structures and traditions (Leff *et al.* 1987). In other words, both in Chandigarh and in London the relapse rate appears to be related to EE, but relapses are less frequent in India. This could therefore have been due to lower levels of EE. Using the pooled Indian and London results (Vaughn & Leff 1976, Leff *et al.* 1987), loglinear analysis confirmed that the better outcome in India can be entirely explained by lower levels of EE, and that the effect is of considerable strength (Kuipers & Bebbington 1988). So, not only does EE have predictive value across very different cultures, it may also serve to explain differences in outcome of schizophrenia in those cultures.

However, the explanation of these findings cannot lie in the overt structural differences between families in India and the west. Although there were fewer high EE families in the rural

**Table 6.2** The applicability of the EE measures

| Author | Location | Proportion of relatives rated high on EE (%) | Proportion of households rated high on EE (%) |
|---|---|---|---|
| Brown *et al.* 1962 | S London | NA | 52 |
| Brown *et al.* 1972 | S London | NA | 45 |
| Vaughn & Leff 1976 | S London | NA | 49 |
| Vaughn *et al.* 1984 | Los Angeles | NA | 67 |
| Moline *et al.* 1985 | Chicago | NA | 70 |
| MacMillan *et al.* 1986 | N London | 53 | NA |
| Karno *et al.* 1987 | Los Angeles (Mexican–American) | 28 | 41 |
| Wig *et al.* 1987b | Aarhus, Denmark | NA | 54 |
| Leff *et al.* 1987 | Chandigarh, India | 23 30 urban 8 rural | 23 |
| McCreadie & Robinson 1987 | Nithsdale, Scotland | 43 | 42 |
| Tarrier *et al.* 1988b | Salford, UK | 73 | 77 |
| Parker *et al.* 1988 | Sydney, Australia | NA | 74 |
| Barrelet *et al.* 1990 | Geneva, Switzerland | NA | 66 |
| Vaughan *et al.* 1992a | Sydney Australia | NA | 53 |
| M. Rostworoska 1987, personal communication | Cracow, Poland | NA | 53 |
| Martins *et al.* 1992, personal communication | Porto Alegre, Brazil | 59 | 63 |

than in the urban areas studied in Chandigarh, there appeared to be no relationship between EE levels and the type of gross family structure (i.e. extended versus nuclear). The uniformly low EE levels in Indian families must therefore arise from other family attributes.

THE LINK BETWEEN ADVERSE HOME
ENVIRONMENT AND RELAPSE

It is reasonable to assume that the home environment characterized by high EE represents a form of psychosocial stress. How then is relapse mediated? One possibility is that it operates via physiological arousal.

Psychophysiological studies now provide con-

siderable evidence in line with this suggestion. Patients seem to be physiologically aroused when with high EE relatives, but not with low EE relatives (Tarrier *et al.* 1979, 1988b, Sturgeon *et al.* 1984). Indeed, Tarrier & Barrowclough (1987) demonstrated a differential psychophysiological effect in a man living with one high and one low EE parent, depending on which was present. The arousal provoked by critical relatives seems to be non-specific, and has been observed in non-schizophrenic disturbed adolescents (Valone *et al.* 1984).

However, changes in EE due to a successful social intervention programme failed to engender concomitant changes in psychophysiological ratings of patients (Leff *et al.* 1982). This turned out to be independently related to relapse. In other words, the benefit from changes in EE does not appear to work through changes in levels of arousal. This research has been reviewed in more detail elsewhere (Kuipers & Bebbington 1988, Turpin *et al.* 1988).

Leff and his colleagues (1983) used these ideas about arousal and material from their intervention study to construct an overall model of relapse in schizophrenia. They concluded that patients unprotected by medication might relapse in response *either* to a life event *or* to living with a high EE relative. Patients taking medication, on the other hand, required exposure to both factors before they would relapse, implying a bigger 'dose' of psychosocial stress. In this model, medication operates generally to raise the threshold for the psychosocial provocation of relapse, suggesting that life events and EE might perhaps have a common mechanism.

## CRITICISM AND OVERINVOLVEMENT

The EE measure is a composite. It covers two attributes of relatives that at first sight seem distinctly different. Criticism and hostility are similar, and easily distinguishable from the other attribute of EE, that is, emotional overinvolvement. Criticism is seen frequently in both spouses and parents of those with schizophrenia, whereas spouses are less likely to be overinvolved than parents. Are these two aspects of EE inherently different, and if so in what sense?

Koenigsberg & Handley (1986) adhere to the principle of keeping them distinct. There may well be differences in their associations: for instance, emotional overinvolvement may be particularly associated with poor premorbid social functioning (Brown *et al.* 1972, Miklowitz *et al.* 1983). However, the two patterns of behaviour cannot be distinguished from the patients' psychophysiological responses to the presence of a relative (Tarrier *et al.* 1988b). Moreover, where studies give results separately for criticism and emotional overinvolvement, they show a similar ability to predict relapse, although it is relatively rare for the latter to be present alone (Brown *et al.* 1972, Vaughn *et al.* 1984, Leff *et al.* 1987). Thus,

although the attitudes look very different and may have different origins, they may actually work in the same way. Criticism and overinvolvement may both be strategies reflecting a need to control situations (Hooley 1985). Is it useful to emphasize the similarities in this way? It is probably worth retaining some separation of the two measures for clinical reasons: we think that emotional overinvolvement and criticism clearly demand different therapeutic strategies (Kuipers & Bebbington 1990).

## EE AS AN INDICATOR OF FAMILY RELATIONSHIPS

EE uses an individual relative's behaviour at a single time to predict the likelihood of a subsequent relapse in the schizophrenic patient with whom that relative lives. What does the measure actually mean in terms of the interplay between members of the patient's family?

It has always been presumed that EE is predictive because it indicates either some continuing feature of the interaction between the relatives, or their capacity to deal with crises (Kuipers 1979). Certainly, relatives who made frequent critical comments when interviewed alone behave similarly in the presence of the patient, although they are usually more restrained (Brown & Rutter 1966, Rutter & Brown 1966).

There is now further evidence for the generalization of relatives' behaviour. The Affective Style coding system can be used to assess families taking part in a standardized task designed to recreate interaction in a laboratory setting (Goldstein *et al.* 1968, Doane *et al.* 1981). Negative Affective Style in these direct interactions is consistently highly correlated with EE measured in the usual way (Strachan *et al.* 1986, Miklowitz *et al.* 1989). Hubschmid & Zemp (1989) have shown that high EE relatives engender a more negative emotional climate, a conflict-prone structure, and more rigid patterns of interaction.

Kuipers and her co-workers (1983) also found it possible to distinguish between high and low EE relatives in discussions that included the patient: high EE relatives talked for longer and were poorer listeners than low EE relatives. Moreover, critical relatives also appear to provide an unpredictable home environment for schizophrenic patients (MacCarthy *et al.* 1986).

High EE also appears to be associated with fears and anxieties on the part of relatives, particularly when they do not attribute the patient's behaviour to illness (Greenley 1986). Preliminary results of a study of attribution in the relatives of schizophrenic patients suggest that causal beliefs are systematically related to the relatives' emotional characteristics. Critical and hostile relatives tended to attribute negative outcomes to causes that were more identified with and controllable by the patient (Brewin *et al.* 1991).

A study of depressed spouses incidentally throws light on the behavioural counterparts of EE. Hooley & Hahlweg (1986) reported sequential analyses of interaction patterns between 44 couples where one partner was depressed. They found that high EE couples had a varied but largely negative style of interaction. Low EE spouses typically provided a continuous positive exchange. It was also possible to distinguish between the high and low EE samples on levels of warmth and marital satisfaction.

High EE also seems to be associated with less effective coping responses (Kuipers 1983, Bledin *et al.* 1990, B. MacCarthy 1989, personal communication). High EE carers of demented elderly people used strategies such as distraction, avoidance, overeating and denial, rather than more positive approaches like problem solving and seeking social support (Bledin *et al.* 1990).

Birchwood & Smith (1987) have investigated the relationship between families' coping behaviour and coping styles and the outcome of disorder in terms of relapse, social adjustment and psychopathology. Although their results cannot be directly related to EE, they suggest that poor coping in relatives has similar effects to high levels of EE.

Interestingly, patients who live with low EE relatives give vent to significantly fewer critical statements and more autonomous statements than those from high EE families. In other words, criticism is reciprocated. This finding is independent of the level of symptoms experienced by the patients (Strachan *et al.* 1989).

Finally, it is clear that the attitudes and behaviours represented by EE seem to characterize the relatives of those who suffer from a number of other conditions in addition to schizophrenia. These include depression (Vaughn & Leff 1976, Hooley *et al.* 1986), bipolar disorder (Miklowitz *et al.* 1988), obesity (Fischman-Havstad & Marston 1984), anorexia (Szmukler *et al.* 1987), mental handicap (Greedharry 1987), Parkinson's disease (B. MacCarthy 1988, personal communication), inflammatory bowel disease (C. Vaughn 1989, personal communication) and senile dementia (Gilhooly & Whittick 1989, Bledin *et al.* 1990). While much theoretical and clinical interest remains in the use of EE in schizophrenia, the measure itself appears to tap difficulties common to the care of many disabling problems. High EE ratings have also been noted in the key workers of long-term patients with schizophrenia (Watts 1988, Moore *et al.* 1992).

The findings linking EE to family behaviour and attitudes are summarized in Table 6.3.

## HOW ARE FAMILY ATTITUDES TOWARDS MENTALLY ILL RELATIVES FORMED?

The EE measure therefore probably taps a variety of attitudes and behaviours referring the family's response to chronically disturbed relatives. What is the origin of these characteristics?

**Table 6.3** Behaviour and attitudes characteristic of high EE families

A)  Carers
    Fears and anxieties
    Negative affective style
    Poor listening
    Non-illness attributions
    Attribution of negative outcomes to patient
    Maladaptive coping

B)  Patients
    More critical
    Less autonomous

C)  Interaction
    Negative
    Rigid
    Conflict ('conflict-prone structure') structure
    Unpredictable

Birchwood & Smith (1987) have argued that the original workers were wrong in thinking that EE reflects some enduring trait of relatives. They claim that high EE develops as the response of some relatives to the burdens of living with someone who has schizophrenia. They based their argument on the fact that high EE is less apparent in relatives of those experiencing first rather than subsequent admissions for schizophrenia. There is certainly a lower relapse rate in first admission when compared to subsequently admitted patients (e.g. Leff & Brown 1977), although there are alternative explanations for this. Brown and his colleagues (1972) showed that differences in outcome persisted after controlling for the patients' previous work impairment and behavioural disturbance, but recent work has suggested that at least some components of high EE are associated with abnormalities of various sorts in the patient (Miklowitz *et al.* 1983, Mavreas *et al.* 1991). However, the causal direction is as usual unclear.

The model put forward by Birchwood & Smith postulates that families' coping efficacy and coping style develops over time, along with other predictors such as the quality of family relationships. There seems little to argue with in this. It must be virtually axiomatic that the characteristics of high EE arise from an interaction between the attributes of relative and patient.

One obvious way of examining this interaction is to relate levels of EE to the 'burden' experienced by relatives. Researchers have hardly ever done this, although the literature on burden is now substantial (Fadden *et al.* 1987, Schene 1990). It seems likely that relatives with high levels of EE will find the same behaviour much more burdensome than those who are low on EE. This is also probably related to coping styles. Bledin and his colleagues (1990) have recently shown that high levels of strain, EE, and maladaptive coping strategies tended to be associated in those caring for demented elderly persons.

The data on social contact from the British studies are open to more than one interpretation. They may indicate that greater social contact with a high EE relative is more stressful. However, the schizophrenic patients most vulnerable to stress may be precisely those who are least able to

control and manage their social relationships – unable to process information effectively because of their cognitive defects, they allow themselves to become overloaded (Hemsley 1987). Those with overinvolved relatives are often the most impaired socially (Brown *et al.* 1972, Miklowitz *et al.* 1983) and may be most at risk, either because of their intrinsic problems or because an overinvolved relative is harder to get away from. Mavreas and his colleagues (1992) make an interesting claim in this context: that behavioural abnormalities are more common in schizophrenic patients when *none* of the relatives in the household is rated low in EE.

## EE OVER TIME

The value of EE assessment may be crucially related to the fact that the relative is dealing with the upheaval surrounding the patient's admission to hospital. As the disturbance settles, at least some high EE relatives become less critical (Brown *et al.* 1972, Dulz & Hand 1986, Hogarty *et al.* 1986, Tarrier *et al.* 1988a, Favre *et al.* 1989). Initial assessments have therefore been made during the admission period. Low EE relatives tend to stay low, although Tarrier and his colleagues (1988a) did report a minority who changed to high levels. There is relatively little other evidence as to the stability of EE measures over time. In the studies of Leff and his colleagues (1982, 1985), the high EE control group showed no significant overall changes in EE over the intervention time of nine months, although 2 of the 12 relatives did spontaneously become low EE.

We think that three groups of relatives can be identified. At one extreme, there are the very low EE relatives, who cope well whatever the circumstances. At the other extreme are very high EE relatives with many problems, which they cope with badly. The intermediate group may change category spontaneously or through the intervention of others, depending on their ability to learn new coping skills, and to use them in surmounting crises. If the new skills are insufficient, they may display reduced EE at one assessment, but revert when there is a crisis that they are unable to manage. Some confirmation of this comes from a study of the stability of EE over a nine-month period in 35 relatives of 22 patients with schizo-phrenia (Favre *et al.* 1989). They found stable high and low EE relatives, but also a proportion of unstable relatives who typically displayed fewer critical comments (six to ten) than the stable high EE group. The authors noted that the relatively few changes observed in EE levels seemed to depend on factors other than the clinical state of the patients.

### Intervention studies

Once it became apparent that particular attrib-utes of family interaction might have a deleterious effect on the course of schizophrenia, intervening to change these attributes became a logical next step. Several reports of social intervention with the relatives of patients with schizophrenia have now been published, and others are nearing completion.

Intervention studies are important both clini-cally and theoretically. We have reviewed these studies in detail and explored their clinical impli-cations elsewhere (Kuipers & Bebbington 1990). Their theoretical significance emerges from what they imply about the causal role of family atmos-phere in provoking relapse. We have noted the occasional contrary findings from the prospective studies listed in Table 6.1, and there are obvious gaps in our knowledge of mechanism. The critics of EE research must however contend with the generally positive results of intervention: the ability to change outcome by changing family atmosphere is highly suggestive of a causal link.

The early studies by Leff and his colleagues (1982, 1985) in London, Falloon and his col-leagues (1982, 1985) in Los Angeles, and Hogarty and his co-workers (1986) in Pittsburg were all successful in reducing the relapse rate. In the intervention group, this became no greater than would be expected in patients from low EE homes. Success was largely but not absolutely related to improved family atmosphere. The techniques used may also be effective in improving the social per-formance of patients (Doane *et al.* 1985, Hogarty *et al.* 1986) and reducing the subjective burden on their families (Falloon & Pederson 1985).

Further interventions by Wallace & Liberman (1985), Tarrier and his colleagues (1988a), Leff and his co-workers (1989), and Kuipers and her associates (Kuipers *et al.* 1989, MacCarthy *et al.* 1989) have also proved effective. Three studies however have reported a failure to improve the lot of patients through intervening with their families (Köttgen *et al.* 1984, McCreadie *et al.* 1991, Vaughan *et al.* 1992b). It is not quite clear why these should have been unsuccessful. The Hamburg study of Köttgen and her colleagues (1984) involved a psychodynamic approach to treatment, and this may have been experienced by the patients as intrusive and upsetting (Strachan 1986). The other two studies used techniques very similar to the previous studies: failure may have been the result of a lack of experience in the therapist or of particular attributes of the client group. In the Sydney study (Vaughan *et al.* 1992b), patients in both intervention and control groups were not very compliant with medication. The intervention in the Nithsdale study (McCreadie *et al.* 1991), which had limited success in engaging families, was also unsuccessful in lowering EE, although even here the total number of relapses was reduced somewhat for patients whose families accepted the intervention.

What do the intervention studies tell us about the causal significance of the family environment in engendering relapse? The success of some inter-ventions has been associated with their effective-ness in reducing EE, contact, or negative affective style (Leff *et al.* 1982, 1990, Falloon *et al.* 1982), and the less successful interventions of Köttgen and her colleagues (1984) and of McCreadie *et al.* (1991) did not manage to reduce EE. Too few reassessments of EE were carried out in Sydney for valid analysis. This suggests that high EE may indeed be a marker of a family environment that adversely affects the course of schizophrenia. However, in the Pittsburg study (Hogarty *et al.* 1986), good outcome in the combined treatment group did not require reduction in EE.

There are other reasons for reserving judgement on the causal role of the family environment. For instance, many studies have involved small numbers. It is also possible that, when interven-tions involve working with patients and their families together, reductions in EE are secondary to improvement in patient behaviour, rather than due to primary and beneficial changes in the behaviour of the relatives. However, the study of Tomaros and his colleagues (1988) is somewhat against this interpretation, as direct improvement of negative symptoms and social function by vocational training and social therapy had little effect on family atmosphere, at least in the short term. Furthermore, in the recent intervention study by Leff *et al.* (1990) working with the relatives alone produced as great a reduction in the relapse rate over two years as family sessions including the patient.

The results of the interventions, taken together with the impressive consensus from the predictive studies, therefore provide a strong indication that EE does indeed reflect a causal process. However, we still need to know how changes in EE relate to changes in the patient, and final clarification requires longitudinal study of the stability of EE and its relationship to relapse in a large sample.

## Social influences on the negative symptoms of schizophrenia

Evidence for a significant environmental influence on the negative symptoms of schizophrenia has long been established. This is of particular significance, as it accepted that such symptoms are relatively resistant to modification by psychopharmacological means (Crow 1989). Belknap (1956), Dunham & Weinberg (1960), and, perhaps most famously, Goffman (1961) propounded with force the clinical opinion that large and environmentally impoverished mental institutions had a damaging effect on long-term inmates. They were able to do this because an association between the institutional environment and the impaired social behaviour of many of those accommodated in them was quite obvious.

However, they did not consider the possibility that individuals handicapped by the chronic effects of severe psychiatric illness might themselves contribute to their own environment. This is apparent from the work of Wing & Freudenberg (1961) who arranged for nurses to provide extra social stimulation for long-term schizophrenic patients. The patients slowly improved, but when the stimulation was withdrawn they deteriorated again. This strongly suggests that improvement in the patients would have to come about by the continuous provision of stimulation from an external source.

The results of this experiment led Wing & his colleagues to mount a further study (Wing & Brown 1970). Three area mental hospitals were selected on the basis that they provided demonstrably different environments for the patients they housed. A sample of female residents with longstanding schizophrenia was studied in each hospital. Measures of the social environment provided by the hospitals confirmed differences between them in terms of the range of the patients' personal possessions, the attitudes of the nurses towards them, the amount of contact with the community outside, the restrictiveness of ward regimes, and the amount of time the patients spent doing nothing. It was hypothesized that these characteristics would be associated with equivalent clinical differences between the patient samples. This was corroborated by the results, which showed in particular that an impoverished and restricted ward environment was associated with prominent negative symptoms.

This cross-sectional association does not guarantee causal direction, but the three groups were followed up over an eight-year period. Improvements in the social environment externally induced were associated with improvements in the patients, and this was independent of medication policies. Although negative symptoms rarely disappeared entirely, the degree of improvement was clinically significant. These effects of the social environment have now been confirmed by other studies located outside large institutions (Tidmarsh & Wood 1972, Hewitt *et al.* 1975).

Although the Three Hospitals Study is a classic of careful investigation which had a major impact on the management of long-term mental illness, no attempt to replicate it has been made until very recently (Curson *et al.* 1990, Barnes, personal communication 1990). These authors examined the relationship between social and clinical poverty in long-stay patients with schizophrenia at a fourth British hospital. The patients were less than 60 years of age and had been resident for over

2 years. All had a DSM-III diagnosis of schizophrenia. Assessments were made with the same instruments as in the Wing & Brown (1970) study. Levels of disability seemed comparable in the two studies.

In the earlier study, the time the patients spent doing nothing was a particularly important predictor of negative symptoms. Despite the fact that the nurse–patient ratio was two and a half times greater in the later study, the patients spent almost two hours *more* doing nothing than in the least stimulating of the three hospitals in the earlier study. Overall, there was a relationship between environmental understimulation and negative symptoms, but the relationship was much weaker than that obtained by Wing & Brown (1970). However, this may reflect a constriction in the variability of the environment rather than unsatisfactory replication: the patients in this study were very much a residual group. The authors also found that there was a relationship between an impoverished social environment and *florid* symptoms. The definitive results of this study are awaited with interest.

As a result of these studies there is little doubt that, while social disablement in schizophrenia to some extent represents an intrinsic part of the disease process, it should respond considerably to enlightened clinical intervention.

## Conclusion

The very extensive literature that we have reviewed here is consistent in supporting a major effect of the social environment on the course and outcome of schizophrenia, and social influences probably have an effect on the first emergence of the condition, at least on its timing. Social factors operate on the condition as a whole, whether expressed in the usually acute florid symptoms, or the more prolonged negative symptoms.

This has enormous implications for the rational clinical management of schizophrenia. In particular, management must be based on a proper attention to the social environment, especially for patients with a history of several relapses, and should be provided continuously by clinicians with special expertise.

## References

Al Khani M.A.F., Bebbington P.E., Watson J.P. & House F. (1986). Life events and schizophrenia: a Saudi Arabian study. *British Journal of Psychiatry*. 148, 12–22.

Barrelet L., Ferrero F., Szigetty L., Giddey C. & Pellizzer G. (1990) Expressed emotion and first admission schizophrenia: nine month follow-up in a French cultural environment. *British Journal of Psychiatry* 156, 357–362.

Bateson G., Jackson D.D., Hally J. & Weakland J.H. (1956) Towards a theory of schizophrenia. *Behavioural Science* 1, 251–64.

Bebbington P.E., Wilkins S., Jones P. *et al.* (1992) Life events and psychosis: initial results from the Camberwell Collaborative Psychosis Study. *British Journal of Psychiatry* (in press).

Belknap I. (1956) *Human Problems of a State Mental Hospital*. McGraw-Hill, New York.

Birchwood M. & Smith J. (1987) Schizophrenia in the family. In: J. Orford (ed.) *Coping with Disorder in the Family*. Croom Helm, London.

Bledin K., MacCarthy B., Kuipers L. & Woods R. (1990) Daughters of people with dementia: Expressed Emotion, strain and coping. *British Journal of Psychiatry* 157, 221–227.

Brewin C.R., MacCarthy B., Duda K. & Vaughn C.E. (1991) Attribution and Expressed Emotion in the relatives of patients with schizophrenia. *Journal of Abnormal Psychology* 100, 546–554.

Brown G.W. (1959) Experiences of discharged chronic schizophrenic mental hospital patients in various types of living group. *Millbank Memorial Fund Quarterly* 37, 105–131.

Brown G.W. (1974) Meaning, measurement and stress of life events. In: B.S. Dohrenwend & B.P. Dohrenwend (eds) *Stressful Life Events: Their Nature and Effects*. John Wiley, New York.

Brown G.W. & Birley J.L.T. (1968) Crises and life changes and the onset of schizophrenia. *Journal of Health and Social Behaviour* 9, 203–214.

Brown G.W., Birley J.L.T. & Wing J.K. (1972) Influence of family life on the course of schizophrenic disorders: a replication. *British Journal of Psychiatry* 121, 241–258.

Brown G.W., Carstairs G.M. & Topping G.C. (1958) The post hospital adjustment of chronic mental patients. *Lancet* ii, 685–689.

Brown G.W. & Harris T.O. (1978) *Social Origins of Depression*. Tavistock, London.

Brown G.W., Harris T.O. & Peto J. (1973) Life events and psychiatric disorders. Part 2: Nature of causal link. *Psychological Medicine* 3, 159–176.

Brown G.W., Monck E.M., Carstairs G.M. & Wing J.K. (1962) Influence of family life on the course of schizophrenic illness. *British Journal of Preventive and Social Medicine* 16, 55–68.

Brown G.W. & Rutter M.L. (1966) The measurement of

family activities and relationships. *Human Relations* 19, 241–263.

Budzyna-Dawidowski P., Rostworowska M. & de Barbaro B. (1989) Stability of Expressed Emotion. A 3 Year Follow-up Study of Schizophrenic Patients. Paper presented at the 19th Annual Congress of the European Association of Behaviour Therapy, Vienna, 10–24 September.

Canton G. & Fraccon I.G. (1985) Life events and schizophrenia: a replication. *Acta Psychiatica Scandinavica* 71, 211–216.

Cazzullo C.L., Bertrando P., Bressi C., Clerici M., Beltz J. & Invernizzi G. (1989) Expressed Emotion in Italian families: A Comparison Between Schizophrenics and Other Patients. Paper presented at the 19th Annual Congress of the European Association of Behaviour Therapy, Vienna, 20–24 September.

Chung R.K., Langeluddecke P. & Tennant C. (1986) Threatening life events in the onset of schizophrenia, schizophreniform psychosis and hypomania. *British Journal of Psychiatry* 148, 680–686.

Crow T.J. (1989) A current view of the Type II syndrome: age of onset, intellectual impairment and the meaning of structural changes in the brain. *British Journal of Psychiatry* 155, suppl. 7, 10–14.

Curson D., Pantelis C., Ward J. & Barnes T.R.E. (1990) A study of the social environment and clinical poverty in long-stay chronic schizophrenic patients in a British mental hospital in 1988. A reassessment of institutionalism and schizophrenia. *Schizophrenia Research* 3, 7–8.

Day R., Neilsen J.A., Korten A. *et al.* (1987) Stressful life events preceding the acute onset of schizophrenia: a cross-national study from the World Health Organization. *Culture, Medicine and psychiatry* 11, 123–206.

Doane J.A., Falloon I.R.H., Goldstein M.J. & Mintz J. (1985) Parental affective style and the treatment of schizophrenia: predicting course of illness and social functioning. *Archives of General Psychiatry* 42, 34–42.

Doane J.A., West K.L., Goldstein M.J., Rodnick E.H. & Jones J.E. (1981) Parental communication deviance and affective style: predictors of subsequent schizophrenic spectrum disorders in vulnerable adolescents. *Archives of General Psychiatry* 38, 679–685.

Dohrenwend B.S., Krasnoff L., Askenasy A.R. & Dohrenwend B.P. (1978) Exemplification of a method for scaling life events: the PERI life events scale. *Journal of Health and Social Behaviour* 19, 205–229.

Drake R.E. & Sederer L.I. (1986) The adverse effects of intensive treatment of chronic schizophrenia. *Comprehensive Psychiatry* 27, 313–326.

Dulz B. & Hand I. (1986) Short term relapse in young schizophrenics: can it be predicted and affected by family (CFI), patient, and treatment variables? An experimental study. In: Goldstein M.J., Hand I. and Hahlweg K. (eds) *Treatment of Schizophrenia: Family Assessment and Intervention.* Springer, Berlin.

Dunham, H.W. & Weinberg, S.K. (1960) *Culture of the State Mental Hospital,* Detroit, Wayne State University Press.

Fadden G.B., Bebbington P.E. & Kuipers L. (1987) The burden of care: the impact of functional psychiatric illness on the patient's family. *British Journal of Psychiatry* 150, 285–292.

Falloon I.R.H., Boyd J.L., McGill C.W., Razani J., Moss H.B. & Gilderman A.M. (1982) Family management in the prevention of exacerbations of schizophrenia. A controlled study. *New England Journal of Medicine* 306, 1437–1440.

Falloon I.R.H., Boyd J.L., McGill C.W. *et al.* (1985) Family management in the prevention of morbidity of schizophrenia. Clinical outcome of a two year longitudinal study. *Archives of General Psychiatry* 42, 887–896.

Falloon I.R.H. & Pederson J. (1985) Family management in the prevention of morbidity of schizophrenia. Adjustment of the family unit. *British Journal of Psychiatry* 147, 156–163.

Favre S., Gonzales C., Lendais G. *et al.* (1989) Expressed Emotion (EE) of Schizophrenic Relatives. Paper presented at VIIIth World Congress of Psychiatry, Athens, 12–19 October.

Ferrera J.A. & Vizarro C. (1989) Expressed Emotion and Course of Schizophrenia in a Spanish Sample. Paper presented at the 19th Annual Congress of the European Association of Behaviour Therapy, Vienna, 20–24 September.

Fischman-Havstad L. & Marston A.R. (1984) Weight loss maintenance as an aspect of family emotion and process. *British Journal of Clinical Psychology* 23, 265–271.

Gilhooly M. & Whittick J.(1989) Expressed Emotion in caregivers of the dementing elderly. *British Journal of Medical Psychology* 62, 265–272.

Goffman E. (1961) *Asylums.* Anchor Books, New York.

Goldberg S.C., Schooler N.R., Hogarty G.E. & Roper M. (1977) Prediction of relapse in schizophrenic outpatients treated by drug and sociotherapy. *Archives of General Psychiatry* 34, 171–184.

Goldstein M. (1985) Family factors that antedate the onset of schizophrenia and related disorders: the results of a 15 year prospective longitudinal study. *Acta Psychiatrica Scandinavica* 71, suppl. 319, 7–18.

Goldstein M. (1987) The UCLA High-risk project. *Schizophrenia Bulletin* 13, 505–514.

Goldstein M., Judd L.L., Rodnick E.H., Alkire A. & Gould E. (1968) A method for studying social influence and coping patterns within families of disturbed adolescents. *Journal of Nervous and Mental Disease* 147, 233–251.

Greedharry D. (1987) Expressed Emotion in the families of the mentally handicapped: a pilot study. *British Journal of Psychiatry* 150, 400–402.

Greenley J.R. (1986) Social control and Expressed Emotion. *Journal of Nervous and Mental Disease* 174, 24–30.

Hemsley D.R. (1987) Psychological models of schizophrenia. In: E. Miller and P. Cooper (eds) *Textbook of Abnormal Psychology.* Churchill Livingstone, Edinburgh.

Hewitt S., Ryan P. & Wing J.K. (1975) Living without the mental hospitals. *Journal of Social Policy* 4, 391–404.

Hirsch S.R. Gaind R., Rohde P.D., Stevens B.C. & Wing J.K. (1973) Outpatient maintenance of chronic schizophrenic patients with long acting fluphenazine: double blind placebo trial. *British Medical Journal* i, 633–637.

Hirsch S.R. & Leff J.P. (1975) *Abnormalities in the Parents of Schizophrenics. Maudsley Monograph No. 22.* Oxford University Press, Oxford.

Hogarty G.E. (1985) Expressed Emotion and schizophrenic relapse: implications from the Pittsburg Study. In: Alpert M. (ed.). *Controversies in Schizophrenia.* Guilford Press, New York.

Hogarty G.E., Anderson C.M. Reiss D.J. *et al.* (1986) Family psycho-education, social skills training and maintenance chemotherapy in the aftercare treatment of schizophrenia. I. One year effects of a controlled study on relapse and Expressed Emotion. *Archives of General Psychiatry* 43, 633–642.

Hooley J.M. (1985) Expressed Emotion: a review of the critical literature. *Clinical Psychology Review* 5, 119–139.

Hooley J.M. & Hahlweg K. (1986) The marriages and interaction patterns of depressed patients and their spouses: comparison of high and low EE dyads. In Goldstein M.J., Hand I. and Hahlweg K. (eds) *Treatment of Schizophrenia: Family Assessment and Intervention.* Springer, Berlin.

Hooley J.M., Orley J. and Teasdale J. (1986) Levels of Expressed Emotion and relapse in depressed patients. *British Journal of Psychiatry* 148, 642–647.

Hubschmid T. & Zemp M. (1989) Interactions in high- and low-EE families. *Social Psychiatry and Psychiatric Epidemiology* 24, 113–119.

Ivanovic M. & Vuletic Z. (1989) Expressed Emotion in the Families of Patients with a Frequent Type of Schizophrenia and its Influence on the Course of illness. Paper presented at the 19th Annual Congress of the European Association of Behaviour Therapy, Vienna, 20–24 September.

Jacobs S. & Myers. J. (1976) Recent life events and acute schizophrenic psychosis: a controlled study. *Journal of Nervous and Mental Disease* 162, 75–87.

Karno M., Jenkins J.H., de la Selva A. *et al.* (1987) Expressed Emotion and schizophrenic outcome among Mexican–American families. *Journal of Nervous and Mental Disease* 175 143–151.

Koenigsberg H.W. & Handley R. (1986) Expressed Emotion: from predictive index to clinical construct. *American Journal of Psychiatry* 143, 1361–1373.

Köttgen C., Sonnichsen I., Mollenhauer K. & Jurth R. (1984) Group therapy with the families of schizophrenic patients: results of the Hamburg Camberwell Family Interview Study III. *International Journal of Family Psychiatry* 5, 84–94.

Kuipers L. (1979) Expressed Emotion: a review. *British Journal of Social and Clinical Psychology* 18, 237–243.

Kuipers L. (1983) Family Factors in Schizophrenia: An Intervention Study. PhD Thesis. University of London.

Kuipers L. & Bebbington P.E. (1988) Expressed Emotion research in schizophrenia: theoretical and clinical implications. *Psychological Medicine* 18, 893–910.

Kuipers L. & Bebbington P.E. (1990) *Working in Partnership: Clinicians and Carers in the Management of Longstanding Mental Illness.* Heinemann Medical, Oxford.

Kuipers L., MacCarthy B., Hurry J. & Harper R. (1989) Counselling the relatives of the long term mentally ill. II. A low-cost supportive model. *British Journal of Psychiatry* 154, 775–782.

Kuipers L., Sturgeon D., Berkowitz R. & Leff J.P. (1983) Characteristics of Expressed Emotion: its relationship to speech and looking in schizophrenic patients and their relatives. *British Journal of Clinical Psychology* 22, 257–264.

Laing R.D. & Esterson A. (1964) *Sanity, Madness and the Family.* Penguin, Harmondsworth.

Leff J., Berkowitz R., Shavit N., Strachan A., Glass I. & Vaughn C. (1989) A trial of family therapy v. a relatives' group for schizophrenia. *British Journal of Psychiatry* 154, 58–66.

Leff J., Berkowitz R, Shavit N., Strachan A., Glass I. & Vaughn C. (1990) A trial of family therapy versus a relatives' group for schizophrenia. Two-year follow-up. *British Journal of Psychiatry* 157, 571–577.

Leff J.P. & Brown G.W. (1977) Family and social factors in the course of schizophrenia (letter). *British Journal of Psychiatry* 130, 417–420.

Leff J.P., Kuipers L., Berkowitz R., Eberlein-Fries R. & Sturgeon D. (1982) A controlled trial of social intervention in schizophrenic families. *British Journal of Psychiatry* 141, 121–134.

Leff J.P., Kuipers L., Berkowitz R. & Sturgeon D. (1985) A controlled trial of social intervention in the families of schizophrenic patients: two year follow up. *British Journal of Psychiatry* 146, 594–600.

Leff J.P., Kuipers L., Berkowitz R., Vaughn C.E. & Sturgeon D. (1983) Life events, relatives' Expressed Emotion and maintenance neuroleptics in schizophrenic relapse. *Psychological Medicine* 13, 799–806.

Leff J.P. & Vaughn C.E. (1981) The role of maintenance therapy and relatives' Expressed Emotion in relapse of schizophrenia: a two year follow up. *British Journal Psychiatry* 139, 102–104.

Leff J.P. & Vaughn C. (1985) *Expressed Emotion in Families.* Guilford Press, New York.

Leff J.P., Wig N., Ghosh A. *et al.* (1987) Influence of relatives' Expressed Emotion on the course of schizophrenia in Chandigarh. *British Journal of Psychiatry* 151, 166–173.

Lidz T., Cornelison A.R., Fleck S. & Terry D. (1957) The intrafamilial environment of the schizophrenic patient. I. *Psychiatry* 20, 329–342.

MacCarthy B., Hemsley D., Schrank-Fernandez C., Kuipers L. & Katz R. (1986) Unpredictability as a correlate of Expressed Emotion in the relatives of schizophrenics.

*British Journal of Psychiatry* 148, 727–730.

MacCarthy B., Kuipers L., Hurry J., Harper R. & Lesage A. (1989) Counselling the relatives of the long term mentally ill. I. Evaluation. *British Journal of Psychiatry* 154, 768–775.

McCreadie R.G. & Phillips K. (1988) The Nithsdale Schizophrenia Survey: VII. Does relatives' high Expressed Emotion predict relapse? *British Journal of Psychiatry* 152, 477–481.

McCreadie R.G., Phillips K., Harvey J.A., Waldron G., Stewart M. & Baird D. (1991) The Nithsdale Schizophrenia Surveys VIII. Do relatives want family intervention and does it help? *British Journal of Psychiatry* 158, 110–113.

McCreadie R.G. & Robinson A.T.D. (1987) The Nithsdale Schizophrenia Survey: VI. Relatives' Expressed Emotion: prevalence, patterns and clinical assessment. *British Journal of Psychiatry* 150, 640–644.

MacMillan J.F., Gold A., Crow T.J., Johnson A.L. & Johnstone, E.C. (1986) The Northwick Park Study of First Episodes of Schizophrenia. IV. Expressed Emotion and relapse. *British Journal of Psychiatry* 148, 133–143.

Malla A.K., Cortese L., Shaw T.S. & Ginsberg B. (1990) Life events and relapse in schizophrenia: a one year prospective study. *Social Psychiatry and Psychiatric Epidemiology* 25, 221–224.

Malzacher M., Merz J. & Ebnother, D. (1981) Einschneidende Lebensereignisse im Vorfeld akuter schizophrener Episoden: Erstmals erkrankte Patienten im Vergleich mit einer Normalstichprobe. *Archiv für Psychiatrie und Nervenkrankheiten* 230, 227–242.

Martins C., de Lemos A.I. & Bebbington P.E. (1992) A Portugese/Brazilian Study of Expressed Emotion. *Social Psychiatry and Psychiatric Epidemiology* 27, 22–27.

Mavreas V., Tomaros V., Carydi N., Economou M., Ioanovich I. & Stephanis C. (1992) Expressed Emotion in families of chronic schizophrenics and its association with clinical measures. *Social Psychiatry and Psychiatric Epidemiology* 27, 4–9.

Michaux W., Gansereit K., McCabe O. & Kurland A. (1967) The psychopathology and measurement of environmental stress. *Community Mental Health Journal* 3, 358–371.

Miklowitz D.J., Goldstein M.J., Doane J.A. *et al.* (1989) Is Expressed Emotion an index of a transactional process? I. Parent's Affective Style. *Family Process* 28, 153–167.

Miklowitz D.J., Goldstein M.J. & Falloon R.H. (1983) Premorbid and symptomatic characteristics of schizophrenics from families with high and low levels of Expressed Emotion. *Journal of Abnormal Psychology* 92, 359–367.

Miklowitz D.J., Goldstein M.J., Nuechterlein K.H., Snyder K.S. & Mintz J. (1988) Family factors and the course of bipolar affective disorder. *Archives of General Psychiatry* 45, 225–231.

Moline R.A. Singh S., Morris A. & Meltzer H.Y. (1985) Family Expressed Emotion and relapse in schizophrenia in 24 urban American patients. *American Journal of Psychiatry* 142, 1078–1081.

Moore E., Ball R. & Kuipers L. (1992) Expressed Emotion in staff working with the long-term adult mentally ill. *British Journal of Psychiatry* (in press).

Mozny P. (1989) Expressed Emotion and Rehospitalization Rates of Schizophrenics in the Psychiatric Hospital, Kromeriz, CSSR. Paper presented at the 19th Annual Congress of the European Association of Behaviour Therapy, Vienna, 20–24 September.

Nuechterlein K.H. Snyder K.S., Dawson M.E., Rappe S., Gitlin M. & Fogelson D. (1986) Expressed Emotion, fixed-dose fluphenazine decanoate maintenance, and relapse in recent onset schizophrenia. *Psychopharmacology Bulletin* 22, 633–639.

Parker G., Johnston P. & Hayward, L. (1988) Parental 'Expressed Emotion' as a predictor of schizophrenic relapse. *Archives of General Psychiatry* 45, 806–813.

Paykel E.S. (1979) Recent life events in the developments of the depressive disorders. In: Depue R.A. (ed.) *The Psychobiology of the Depressive Disorders: Implications for the Effects of Stress*. Academic Press, New York.

Rutter M.L. & Brown G.W. (1966) The reliability and validity of measures of family life and relationships in families containing a psychiatric patient. *Social Psychiatry* 1, 38–53.

Salokangas R.K.R. (1983) Prognostic implications of the sex of schizophrenic patients. *British Journal of Psychiatry* 142, 145–151.

Schene A.H. (1990) Objective and subjective dimensions of family burden: towards an integrative framework for research. *Social Psychiatry and Psychiatric Epidemiology* 25, 289–297.

Shakow D. (1973) Some thoughts about schizophrenic research in the context of high risk studies. *Psychiatry* 36, 353–365.

Stevens B.C. (1973) Evaluation of rehabilitation for psychotic patients in the community. *Acta Psychiatica Scandinavica* 46, 136–140.

Strachan A.M. (1986) Family intervention for the rehabilitation of schizophrenia. *Schizophrenia Bulletin* 12, 678–698.

Strachan A.M., Feingold D., Goldstein M.J., Miklowitz D.J. & Nuechterlein K.H. (1989) Is Expressed Emotion an index of a transactional process II. Patient's coping style. *Family Process* 28, 169–181.

Strachan A.M., Leff J.P., Goldstein M.J., Doane A. & Burrt C. (1986) Emotional attitudes and direct communication in the families of schizophrenics: a cross-national replication. *British Journal of Psychiatry* 149, 279–287.

Stricker K., Rook A. & Buchkremer G. (1989) Expressed Emotion and Course of Disease in Schizophrenic Outpatients: Results of a Two Year Follow-up in a German Study. Paper presented at the 19th Annual Congress of the European Association of Behaviour Therapy, Vienna, 20–24 September.

Sturgeon D., Turpin D., Kuipers L., Berkowitz R. & Leff J. (1984) Psychophysiological responses of schizophrenic patients to high and low Expressed Emotion relatives:

*Chapter 6*

a follow-up study. *British Journal of Psychiatry* 145, 62–69.

Szmukler G.I., Berkowitz R., Eisler I., Leff J. & Dare C. (1987) Expressed Emotion in individual and family settings: a comparative study. *British Journal of Psychiatry* 151, 174–178.

Tarrier N. & Barrowclough C. (1987) A longitudinal psychophysiological assessment of a schizophrenic patient in relation to the Expressed Emotion of his relatives. *Behavioural Psychotherapy* 15, 45–57.

Tarrier N., Barrowclough C., Porceddu K. & Watts S. (1988a) The assessment of psychophysiological reactivity to the Expressed Emotion of the relatives of schizophrenic patients. *British Journal of Psychiatry* 153, 532–542.

Tarrier N., Barrowclough C., Vaughn C. *et al.* (1988b) The community management of schizophrenia: a controlled trial of a behavioural intervention with families to reduce relapse. *British Journal of Psychiatry* 153, 532–542.

Tarrier N., Vaughn C.E., Lader M.H. & Leff J.P. (1979) Bodily reactions to people and events in schizophrenics. *Archives of General Psychiatry* 36, 311–315.

Tidmarsh D. & Wood S. (1972) Psychiatric aspects of destitution. In: J.K. Wing and A.M. Hailey (eds) *Evaluating a Community Psychiatric Service*. Oxford University Press, London.

Tomaros V., Vlachonikolis I.G., Stefanis C.N. & Madianos M. (1988) The effect of individual psychosocial treatment on the family atmosphere of schizophrenic patients. *Social Psychiatry* 23, 256–261.

Turpin G., Tarrier N. & Sturgeon D. (1988) Social psychophysiology and the study of biopsychosocial models of schizophrenia. In: Wagner H. (ed.) *Social Psychophysiology: Theory and Clinical Applications*. Wiley, Chichester.

Valone K., Goldstein M.G. & Morton J.P. (1984) Parental Expressed Emotion and psychophysiological reactivity in an adolescent sample at risk for schizophrenic spectrum disorders. *Journal of Abnormal Psychology* 93, 448–457.

Vaughan K., Doyle M., McConaghy N., Blaszczynski A., Fox A. & Tarrier N. (1992a) The relationship between relative's Expressed Emotion and schizophrenic relapse: an Australian replication. *Social Psychiatry and Psychiatric Epidemiology* 27, 10–15.

Vaughan K., Doyle M., McConaghy N., Blaszczynski A., Fox A. & Tarrier N. (1992b) The Sydney Intervention Trial: a controlled trial of relatives' counselling to reduce schizophrenic relapse. *Social Psychiatry and Psychiatric Epidemiology* 27, 16–21.

Vaughn C. (1986) Patterns of emotional response in the families of schizophrenic patients. In: Goldstein M.J., Hand I. and Hahlweg K. (eds) *Treatment of Schizophrenia: Family Assessment and Intervention*. Springer, Berlin.

Vaughn C.E. (1989) Annotation: Expressed Emotion in family relationships. *Journal of Child Psychology* 30, 13–22.

Vaughn C. & Leff J.P. (1976) The influence of family and social factors on the course of psychiatric illness: a comparison of schizophrenic and depressed neurotic patients. *British Journal of Psychiatry* 129, 125–137.

Vaughn C.E., Snyder K.S., Jones S., Freeman W.B. & Falloon I.R.H. (1984) Family factors in schizophrenic relapse: replication in California of British research in Expressed Emotion. *Archives of General Psychiatry* 41, 1169–1177.

Venables P. (1977) Psychophysiological High Risk Strategy with Mauritian Children: Methodological Issues. Paper read at the Psychophysiological Conference, London.

Ventura J., Nuechterlein K.H., Lukoff D. & Hardisty J.P. (1989) A prospective study of stressful life events and schizophrenic relapse. *Journal of Abnormal Psychology* 98, 407–411.

Wallace C.J. & Liberman R.P. (1985) Social skills training for patients with schizophrenia: a controlled clinical trial. *Psychiatry Research* 15, 239–247.

Watts S. (1988) A Descriptive Investigation of the Incidence of High EE in Staff Working with Schizophrenic Patients in a Hospital Setting. Unpublished dissertation. Diploma in Clinical Psychology, British Psychological Society.

Wig N.N., Menon D.K., Bedi H. *et al.* (1987a) The cross-cultural transfer of ratings of relatives' Expressed Emotion. *British Journal of Psychiatry* 151, 156–160.

Wig N.N., Menon D.K., Bedi H. *et al.* (1987b) The distribution of Expressed Emotion components among relatives of schizophrenic patients in Aarhus and Chandigarh. *British Journal of Psychiatry* 151, 160–165.

Wing J.K., Bennett D.H. & Denham J. (1964) *The Industrial Rehabilitation of Long Stay Schizophrenic Patients*. Medical Research Council Memo No. 42. HMSO, London.

Wing J.K. & Brown G.W. (1970) *Institutionalism and Schizophrenia. A Comparative Study of Three Mental Hospitals 1960–68*. Cambridge University Press, Cambridge.

Wing J.K. & Freudenberg R.K. (1961) The response of severely ill chronic schizophrenic patients to social stimulation. *American Journal of Psychiatry* 118, 311–322.

World Health Organization (1979) *Schizophrenia: An International Follow-up Study*. John Wiley, Chichester.

Wynne L.C. & Singer M. (1963) Thought disorder and family relations of schizophrenics. I. *Archives of General Psychiatry* 9, 191–206.

Wynne, L.C. & Singer, M. (1965) Thought disorder and family relations of schizophrenics. II. *Archives of General Psychiatry* 12, 187–212.

# Chapter 7
## Social Factors in the Onset and Maintenance of Depression

Z. COOPER & E.S. PAYKEL

## Introduction

In this chapter evidence will be reviewed concerning the effects of the social environment on the development, maintenance and relapse of depressive disorders. The discussion will be divided into two main sections: a consideration of the role of recent major changes in the environment, that is, life events, in psychiatric disorder, and a consideration of social support as a factor modifying the effects of these stressful life events.

The notion that a variety of negative and stressful life experiences may adversely affect psychological well-being and even precipitate psychiatric disorder has a long history. Since the 1960s there has been a large volume of systematic research on the role of recent life events in psychiatric disorder. This literature is now sufficiently extensive for it to be clear that the risk of depression is considerably increased following stressful life events. Nevertheless, most people do not become clinically depressed even when exposed to such stressful events (Paykel 1978). More recently, this observation has led to the search for other social factors: those which both protect individuals against life stress and those which make them vulnerable to it. Quite apart from the gain in theoretical understanding to be obtained from such a search for the modifying factors which might explain individual differences in response to stress, there are also practical implications of this strategy. Whereas many threatening life events of the type likely to precipitate depression are environmental events over which the individual and the clinician have no control, it has been noted (Andrews *et al.* 1978) that the social factors which modify vulnerability to life events may be potentially amenable to therapeutic intervention.

## Theoretical and methodological issues

### The nature of life events and social support

Most discussions of the effects of life events assume that there is consensus as to what the term means. It is nevertheless necessary to give an explicit definition of the term. Life events refer to a change in the external environment which occurs sufficiently rapidly to be approximately dated. This involves several elements: change which is relatively abrupt rather than slow, and which involves the external, usually social, environment. An event should usually be external and potentially verifiable. This definition does not quite capture the full range of life events. The development of a personal physical illness is potentially verifiable and has implications similar to those of major changes in the social environment. It is not however an external event, but an internal change. Nevertheless, it is usually accepted as a life event (also see Chapter 10).

The work of Brown and colleagues has also included the concept of 'difficulties' defined as problems which last for at least four weeks. This refers to a more chronic form of stress than is usually included in the notion of a life event. However, in most studies difficulties have been amalgamated with life events as 'provoking agents' and have not been analysed separately. Such difficulties may not be conceptually distinct from life events and may simply represent the ongoing chronic effects of a previous life event. There is a further problem of conceptual overlap between 'difficulties' and what Brown has termed vulnerability factors, that is, ongoing problematical situations which increase an individual's vulnerability to disorder in the presence of a life event.

In contrast to life events, few investigators have provided a conceptual definition of social support or attempted to use such a definition to develop reliable and valid measures of support. Others have provided definitions of a kind which leave key terms undefined and use the terms to be defined in the definition they provide. For example, Kaplan *et al.* (1977) suggest that 'support is defined by the relative presence or absence of psychosocial support resources from significant others'. However, the term 'support resources' is left unexplained (see also Chapter 30).

More detailed and less obviously unsatisfactory definitions have also been provided. Cobb (1976) defines social support as 'information leading the subject to believe (i) that he is cared for and loved, (ii) is esteemed and valued, and (iii) belongs to a social network of communication and mutual obligation'. This definition focuses only on emotional support, but at least does not use the terms to be defined in the definition itself. In a later paper, Cobb (1979) offers descriptions of other kinds of support which include instrumental support, active support, and material support. House (1981) suggests that social support is an interpersonal transaction involving one or more of the following:

1 Emotional concern (liking, love, empathy).
2 Instrumental aid (goods or services).
3 Information (about the environment).
4 Appraisal (information relevant to self-evaluation).

This again offers a more detailed attempt to define support without using the terms to be defined. It is also a fairly comprehensive definition capable of being operationalized for the purpose of measurement.

Despite a wide variety of definitions there is some consensus that social support is a multi-dimensional concept. Thoits (1985) suggests that it refers to helpful functions performed for an individual by significant others, such as family members, friends, co-workers, relatives and neighbours. The functions may include: socio-emotional aid, such as demonstration of love, caring, esteem, value, empathy, sympathy, and/or group belonging; instrumental aid such as actions and materials that enable fulfilment of everyday responsibilities and obligations, and informational aid which refers to communications such as advice, personal feedback and job information.

Clearly measures for the various functions listed above may assess the objective presence and availability of such aid and its utilization or the agent's subjective perception of the availability of the possibility of such aid, and these two forms of measurement may not yield the same result. Whether it is subjective perception of support or the objective availability of such support which is more critical for subsequent disorder is an empirical question to which we shall return later.

Quite apart from the failure of a general conceptual definition in this area and the failure of investigators to develop valid and reliable measures of the concepts so defined, there appears to be an even more serious problem in the definition of social support. The problem is that social support may be confounded with the occurrence of life events and it may be that many studies are not measuring two distinct phenomena. Many life events may be seen as losses and gains of social support (e.g. divorce, death of spouse, marriage, etc.). These events may not be conceptually distinct from social support changes, which may simply be a reflection of prior life events. Furthermore, events may themselves provoke further changes in social support. Clearly if support is not conceptually distinct from life events, this will have major implications for the debate about whether social support (or its lack) directly influences subsequent disorder (Thoits 1985) acting, as it were, simply as a life event, or does so only indirectly by acting as a buffer between adverse life events and subsequent disorder.

### Measures of life events and social support

The earliest studies of life events and psychiatric disorder used pencil and paper checklists where subjects were simply required to report which of a list of life events had occurred in a defined time period (Holmes & Rahe 1967). Although at the time such self-report questionnaires represented a considerable advance in method, it is now clear that life event research involves a number of problems which this method cannot satisfactorily resolve. Questionnaires do not usually enable full definitions to be given of what is to count as a rateable event. Since life events by their very nature have to be reported retrospectively, accuracy of recall is an issue. There are two aspects to this problem. The inherent inaccuracies of recall over fairly long periods may lead to events being reported which have occurred outside the study period. Also events may be overreported or exaggerated by people who experience subsequent psychiatric disorder in an attempt to explain the disorder in terms of previous life stress. In an interview, in contrast to a questionnaire, the researcher can obtain sufficient detailed knowledge of the subject's circumstances to avoid the tendency to an 'effort after meaning' as the phenomenon of overreporting to explain disorder has been termed, and can cross check the reported timing of events.

The difficulties outlined above have led to the development of semi-structured interview schedules which allow the interviewer to obtain more detailed information about the circumstances of the subject's life. Two such interviews are the Bedford College Life Events and Difficulties Schedule (LEDS) (Brown & Harris 1978) and the Interview for Recent Life Events (Paykel 1983). Both interviews allow detailed timing of events, so that attention can be focused on a specific period prior to disorder, have associated procedures for quantification of stress, and a provision for the exclusion of events probably due to illness. A review of studies of reliability and validity (Paykel 1983) has shown adequate performance for interviews of this kind, with rather lower figures for self-report questionnaires.

There is no generally accepted measure of social support, despite the development of numerous self-report questionnaires (Blazer 1983, Waring & Patton 1984, Billings & Moos 1985) and the existence of some interview methods of assessment (Brown & Harris 1978, Henderson 1981, Brown *et al.* 1986). Assessments of social support therefore tend to vary from study to study, with a few investigators attempting to assess a multidimensional concept (e.g. Ullah *et al.* 1985, Parry & Shapiro 1986), while others assess only one or two aspects of social support such as, for example, the presence of an intimate confiding relationship with a spouse or lover (Campbell *et al.* 1983, Bebbington *et al.* 1984). Some studies use self-report questionnaires while others prefer to use interview methods. While self-report questionnaires may be adequate for assessing the respondent's subjective perception of the quality and availability of social support, it is rather more doubtful that they are able to assess the objective quality or availability of such support. To obtain accurate information on so complex a topic it may be necessary to use investigator-based interviews where the interviewer is able to make judgements and ratings on the basis of information obtained, and not simply accept the informant's view of the situation. Whatever form of assessment is used, there are also always issues about the reliability and validity of the measures used. In the area of social support, where so many different measures of support are used, this is of particular concern.

### Sampling issues and uniformity of results

The choice of samples is an important issue of method in relation to life events and depression. Depression is common in the general population and it may be that those who receive psychiatric treatment are not representative of the entire depressed population. Depression in the general population may be milder and different in quality from that experienced by those receiving psychiatric care (Sireling *et al.* 1985). One of the possible differences may be that milder depressions have a closer link with social stress (Bebbington *et al.* 1981). Thus conclusions as to factors linked to the onset and maintenance of depression may differ in different population groups.

For studies of life events the choice of a control group is also an important issue. Early studies compared the rate of events in psychiatric patients with medical and surgical patients. However, event rates may be raised in such physically ill subjects either by the occurrence of events which are consequences of illness or because events may be associated with the worsening of their medical condition and the need for hospitalization. It is therefore preferable that psychiatric patients are compared with normal controls, matched on factors such as age, gender, marital status and social class which are known to relate to the frequency of events. Comparisons between groups of patients with different psychiatric disorders are also necessary if the issue of the specificity of the effects of events in different disorders is to be explored.

There is a similar problem of choice of samples in the research aimed at understanding the role of social support in protecting individuals against disorder. Underlying the extensive research literature in this area there is an assumption that however social support functions to protect individuals against disorder, it does so in a uniform way. This uniformity is not only assumed across individuals, but also across different groups of individuals. Empirical studies have investigated support and its protective role in patient samples and community samples, in groups of women only and in mixed gender groups, and drawn conclusions on the basis of one particular group about the role of social support generally. Few studies have compared results obtained from different groups in an attempt to understand whether social support may play a different role in, for example, a patient sample as compared to a community sample. Recently, there has been some interest in gender differences in social support (Salokangas *et al.* 1988, Emmerson *et al.* 1989, Brugha *et al.* 1990). It may be that certain types of support are more significant for women than for men, or that the way social support exerts its protective function is totally different in men and women. Similar considerations apply also to social support in patient and community groups. There have been suggestions in the literature that social support may be more important in community groups in protecting individuals against the development of disorder than in patient groups. It is necessary therefore in evaluating empirical studies to be clear about the particular group under investigation and to be cautious when generalizing results to other groups of individuals on the assumption that support functions in a uniform manner across various groups.

### Causal inference

Events occur in the context of an individual's life and may well be the result rather than the precipitant of disorder. It is necessary therefore to establish that events are independent of subsequent disorder. This is done by careful dating of events and disorder as well as by ratings of independence (Brown & Harris 1978) of the event from the disorder.

The problem of independence is more acute when studying social support. Support is not a dateable event and occurs over a period of time. Many studies of social support are cross-sectional. They employ multivariate analyses of all variables as they interact at one point in time and therefore cannot provide information about the direction of causal influences or the influence of protective factors. Although data from cross-sectional studies are consistent with aetiological hypotheses, they cannot test these hypotheses. Clearly, at the very least, longitudinal data which incorporate measurements of key variables at two points in time are required in order to claim that poor social support together with adverse life events causes or maintains depressive disorder. Without such data, it would be impossible to rule out the possibility that the disorder brought about the poor social support and adverse life events. Although cross-sectional studies often take great care in dating onset of disorder and measuring life stress both independently of disorder and prior to it, the problems in employing a similar strategy for the measurement of social support are more severe. It is not easy to be certain that one is measuring support before onset of disorder and there are also all the well-known difficulties of retrospective reporting. In addition, measuring social support when the subject is depressed may result in a biased estimate of both current and previous social support as a result of the individual's present negative assessment of circumstances. This may be a particular problem when assessment is done by questionnaire. Despite these difficulties many studies do not attempt to assess social support at any time other than currently.

A further complicating issue about claims for

the aetiological role of social support is the debate about whether the role of social support is direct or indirect. Two different views have been proposed, and both have gained some support from the literature, although until recently there has been a paucity of longitudinal data on which to base conclusions. One view proposes that lack of social support only increases the risk of subsequent disorder in the face of adversity. Thus, the presence of support serves as a protective buffer between adverse life events and subsequent disorder. This is usually termed the buffer theory of social support, or the buffering hypothesis (Thoits 1982, Cohen & Wills 1985, Alloway & Bebbington 1987). The alternative view is that lack of social support increases the risk of disorder irrespective of the presence of other life stress (Aneshensel & Stone 1982, Cohen & Wills 1985). This claim about the direct role of social support has been termed the main effect hypothesis or model.

Difficulties of conceptual overlap which might arise when life events result in changes in social support, and changes in support alter the likelihood of the occurrence of life events, can only be overcome with longitudinal data. Independent measures of support, life events and disorder at various points in time are required. Only with such data is it possible to test various possible sources of causal influence and to test whether independently determined levels of social support persisting over time do indeed buffer against adverse life experiences or whether support directly influences subsequent disorder (see also Chapter 4).

## Data analysis

A much debated question in the literature, in particular that on the buffer theory of social support, has been the question of the appropriate statistical model which should be used to test for the hypothesized buffering effect. A detailed discussion of this issue is beyond the scope of this chapter. The term 'buffering effect' may be used to describe at least two kinds of interaction effect, a multiplicative interaction or an additive one.

Often it is assumed that interaction in this area is synonymous with a statistical interaction effect as determined by most traditional multivariate analyses. This effect is a multiplicative interaction which is the most extreme type of interaction whereby one variable multiplies the effect of the relationship between two other variables. There are however other forms of synergistic effects whereby one variable potentiates the effect of another, but the effect does not amount to multiplication. In such cases a variable adds to the strength of a relationship between two variables. This is called an additive interaction. Neither model of buffering is correct and Rutter (1983) has argued persuasively that the choice of a method of analysis should depend on the hypothesized mechanisms of interaction. Another strategy is to test both additive and multiplicative concepts of buffering, stating clearly the model one is testing (Paykel *et al.* 1980, Costello 1982, Solomon & Bromet 1982).

## Empirical studies

### Life events and onset of depression

Studies of life events and onset of depressive episodes have been particularly extensive. Table 7.1 summarizes findings of 27 published retrospective comparisons (one employing two comparison groups) of psychiatrically treated depressed patients with control groups. Sixteen studies, from the USA, England, Eire, Italy, Spain, Poland, The Netherlands, Kenya and India, employed general population controls, including two studies of elderly patients (Murphy 1982, Emmerson *et al.* 1989). All found more events reported prior to the onset of depression although in one study, with small numbers, the difference did not reach significance. Two studies compared depressed patients with medical patient controls, and found more events reported by depressed patients. The differences were not very striking and as already mentioned, it is difficult to interpret results using this kind of control group.

Comparisons of depressed patients and other psychiatric patients are also summarized in Table

**Table 7.1** Controlled comparisons of life events on onset of clinical depression

| Nature of controls | Author | Excess any events | Excess separations | Excess other types of events |
|---|---|---|---|---|
| *General population* | Paykel *et al.* 1969 | Yes | Yes | Various especially undesirable events |
| | Thompson & Hendrie 1972 | Yes | Not reported | More stress overall |
| | Cadoret *et al.* 1972 | Suggestive | Suggestive | Not reported |
| | Brown *et al.* 1973 | Yes | Not reported | Markedly and moderately threatening events |
| | Fava *et al.* 1981 | Yes | Yes | Undesirable, negative impact |
| | Vadher & Ndetei 1981 | Yes | Yes | Suggestive only |
| | Chatterjee *et al.* 1981 | Yes | Yes | Health, interpersonal |
| | Bebbington *et al.* 1981 | Yes, males only | Not reported | Events of severe and moderate threat |
| | Murphy 1982 | Yes | Suggestive | Health |
| | Billings *et al.* 1983 | Yes | Yes | Various negative events |
| | Faravelli & Ambonetti 1983 | Yes | Not reported | Undesirable, exit and severe |
| | Bidzinska 1984 | Yes | No | Marital and family conflicts, work overload, failures |
| | Roy *et al.* 1985 | Yes | No | Undesirable events |
| | Brugha & Conroy 1985 | Yes | Not reported | Undesirable, threatening. Not independent, uncontrolled |
| | Ezquiaga *et al.* 1987 | Yes | Not reported | Threatening, independent |
| | Emmerson *et al.* 1989 | Yes | Not reported | Severely threatening |
| | Cornelis *et al.* 1989 | Yes | No | Undesirable, higher stress |
| *Medical patients* | Forrest *et al.* 1965 | Yes, weak | No | Social factors |
| | Hudgens *et al.* 1967 | Yes, weak | No | Moves, interpersonal discord |
| *Other psychiatric patients* | *Schizophrenics* | | | |
| | Beck & Worthen 1972 | Yes | Suggestive | Events of higher rated hazard |
| | Brown *et al.* 1973 | Yes | Not reported | Events/moderate and marked threat over longer time |
| | Jacobs *et al.* 1974 | Yes | Yes | Undesirable, health financial interpersonal discord |
| | Leff & Vaughn 1980 | Suggestive | Not reported | Not for undesirable events |
| | *Suicide attempters* | | | |
| | Paykel *et al.* 1975 | Fewer events in depressives | No | Fewer events in depressives, especially undesirable, upsetting |
| | Slater & Depue 1981 | Fewer events in depressives | No Fewer exits | Fewer independent events |
| | Cohen-Sandler *et al.* 1982 | Fewer events in depressives | Fewer deaths, separations | Casenote study in children |
| | *Mixed psychiatric patients* | | | |
| | Sethi 1964 | Yes | Yes | Not reported |
| | Levi *et al.* 1966 | Yes | Yes | Not reported |
| | Malmquist 1970 | No | No | No |
| | Uhlenhuth & Paykel 1973 | No | No | No |

7.1. Depressed patients reported more events than schizophrenic patients in all but one study (Leff & Vaughn 1980) where differences for independent events were suggestive but not significant.

Comparisons between depressed patients and groups of mixed psychiatric patients have produced inconsistent results. Three comparisons of those who attempt suicide with depressed patients found more events in suicide attempters. Evidence from other studies comparing patient groups with general population controls confirms that the largest patient-control differences are for suicide attempts. Much smaller effects have been found for schizophrenia, and depression is intermediate between these two groups (Paykel & Cooper 1990).

Similar findings have been reported for children. Goodyer and colleagues have studied effects of life events in children attending a child psychiatry clinic (Goodyer *et al.* 1985, 1987). In comparison with community controls, children reported more events of severe negative impact in the 12 months before onset. These effects were apparent in four diagnostic groups: conduct disorder, severe mood disorder, mild mood disorder, and neurotic disorder. Marital and family and accident and illness events appeared to be more important for conduct disorder and mild mood disorder, and exit events for severe mood disorder. The effects extended across the full year, but tended to be more marked in the immediate preceding 16 weeks. In a further study in a new sample (Goodyer *et al.* 1990), events and poor friendships exerted independent effects and showed an additive interaction.

Epidemiological studies have also been used to study effects of life events. Since the literature on patient groups is extensive, the epidemiological literature will not be reviewed in detail. Among studies showing association of life events and minor psychiatric disorder are those of Myers *et al.* (1971), Dohrenwend (1973a,b), Uhlenhuth *et al.* (1974) and Bebbington *et al.* (1988). The major studies by Brown and colleagues, which have also predominantly been based on community samples, will be discussed further in later sections.

## SPECIFICITY OF LIFE EVENTS

As can be seen from Table 7.1, life events play some role in the onset of disorder other than depression. Life events as such are not therefore specific to depression. However, it is possible that certain types of life event are most likely to lead to depression. Most prominent in the literature is the role of loss. The concept of loss is somewhat loosely defined, often including interpersonal separations and deaths, loss of self-esteem, and loss of valued ideas.

Interpersonal losses of various kinds have received the most study. Findings from the studies are summarized in Table 7.1. Twenty-one studies have reported specifically on recent separations. In 11, depressed patients reported more separations than general population controls and than other psychiatric patient controls. There was, however, no excess of separations as compared to medical patients. Two studies not only found exit events related to depression but also found that their converse, entrance events, were not (Paykel *et al.* 1969, Fava *et al.* 1981). However, one study (Slater & Depue 1981) found that primary depressed patients making a suicide attempt had experienced more exits than those that did not, indicating that the relationship between exit events and suicide attempts might be stronger than that between exit events and depression. As can be seen from Table 7.1, a wide variety of events is involved in depression. In general the studies produce only weak evidence for a specific link between event types and depression. There is some relationship between depression and interpersonal losses, but these also precede other disorders, and many depressions are not preceded by them. The strongest relationship between events and depression appears when events are categorized in rather broad terms such as 'threatening' or undesirable. However, this covers a wide range of events.

Brown and colleagues in recent studies of women in the community have attempted to refine their definitions of 'threatening' or severe events in a way that will greatly increase the size of the association between the events so defined and subsequent depression. In a prospective study Brown *et al.* (1987) found that by taking into account various ways in which an event can 'match' the characteristics of an individual present before the occurrence of the event or the onset of depression, the association between events and depression can be strengthened by at least a factor of three.

Studies of specific events and depression produced differing results. Studies of hysterectomy and childbirth indicate that these events in themselves do not appear to lead to the onset of depression (Paykel *et al.* 1980, Gath *et al.* 1982, O'Hara *et al.* 1984, Cooper & Stein 1989). Recent loss of a parent, particularly of the opposite sex to the patient, is more frequent in depressed patients than in a control population (Birtchnell 1975).

## Life events and specific symptom patterns

The discussion so far suggests that there is a rather weak relationship between specific classes of life event and depression, although the work by George Brown on matching suggests that further detailed description of events may strengthen the association between events and depression. Another way in which the specificity of the association between events and depression might be explored is to examine whether events are particularly related to specific symptom patterns in depression. A proportion of depressive episodes, perhaps about 20% in the controlled studies, are not preceded by life events. It has been claimed that these episodes are endogenous in terms of symptom pattern, and that it is episodes with more endogenous or psychotic features which are not preceded by life events.

Several recent studies using careful life event methods have shown that life events and symptom pattern are only weakly related. Paykel (1974) reported a study in which symptoms were rated by one rater and life event information collected blind by another. Absence of life stress showed only a low correlation, although in the predicted direction, with endogenous symptoms. In a subsequent study (Paykel 1979) using a more crude clinical judgement as to whether the depression was precipitated, there was no relationship with symptom pattern. In a third study (Paykel *et al.*

1984) the relationship between life stress, obtained at systematic interview, and symptom pattern, rated independently, was examined in a sample of depressed outpatients. Again, only a very weak relationship between symptom pattern and life stress was found.

Brown *et al.* (1979) in one of the early event studies found that depressed patients characterized as psychotic or neurotic on the basis of their symptoms showed only a very small difference in the proportions whose illnesses had been preceded by a severe event or major difficulty. When the depressions were divided into those with and without such an event or difficulty relatively few individual symptoms distinguished the groups. Benjaminsen (1981) compared neurotic and non-neurotic depressed patients and found that almost equal proportions had experienced a stressful event. Katschnig & Berner (1984) obtained similar findings, as did Monroe *et al.* (1985). Matussek & Neuner (1981), using a lengthy and probing interview, found differences between neurotic and endogenous depression only for separations from an important partner. Dolan *et al.* (1985) found antecedent life events associated with more severe illness but not with any less evidence of endogenous symptoms. Brugha & Conroy (1985) found greater patient-control life event differences for CATEGO R (retarded or endogenous) depressed patients than for CATEGO N (neurotic) patients. Bebbington *et al.* (1981) in a small study did find fewer life events in patients with an endogenous symptom pattern, but found little evidence of this in a larger sample (Bebbington *et al.* 1988). However in this sample Brugha *et al.* (1987) found that, although neurotic and endogenous depressed patients did not differ in social network and social support, absence of support was more strongly related to poor outcome at four months in the former than the latter. Roy *et al.* (1985) compared the frequency of life events in endogenous and neurotic depressed patients, and a third group of normal controls who were matched on age and sex. When the depressed group were taken together and compared with the control group, those who were depressed showed more life events than controls. A further analysis looked at the subcategories of the depressed group and found that the neurotic group had significantly more life events than the endogenous group and were responsible for the excess over the controls.

Overall it would appear that life events bear only a weak relationship to symptom pattern, and that the latter is predominantly determined by some other mechanism.

Events concurrent with treatment might be expected to have greater effects on outcome than those occurring prior to onset. In the study cited earlier, Lloyd *et al.* (1981) found that patients who had a poor outcome after four weeks were more likely to have experienced undesirable events, physical illnesses, illnesses in family members, and events outside the patient's control in that period. Rowan *et al.* (1982) found that events occurring during a six-week treatment period had no significant effect on outcome, but few major independent events occurred. Tennant *et al.* (1981), in a study of community cases, found that remission was more likely over a one-month period if a 'neutralizing' event had taken place. They defined a neutralizing event as one which caused minimal threat, but which counteracted the effect of an earlier threatening event or chronic difficulty.

Three studies have examined concurrent events over follow-up periods of between three and nine months. The first (Surtees 1980) used a mixed sample of depressed patients and found that greater event stress was associated with worse outcome. The second (Paykel & Tanner 1976) examined relapse. The patients were women who had responded to amitriptyline and were then either continued on or withdrawn from medication. Life events were assessed concurrently and relapse was found to be associated with undesirable life events in the previous three months. These relapses appeared to be separate from those related to drug withdrawal. Monroe *et al.* (1985) failed to find outcome influenced by concurrent events.

Among longer-term follow-up studies in patients Murphy (1983) and Giel *et al.* (1978) both found worse outcome where threatening events had occurred. In women in the community Brown *et al.* (1988) found recovery from chronic

depression preceded by reduction in ongoing difficulties and occurrence of events, implying a fresh start towards a better future. In a seven-year follow-up Wittchen (1987) found events, and particularly loss events, over the whole period excluding the last year to predict worse outcome. However, in a 12-month follow-up of a small sample of patients on maintenance therapy Mendlewicz *et al.* (1986) found no overall effect of life events on relapse, although there was a non-significant association with bereavement.

The picture emerging from these studies is that life events at onset do not greatly effect outcome, although there is a weak trend to better outcome where there have been antecedent events. However, where events occur concurrently with treatment, negative events lead to worse outcome, and neutralizing or fresh start events to better outcome.

### Prospective studies and magnitude of effect

The effects of life events may be examined in a prospective study in which all subjects undergoing a specific event are followed up. This is an excellent strategy for examining the proportions of subjects affected adversely by an event, and also the effects of modifying factors. Among a number of events which have been studied in this manner are bereavement, loss of employment (Kasl *et al.* 1975), mastectomy (Maguire *et al.* 1978) and effects of other physical illnesses. Such studies indicate that, while many subjects undergo considerable distress, relatively few develop overt clinical depression and even fewer seek psychiatric help. Clayton's studies of bereavement are instructive. Among 40 bereaved subjects followed (Clayton *et al.* 1968), the majority developed depressed mood, sleep disturbance and crying, but ideas of guilt and suicidal thoughts were uncommon. Although 25% consulted a physician for symptoms related to grief, only one subject saw a psychiatrist. In a second study of a new sample, 35% showed symptoms of depression after one month, 17% after a year, but none saw a psychiatrist (Bornstein *et al.* 1973).

Prospective studies form a useful balance to

case-control studies, which ignore base rates for events and disorder in the general population. The majority of events experienced by depressed patients, although stressful, are not of catastrophic magnitude. They are not uncommon in the general population and are often experienced without overt disorder following.

There have been several attempts to quantify the extent to which life events cause depression. Brown *et al.* (1973) used the concept of 'brought forward time': an estimate of the average time from an onset brought about by an event to the time a spontaneous onset would have occurred if no event were present. They concluded that the effect was large in magnitude and formative for depression but smaller and only triggering for schizophrenia.

Paykel (1978) used an epidemiological measure, the relative risk. This is the ratio of the rate of disease among those exposed to a putative causal factor to the rate among those not exposed. It can be applied to the control studies using as an approximation relative odds. When this was applied to some published studies, it was found that the risk of developing depression in the six months after the most stressful classes of events was approximately 6:1, falling off rapidly with time after the event. The relative risks for schizophrenia were much lower at only two to three over six months, but for suicide attempts they were higher.

Cooke (1987) has used an alternative epidemiological measure, the population attributable risk, expressed as a percentage. This is an estimate of the proportion of disorder caused by life events, and is most easily applied to epidemiological general population studies. Applying this to a number of published studies of depression he obtained values ranging from 29% to 69% and in general around 40%.

Relative and attributable risks of this magnitude indicate effects which are important, but not exclusive. They suggest disorders with multifactorial causation, in which any single factor may account for only a relatively small proportion of the variance. Although events are important, a large part in determining whether an event is followed by disorder must be attributed to other modifying factors. There may be a whole host of these, both genetic and environmental.

## Social support and depression

### CROSS-SECTIONAL STUDIES

There is a fairly extensive literature relating psychiatric disorder to lack of social support. Table 7.2 provides a brief summary of 24 recent cross-sectional studies of social support. As can be seen, life stress and life events are usually measured together with social support. Only eight studies do not formally assess life stress or life events at the same time as measuring social support. Some of these studies have made use of a naturally occurring stressful event such as unemployment, retirement, or the nuclear accident at Three Mile Island (see Solomon & Bromet 1982, Ullah *et al.* 1985, Salokangas *et al.* 1988). Most of the studies investigated social support in community samples, although there are a number of studies which have investigated these issues in patient samples (e.g. Brugha *et al.* 1982, Murphy 1982, Emmerson *et al.* 1989). The samples investigated were mainly of mixed gender, although a number of studies have confined their samples to women (e.g. Brown & Harris 1978, Brown & Prudo 1981, Solomon & Bromet 1982, Campbell 1983). Only two studies (Andrews *et al.* 1978, Lin *et al.* 1979) investigated the dependent variable, mental state or psychological functioning, by questionnaire only, and most studies used a semi-structured interview, in particular the Present State Examination (PSE). Other studies required subjects to meet well recognized diagnostic criteria such as DSM-III or Research Diagnostic Criteria (RDC) without specifying exactly what form the interview took (Hallstrom 1986, Emmerson *et al.* 1989).

Measures of social support varied rather more than the measurement of mental state, although approximately half the studies measured intimacy of some form or other, while others measured degree of social integration (Brown & Prudo 1981), community participation (Andrews *et al.* 1978, Lin *et al.* 1979), size of social network (Aneshensel & Stone 1982, Brugha *et al.* 1982), and availability of good friends (Birtchnell 1988).

The range of different kinds of support measured clearly reflects the variety of different conceptions of social support in the literature. It is also apparent from these studies that not only are different aspects of social support being measured in different studies, but also that a variety of assessment techniques are being used to measure it. In this regard, the study of Vaughn & Leff (1976) deserves particular mention in regard to what is being measured as social support. This study assessed Expressed Emotion rather than social support. However, inasmuch as expressed emotion is an assessment of the quality of close family relationships, it can be regarded as a special case of a measure of intimacy. In the study of depression in particular, Expressed Emotion is generally assessed between spouses and its main component is the number of critical comments made about the ill relative. Thus it can be regarded as one means of measuring the quality of intimate relationships. Although the main component of the Expressed Emotion construct is critical comments and indeed it is this that has been related to relapse, warmth and positive remarks are also measured.

Studies rarely measured a range of different aspects of social support within one study, and thus do not reflect the multidimensional nature of support. A few studies (e.g. Ullah *et al.* 1985, Parry & Shapiro 1986) did explicitly attempt to measure a range of aspects of social support such as instrumental support, expressive support, social contacts and intimacy as part of one study. Only three studies (Andrews *et al.* 1978, Flaherty *et al.* 1983, Merikangas *et al.* 1985) measured social support solely by questionnaire. The issue of whether studies measured perceived or objective support is not so clear. Although most studies employed interviews, many do not state explicitly whether they were measuring perceived support or objective support, nor indeed what measures were taken to establish whether the information obtained could be regarded as objective.

Only six studies (Henderson *et al.* 1978, Leff & Vaughn 1980, Brugha *et al.* 1982, Roy & Kennedy 1984, Merikangas *et al.* 1985, Friedman *et al.* 1988) specified precisely the time period over which social support was being measured, and

in all but two studies (Roy & Kennedy 1984, Merikangas *et al.* 1985) this period was more or less contemporaneous with the time of the assessment of mental state. More importantly, no attempt was made to establish the temporal relationships between social support and the onset of depression. One study assessed social support a year before the onset of depression (Roy & Kennedy 1984) and one assessed it after recovery from an acute episode (Merikangas *et al.* 1985). As a result, it is not clear whether the level of social support found in most of these studies is a function of current mental state, a result of previous life stress, a pre-existing vulnerability factor, or indeed a causal factor in its own right.

The results of these cross-sectional studies discussed above are also briefly summarized in Table 7.2. In attempting to draw conclusions from these studies, caution is needed both because the studies are cross-sectional in nature and because there are numerous other methodological problems. On a very general level, there is clearly an association between lack of social support broadly defined and psychological distress or disorder. This relationship appears to hold in both community and patient samples and in both mixed gender groups and groups of women only. Only two studies which investigated mixed gender samples reported specific gender differences. In the study by Salokangas *et al.* (1988) the well-documented findings for the importance of intimate relationships held across gender as in other studies. However, the significance of having a close friend seemed to depend on gender. It was associated with a less than average symptom level in men who were not married, while it was associated with a high level of symptoms in women. The authors interpret this as women having the ability to retain close friends despite psychiatric difficulties. A recent study by Emmerson *et al.* (1989) challenges the widespread finding of an association between lack of intimacy and depression in both men and women. In this study, the lack of a confiding relationship was associated with depression in men only, but not women. The evidence for lack of support as an aetiological factor is unclear from these studies and indeed it would be difficult to establish in cross-sectional studies of

**Table 7.2** Cross-sectional studies of social support and disorder

| Authors | No. | Sex | Dependent variable | Quest/interview | Social support measure content | Quest/interview | Time period | Life events | Result |
|---|---|---|---|---|---|---|---|---|---|
| *Community samples* | | | | | | | | | |
| Andrews et al. 1978 | 863 | Mixed | GHQ | Q | Postal survey Crisis support Neighbourhood interaction Community participation | Q | Not specified | Questionnaire 2–13 months prior to survey | Relationship between social support and impairment independent of life event stress |
| Brown & Harris 1978 | 458 | Women | Judgement of caseness based on PSE | I | LEDS Intimacy | I | 12 months prior to onset? – not specified | LEDS year before interview | Lack of social support, increased vulnerability to disorder in presence of life events |
| Lin et al. 1979 | 170 | Mixed | Self-report symptom scale | Q | Scale of interaction and involvement with neighbours and community and social adjustment | I | Not specified | Holmes & Rahe scale 6 months prior to interview | Relationship between events and illness and between social support and absence of illness – no interaction or buffering |
| Paykel et al. 1980 | 120 | Women postpartum | Clinical interview for depression | I | Support from husband | I | Not specified | Interview for recent life events prior 10½ months | Poor support vulnerability factor in presence of stressful life event |
| Brown & Prudo 1981 | 335 | Women | Judgement of caseness based on PSE | I | LEDS – intimacy Social integration | I | 12 months prior to onset? | LEDS 12 months prior to interview | Provoking agent plus lack of intimacy, 3 children <14 and regular churchgoing increase risk of depression |
| Solomon & Bromet 1982 | 435 | Women | Mental state RDC for depression and anxiety SADS | I | Social network interview – intimacy | I | Not specified | Three Mile Island incident and life event scale 12 months prior to interview | No confidant associated with increased affective disorder in those who had experienced stress |

| Aneshensel & Stone 1982 | 1000 | Mixed | Current depressive symptomatology, especially depressed mood | 1 | Number of close relationships, perceived social support | 1 | Not specified | Life events in past year, perceived strain | Life events and strain associated with depression. Close relationships and perceived support negatively related to depression. Effects direct – no interaction |
| Costello 1982 | 449 | Women | PSE Mental state | 1 | LEDS – intimacy | 1 | Not specified | LEDS 12 months prior to interview | Lack of intimacy increased risk of depression. Severe events and difficulties associated with depression. No interactions |
| Campbell et al. 1983 | 110 | Women | Mental state PSE | 1 | LEDS – intimacy | 1 | Not specified | LEDS 12 months prior to interview | Lack of confiding relationship increased risk of disorder in face of provoking agent |
| Ullah et al. 1985 | 1150 | Mixed 17 year olds | GHQ Zung scale depression and anxiety | 1 | Support – information, emotional, instrumental, social contacts | 1 | Not specified | Not assessed but all subjects unemployed | Only lack of instrumental support associated with psychological distress. Only partial support for stress buffering |
| Bebbington et al. 1984 | 310 | Mixed | Mental state PSE | 1 | LEDS – intimacy | 1 | Not specified | LEDS 10 months before onset or interview | Lack of confidant associated with disorder. No confirmation for vulnerability model. No interaction with events |

*continued on p. 112*

**Table 7.2** (*continued*)

| Authors | No. | Sex | Dependent variable | Quest/interview | Social support measure content | Quest/interview | Time period | Life events | Result |
|---|---|---|---|---|---|---|---|---|---|
| Hallstrom 1986 | 800 | Women | Mental state DSM-III | I | Intimacy – assumed not present in never married, divorced, widowed, as well as those who reported lack of intimacy | I | No period specified | Interview covering 10 defined stressors 1 year prior to onset | Lack of intimacy increased risk of depression without provoking agent |
| Parry & Shapiro 1986 | 193 | Women | Mental state PSE | I | Instrumental support Expressive support Intimacy | I | Some aspects 7 days prior to interview | LEDS 12 months prior to interview | Life events and support have independent effects on distress. No interactions |
| Friedman et al. 1988 | 4913 | Mixed | Major depressive disorder – DIS | I | Social contacts Social activities Satisfaction with work | I | 2 weeks prior to interview | Not assessed | Poorer intimate relationships for those currently depressed vs. past disorder, other disorder and no disorder |
| Salokangas et al. 1988 | 389 | Mixed | GHQ | Q & I | Married intimate vs. married non-intimate vs. unmarried non-intimate | I | Not specified | Not formally assessed: about to retire or retired | Married intimate > non-married intimate > non-intimate in terms of lack of depressive symptoms gender differences |
| Birtchnell 1988 | 50 | Women | Mental state PSE | I | Social integration Presence of close friend | I | Not specified | Not assessed | Those with fewer friends had higher scores on PSE |
| *Patient samples* | | | | | | | | | |
| Henderson et al. 1978 | 50 | Mixed | GHQ PSE | I | Interview Schedule for Social Interaction | I | Week prior to interview | Life events schedule | Patients had fewer good friends and fewer contacts outside home than controls. No difference in life events |
| Leff & Vaughn 1980 | 30 | Mixed | Mental state PSE | I | CFI Expressed Emotion – measure of criticism of close relative usually spouse | I | Present level of EE | Brown & Birley schedule 3 months prior to onset | Combination of threatening life event and high EE more susceptible to depression |

| Study | n | Sample | Depression measure | | Social support/marital measure | | Timing | Life events | Findings |
|---|---|---|---|---|---|---|---|---|---|
| Murphy 1982 | 119 | Mixed (168 controls) | PSE Mental state | I | LEDS – intimacy | I | Not specified 12 months prior to onset | LEDS 12 months prior to onset or prior to interview | Severe event without intimacy increased risk of depression |
| Brugha et al. 1982 | 50 | Mixed | PSE Mental state | I | Interview Schedule for Social Interaction Size of network Number of social contacts, quality of social interactions | I | Past week | Not assessed | Patients had less contacts, close relatives, good friends than controls |
| Flaherty et al. 1983 | 44 | Mixed | HRSD SAS – self-report marital familial functioning | I | Social support network – support received from five closest members | Q | Not specified | Schedule of recent events for last year | Patients with high social support scores on HRSD. No effect for life events |
| Roy & Kennedy 1984 | 72 | Mixed | GHQ – short psychiatric interview | Q & I | Marital interview (Quinton) | I | Year before onset of depression | Not assessed | Lack of good marital relationship associated with depression |
| Merikangas et al. 1985 | 45 | Mixed | RDC for major depression | I | Self-report marital questionnaire | Q | Measured after recovery from acute episode | Not measured | Marriages of depressed patients worse in all areas than controls |
| Emmerson et al. 1989 | 186 Depressed patients, n = 101 Community residents n = 85 Mixed | | DSM-II at least 4 weeks | I | ISSI and LEDS modified intimacy | I | Not specified 12 months prior to onset? | LEDS 12 months prior to onset | Lack of confiding relationship associated with depression in men but not women. No association of life events with depression |

Abbreviations: CFI, Camberwell Family Interview; DIS, Diagnostic Interview Schedule; GHQ, General Health Questionnaire; HRSD, Hamilton Rating Scale for Depression; LEDS, Life Events and Difficulties Schedule; PSE, Present State Examination; RDC, Research Diagnostic Criteria; SADS, Schedule for Affective Disorders and Schizophrenia; SAS, Social Adjustment Scale; ISSI, Interview for Social Interaction.

this kind. The majority of studies do not support the stress-buffering view of social support but found independent effects for social support (Andrews *et al.* 1978, Henderson *et al.* 1978, Lin *et al.* 1979, Aneshensel & Stone 1982, Flaherty *et al.* 1983, Bebbington *et al.* 1984, Hallstrom 1986, Parry & Shapiro 1986, Emmerson *et al.* 1989). On the other hand at least seven studies produced support for some form of the Brown and Harris vulnerability model (Brown & Harris 1978, Paykel *et al.* 1980, Leff & Vaughn 1980, Brown & Prudo 1981, Murphy 1982, Solomon & Bromet 1982, Campbell *et al.* 1983). However, these conclusions must be seen in the light of the limitations of methodology discussed earlier and it must be borne in mind that the majority of studies did not test both multiplicative and additive models of interaction.

LONGITUDINAL STUDIES

There are far fewer longitudinal studies than cross-sectional studies of social support. These studies also suffer from many of the problems of method noted in the previous sections. The studies fall into two categories: those that attempt to relate social support at the time of distress or disorder to subsequent outcome (e.g. Waring & Patton 1984, Miller *et al.* 1987, George *et al.* 1989, Brugha *et al.* 1990) and those which attempt to measure social support prior to onset and investigate its subsequent role in onset (Henderson 1981, Bolton & Oatley 1987, Brown *et al.* 1986). Studies in the first category are studies of maintenance rather than onset and it cannot necessarily be inferred that a variable which plays a significant role in maintenance will also be important in onset.

As can be seen from Table 7.3, the longitudinal studies divide almost equally between community studies and patient studies. In general, in both community and patient samples, various forms of lack of social support while individuals are depressed predict subsequent poor outcome. In all, nine such studies are listed in Table 7.3. The research strategy in the majority of these studies has been to attempt to identify those aspects of social support at the time when the individual is

depressed which predict the subsequent outcome of the depression. While this strategy allows the identification of factors which may predict persistence, remission, recovery, or relapse of disorder, it does not necessarily elucidate factors that produce onset. Thus the finding that poor social support is associated with worse outcome, is consistent with poor support producing and contributing to depression as well as depression producing poor support and further subsequent depression. It also cannot be assumed that maintaining factors are those involved in onset.

Only three studies (Henderson 1981, Brown *et al.* 1986, Bolton & Oatley 1987) are truly prospective in that they identify deficiencies in social support prior to the onset of disorder which is then related to subsequent disorder. Two of these (Brown *et al.* 1986, Bolton & Oatley 1987) support a buffering or interactive view of social support, while the third provides some evidence for the direct effects of social support. In all three cases, the samples studied were drawn from the community.

Brown *et al.* (1986) carried out a large prospective study of 400 largely working class women with children living at home. Social support was assessed in order to predict the risk of depression in the following year once a stressor had occurred. Actual support at the time of a crisis was also measured. Lack of support from a core tie (husband, lover or very close friend) was associated with an increased risk of subsequent depression once a stressor had occurred, as was lack of support at the time of the crisis.

Bolton & Oatley (1987) reported on a six- to eight-month follow-up of 49 unemployed men and a matched control group who were employed. They found that depression scores at follow-up were higher for those who remained unemployed and who had had little social contact before losing their jobs.

Henderson (1981) in a large prospective study found that deficiencies in social relationships, both perceived and actual, predicted neurotic symptoms four months later.

These studies do not however provide strong support for the role of social support as usually conceived. The Henderson study found the

**Table 7.3** Longitudinal studies of social support and disorder

| Authors | No. | Sex | Dependent variable | Quest/ interview | Social support measure content | Quest/ interview | Life events | Assessment points | Result |
|---|---|---|---|---|---|---|---|---|---|
| *Community samples* | | | | | | | | | |
| Myers *et al.* 1975, Eaton 1978 (reanalysis) | 720 | Mixed | Psychiatric disorder Gurin index | I | Not clearly specified Social integration | I | Life crises not clearly specified | Initial 2-year follow-up | Those with high symptom levels and few life events were less integrated in community than few symptoms and many life events |
| Henderson 1981 | 323 | Mixed | GHQ – 30 item | Q | ISSI Close bonds and diffuse ties | I | List of recent experiences interview for adverse events | Four waves at 4-month intervals | Deficiencies in personal relationships and perceived inadequacy associated with development of neurotic symptoms under adversity |
| Blazer 1983 | 331 | Mixed | 18-item depression scale | Q | Duke questionnaire | Q | Not assessed | Initial assessment; 30-month follow-up | Depression at time I associated with improvement of social support at time II |
| Parker & Blignault 1985 | 66 | Mixed | Zung depression scale PSE | Q & I | Social relationships; intimacy | I | LEDS | Initial assessment; 6 week follow-up; 20-weeks follow-up | Improvement at 6 and 20 weeks predicted by break up of intimate relationship in preceding 12 months |
| Brown *et al.* 1986 | 400 | Women | Caseness based on PSE | I | Intimacy SESS | I | LEDS | Initial assessment; 1-year follow-up | Negative evaluation of self and other indices of lack of support from a core tie at first interview were associated with increased risk of subsequent depression once a stressor occurred. Lack of support from core tie at time of crisis particularly highly associated with increased risk |
| Miller *et al.* 1987 | 415 | Women | Psychiatric assessment schedule | I | Social support interview | I | LEDS | Initial assessment; 6-month follow-up; 1-year follow-up | Impaired relationships went with continuing illness |

*continued on p. 116*

Table 7.3 *(continued)*

| Authors | No. | Sex | Dependent variable | Quest/ interview | Social support measure content | Quest/ interview | Life events | Assessment points | Result |
|---|---|---|---|---|---|---|---|---|---|
| Bolton & Oatley 1987 | 49 unemployed | Men | BDI | Q | Semi-structured interview Quantity of social interaction, emotional support, material assistance, evenings out | I | Recent unemployment Social Readjustment Rating Scale | Initial assessment; 6–8-month follow-up | Depression scores at follow-up higher for those who remained unemployed and who had little social contact prior to being unemployed |
| *Patient samples* | | | | | | | | | |
| Vaughn & Leff 1976 | 32 | Depressed Mixed | Relapse of depression PSE | I | Level of critical comments of relative, usually spouse | I | Not assessed | EE measured at index episode | Level of EE in key relative at index episode predicted subsequent relapse of depression |
| Surtees 1980 | 80 | Depressed Mixed | HRSD semi-structured version | I | Support – close and diffuse | I | LEDS | Index episode; 28-week follow-up | Social support conferred partial immunity against recurrence of symptoms |
| Waring & Patton 1984 | 75 | Depressed Mixed | BDI GHQ | Q | Waring intimacy questionnaire | Q | Not assessed | Index episode; 1-month follow-up | Patients with lowest levels of intimacy failed to improve at 1-month follow-up |
| Billings & Moos 1985 | 424 | Depressed Mixed | Depression severity on rating scale: employment, self-esteem, etc. | Q by postal survey | Supportive aspects of family, social resources, stress at work, number of friends, network contacts and close relationships | Q | Life stress by questionnaire | At treatment intake; 12-month follow-up | Life stress and social resources related to functioning at follow-up |
| George et al. 1989 | 150 | Depressed Mixed | CES-D Depression Scale | I | Duke social support index | I | 19-item life event checklist | Index episode 6–32 months later | Size of network and subjective social support predictors of depressive symptoms at follow-up |
| Brugha et al. 1990 | 130 | Depressed Mixed | PSE | I | IMSR – social network and support contacts and quality | I | Adversity measure | Index episode 4-month-follow-up | Recovery associated with social support gender differences |

Abbreviations (refer to notes to Table 7.2): BDI, Beck Depression Inventory; CES-D, Centre for Epidemiologic Studies Depression Scale; IMSR, Interview Measure of Social Relationships; SESS, Self Evaluation and Social Support.

strongest relationships for perceived support rather than objective support and subsequent onset, while the Brown study found the strongest relationship between support in a crisis, retrospectively assessed and subsequent onset. Thus, only the Bolton & Oatley study provides unequivocal support for social support as a predictor of subsequent disorder.

In general, these longitudinal studies have investigated a range of different concepts of social support measured in a variety of ways. Most studies have investigated intimacy or close support in some form but other dimensions of support such as social integration and expressed emotion have also been assessed.

Almost all of the longitudinal studies are of mixed gender groups, with only two studies investigating women exclusively (Brown *et al.* 1986, Miller *et al.* 1987). While all other studies were of mixed gender groups, only one (Brugha *et al.* 1990) reports gender differences. In this study, the association between personal relationships and recovery varied with gender. In women the significant predictor of recovery appeared to be the number of primary group members named and contacted and satisfaction with social support. In men, on the other hand, negative social interaction with members of the primary group and living as married were associated with recovery.

Conclusions for these longitudinal studies must be cautiously drawn. Studies vary in their definition of social support, their methods of assessing it and the precise timing of these assessments. They vary too in the way the dependent variable, the individual's psychological or mental state, is assessed.

Although precise conclusions are difficult to draw, the results of these studies generally support the view that social support at the time of disorder is related to subsequent course. There is also some suggestion that social support may be independent of disorder and a causal factor in its precipitation. The evidence for a buffering view of social support as opposed to a direct effects view is even less conclusive, and the issue of the exact role of social support in depressive disorder remains an open one.

## Future directions

It is worth considering briefly the requirements for future studies so that they might avoid some of the problems of method of the studies reviewed. Psychiatric status should be established by a standard interview in which well-defined symptoms are assessed. Symptoms elicited thus can be used both to provide a continuous measure of mental state as well as to define a given level of severity as a 'case' of psychiatric disorder. Onset of disorder should be rated as accurately as possible. Social support should be clearly defined and a valid and reliable interview method of assessing it should be used. The next crucial requirement of any future study is that it is designed in a way such that the role of social support in the onset and maintenance of disorder can be assessed. Testing whether the role of social support is direct or stress buffering requires the accurate assessment and dating of life events. In order to establish the exact role of support in onset and maintenance of disorder, careful attention must be paid to the timing of the assessment of support. To test an onset theory, social support should be assessed independently of disorder and prior to its onset. It may be possible to achieve this using retrospective assessment techniques, but ideally a prospective study along the lines reported by Brown *et al.* (1986) should be undertaken. Frequent serial assessments of support and disorder would allow changes in support to be related to onset and subsequent maintenance of disorder. With further evidence about the relationships between support and disorder it might even be possible to design an intervention study to assess whether by changing levels of support, subsequent disorder may be prevented or at least made less severe. Such a study would provide an experimental method of testing the aetiological role of social support as well as assessing the efficacy of an approach to treatment.

In addition to the detailed requirements for future studies, it is also worth considering briefly the future general directions of the field. The relationship between life events and depression is now well established both in patient and general population groups. Life events precede and appear to contribute to a substantial proportion of depressions. They do not however precede all depressions, nor do they occur only in depression. Clearly, therefore, life events are only one of many factors involved in an individual becoming depressed. There is also clearly an association between lack of social support and depression in both patient and community samples. Whether lack of support or poor support precedes depression and contributes to its onset is less clear. In some studies social support has been shown to have direct effects on depression while in others only indirect stress buffering effects have been found. As yet, this issue of the role of social support also remains unresolved, but it may be that social support can have both effects depending on particular circumstances. Life events together with social support as either an independent contributor to depression or as a vulnerability factor will still not provide a complete account of the onset of depression. There are clearly many other factors, such as cognitive, personality and biological vulnerabilities, which also contribute to the onset of depression. The challenge to future research is to understand how these factors interact with each other in the onset of depression. In particular, an understanding of the relationship between psychological and social factors and biological factors is required.

## References

Alloway R. & Bebbington P.E. (1987) The buffer theory of social support: a review of the literature. *Psychological Medicine* 17, 91–108.

Andrews G., Tennant C., Hewson D. & Schonell M. (1978) The relation of social factors to physical and psychiatric illness. *American Journal of Epidemiology* 108, 27–35.

Aneshensel C.S. & Stone J.D. (1982) Stress and depression: a test of the buffering model of social support. *Archives of General Psychiatry* 39, 1392–1396.

Bebbington P.E., Hurry J. & Tennant C. (1988) Adversity and the symptoms of depression. *International Journal of Social Psychiatry* 34, 163–171.

Bebbington P.E., Sturt E., Tennant C. & Hurry J. (1984) Misfortune and resilience: a replication of the work of Brown and Harris. *Psychological Medicine* 14, 347–363.

Bebbington P.E., Tennant C. & Hurry J. (1981) Adversity and the nature of psychiatric disorder in the community. *Journal of Affective Disorders* 3, 345–366.

Beck J.C. & Worthen K. (1972) Precipitating stress, crisis theory and hospitalization in schizophrenia and depression. *Archives of General Psychiatry* 26, 123–129.

Benjaminsen S. (1981) Stressful life events preceding the onset of neurotic depression. *Psychological Medicine* 11, 369–378.

Bidzinska E.J. (1984) Stress factors in affective diseases. *British Journal of Psychiatry* 144, 161–166.

Billings A.G., Cronkite R.C. & Moos R.H. (1983) Social-environment factors in unipolar depression: comparisons of depressed patients and nondepressed controls. *Journal of Abnormal Psychology* 92, 119–133.

Billings A. & Moos R.H. (1985) Psychosocial processes of remission in unipolar depression: comparing depressed patients with matched community controls. *Journal of Consulting and Clinical Psychology* 53, 314–325.

Birtchnell J. (1975) Psychiatric breakdown following recent parent death. *British Journal of Medical Psychology* 48, 379–390.

Birtchnell J. (1988) Depression and life circumstances: a study of young, married women on a London housing estate. *Social Psychiatry and Psychiatric Epidemiology* 23, 240–246.

Blazer D.G. (1983) Impact of late-life depression on the social network. *American Journal of Psychiatry* 140, 162–166.

Bolton W. & Oatley K. (1987) A longitudinal study of social support and depression in unemployed men. *Psychological Medicine* 17, 453–460.

Bornstein P.E., Clayton P.J., Halikas J.A., Maurice W.L. & Robins E. (1973) The depression of widowhood after thirteen months. *British Journal of Psychiatry* 122, 561–566.

Brown G.W., Adler Z. & Bifulco A. (1988) Life events, difficulties and recovery from chronic depression. *British Journal of Psychiatry* 152, 487–498.

Brown G.W., Andrews B., Harris T., Adler Z. & Bridge L. (1986) Social support, self-esteem and depression. *Psychological Medicine* 16, 813–831.

Brown G.W., Bhrolchain N.I.M. & Harris T.O. (1979) Psychotic and neurotic depression. Part 3. Aetiological and background factors. *Journal of Affective Disorders* 1, 195–211.

Brown G.W., Bifulco A. & Harris T.O. (1987) Life events, vulnerability and onset of depression. *British Journal of Psychiatry* 150, 30–42.

Brown G.W. & Harris T. (1978) *The Social Origins of Depression: A Study of Psychiatric Disorder in Women.* Tavistock, London.

Brown G.W., Harris T.O. & Peto J. (1973) Life events and psychiatric disorders. Part 2. Nature of causal link. *Psychological Medicine* 3, 159–176.

Brown G.W. & Prudo R. (1981) Psychiatric disorder in a rural and an urban population: aetiology of depression. *Psychological Medicine* 11, 581–599.

Brugha T., Bebbington P.E., MacCarthy B., Potter J., Sturt E. & Wykes T. (1987) Social networks, social support and the type of depressive illness. *Acta Psychiatrica Scandinavica* 76, 664–673.

Brugha T.S., Bebbington P.E., MacCarthy B., Sturt E., Wykes T. & Potter T. (1990) Gender, social support and recovery from depressive disorders: a prospective clinical study. *Psychological Medicine* 20, 147–156.

Brugha T.S. & Conroy R. (1985) Categories of depression: reported life events in a controlled design. *British Journal of Psychiatry* 147, 641–646.

Brugha T.S., Conroy R., Walsh N. *et al.* (1982) Social networks, attachments and support in minor affective disorders: a replication. *British Journal of Psychiatry* 141, 249–255.

Cadoret R.J., Winokur G., Dorzab J. & Baker M. (1972) Depressive disease: life events and onset of illness. *Archives of General Psychiatry* 26, 133–136.

Campbell E.A. (1983) Depression in Women: The Role of Life Events, Social Factors and Psychological Vulnerability. Unpublished DPhil Thesis, University of Oxford.

Campbell E., Cope S. & Teasdale J. (1983) Social factors and affective disorder: an investigation of Brown and Harris's model. *British Journal of Psychiatry* 143, 548–553.

Chatterjee R.N., Mukherjee S.P. & Nandi D.N. (1981) Life events and depression. *Indian Journal of Psychiatry* 23, 333–337.

Clayton P., Desmarais L. & Winokur G. (1968) A study of normal bereavement. *American Journal of Psychiatry* 125, 168–178.

Cobb S. (1976) Social support as a moderator of life stress. *Psychosomatic Medicine* 38, 300–315.

Cobb S. (1979) Social support and health through the life course. In: Riley M.W. (ed.) *Aging from Birth to Death: Interdisciplinary Perspectives*, pp. 147–188. American Association for the Advancement of Science, Washington DC.

Cohen S. & Wills T.A. (1985) Stress, social support and the buffering hypothesis. *Psychological Bulletin* 98, 310–357.

Cohen-Sandler R., Berman A.L. & King R.A. (1982) Life stress and symptomatology: determinants of suicidal behaviour in children. *Journal of American Academy of Child Psychiatry* 21, 178–186.

Cooke D.J. (1987) The significance of life events as a cause of psychological and physical disorder. In: Cooper B. (ed.) *Psychiatric Epidemiology*, pp. 67–80. Croom Helm, London.

Cooper P.J. & Stein A. (1989) Life events and postnatal depression: the Oxford study. In: Cox J.L., Paykel E.S. & Page M.L. (eds) *Childbirth as a Life Event*. Duphar Medical Relations, Southampton.

Cornelis C.M., Ameling E.H. & de Jonghe F. (1989) Life events and social network in relation to the onset of depression. A controlled study. *Acta Psychiatrica Scandinavica* 88, 174–179.

Costello C.G. (1982) Social factors associated with depression: a retrospective community study. *Psychological Medicine* 12, 329–339.

Dohrenwend B.S. (1973a) Life events as stressors: a methodological inquiry. *Journal of Health and Social Behavior* 14, 167–175.

Dohrenwend B.S. (1973b) Social status and stressful life events. *Journal of Personality and Social Psychology* 28, 225–235.

Dolan R.J., Calloway S.P., Fonagy P., De Souza F.V.A. & Wakeling A. (1985) Life events, depression and hypothalamic-pituitary-adrenal axis function. *British Journal of Psychiatry* 147, 429–433.

Eaton W.W. (1978) Life events, social supports, and psychiatric symptoms: a re-analysis of the New Haven data. *Journal of Health and Social Behavior* 19, 230–234.

Emmerson J.P., Burvill P.W., Finlay-Jones R. & Hall W. (1989) Life events, life difficulties and confiding relationships in depressed elderly. *British Journal of Psychiatry* 155, 787–792.

Ezquiaga E., Gutierrez J.L.A. & Lopez A.G. (1987) Psychosocial factors and episode number in depression. *Journal of Affective Disorders* 12, 135–138.

Faravelli C. & Ambonetti A. (1983) Assessment of life events in depressive disorders. A comparison of three methods. *Social Psychiatry* 18, 51–56.

Fava G.A., Munari F., Pasvan L. & Kellner R. (1981) Life events and depression. A replication. *Journal of Affective Disorders*, 3, 159–165.

Flaherty J., Gaviria M. & Black E. (1983) The role of social support in the functioning of patients with unipolar depression. *American Journal of Psychiatry* 140, 473–476.

Forrest A.D., Fraser R.H. & Priest R.G. (1965) Environmental factors in depressive illness. *British Journal of Psychiatry* 111, 243–253.

Friedman L., Weissman M.M., Leaf P.J. & Bruce M.L. (1988) Social functioning in community residents with depression and other psychiatric disorders: results of the New Haven Epidemiologic Catchment Area Study. *Journal of Affective Disorders* 15, 103–112.

Gath D., Cooper P. & Day A. (1982) Hysterectomy and psychiatric disorder: I. Levels of psychiatric morbidity before and after hysterectomy. *British Journal of Psychiatry* 140, 335–350.

George L.K., Blazer D.G., Hughes D.C. & Fowler N. (1989) Social support and outcome of major depression. *British Journal of Psychiatry* 154, 478–485.

Giel R., Ten Horn G.H.M.M., Ormel J., Schudel W.J. & Wiersma O. (1978) Mental illness, neuroticism and life events in a Dutch village sample: a follow-up. *Psychological Medicine* 8, 235–243.

Goodyer I., Kolvin I. & Gatzanis S. (1985) Recent undesirable life events and psychiatric disorder in childhood and adolescence. *British Journal of Psychiatry* 147, 517–523.

Goodyer I.M., Kolvin I. & Gatzanis S. (1987) The impact of recent undesirable life events on psychiatric disorders in childhood and adolescence. *British Journal of Psychiatry* 151, 179–184.

Goodyer I., Wright C. & Altham P. (1990) The friendships and recent life events of anxious and depressed school-age children. *British Journal of Psychiatry* 156, 689–698.

Hallstrom T. (1986) Social origins of major depression: the role of provoking agents and vulnerability factors. *Acta Psychiatrica Scandinavica* 73, 383–389.

Henderson S. (1981) Social relationships, adversity and neurosis: an analysis of prospective observations. *British Journal of Psychiatry* 138, 391–398.

Henderson S., Duncan-Jones P., McAuley H. & Ritchie K. (1978) The patient's primary group. *British Journal of Psychiatry* 132, 74–86.

Holmes T.H. & Rahe R.H. (1967) The social readjustment rating scale. *Journal of Psychosomatic Research* 11, 213–218.

House J.S. (1981) *Work Stress and Social Support.* Addison-Wesley, Reading, MA.

Hudgens R.W., Morrison J.R. & Barchha R. (1967) Life events and onset of primary affective disorders. A study of 40 hospitalised patients and 40 controls. *Archives of General Psychiatry* 16, 134–145.

Jacobs S.C., Prusoff B.A. & Paykel E.S. (1974) Recent life events in schizophrenia and depression. *Psychological Medicine* 4, 444–453.

Kaplan B.H., Cassel J.C. & Gore S. (1977) Social support and health. *Medical Care* 15, 47–58.

Kasl S.V., Gore S. & Cobb S. (1975) The experience of losing a job: reported changes in health, symptoms and illness behaviour. *Psychosomatic Medicine* 37, 106–122.

Katschnig H. & Berner P. (1984) The poly-diagnostic approach in psychiatric research. In *Proceedings of the International Conference on Diagnosis and Classification of Mental Disorder and Alcohol and Drug Related Problems* (Copenhagen, 13–17 April 1982). World Health Organization, Geneva.

Leff J.P. & Vaughn C. (1980) The interaction of life events and relatives' expressed emotion in schizophrenia and depressive neurosis. *British Journal of Psychiatry* 136, 146–153.

Levi L.D., Fales C.H., Stein M. & Sharp V.H. (1966) Separation and attempted suicide. *Archives of General Psychiatry* 15, 158–165.

Lin N., Ensel W., Simeone R. & Kuo W. (1979) Social support, stressful life events and illness: a model for an empirical test. *Journal of Health and Social Behavior* 20, 108–119.

Lloyd C., Zisook S., Click M. & Jaffe K.E. (1981) Life events and response to antidepressants. *Journal of Human Stress* 7, 2–15.

Maguire G.P., Lee E.G., Bevington D.J., Kuchemann C.S., Crabtree R.J. & Cornell C.E. (1978) Psychiatric problems in the first year after mastectomy. *British Medical Journal* 1, 963–965.

Malmquist C.P. (1970) Depression and object loss in psychiatric admissions. *American Journal of Psychiatry* 126, 1782–1787.

Matussek P. & Neuner R. (1981) Loss events preceding endogenous and neurotic depressions. *Acta Psychiatrica Scandinavica* 64, 340–350.

Mendlewicz J., Charon F. & Linkowski P. (1986) Life events and the dexamethasone suppression test in affective illness. *Journal of Affective Disorders* 10, 203–206.

Merikangas K.R., Prusoff B.A., Kupfer D.J. & Frank E. (1985) Marital adjustment in major depression. *Journal of Affective Disorders* 9, 5–11.

Miller P. McC., Ingham J.G., Kreitman N.B., Surtees P.G. & Sashidharan S.P. (1987) Life events and other factors implicated in onset and remission of psychiatric illness in women. *Journal of Affective Disorders* 12, 73–88.

Monroe S.M., Thase M.E., Hersen M., Himmelhoch J.M. & Bellack A.S. (1985) Life events and the endogenous-nonendogenous distinction in the treatment and post-treatment course of depression. *Comprehensive Psychiatry* 26, 175–186.

Murphy E. (1982) Social origins of depression in old age. *British Journal of Psychiatry* 141, 135–142.

Murphy E. (1983) The prognosis of depression in old age. *British Journal of Psychiatry* 142, 111–119.

Myers J.K., Lindenthal J.J. & Pepper M.P. (1971) Life events and psychiatric impairment. *Journal of Nervous and Mental Diseases* 152, 149–157.

Myers J.K., Lindenthal J.J. & Pepper M.P. (1975) Life events, social integration and psychiatric symptomatology. *Journal of Health and Social Behavior* 16, 421–427.

O'Hara M.W., Nennaber D.J. & Zekoski E.M. (1984) Prospective study of post partum depression. Prevalence, course and predictive factors. *Journal of Abnormal Psychology* 93, 158–171.

Parker G. & Blignault I. (1985) Psychosocial predictors of outcome in subjects with untreated depressive disorder. *Journal of Affective Disorders* 8, 73–81.

Parry G. & Shapiro D.A. (1986) Social support and life events in working-class women: stress buffering or independent effects? *Archives of General Psychiatry* 43, 315–323.

Paykel E.S. (1974) Life stress and psychiatric disorder: application of the clinical approach. In Dohrenwend B.S. & Dohrenwend B.P. (eds) *Stressful Life Events: Their Nature and Effects*, pp. 135–149. John Wiley, New York.

Paykel E.S. (1978) Contribution of life events to causation of psychiatric illness. *Psychological Medicine* 8, 245–253.

Paykel E.S. (1979) Recent life events in the development of the depressive disorders. In Depue R.A. (ed.) *Psychobiology of the Depressive Disorders: Implications for the Effects of Stress*, pp. 245–262. Academic Press, New York.

Paykel E.S. (1983) Methodological aspects of life events research. Journal of Psychosomatic Research 27: 341–352.

Paykel E.S. & Cooper Z. (1990) Recent life events and

psychiatric illness. In Seva A. (ed.) *European Handbook of Psychiatry and Mental Health*. University Press of Zaragoza, Zaragoza, Spain (in press).

Paykel E.S., Emms E.M., Fletcher J. & Rassaby E.S. (1980) Life events and social support in puerperal depression. *British Journal of Psychiatry* 136, 339–346.

Paykel E.S., Myers J.K. & Dienelt M.N. (1969) Life events and depression: a controlled study. *Archives of General Psychiatry* 21, 753–760.

Paykel E.S., Prusoff B.A. & Myers J.K. (1975) Suicide attempts and recent life events: a controlled comparison. *Archives of General Psychiatry* 32, 327–333.

Paykel E.S., Rao B.M. & Taylor C.M. (1984) Life stress and symptom pattern in out-patient depression. *Psychological Medicine* 14, 559–568.

Paykel E.S. & Tanner J. (1976) Life events, depressive relapse and maintenance treatment. *Psychological Medicine* 6, 481–485.

Rowan P.R., Paykel E.S. & Parker R.R. (1982) Phenelzine and amitriptyline: effects on symptoms of neurotic depression. *British Journal of Psychiatry* 140, 475–483.

Roy A., Breier A., Doran A.R. & Pickar D. (1985) Life events in depression. Relationship to subtypes. *Journal of Affective Disorders* 9, 143–148.

Roy A. & Kennedy S. (1984) Risk factors for depression in Canadians. *Canadian Journal of Psychiatry* 29, 11–13.

Rutter M. (1983) Statistical and personal interactions: facets and perspectives. In Magnusson D. & Allen V. (eds) *Human Development: An Interactional Perspective*. Academic Press, London.

Salokangas R.K.R., Mattila V. & Joukamaa M. (1988) Intimacy and mental disorder in late middle age. *Acta Psychiatrica Scandinavica* 78, 555–560.

Sethi B.B. (1964) Relationship of separation to depression. *Archives of General Psychiatry* 10, 186–195.

Sireling L.I., Freeling P., Paykel E.S. & Rao B.M. (1985) Depression in general practice: clinical features and comparison with out-patients. *British Journal of Psychiatry* 147, 119–126.

Slater J. & Depue R.A. (1981) The contribution of environmental events and social support to serious suicide attempts in primary depressive disorder. *Journal of Abnormal Psychology* 90, 275–285.

Solomon Z. & Bromet E. (1982) The role of social factors in affective disorder: an assessment of the vulnerability model of Brown and his colleagues. *Psychological Medicine* 12, 123–130.

Surtees P.G. (1980) Social support, residual adversity and depressive outcome. *Social Psychiatry* 15, 71–80.

Tennant C., Bebbington P. & Hurry J. (1981) The short-term outcome of neurotic disorders in the community: the relation of remission to clinical factors and to 'neutralizing' life events. *British Journal of Psychiatry* 139, 213–220.

Thoits P.A. (1982) Conceptual, methodological and theoretical problems in studying social support as a buffer against life stress. *Journal of Health and Social Behavior* 23, 145–159.

Thoits P.A. (1985) Social support processes and psychological well-being: theoretical possibilities. In Sarason I.G. & Sarason B. (eds) *Social Support: Theory, Research and Applications*. Martinus Nijhof, The Hague.

Thompson K.C. & Hendrie H.C. (1972) Environmental stress in primary depressive illness. *Archives of General Psychiatry* 26, 130–132.

Uhlenhuth E.H., Lipman R.S., Balter M.B. & Stern M. (1974) Symptom intensity and life stress in the city. *Archives of General Psychiatry* 31, 759–764.

Uhlenhuth E.H. & Paykel E.S. (1973) Symptom configuration and life events. *Archives of General Psychiatry* 28, 743–748.

Ullah P., Banks M. & Warr P. (1985) Social support, social pressures and psychological distress during unemployment. *Psychological Medicine* 15, 283–295.

Vadher A. & Ndetei D.M. (1981) Life events and depression in a Kenyan setting. *British Journal of Psychiatry* 139, 134–149.

Vaughn C.E. & Leff J.P. (1976) The influence of family and social factors on the course of psychiatric illness. *British Journal of Psychiatry* 129, 125–137.

Waring E.M. & Patton D. (1984) Marital intimacy and depression. *British Journal of Psychiatry* 145, 641–644.

Wittchen H.U. (1987) Chronic difficulties and life events in the long-term course of affective and anxiety disorders: results from the Munich follow-up study. In Angermeyer M.C. (ed.) *From Social Class to Social Stress*, pp. 176–196. Springer-Verlag, Berlin.

# Chapter 8
# Social Factors and the Classification of Personality Disorder

PETER TYRER

Personality disorder constitutes a separate axis of classification, Axis II in the USA (American Psychiatric Association 1980, 1987), and so is in a different domain of measurement and function from mental state problems (Axis I Disorders). Social functioning is more intimately concerned with personality disorder than mental state disorders because social function in its broadest aspects, relationships with other people, determines the diagnosis of personality disorder. Schneider (1923) elegantly defined personality disorder as a condition from which 'the patient suffers and society has to suffer' and this distinguishes it from all other disorders in that the effect on society is an integral part of the definition, and thus involves assessment of social factors in making the diagnosis. However, there have been some changes in classification in the most recent description, DSM-III-R (American Psychiatric Association 1987) and ICD-10 (World Health Organization 1992), that have altered the significance of social factors in personality disorder. The general descriptions of personality disorder in these two classifications are shown in Table 8.1.

Because social function is so important in assessing personality disorder it makes it more difficult to decide whether social factors are aetiological precursors of personality disorder or predictable consequences of the disturbed personality. Although there have been many studies since Lee Robins' seminal work (1966) first demonstrated the link between social deprivation, conduct disorder in childhood and adult antisocial personality disorder (see Chapter 13), it is important to realize that this association does not apply across the range of personality disorders. Epidemiological studies show that although antisocial personality disorder is more common in deprived inner city areas, this is compensated by a greater proportion of anankastic (obsessive-compulsive) personality disorders in better-off rural areas (Casey & Tyrer 1990) and the total prevalence of personality disorder is similar in both populations.

In acknowledging the role of social factors in assessing personality disorder it is important to stress that only some aspects are consistently emphasized. In particular, the disruption of personal relationships has always been a key element in the recognition of personality disorder although, as we shall see later, this has not always been applied consistently and other aspects of social function are also incorporated at times. In both ICD-10 and DSM-III-R classifications the possibility that personality disorder can lead only to personal distress without any significant impairment of social function is allowed. This signifies an important change in attitudes towards the diagnosis of personality disorder in recent years. In the first 60 years of this century personality disorder was often equated with psychopathy, and it is of interest that early writers such as Schneider & Kretschmer described all personality disorder under this heading. This attached much greater importance to the deleterious effects of the personality on society at large (not just the immediate intimates of the patient) and usually implied that personal distress was a consequence of this general social disruption rather than an intrinsic part of the personality disorder. The new concept allows for the possibility that individuals with personality disorder *perform* adequately in all social relationships but only do so at the expense of considerable internal distress and pain. It also allows for the possibility of individuals

**Table 8.1** General description of personality disorder in ICD-10 and DSM-III-R classifications

**ICD-10**

The diagnostic criteria for the Personality Disorders refer to behaviours or traits that are characteristic of the person's recent (past year) and long-term functioning (generally since adolescence or early adulthood). The constellation of behaviours or traits causes either significant impairment in social or occupational functioning or subjective distress. Behaviours or traits limited to episodes of illness are not considered in making a diagnosis of Personality Disorder

**DSM-III-R**

These types of conditions comprise deeply ingrained and enduring behaviour patterns, manifesting themselves as inflexible responses to a broad range of personal and social situations. They represent either extreme or significant deviations from the way the average individual in a given culture perceives, thinks, feels, and particularly, relates to others. Such behaviour patterns tend to be stable and to encompass multiple domains of behaviour and psychological functioning. They are frequently, but not always, associated with various degrees of subjective distress and impaired social functioning

avoiding many aspects of personal relationships because of their personality disorder. The best examples of this are avoidant personality disorder in DSM-III-R and anxious personality disorder in ICD-10.

## Assessment of social functioning in personality disorder

### General issues

Although social function is incorporated into the definition of personality disorder it is also impaired in almost all other psychiatric disorders. For purposes of classification such impairment is often not taken into account but increasingly is being recognized as a secondary diagnostic feature. For example, in ICD-10 depressive disorders are separated into single and recurrent episodes and further subdivided into mild, moderate or severe. The degree of social impairment produced by the depression is important in classifying an individual patient into one of these

three major groups (World Health Organization, 1992). When social function is compared in patients with mental state and personality disorders the impairment is roughly similar in both groups (Casey *et al.* 1985), although in some conditions, particularly the depressive disorders, social function can show greater impairment (Casey *et al.* 1985, Cassano *et al.* 1990).

Matters are also complicated by the frequent overlap between personality disorders and mental illness; between one-third and two-thirds of all mental state diagnoses are accompanied by an additional personality disorder diagnosis (Tyrer *et al.* 1988b). It is, therefore, hard to know how much the personality rather than the mental state abnormality contributes to social impairment. It is, therefore, clear that the measurement of social function, at least in the short term, cannot be used to distinguish personality disorder from mental illness.

When assessing personality disorder it is therefore customary to subtract any episodes of mental illness from the personality disorder assessment, as is illustrated in Table 8.1. Although this is stated clearly in all measuring instruments for personality disorder it is not always easy in practice to identify the boundary between long-standing personality and social functioning on the one hand and (allegedly discrete) episodes of mental illness on the other. This is particularly difficult with chronic psychiatric disorders such as schizophrenia which may begin early in life and continue for many years. Schizophrenia also presents a problem because the disorder itself creates personality change and so even after recovery from the major mental symptoms there is a different personality from what existed before. When one adds to this the difficulty in deciding when the prodrome of schizophrenia begins (as in the early stage of schizophrenia there may also be personality disturbance), it is understandable why the assessment of personality disorder in some mental illnesses is almost impossible! However, for other mental disorders these difficulties are not nearly so pronounced and the persistence of social dysfunction over a long time-scale may be useful as a marker in deciding whether or not personality disorder is present. In the case of mental state disorders such as depressive illness, social functioning improves as mental state improves (Cassano *et al.* 1990) and thereby can be distinguished from personality disorder.

The major impact of personality disorder is on relationships with others. This, however, is only one part of social functioning. The others, including work and domestic performance, finances, self-care and spare-time activities, do not necessarily involve significant relationships. It is therefore possible to envisage patients with personality disorder having significant problems in their personal relationships but achieving reasonable social performance. This does not happen if social function is defined adequately, and this is discussed later in this chapter.

Another important issue is the possibility that problems in social functioning quite independent of personality disorder might be wrongly construed as created by personality abnormality. This includes a range of situations, from therapists not liking their patients (and vice versa) to economically deprived circumstances which preclude proper use of occupational, social and leisure activities. This inappropriate attribution is one of the reasons why many remain unhappy about the diagnosis of personality disorder and regard it as a diagnosis of prejudice rather than one based on fact (Blackburn 1988, Lewis & Appleby 1988).

Although this viewpoint is acknowledged it is not difficult to solve in clinical practice. Both subjects and close informants are quite able to distinguish independent social factors from those aspects of social and personality function that are a consequence of their own behaviour. There are some exceptions, particularly with paranoid personality disorder, in which the mental mechanism of projection means that most personal failings are blamed on other people, but the problem is usually surmountable without much difficulty. Another problem, which runs throughout the literature on social functioning, is what constitutes 'normal' social adjustment. This has been discussed elsewhere in more detail (Platt 1981, Tyrer 1990) and the full arguments will not be repeated here. In summary, since the introduction of the first social functioning schedule 35

years ago (Barrabee *et al.* 1955), there has been concern that normal functioning is determined by some hypothetical middle-class norm that is only representative of the people devising the instruments. This takes no account of people's different roles in society and of subcultures within the larger macrocosm of society.

The arguments for and aganist having a common measure of social function are presented in Table 8.2 and could easily be reworded slightly and requoted similarly for the assessment of personality disorder. It is understandable for nosologists to look for common measurements that apply across the world. The classification of the plant and animal kingdom is a good example. These classifications are common to all parts of the world and it would be ludicrous to suggest that they should differ between countries. Unfortunately, however, social functioning is closely involved with human behaviour, which shows little sign of commonality. Even in the animal and plant kingdoms selective breeding has led to varieties of plants and animals that do not fit current classifications except by introducing a category beyond the level of species. The author is firmly against a common measure of social functioning or of personality.

**Table 8.2** Advantages and disadvantages of a common (norm-based) definition of social function

| Advantages | Disadvantages |
|---|---|
| Better interrater reliability of measurement | Poor cross-cultural reliability as norms vary from society to society |
| Comparisons made with expectations of behaviour that are common to society at large | No allowance made for differing roles in society |
| Common targets for good social function (cf. DSM-III) | Imposes an Orwellian society in which individuals have no say in what is regarded as normal |
| Consistent yardsticks of measurement | There is no common measure of social function as it is determined by adjustment within groups that are inherently different |

Although society is capable of imposing apparent norms for the whole population to follow (exemplified by 'Victorian values' and the American 'enterprise society'), these norms do not extend across cultures and are not temporally consistent even within a single society. Both personality disorders and social dysfunction are therefore manifest by individuals demonstrating persistent attitudes and behaviour that are incompatible with those of *immediate* society, which includes family members, friends, neighbours, work colleagues and leisure companions. Wider society may also be important, as in the area of antisocial (sociopathic) personality disorder, but few individuals have such severe personality disorder that society as a whole is affected. It is quite inappropriate to expect people to follow a common norm of behaviour in all societal settings. If variation was not allowed there would have to be a common social role and this would clearly be inappropriate for the whole population. In trying to resolve disputes in psychotherapeutic settings it is common to invoke role playing to illustrate the different standpoints that people adopt in their relationships with others. If role playing is so important among intimates how much more important it must be for people in wider society.

The last general issue concerns the role of subjects and informants in assessing social function and in personality disorder. Although it is common to assess social function with subjects only (Tyrer 1990), there is a good case for asking informants for assessments also. Obviously if an individual is showing acceptable social functioning to others it does not necessarily mean that he or she is not stressed in this role. Most social function schedules take this into account by assessing behaviour and stress in separate sections. However, it is equally true that some subjects may regard their social function as normal but their close informants may have a completely different view. This divergence of opinion is shown most strongly in the field of antisocial behaviour, in which it has often been recognized as a core feature that such individuals act without consideration of others and do not think of the impact of their behaviour on people at large. This assumes more importance than the assessment of personality disorder because as is clear from the definitions in Table 8.1, the separate suffering of society is an important diagnostic element and can occur independently of personal suffering or social dysfunction. Of course, in the end, like a typical Western film, the antisocial person will suffer for his or her past misdeeds, but this may be many years in coming.

### Specific issues in measuring social function and personality disorder

The problem with personality is that it is as unique as a fingerprint. It is, therefore, difficult to classify personality types in a way that does not ride roughshod over individual differences that are so important in making the study of humans so interesting. It is possible to argue that personality disorder is more stereotyped and can be classified appropriately and, indeed, it is generally true that as the severity of psychiatric disturbance increases the number of conditions manifest by the disorder get smaller. The simple relationship between social function and personality disorder becomes more complicated when categorization of personality takes place. The current classification is summarized in Table 8.3 and shows good concordance between ICD-10 and DSM-III-R classifications. The categories derive from different sources. The classical phenomenologists of the German school introduced anankastic, paranoid, schizoid, histrionic and antisocial personality disorders, American psychotherapists were mainly responsible for the introduction of narcissistic and borderline personality disorders, and avoidant personality disorder comes from psychological constructs. The others derive from empirical work and renaming of former categories, such as impulsive for explosive and dependent for asthenic in the ICD classification. Self-defeating personality disorder began life under the adjective 'masochistic', but came under heavy fire from feminists in the USA and so was renamed using a slightly more acceptable adjective.

It can be guessed immediately that these different personality disorders affect different aspects of social function, although all should affect

**Table 8.3** Comparison of current classification of personality disorder

| ICD-10 | | DSM-III-R | |
|---|---|---|---|
| Description | Code | Description | Code |
| Paranoid – excessive sensitivity, suspiciousness, preoccupation with conspiratorial explanation of events, with a persistent tendency to self-reference | F60.0 | Paranoid – interpretation of people's actions as deliberately demeaning or threatening | 301.00 |
| Schizoid – emotional coldness, detachment, lack of interest in other people, eccentricity and introspective fantasy | F60.1 | Schizoid – indifference to relationships and restricted range of emotional experience and expression | 301.20 |
| No equivalent | | Schizotypal – deficit in interpersonal relatedness with peculiarities of ideation, appearance and behaviour | 302.22 |
| Anankastic – indecisiveness, doubt, excessive caution, pedantry, rigidity and need to plan in immaculate detail | F60.5 | Obsessive-compulsive – pervasive perfectionism and inflexibility | 301.40 |
| Histrionic – self-dramatization, shallow mood, egocentricity and craving for excitement with persistent manipulative behaviour | F60.4 | Histrionic – excessive emotionally and attention-seeking | 301.50 |
| Dependent – failure to take responsibility for actions, with subordination of personal needs to those of others, excessive dependence with need for constant reassurance and feelings of helplessness when a close relationship ends | F60.7 | Dependent – persistent dependent and submissive behaviour | 301.60 |
| Dyssocial – callous unconcern for others, with irresponsibility, irritability and aggression, and incapacity to maintain enduring relationships. | F60.2 | Antisocial – evidence of repeated conduct disorder before the age of 15 | 301.70 |
| No equivalent | | Narcissistic – pervasive grandiosity, lack of empathy, and hypersensitivity to the evaluation of others | 301.81 |
| Anxious – persistent tension, self-consciousness, exaggeration of risks and dangers, hypersensitivity to rejection, and restricted lifestyle because of insecurity | F60.6 | Avoidant – pervasive social discomfort, fear of negative evaluation and timidity | 301.82 |
| Impulsive – inability to control anger, to plan ahead, or to think before acts, with unpredictable mood and quarrelsome behaviour | F60.30* | No equivalent | |
| Borderline – unclear self-image, involvement in intense and unstable relationships | F60.31* | Borderline – pervasive instability of mood, and self-image | 301.83 |
| No equivalent | | Passive-aggressive – pervasive passive resistance to demands for adequate social and occupational performance | 301.84 |

* Included under heading of emotionally labile personality disorder.

**Table 8.4** Mean social function scores in 163 patients
with conspicuous psychiatric morbidity in primary care
separated by personality status

| Personality disorder | Mean social function score (Social Functioning Schedule) |
|---|---|
| Normal | 21.47 |
| Schizoid | 33.12 |
| Explosive | 30.13 |
| Anankastic | 33.69 |
| Hysterical | 29.45 |
| Asthenic | 33.57 |
| Sociopathic | 19.80 |
| Other | 20.17 |

From Casey *et al.* 1985.

interpersonal relationships. Thus dependent personality disorders create problems by clinging on to key figures in their lives, histrionic ones manipulate them and schizoid ones try hard to pretend they do not exist. What is interesting is that, despite the different categories of personality disorder, social function between the main groups of personality disorder is roughly similar in all of them (Table 8.4) (Casey *et al.* 1985).

In Table 8.4 the mean social function scores of patients with different personality disorders are compared with each other and with non-personality disordered patients with other mental state illnesses. All the patients concerned were interviewed in an epidemiological study to determine the prevalence of psychiatric disorder in patients recognized as having primary psychiatric problems in general practice (sometimes described as conspicuous psychiatric morbidity) (Kessel 1960). Although it might have been expected that antisocial personality disorder would produce greater social dysfunction, it is equally possible to argue that the wider spread of social disruption caused by such personality disorders leads to a lower threshold of diagnosis than others. However, it is fair to add that this study was carried out with an instrument, the Personality Assessment Schedule (PAS; Tyrer & Alexander 1979), which is more closely linked to the assessment of social function than other personality disorder schedules and questionnaires. It is possible to

argue that all the categories of personality disorders in Table 8.3 have only 'earned their spurs' when patients satisfying the criteria for them have consistently greater social impairment than others who differ by not having the named personality disorder concerned.

## Operational criteria

Although the definitions given in Table 8.1 at the beginning of this chapter suggest that social dysfunction is an essential part of personality disorder, it has largely been forgotten in defining personality disorders in both ICD-10 and DSM-III-R classifications. This is because the attraction of operational criteria in DSM-III-R (diagnostic criteria in ICD-10) has proved too hard to resist. Operational criteria were first introduced into DSM-III in 1980 and were themselves based on other data, particularly Research Diagnostic Criteria established for depression and schizophrenia. When sufficient data were not available to introduce operational criteria the classifiers did not get too concerned, they just made up some criteria that seemed to fit the requirements. This is not necessarily unsatisfactory, because it has always been stated the classifications proposed in DSM are provisional, serving to test hypotheses so that they can eventually be improved. Unfortunately, however, such has been the success of DSM-III that most of the diagnoses included in it, and modified in DSM-III-R, are given undue authority and are seldom challenged (Tyrer 1988). Because the introduction of operational criteria has been so successful in categorizing mental state disorders it was also assumed that the technology could be exported equally successfully to personality disorders. Again I have argued elsewhere that this is inappropriate (Tyrer 1988), because personality does not lend itself to the precise definition necessary for operational criteria. The diagnosis of personality disorder requires some skill that cannot be replaced by a list of operational criteria and, in particular, requires a longitudinal assessment of the characteristics in question with appropriate subtraction for times when the patient has been significantly ill with a mental state disorder. It is extremely difficult to incorporate these aspects into the necessarily tight definitions of operational criteria. Thus it is not surprising that the items chosen do not match up with the general statement about personality disorder given at the beginning of each of these classifications (reproduced in Table 8.1).

The hope has been that certain items of behaviour can be regarded as so characteristic of a single personality disorder that they are 'prototypical acts' that exemplify the personality disorder concerned. However, despite efforts to define such prototypical behaviours (Blashfield *et al.* 1985), the exercise has not been conspicuously successful.

The advantages of operational criteria are that they can be applied universally and are not subject to the vagaries of culture and national characteristics. However, many of them can be satisfied without producing any impairment of social or personality functioning. It is possible to take many of the diagnostic guidelines from ICD-10 (which are less restrictive than DSM-III-R) for each of the major personality disorders and find examples of this. Thus 'a tendency to experience excessive self-importance, manifest in a persistent self-referential attitude' is very common in aspiring young people (often collectively numbered among the 'Yuppies'), and these pocket Napoleons often do not cause distress to themselves or others, yet the item is one of the key guidelines for paranoid personality disorder. Similarly, one of the characteristics of schizoid personality disorder is 'little experience in having sexual experiences with another person (taking into account age)'. This brings us back to the problem of imposing normative social functioning on the population at large. There are many extremely worthy people who make a major contribution to society but who still satisfy this schizoid criterion. Psychoanalysts have argued for years that the sexual drives of such individuals are sublimated into other works. Whether or not this is true, the frequency of sexual intercourse should not be a criterion for deciding what constitutes personality disorder. One of the guidelines for histrionic personality disorder is 'persistent manipulative behaviour to achieve own needs'. There are many highly successful individuals, particularly in

politics, commerce and industry, whose success depends on such manipulative behaviour, which would often be described as a positive personality attribute rather than a personality disorder.

Of course it may be pointed out that it is only when these characteristics become persistent and apply across a wide range of situations, both appropriate and inappropriate, that the condition constitutes a personality disorder. However, what tends to happen in practice is that the particular characteristics identified by each of the guidelines 'rings the bell' of recognition and, once this connection has been made, it is easy to see how the operational criterion can become the driving force in making the diagnosis, rather than the (more important) impairment of social functioning caused by the attribute in question.

## Type of social functioning and its influence on personality disorder

Weissman and her colleagues (1981) have pointed out that social function comprises at least five separate elements:

1 Social supports and networks.
2 Social attachments.
3 Social competence.
4 Social status.
5 Social role performance.

It is difficult to know which of these are considered important in making the assessment of personality disorder, but the suspicion must be that the last of these, social role performance, is uppermost. For example, in the criteria for diagnosing specific personality disorders there needs to be 'evidence that the individual's characteristic and enduring patterns of inner experience and behaviour deviate markedly as a whole from the culturally expected and accepted range (or "norm")' (World Health Organization 1990).

Certainly this is the area of social dysfunction which has the widest impact on relationships with others. However, the wording of individual operational criteria suggests that other elements of social functioning are also taken into account. For example, the lack of 'close, confiding personal relationships' in DSM-III-R and ICD-10 as one of the criteria for schizoid personality disorder suggests that the absence of social support is a criterion in personality disorder. The same comment also applies to social attachments. The area of social competence appears to be included under items such as 'pedantry and conventionality with limited capacity to express warm emotion' under the characteristics in ICD-10 for anankastic personality disorder.

It is pleasing to note that social status does not appear to enter into any of the diagnostic guidelines or operational criteria. However, the absence of any reference to social status does not mean that it is not taken into account by an assessor when making assessments of personality status. For example, one of the criteria for antisocial personality disorder in DSM-III-R is 'significant unemployment for six months or more within five years when expected to work and work was available'. The interpretation of the last two clauses could be influenced by social status. In particular, a professional middle-class assessor may have a completely different view of 'available work' than a tramp on the streets. What is perceived by one as a statistical work vacancy is viewed as demeaning drudgery by the other, and much less acceptable than unemployment.

The personality norms set by society are also influenced insidiously by social status, so that 'acceptable' behaviour may be too closely linked to middle-class expectations, and therefore subject to the same criticisms as 'normative social function' mentioned earlier. Attempts to ensure that assessment is 'social status-proof' are still needed.

## Assessment of personality disorder in practice

A good assessment of personality disorder should avoid prejudice and criticism but it is usually possible to see evidence of both these qualities by visiting any clinical setting and examining the criteria that seem to go towards recording personality disorder. Unfortunately, because there is no clear form of assessment to determine personality disorder (apart from structured clinical interviews) much of the assessment of personality is conducted piecemeal and may extend over many weeks after first contact with the patient. Thus characteristics such as the therapist disliking the patient (with the patient reciprocating), the failure to respond to treatment, disruption in either outpatient or hospital settings, the patient challenging decisions made by psychiatric staff, and the apparent need to consume a large amount of therapeutic time, all appear to contribute to an impressionistic diagnosis of personality disorder that often blends into a formal one. Similarly the identification of social and cultural circumstances that differ from normative expectations (e.g. this patient only eats food which is not available on the hospital menu) can easily be attributed to personality disorder. It is possible to avoid these value judgements by assessing personality disorder early in contact with patients. This not only helps to assess personality but also puts any concurrent mental illness into perspective. A formal assessment of personality involves collecting information from as many sources as possible, but certainly including the patient and a reliable informant, presumably a close one. It is not normally necessary to assess social function as well, not least because of the high correlation between social malfunction and mental state disturbance as independent of personality.

Although formal assessment of personality disorders have their attractions, particularly in research studies, they are far from satisfactory. Many of them are linked closely to the DSM classification and follow operational criteria slavishly. This can lead to long interviews that are not easy to carry out since all the questions refer to attributes that are socially undesirable. The main instruments being used are the Personality Assessment Schedule (Tyrer & Alexander 1979, Tyrer *et al.* 1988a), the Standardized Assessment of Personality (SAP) (Mann *et al.* 1981), the Structured Interview for DSM-III Personality Disorders (SIDP) (Pfohl *et al.* 1982), and the Personality Disorder Examination (PDE) (Loranger *et al.* 1985).

The main interview schedules for recording personality disorder are shown in Table 8.5. Although there are self-rating instruments (which have major attractions because of the length of time that it takes to assess personality disorder), there is insufficient information about the correlations between self-rating and interview instru-

**Table 8.5** Instruments for measuring personality disorders

| Instrument | Authors | Main features |
|---|---|---|
| Personality Assessment Schedule (PAS) | Tyrer & Alexander 1979, Tyrer *et al.* 1988a | Assesses 24 key personality traits with scores determined by degree of social dysfunction. Computer classification yields four main personality disorders and nine subcategories. Personality separated into five bands of severity ranging between personality difficulty and gross personality disorder. Subject and informant versions (20–45 minutes). ICD-10 version also available |
| Standardized Assessment of Personality (SAP) | Mann *et al.* 1981 | Original version yielded ICD-9 diagnoses with two others (anxious and self-conscious), now revised to yield ICD-10 diagnoses. Informant only interviewed (15–30 minutes) |
| Structured Interview for DSM-III Personality Disorders (SID-P) | Pfohl *et al.* 1982 | Originally made DSM-III diagnoses, now revised to include DSM-III-R. Interviews mainly with subject but can also use informant information (45–75 minutes) |
| Personality Disorder Examination (PDE) (recently amplified to International Personality Disorder Examination) (IPDE) | Loranger *et al.* 1985 | PDE yields DSM-III-R diagnoses and IPDE yields both DSM-III-R and ICD-10 diagnoses. Subject version only (2–4 hours) |
| Structured Clinical Interview for DSM-III-R Personality Disorders (SCID-II) | Spitzer *et al.* 1987 | Yields DSM-III-R diagnoses and is simple to administer but has had less validation carried out than some other instruments. Subject version only (20–45 minutes) |

ments to judge whether any self-rating instrument could be used instead of formal interview schedules. At present they are probably best regarded as screening instruments and there is probably room for considerable shortening if they were used for this function.

Almost all these instruments derive a number of personality disorders simultaneously. There are no rules for deciding which is the major personality disorder when several coexist after formal classification. The exception is the Personality Assessment Schedule in which the primary personality disorder is the one that causes the greatest social dysfunction when the Schedule is scored (see Appendix to this chapter). Because of the confusion engendered by multiple personality disorders it is common for investigators to concentrate on three main groups: flamboyant (including antisocial, narcissistic, histrionic and borderline personalities), the withdrawn (schizoid, schizotypal, paranoid), and a timid, fearful group (avoidant, anankastic (obsessive-compulsive), dependent).

## Summary

Social factors, social function and personality disorder are closely related and it is difficult to determine how each influences the others. Although it is easy to fall back to the common hypothesis that constitutional factors create vulnerability to personality disorder that is then made explicit by social factors, this is probably wrong. The main characteristic of personality disorders is that they create persistent dysfunction independent of setting and so it is possible to argue that most social factors are effects rather than causes. The recent demonstration that patients with antisocial and dependent personality disorders have higher rates of life events than others (Seivewright 1987) supports the view that people with these personality disorders create the circumstances for adverse

**Appendix 8.1** Extract from ICD-10 version of Personality Assessment Schedule – informant version

| | Score | | |
|---|---|---|---|
| | 0 | 1 | 2 |
| Paranoid personality disorder | No | Yes, but no social impairment | Yes, with social impairment |
| 1 Is S(subject) excessively sensitive to things that go wrong in his/her life? | ☐ | ☐ | ☐ |
| 2 Does S find it difficult to forgive others, so that he/she bears grudges against them? | ☐ | ☐ | ☐ |
| 3 Is S abnormally suspicious and thinks people are against him/her when they are just acting normally? | ☐ | ☐ | ☐ |
| 4 Is S excessively concerned about his/her personal rights? | ☐ | ☐ | ☐ |
| 5 Is S abnormally jealous? | ☐ | ☐ | ☐ |
| 6 Does S act and talk as if he/she was an important person who attracts special attention from others? | ☐ | ☐ | ☐ |
| 7 Does S tend to think that people are plotting against him/her persistently? | ☐ | ☐ | ☐ |

A score of 7 or more with social impairment manifest for at least three questions indicates a paranoid personality disorder.

(Note: For the purposes of assessment social impairment is defined as persistent difficulties in occupational, leisure or personal relationships occurring as a consequence of the personality attribute in question.)

social circumstances rather than being unwitting victims.

Although it is recognized that personality disorder creates social dysfunction, investigators have been seduced by the attractions of operational criteria in defining personality disorders and have tended to ignore the general effects of disorder on social functioning. There has also been confusion over the different roles and definitions of social functioning in understanding personality disorder.

It is tempting to argue that better definition of behaviours characteristic of personality disorders is possible and attainable. This may prove to be an elusive goal as few personality disorders demonstrate such stereotypes of behaviour in such a persistent way that they could be regarded as typical of personality disorder.

The approach linking the assessment of social functioning and personality disorder has always been the most attractive in personal work because

this reflects the impact of personality disorder on personal functioning and that of society. It offers the opportunity to match current classification practice, which in my view is too dependent of operational criteria, with clinical practice, in which assessment is made from many more sources of information. An example of this is shown in Appendix 8.1 where part of the ICD-10 version of the PAS is illustrated.

### References

American Psychiatric Association (1980) *Diagnostic and Statistical Manual of Mental Disorders*, 3rd edn. American Psychiatric Association, Washington DC.

American Psychiatric Association (1987) *Diagnostic and Statistical Manual of Mental Disorders*, 3rd edn revised. American Psychiatric Association, Washington DC.

Barrabee R., Barrabee E.L. & Finesinger J.E.F. (1955) A normative social adjustment scale. *American Journal of Psychiatry* 112, 252–259.

Blackburn R. (1988) On moral judgements and personality disorders. The myth of psychopathic personality revisited. *British Journal of Psychiatry* 153, 505–512.

Blashfield R., Sprock J., Pinkston K. & Hodgin J. (1985) Exemplar prototypes of personality disorder diagnoses. *Comprehensive Psychiatry* 26, 11–21.

Casey P. & Tyrer P. (1990) Personality disorder and psychiatric illness in general practice. *British Journal of Psychiatry* 156, 261–265.

Casey P.R., Tyrer P.J. & Platt S. (1985) The relationship between social functioning and psychiatric symptomatology in primary care. *Social Psychiatry* 20, 5–9.

Cassano G.B., Perugi G., Maremmani I. & Akiskal H.S. (1990) Social adjustment in dysthymia. In Burton S. & Akiskal H.S. (eds) *Dysthymic Disorder*, pp 78–85. Gaskell Books, London.

Kessel N. (1960) Psychiatric morbidity in a London general practice. *British Journal of Preventive and Social Medicine* 14, 16–22.

Lewis G. & Appleby L. (1988) Personality disorder: the patients psychiatrists dislike. *British Journal of Psychiatry* 153, 44–49.

Loranger A.W., Susman V.L., Oldham J.M. & Russakoff L.M. (1985) *Personality Disorder Examination (PDE). A Structured Interview for DSM-III-R and ICD-9 Personality Disorders.* WHO/ADAMHA pilot version. The New York Hospital, Cornell Medical Center, Westchester Division, Whit Plains, New York.

Mann A.H., Jenkins R., Cutting J.C. & Cowen P.J. (1981) The development and use of a standardized assessment of abnormal personality. *Psychological Medicine* 11, 839–847.

Pfohl B., Stangl D. & Zimmerman M. (1982) *Structured Interview for DSM-III Personality Disorders (SID-P).* Iowa City, University of Iowa Hospitals and Clinics.

Platt S. (1981) Social Adjustment as a criterion of treatment success: just what we were measuring? *Psychiatry* 44, 95–112.

Robins L.N. (1966) *Deviant Children Grown Up.* Williams & Wilkins, Baltimore.

Schneider K. (1923) *Die Psychopathischen Personlichkeiten.* Springer, Berlin.

Seivewright N. (1987) Relationship between life events and personality in psychiatric disorder. *Stress Medicine* 3, 163–68.

Spitzer R., Williams J.B.W. & Gibbon M. (1987) *Structured Interview for DSM-III-R Personality Disorders.* Biometrics Research Department, New York State Psychiatric Institute, New York.

Tyrer P. (1988) What's wrong with DSM-III personality disorders? *Journal of Personality Disorders* 2, 281–291.

Tyrer P. (1990) Personality disorder and social functioning. In Peck D. & Shapiro C. (eds), *Measuring Human Problems: A Practical Guide*, pp. 119–142. John Wiley, Chichester.

Tyrer P. & Alexander J. (1979) Classification of personality disorder. *British Journal of Psychiatry* 135, 163–167.

Tyrer P., Alexander J. & Ferguson B. (1988a) Personality assessment schedule. In Tyrer P. (ed.) *Personality Disorders: Diagnosis, Management and Course*, pp. 140–167. Wright (an imprint of Butterworth-Heinemann), Oxford.

Tyrer P., Casey P. & Ferguson B. (1988b) Personality disorder and mental illness. In Tyrer P. (ed.) *Personality Disorders: Diagnosis, Management and Course*, pp. 93–104. Wright (an imprint of Butterworth-Heinemann), Oxford.

Weissman M.M., Sholomskas D. & John K. (1981) The assessment of social adjustment: an update. *Archives of General Psychiatry* 38, 1250–1258.

World Health Organization (1990) *Mental and Behavioural Disorders: Diagnostic Criteria for Research*, draft version. WHO, Geneva.

World Health Organization (1992) *The ICD-10 Classification of Mental and Behavioural Disorders: Clinical Descriptions and Diagnostic Guidelines.* WHO, Geneva.

# Chapter 9
## Social Factors in Phobias and Obsessions

M.J.POWER

## Introduction

Born from an extramarital affair between Aphrodite, the goddess of desire, and Ares, the god of war, Phobus was the son who was frightened of his enemies. The origins of the term 'phobia', therefore, emphasize its social nature, though with friends like Aphrodite and Ares, who needs enemies?

In this chapter, the emphasis will be placed on social factors and how they interact with psychological characteristics in the onset, maintenance, and recovery of individuals with phobias and obsessions. An attempt will be made to look at a broad range of psychological factors from a lifespan perspective; for example, the data collected about the age of onset of different types of phobias and obsessions reveals striking differences that may relate to the developmental stage and normative social transitions with which the individual is faced. The term 'social' will be interpreted broadly to consider not only family and relationship factors relevant to the onset of a condition, but also the importance of the therapeutic relationship, and the cultural and community context in which these disorders occur.

Perhaps one question that should be clarified from the beginning is whether there is any similarity between phobias and obsessions that warrants their joint consideration. In his original seduction theory Freud (e.g. 1896) linked phobias and obsessions, the difference being that whereas phobias arose from the experience of a passive seduction in childhood, obsessions purportedly arose when the child was actively involved in the seduction of the adult. Although Freud subsequently rejected this seduction theory, it served to highlight the central role of anxiety in ob-

sessional disorders. In fact, the proposal that the obsessional rituals serve to defend the individual against an ego-alien wish or impulse that gives rise to anxiety has recently resurfaced in the cognitive model of obsessions presented by Salkovskis (1985). Modern classificatory systems such as DSM-III, therefore, view obsessional disorders as a variant of an anxiety disorder. In a similar manner, the behavioural treatment emphasizes *exposure* to the feared or avoided stimulus in both conditions. As an interesting addendum, it might be noted that both psychoanalysis and behaviourism have mythologized their animal phobics: Freud's (1909) classic case of Little Hans has more recently been considered to have been a horse phobic (e.g. Rachman 1990a), whereas J.B. Watson's furry-animal phobic Little Albert (Watson & Rayner 1920) seems to have reacted to animals in a way that few subsequent Little Alberts have.

## Epidemiology

The prevalence of phobias in a population depends on a number of factors, including the severity at which a mild fear is considered to become a phobia; thus, Myers *et al.* (1984) in their large epidemiological study of psychiatric disorders in the community found an average of 5.9 per 100 for mild levels of phobic disorder, with a preponderance amongst women at 8.0 per 100 compared to 3.4 per 100 for men. However, they found that only 2.2 cases per 1000 would be considered disabling. Mild obsessional problems showed a prevalence of about 1–2 per 100 (Myers *et al.* 1984), though again only a small proportion of them are disabling and come to the attention of psychiatric services. Indeed, Rachman

**Table 9.1** Mean age of onset of different types of phobias (based on Ost 1987) and obsessional disorders (based on Minichiello *et al.* 1990)

| | Age (years) | | | | | | |
|---|---|---|---|---|---|---|---|
| | 0 | 5 | 10 | 15 | 20 | 25 | 30 |
| Simple phobias | | Animal Blood | Dental | | Claustrophobia | | |
| Other phobias | | | | Social phobia | | | Agoraphobia |
| Obsessional disorders | | | | | Checkers | | Cleaners Ruminators |

& Hodgson (1980) reported that less than 1% of the psychiatric outpatient population have an obsessional compulsive disorder.

Some of the more interesting epidemiological characteristics are revealed when the overall data for age of onset are broken down according to specific conditions. Table 9.1 shows the points for the mean age of onset of a range of phobic and obsessional disorders.

### Phobias

The majority of simple phobias such as animal, blood and dental phobias begin in childhood, with the animal phobias typically arising earliest. It must be noted though that emotional disorders are quite common in childhood and are associated with a range of feared objects and situations. However, these emotional disorders tend to be transient and show only modest continuity across time (e.g. Rutter 1984), but if they do continue into adulthood they are homotypic or consistent in their presentation. As noted earlier, there is a preponderance of phobias in women, but this is especially true of animal phobias, for which Marks (1969) estimated that 95% of those affected were women.

Social phobia tends to occur in the teenage years, with a mean age of onset of 16.3 years reported by Ost (1987) in his study of phobics. Some studies have reported slightly higher incidences of social phobia amongst women, for example, both Marks (1969) and Bourdon *et al.* (1988) found approximately 60% of social phobics to be women. However, the increase for women in the Bourdon *et al.* study was not significant and, given that the sample size was over 18 500, suggests that the sex ratio is approximately equivalent in social phobia. Social phobia tends to be seen less often in the clinic than is agoraphobia, because unlike the latter condition there tends to be few additional symptoms in social phobia and it is not so debilitating (Mannuzza *et al.* 1990).

Claustrophobia has been considered to be a simple phobia (e.g. Ost 1987) but its typical age of onset is about age 20 years, which places it considerably later than the animal, blood and dental phobias. One suggestion, therefore, is that it is more akin to agoraphobia and could be a mild variant of it (Klein 1981).

Agoraphobia is the main phobia seen in the clinic despite its greater rarity than simple phobias, because it is usually associated with a wider range of other psychological problems (e.g. Watts 1988). The majority of agoraphobics are women who constitute 75–90% of cases (Marks 1969); the typical age of onset is in the late twenties. As a number of authors have pointed out, in many respects it is not a true phobia; its literal meaning 'fear of the market-place' does not capture its presentation which is more typically separation from a source of security accompanied by panic attacks (e.g. Hallam 1978, Noyes *et al.* 1986).

**Table 9.2** Percentage of phobics reporting either conditioning or modelling/instruction onsets for their disorders (based on Ost 1987)

|  | Agoraphobia | Social | Claustrophobia | Animal | Blood | Dental |
|---|---|---|---|---|---|---|
| Conditioning | 81% | 58% | 67% | 48% | 45% | 68% |
| Modelling or instruction | 8% | 17% | 17% | 40% | 38% | 19% |

### Obsessional disorders

The typical age of onset of obsessional disorders tends to be in the early twenties, though Minichiello *et al.* (1990) found the onset of checking and mixed obsessional disorders to occur at about 18–19 years, with cleaning and rumination disorders occurring later at about 27 years. The majority of cleaning obsessionals tend to be female, though there is a greater preponderance of males in the small number of childhood onsets (Rachman & Hodgson 1980). If obsessions do arise in childhood, they can be consistent into adulthood (Rutter 1984).

## Current approaches

### Phobias

For some time the dominant psychological model of phobia acquisition and maintenance was the so-called two-factor theory (Mowrer 1939). This theory stated that classical conditioning occurred between a Conditioned Stimulus (CS) and an Unconditioned Stimulus (US) and that this subsequently led to escape from or avoidance of the CS; for example, if a dog (the CS) bit a child, the child might learn to avoid dogs because of the traumatic experience. Although the two-factor theory was found to fit some phobias, it was realized that not all phobias are acquired in this manner. In many cases the individual has had no direct contact with the feared object or situation, such as in the case of snakes or aeroplanes. Nor do traumatic experiences necessarily lead to the development of phobias. A further problem for the conditioning model is that under laboratory conditions fear normally extinguishes rapidly when the CS is presented repeatedly without reinforcement, yet, for example, animal phobics

may have had their phobias for many years without ever having experienced a traumatic conditioning event.

The proposed resolution to the problems with the two-factor theory was that there are three pathways to fear (e.g. Rachman 1990a). The first is through the conditioning method outlined by Mowrer (1939). The second is through vicarious acquisition or modelling, that is, through the observation of another individual acting fearfully in the presence of a particular object or situation. And the third is through the provision of information or instruction that might lead to a fearful reaction. In practice, though, modelling and instruction are likely to occur together and could be considered to be two different aspects of a single mechanism; for example, if a child's mother acts fearfully in the presence of a dog, she is likely to instruct the child about taking precautions in the presence of dogs.

One of the main ways in which the three pathways to fear hypothesis has been tested is through the questioning of phobics about the onset of their disorders. Although there is considerable disagreement between different studies about the relative contributions of the different pathways, the recent data from Hekmat (1987) on the acquisition of animal phobias and from Ost (1987) on a wider range of phobias provide some interesting clues. The figures in Table 9.2 show that individuals are very likely to ascribe the late-onset agoraphobia to an aversive event, whereas early-onset animal and blood phobias were more evenly distributed between conditioning and modelling/instruction explanations. In fact, instruction onsets had the lowest mean age (mean = 9 years), modelling next (mean = 13 years), and last were the conditioning explanations (mean = 19 years). An important point, however, which will be expanded upon later is that even though a phobic or obsessional individual links the onset of the disorder to an aversive event this does not necessarily implicate a conditioning mechanism; care must be taken, therefore, not to accept these interpretations unquestioningly.

In a more detailed study of animal phobias Hekmat (1987) found that only 22.5% of individuals reported aversive encounters, though a further 36% reported that 'being teased' with the appropriate animal was the significant factor. Overall, Hekmat found that 57% of his sample attributed onset to instruction/modelling; 50% of males and 33.3% of females identified the mother as the prime source of the transmission of negative information. This finding is reminiscent of Aubrey Lewis' (1942) classic report to the Medical Research Council on the effects of bombing on the civilian population during World War II, in which he concluded that it was not the bombing itself that led to symptoms but 'frightened mothers who communicated their fears to the children'.

### Obsessional disorders

The evidence relevant to the aetiology of obsessional disorders is sparse. A number of studies have suggested that it is typically a problem arising in late adolescence or early adulthood with a sudden onset following a stressful event. However, the division into the two main varieties of checkers and cleaners reveals some differences. As noted in Table 9.1, checkers tend to be male and have an earlier onset of a more gradual nature, whereas cleaners tend to be female with a later sudden onset (e.g. Rachman & Hodgson 1980). The events associated with sudden onset in women are sometimes connected with first pregnancy and the transition to motherhood, and the gradual onset in men may be connected with increases in responsibility in work or social settings. However, the evidence tends to be of a clinical and anecdotal nature and warrants more systematic research. Rachman & Hodgson (1980) did of course comment on a number of patients who were exceptions to these rules, one of whom reported the gradual onset of a cleaning compulsion in relation to any word or photograph or object

associated with the city of Birmingham.

The types of events (e.g. conditioning events versus life events) and the types of vulnerability may be different for the different disorders; nevertheless, the recognition of the importance of sudden events in the onset of phobias and obsessions provides a strong link with the diathesis-stress models that are frequently considered in medicine in general, and which are almost always implicated in social psychiatry. Since the early work of Adolf Meyer the importance of life events in the onset and maintenance of disorders has been well recognized. Brown and his colleagues (e.g. Brown & Harris 1978) have developed this type of vulnerability model for depression and have shown that the majority of depressions are preceded by the occurrence of severe life events. However, the important point is that of the many people who experience severe events, only a proportion become clinically depressed; these at-risk individuals show a range of current psychosocial vulnerabilities such as lack of an intimate relationship (e.g. Champion 1990), and a range of distal vulnerabilities such as inadequate care in childhood (e.g. Harris *et al.* 1986).

The vulnerability-stress model that has proven very successful in its application to depression has not yet been developed in the area of obsessions and phobias despite the obvious pointers from the pathways to fear approach and from the clinical accounts of these conditions. In their review of life events and anxiety disorders in general, Monroe & Wade (1988) argued that overall there was evidence for *some* association between life events and the occurrence of anxiety disorders, but that the failure so far to look at subtypes of the disorder made it difficult to arrive at any definite conclusions. For example, in a study that needs independent replication Finlay-Jones & Brown (1981) found that life events that were characterized by 'danger' or 'threat' tended to lead to the onset of anxiety, whereas events that involved severe loss were more likely to lead to depression.

In view of the evidence presented earlier (see Table 9.2) of the high proportion of 'conditioning' or traumatic experience explanations offered by agoraphobics, it is not surprising that this is the one disorder where some systematic evidence has been collected. Although this research was separate in origin to life events research, both areas have converged in their focus on the quality of the marital relationship in combination with stress experienced within it. One of the first of the 'poor marriage' interpretations of agoraphobia was offered by Goldstein & Chambless (1978), who found that whereas almost 63% of their group of agoraphobics reported an interpersonal precipitant, only 3% of a group of simple phobics did so. However, although the poor marriage explanation of agoraphobia has been considered as an explanation for both the onset and the maintenance of agoraphobia, the evidence so far would seem equivocal (e.g. Watts 1988). For example, Arrindell & Emmelkamp (1986) assessed 30 female agoraphobics and their partners on a range of measures of marital quality and compared them to non-phobic psychiatric, maritally distressed, and happily married comparison couples. The results showed that the agoraphobic couples rated their marriages overall better than the psychiatic and distressed couples, and sometimes as good as the happily married couples. Perhaps one of the problems that may lead to inconsistent findings is the reliance on clinic attendance for samples; thus, it is clear that less than a quarter of phobics receive treatment, and that there is a considerable overrepresentation of agoraphobics amongst referred phobics (e.g. Boyd *et al.* 1990). A more general interpretation might therefore be offered for agoraphobia which focused on an overall sensitivity to interpersonal stress of which marital stress is one variety. For example, Last (1988) reported that in her study of 58 agoraphobics 81% had a precipitating event; 29% of these events related to the death or serious illness of a significant other, whereas 35% followed a birth, miscarriage or hysterectomy. Indirect evidence in support of a sensitivity to interpersonal stress also comes from the views of Mathews *et al.* (1981) and Rachman (1990a). Mathews and his colleagues argued that agoraphobics have an avoidant–dependent coping style. Rachman, in a separate but related proposal, has argued that the dependency arises from the agoraphobic's core fear that his or her health or well-being is threatened, but the presence of a

trusted other tips the balance in favour of safety over danger.

The question of vulnerability in agoraphobia and other phobias has been addressed even less that the question of the role of stress. Retrospective reports from adult agoraphobics suggest that they have experienced more separation anxiety in childhood (e.g. Monroe & Wade 1988), but as Rutter (e.g. 1984) has pointed out about anxiety disorders in general, there are only modest continuities over time; thus, anxious children can become well adults, and well children can become anxious adults. Nevertheless, there is *some* overall association between family factors and the occurrence of anxiety and obsessional disorders in significant family members. For example, Aubrey Lewis (1942) pointed to two mechanisms noted in his report on war-torn Britain; first, through the mechanism noted earlier that 'frightened mothers communicated their fears to the children'; and, second, that 'the terrors of an actual air-raid have proved less important than the disruption of homes, and other secondary effects of bombing'. Lewis, therefore, identified two social mechanisms, one a potential childhood vulnerability, and the second the disruption of current roles and networks through the experience of severe stress. Both mechanisms also illustrate the fact that it is when acute stress leads to chronic longer-term adversity that disorder is more likely to occur, for example, when the early loss of a significant care-taker is compounded by a subsequent lack of care because no adequate substitute care-taker is available (e.g. Rutter 1984).

Some evidence indirectly supporting these proposals has been obtained from family prevalence studies. Berg (1976) reported that the children of agoraphobic women showed an increase in school phobia (14% at 11–15 years). Last (1988) reported that 83% of mothers of children with separation anxiety disorder had a lifetime history of anxiety disorder, and 57% had an anxiety disorder concurrent with the child's. However, children with school phobia were mostly male, postpubertal, and of a higher socio-economic status than children with separation anxiety, and much lower rates of disorder were found in mothers of school phobics than in mothers of separation anxiety children. Noyes *et al.* (1986) in their family study of 40 agoraphobic probands found that 9.4% of the relatives of agoraphobics also had agoraphobia and 34.7% had an anxiety disorder of some type; however, the increase in morbidity risk was three times greater for female relatives than for males. Finally, Rachman (1990b) reported that, overall, studies of fears in children and their mothers show correlations of between 0.65 and 0.74 in normal circumstances. One of the factors that Rachman points to is that where few other individuals are available to the young child and the relationship with the main caretaker is very close, phobias and obsessions are more likely to be transmitted to the child. Similarly, in such cases children may be given incorrect information about, for example, bodily states that makes them more likely to make catastrophic misinterpretations (Clark 1986) and experience panic attacks.

To summarize, there are a number of converging lines of evidence that provide some clues to the aetiology of phobias and obsessions. Retrospective studies of phobic and obsessional patients suggest that both childhood and recent stressful events play some role, but, in addition, a close tie with an anxious or obsessional individual is also likely to be significant. There are, however, important contributions from the individual's developmental stage: in the next section, therefore, an attempt will be made to link the findings that have been presented so far with the level of psychosocial development that the individual has reached.

### A developmental framework: some speculations

One of the most significant aspects of the epidemiology of phobias and obsessions arises from consideration of the data on gender and age of onset. These patterns prompt questions about the biological, psychological, and social tasks that the individual must face during development and whether different tasks at different stages lead to different risks. This life-span development approach is in many ways still in its infancy, nevertheless, it is possible to make some crude statements about the tasks that individuals face and to speculate about whether there might be any

implications for phobias and obsessional disorders. The argument is not that life-style is the only cause nor even the most important cause, but, rather, that it may contribute to risk or protection and therefore the likelihood of the onset of a disorder.

An important observation of the life-span approach is that the life-cycle includes norms for when certain events or transitions should occur, together with boundaries for their optimum timing; in effect there is a 'social clock' (Neugarten 1979) that defines whether an event or transition occurs at an optimum time or occurs 'off-time'. To give an example, figures for the early transition to motherhood show that there are significant class differences, with 17% of women in classes IV and V having their first child in their teens, but only 2% of women in classes I and II (Joshi 1985). The occurrence of early pregnancy, therefore, is more likely to occur in already disadvantaged groups; it is likely to lead to further restrictions in the options that a woman has in other domains of her life (Maughan & Champion 1991), and it is another step on the road to depression (e.g. Quinton & Rutter 1985, Harris *et al.* 1987).

A useful framework in which to view the importance of transitions has been provided by Champion (e.g. Maughan & Champion 1990, Champion & Power 1992). The proposal is that there are a number of domains such as work, personal relationships, and the capacity for independent living which must be viewed from a life-span perspective: the occurrence of events and transitions in one domain may have significant implications for the remaining domains and may either increase or decrease the available options. Tasks or transitions within domains are socially prescribed, as are moves through the life-course. Each life-stage can be characterized by key transitions in each domain, but the relative importance of each domain varies with life-stage, sex, social class, and so on. Those domains which are most important therefore may contribute most to the risk of certain disorders.

A preliminary application of this framework to the area of phobias and obsessions is presented in Table 9.3. The diagram shows three domains, some of the developmental tasks and transitions

**Table 9.3** A crude outline of the approximate age of transitions in a number of domains, together with some possible associated phobias or obsessions

| Domain | Age (years) | | | | | | |
|---|---|---|---|---|---|---|---|
| | 0 | 5 | 10 | 15 | 20 | 25 | 30 |
| Capacity for independent living | Biological dependency/vulnerability (Animal/blood/dental phobias) | | | | Biological sufficiency/independence | | |
| Personal relationships | Attachment | School peers | Peer attachments (Social phobia) | | Love relationships (Claustrophobia) | Marriage/parenthood (Agoraphobia/cleaning obsessions) | |
| Work | Basic skills | School | | | Work/further education (Checking obsessions) | Work | |

in each domain, and the age of onset data for phobias and obsessions presented earlier in Table 9.1.

The first set of early animal, blood and dental phobias typically occur at a time when the child is biologically dependent on an attachment figure; the combination of biological vulnerability plus the need to develop survival skills makes the mother or other care-taker as significant in the teaching of emotional reactions as in the teaching of, for example, language and communication skills. An additional factor that may be relevant to these fears is Seligman's (1970) concept of 'preparedness', that is, the proposal that there may be innate, possibly species-specific, predisposing factors that contribute to the widespread occurrence and early onset of these fears. Although Seligman's proposal has subsequently received less consideration following a number of unexceptional laboratory experiments, Rachman (1990a) has recently suggested that the idea should be exhumed and given a fairer trial. It is clear that fears of insects and animals decline significantly with age, probably, as Rachman suggests, because the child's own growth in strength and competence leads to a shedding of such fears. An interesting possibility therefore is that the preponderance of adult female animal phobics is not so much due to

different rates of onset of such fears in boys versus girls, but rather that boys are encouraged more in our culture to overcome such early fears because their reactions are not 'boylike'.

The second type of disorder is social phobias. These phobias have an onset in adolescence and may be a consequence of the increasing importance of peer relationships and the relative decrease in emphasis or focus on family relationships in the personal relationships domain. A slightly earlier phobia that is preponderant in boys is school phobia, though as noted earlier these boys are often of higher socioeconomic status. The latter observation would suggest that school phobias are possibly related to the overvaluation of the work domain in higher socioeconomic status families. Indeed, as noted above, the early-onset checking obsessions are also preponderant in males and often occur because of an increase in responsibilities around the time of transitions in the work domain (e.g. Rachman & Hodgson 1980).

The other disorder with an onset in late teens or early twenties is claustrophobia; the onset data suggest that it is not a simple phobia even though it is classified as such. One speculation is that it occurs because of problems in the domain of personal relationships at a time when the normative transition is towards one-to-one love attachments; some evidence that could be interpreted as support for this alternative is that the divorce rates tend to be higher in claustrophobia than in other phobias (Ost 1987). Other related findings are that in contrast to agoraphobics, claustrophobics do not benefit from the presence of a trusted person when they are anxious, and, similarly, they seldom seek professional help for their problems. Rachman (1990a) suggests that like simple phobias there may be an innate or 'preparedness' factor, but the finding that claustrophobia responds quickly in therapy might suggest the contrary. The present proposal does not deny that the main presenting complaints in claustrophobia are fear of suffocation and/or fear of enclosure, but, rather, that a number of other characteristics of the problem demand a more sophisticated account than is typically provided. Indeed, as a tailnote to this putative link, it might be noted that in Erikson's (e.g. 1980) theory of psychosocial development, the stage from 20 years onwards of young adulthood has as its central developmental 'crisis' the resolution of issues of intimacy versus isolation; the conflict between intimacy and suffocation may contribute to the increased appearance of claustrophobia at this stage, though as Rachman (1990a) points out, there is little evidence as yet for this symbolic link.

Both agoraphobia and cleaning obsessions predominate in women and both tend to follow severe events in the interpersonal domain. Although as noted earlier there is a tradition of linking agoraphobia with poor marriages, it is possible that an additional factor may be the transition to parenthood as much as it is to marriage. For example, Last (1988) reported that 35% of the precipitating events in a sample of agoraphobics were births, miscarriages or hysterectomies. Rachman (1990a) also points out that a period of being housebound, which typically occurs after a birth but which could also follow a significant loss, may lead to a weakening of the effectiveness of safety signals and procedures because of lack of repetition and practice. Indeed, it was also noted earlier that cleaning obsessions often have a sudden onset following the transition to parenthood: the normal perinatal increased attention to

cleanliness which occurs in most women presumably catapults the vulnerable woman into an extreme state that is difficult to escape from. In contrast to claustrophobics who have the highest divorce rates, agoraphobics typically have the highest rates for marriage and the lowest rates for being single (Ost 1987); one of the issues for agoraphobics, therefore, may not simply be whether they can remain proximal to an individual who can make them feel secure in the face of threats to their health or well-being, but also whether they in turn can provide safety for an individual who is dependent on them in the way that a child might be.

The purpose of this section has been to raise questions about some of the epidemiological evidence about phobias and obsessions in relation to a life-span developmental perspective. The framework presented is approximate and in need of considerable refinement. Notwithstanding this problem, it seems a useful framework and one onto which a greater range of childhood, adolescent and adult disorders can be mapped in addition to those considered here. For example, conduct disorders, eating disorders, parasuicides and depression all have interesting age of onset and gender differences that could also be mapped onto Table 9.3 in order to provide a fuller picture of how problems in transitions in different domains lead to increased risks of disorders. We must await future research, however, before the details can be filled in.

### Social factors in therapy

It is not the intention of this section to provide a detailed account of social factors in therapy, because such factors are not specific to therapy for phobias and obsessions. Leff (see Chapter 1) has also pointed out that the two original strands of social psychiatry, namely, epidemiology and social therapy, diverged to the point where epidemiology alone became the only true heir. Nevertheless, this section is partly designed as a reminder that the one essential factor that seems to be necessary for successful outcome in therapy is that there is a good therapeutic relationship whatever type of therapy is being considered (e.g.

Frank 1982). The importance of this therapeutic relationship, however, has been traditionally underplayed or even denied in the more technique-oriented behaviour therapies.

Perhaps the most successful application of the behaviour therapies has been to the treatment of obsessions and phobias: meta-analyses of outcome studies show significant clinical improvement in something of the order of 70% of cases. The fact, however, that behaviour therapists have played down the role of the therapeutic relationship is paradoxical even from within behavioural therapy. This paradox stems from the identification by Rachman and others of two of the pathways to fear: namely, modelling by a significant other, and information or instruction typically provided by the mother. For example, in a recent cognitive approach to panic Clark (1986) has emphasized the importance of correcting the patient's catastrophic misinterpretations of internal states. It is likely that incorrect information may have been given to such individuals by significant others (cf. Rachman 1990b), which can only be corrected if the therapist is seen to be both trustworthy and credible. Although it is obviously unethical to study the acquisition of phobias, Mineka's (e.g. Mineka 1987) work with the acquisition of fear in Rhesus monkeys has similarly emphasized that fear is easily acquired through modelling if it is the infant's parent who is reacting in a fearful manner in the presence of a snake.

One of the disorders in which there has been great interest in the importance of social factors in treatment is agoraphobia. The home-based programme devised by Mathews *et al.* (1981) normally includes enlistment of the spouse or a close friend or relative in the treatment; the results show improved outcome particularly over a follow-up period. The involvement of a spouse or friend in therapy obviously provides benefits at a number of levels above and beyond the behavioural treatment itself. A similar improvement in therapeutic effectiveness has been found with the use of group treatment for agoraphobia, especially if the group becomes cohesive (Watts 1988). Again, social factors operate at various levels within cohesive groups; patients are provided with a range of information and instruction, modelling experiences, exposure treatment, and the powerful effects of factors such as 'universality' identified by Yalom (1986). Social influences can of course work in both directions and either facilitate or inhibit fear; thus, in view of the speculations considered earlier about the possible conflicts about intimacy present in claustrophobics, it might be predicted that a group approach would be less successful in their case.

In addition to the social influences within the therapeutic relationship, it is also necessary to look at the social context within which the problem exists and to ask whether therapy can overcome any of these more general problems. The extent of these problems does of course vary with the type of phobia or obsession and with its severity; thus, circumscribed simple phobias need have no effect on the individual's social roles and relationships apart from perhaps limited avoidance of a specific object or situation. In contrast, a severe agoraphobic or obsessional disorder may damage a wide range of personal, family and work roles and relationships. In their summary of the literature, Watts & Bennett (1983) found that although behaviour therapy for obsessional and phobic disorders often had positive effects on work and leisure roles, there was little effect on personal and family relationships when problems already existed in these domains. From his summary of the work with obsessional disorders Reed (1985) concluded that the majority continued to work and have satisfactory social relationships, in particular when there was improvement from therapy. However, the majority of the more severe disorders and those who did not respond to treatment had unsatisfactory social relationships and were unable to sustain a work role. One of the morals of this tale therefore is that the individual's range of available roles and relationships should be carefully assessed in order to determine whether there have been restrictions due to the disorder; for example, part of the rehabilitation of the housebound agoraphobic should include the exploration of meaningful work and leisure roles in addition to tackling the fears about health and well-being.

## Final comments and conclusions

The dominant theories and treatment approaches to phobias and obsessions are psychological in nature. However, a brief look at the types of factors that are implicated in the onset, maintenance and treatment of phobias reveals the importance of social factors and how these interact with psychological ones. For example, the combination of age of onset with the gender differences and data on method of acquisition suggests that there is a significant developmental context in which phobias, obsessions and other disorders may be understood. This approach can at minimum provide a more sophisticated framework for clinical work and research. However, the fact that there is no single pathway to the onset and maintenance of fear must also have implications for treatment; the emphasis within acquisition on the role of significant others as the source of information, modelling and traumatic experiences indicates that the therapist also plays multiple functions in therapy, that effective therapy must occur in the context of a good therapeutic relationship, and that the therapist must also address the social context in which the disorder occurs.

## Acknowledgements

The pathways to temptation are even more numerous than the pathways to fear. I must thank my friends and colleagues Lorna Champion and Fraser Watts for pointing out when my temptations have been excessive, and I take full responsibility for the places where I have ignored their sound advice.

## References

Arrindell W.A. & Emmelkamp P.M.G. (1986) Marital adjustment, intimacy and needs in female agoraphobics and their partners: a controlled study. *British Journal of Psychiatry* 149, 592–602.

Berg I. (1976) School phobia in the children of agoraphobic women. *British Journal of Psychiatry* 128, 86–89.

Bourdon K.H., Boyd J.H., Rae D.S., Burns B.J., Thompson J.W. & Locke B.Z. (1988) Gender differences in phobias: results of the ECA Community survey. *Journal of Anxiety Disorders* 2, 227–241.

Boyd J.H., Rae D.S., Thompson J.W., Burns B.J., Bourdon K., Locke B.Z. & Regier D.A. (1990) Phobia: prevalence and risk factors. *Social Psychiatry and Psychiatric Epidemiology* 25, 314–323.

Brown G.W. & Harris T. (1978) *Social Origins of Depression*. Tavistock, London.

Champion L. (1990) The relationship between social vulnerability and the occurrence of severely threatening life events. *Psychological Medicine* 20, 157–162.

Champion L. & Power M.J. (1992) *Cognitive Approaches to Depression: Towards A New Synthesis* (submitted).

Clark D.M. (1986) A cognitive approach to panic. *Behaviour Research and Therapy* 24, 461–470.

Erikson E.H. (1980) *Identity and the Life Cycle: A Reissue*. W.W. Norton, New York.

Finlay-Jones R. & Brown G.W. (1981) Types of stressful life event and the onset of anxiety and depressive disorders. *Psychological Medicine* 11, 803–815.

Frank J. (1982) Therapeutic components shared by all psychotherapies. In Harvey J.H. & Parks M.M. (eds) *Psychotherapy Research and Behaviour Change*. APA, Washington.

Freud S. (1896) The aetiology of hysteria. In Jones E. (ed.) *The Standard Edition*, vol. 3. Hogarth Press, London.

Freud S. (1909) Analysis of a phobia in a five-year-old boy. In A. Richards (ed.) *The Penguin Freud Library*, vol. 8. Penguin, Harmondsworth.

Goldstein A.J. & Chambless D.L. (1978) A reanalysis of agoraphobia. *Behaviour Therapy* 9, 47–59.

Hallam R.S. (1978) Agoraphobia: a critical review of the concept. *British Journal of Psychiatry* 133, 314–319.

Harris T., Brown G.W. & Bifulco A. (1986) Loss of parent in childhood and adult psychiatric disorder: the role of lack of adequate parental care. *Psychological Medicine* 16, 641–659.

Harris T., Brown G.W. & Bifulco A. (1987) Loss of parent in childhood and adult psychiatric disorder: the role of social class position and premarital pregnancy. *Psychological Medicine* 17, 163–183.

Hekmat H. (1987) Origins and development of human fear reactions. *Journal of Anxiety Disorders* 1, 197–218.

Joshi H. (1985) Motherhood and employment: change and continuity in post-war Britain. In *Measuring Socio-Demographic Change* (Occassional Paper 34). British Society for Population Studies, London.

Klein D.F. (1981) Anxiety reconceptualized. In Klein D.F. & Rabkin J. (eds) *Anxiety: New Research and Changing Concepts*. Raven Press, New York.

Last C.G. (1988) Anxiety disorders in childhood and adolescence. In Last C.G. & Hersen M. (eds) *Handbook of Anxiety Disorders*. Pergamon Press, New York.

Lewis A. (1942) Incidence of neurosis in England under war conditions. *Lancet* 15 August, 175–183.

Mannuzza S., Fyer A.J., Liebowitz M.R. & Klein D.F. (1990) Delineating the boundaries of social phobia: its relationship to panic disorder and agoraphobia. *Journal* of *Anxiety Disorders* 4, 41–59.

Marks I.M. (1969) *Fears and Phobias.* Academic Press, New York.

Mathews A.M., Gelder M.G. & Johnston D.W. (1981) *Agoraphobia: Nature and Treatment.* Guilford Press, New York.

Maughan B. & Champion L. (1990) Risk and protective factors in the transition to young adulthood. In Baltes P.B. & Baltes M.M. (eds) *Successful Ageing: Perspectives from the Behavioural Sciences.* Cambridge University Press, Cambridge.

Mineka S. (1987) A primate model of phobic fears. In Eysenck H.J. & Martin I. (eds) *Theoretical Foundations of Behaviour Therapy.* Plenum Press, New York.

Minichiello W.E., Baer L., Jenike M.A. & Holland A. (1990) Age of onset of major subtypes of obsessive-compulsive disorder. *Journal of Anxiety Disorders* 4, 147–150.

Monroe S.M. & Wade S.L. (1988) Life events. In Last C.G. & Hersen M. (eds) *Handbook of Anxiety Disorders.* Pergamon Press, New York.

Mowrer D.H. (1939) Stimulus response theory of anxiety. *Psychological Review* 46, 553–565.

Myers J.K., Weissman M.M., Tischler G.L. *et al.* (1984) Six-month prevalence of psychiatric disorders in three communities. *Archives of General Psychiatry* 41, 959–967.

Neugarten B.L. (1979) Time, age and life cycle. *American Journal of Psychiatry* 136, 887–894.

Noyes R., Crowe R.R., Harris E.L., Hamra B.J., McChesney C.M. & Chaudhry D.R. (1986) Relationship between panic disorder and agoraphobia: a family study. *Archives of General Psychiatry* 43, 227–232.

Ost L.G. (1987) Age of onset in different phobias. *Journal of Abnormal Psychology* 96, 223–229.

Quinton D. & Rutter M. (1985) Parenting behaviour of mothers raised 'in-care'. In Nicol A.R. (ed.) *Longitudinal Studies in Child Psychology and Psychiatry.* Wiley, New York.

Rachman S. (1990a) *Fear and Courage,* 2nd edn. W.H. Freeman, San Francisco.

Rachman S. (1990b) The determinants and treatment of simple phobias. *Advances in Behaviour Research and Therapy* 12, 1–30.

Rachman S. & Hodgson R. (1980) *Obsessions and Compulsions.* Prentice Hall, Englewood Cliffs, New Jersey.

Reed G.F. (1985) *Obsessional Experience and Compulsive Behaviour: A Cognitive–Structural Approach.* Academic Press, Orlando.

Rutter M. (1984) Psychopathology and development: 1. Childhood antecedents of adult psychiatric disorder. *Australian and New Zealand Journal of Psychiatry* 18, 225–234.

Salkovskis P.M. (1985) Obsessional-compulsive problems: a cognitive-behavioural analysis. *Behaviour Research and Therapy* 23, 571–583.

Seligman M.E.P. (1970) On the generality of the laws of learning. *Psychological Review* 77, 406–418.

Watson J.B. & Rayner P. (1920) Conditioned emotional reactions. *Journal of Experimental Psychology* 3, 1–14.

Watts F.N. (1988) Agoraphobia: the changing face of treatment. In Watts F.N. (ed.) *New Developments in Clinical Psychology,* vol. II. Wiley, Chichester.

Watts F.N. & Bennett D.H. (1983) Neurotic, affective, and conduct disorders. In Watts F.N. & Bennett D.H. (eds) *Theory and Practice of Psychiatric Rehabilitation.* Wiley, Chichester.

Yalom I.D. (1986) *Theory and Practice of Group Psychotherapy,* 3rd edn. Basic Books, New York.

# Chapter 10
# Life Events

FRANCIS CREED

## Introduction

In order to establish that life events cause psychiatric disorder it is necessary to fulfil the following criteria outlined by Cooke (1986) and Maes *et al.* (1987). First, there must be sufficiently clear statistical correlation between the life events and the onset of psychiatric disorder. Second, given such statistical correlation there must be evidence that life events lead to illness not the other way around. Third, a satisfactory theoretical construct must be found, indicating a specific relationship between life events and disorder, and one in which confounding variables, such as demographic or personality factors, are not responsible for the statistical relationship. Fourth, the relationship should hold across different populations at different times. Each of these aspects will be considered in this chapter and the life events prior to specific disorders will be considered.

## Statistical correlation between life events and onset of disorder

This relationship has been studied in two ways. Individual severe life events, such as bereavement, have been shown to be related to the onset of depression and physical disorders (Parkes 1964, Creed 1985). Alternatively recent onset of a psychiatric disorder can be shown to be associated with an excess of recent life events compared to a healthy control group. Such a demonstration requires a clear onset of disorder, a reliable measure of life events and adequate sample size.

The problems of obtaining a reliable measure of events has been the subject of many reviews (Brown & Harris 1978a, Cleary 1980, Paykel 1983, Dohrenwend *et al.* 1987, Brown 1989).

Dohrenwend *et al.* (1987) stated that there were very few case-control life event studies that 'meet even minimal criteria for adequacy', including use of appropriate controls, assessing which events and circumstances occur independently of the subjects' prior mental state and behaviour, and attempting to date the occurrence of events in relation to episodes of illness. Dohrenwend's statement comes about because 90% of life events research has used self-administered questionnaires, which simply ask respondents to tick life events they have experienced over recent months (Cohen & Wills 1985). Such questionnaires make no specific attempt to prompt respondents or check the accuracy of the replies (Jenkins *et al.* 1979); in one study 36% of the events elicited at a life events interview had been missed by a prior self-administered questionnaire (Klein & Rubovits 1987). In addition to this problem of recall, there is also a problem of vaguely worded items, such as 'serious illness in family member', which allows the respondent to use his own definitions of 'serious' and 'family member'. This may lead to biased measurement (see distorted recall below). Not surprisingly, therefore, questionnaires have been shown to be unreliable, with a test-retest reliability sometimes as low as 0.2 (Johnson & Sarason 1978, Steele *et al.* 1980).

The only alternative to these self-administered questionnaires is a life events interview which is usually lengthy and expensive in research time, but has an interinformant reliability of 75–92% (Hudgens *et al.* 1970, Brown *et al.* 1973). The Life Events and Difficulties Schedule (LEDS – Brown & Harris 1978a) is the most established and reliable interview in the UK and forms the basis of most of the research quoted in this chapter.

The criteria by which an instrument may be

**Table 10.1** Criteria for a satisfactory life events inventory as illustrated by the Life Events and Difficulties Schedule (LEDS)

---

1  Observer-based: previously defined criteria for inclusion of each event and research group determined rating of severity
2  Excludes symptoms *and* any illness-related events
3  Considers individual meaning of event using biographical and contextual details
4  Severity scale based on 'threat', both immediate and long term
5  No additivity assumed and subjects categorized as experiencing particular type of event or not
6  Exact timing of events, which can be compared with time of onset
7  Allows fall-off of reporting to be measured
8  Events and difficulties rating as separate aetiological agents

---

judged to provide a reliable measure of life events are listed in Table 10.1. The aspect of reliability to be considered in this section will be accurate recall. Exact dating and independence of events will be dealt with in the next section.

### Accurate recall

Accurate recall can be checked by comparing the number of events recalled over recent weeks with the number recalled over more distant time periods. A considerable 'fall-off' of reported events in the time periods most distant from the interview suggest poor recall. The rate of fall-off with self-administered questionnaires is unacceptable – about 5% per month, which amounts to 30% over a six-month period. This compares with fall-off rates of only 1% per month using the interviews of Paykel (1983) and the LEDS, provided that the interviewer has been adequately trained (Brown & Harris 1982). Training is necessary as in untrained hands the LEDS may have a high rate of fall-off (Schmid *et al.* 1981).

For severe events, which can more readily be remembered, the rate of fall-off is even less – 0.36% per month for a new German interview method (Wittchen *et al.* 1989) and as low as 2.9%

*per year* with the LEDS over a ten-year retrospective study (Neilson *et al.* 1989). Such a low rate of fall-off is possible because interviewers take considerable trouble to prompt the person's memory using probes and reminders (e.g. Brown & Harris 1978a, Wittchen *et al.* 1989). Without aids to memory fewer events are recalled and inconsistencies occur in dating of events and their relevant details (Sobell *et al.* 1990).

Without such accurate recall it is impossible to study life events prior to illness onset and overcome the bias of ill subjects to record more events than a healthy group ('effort after meaning' – see below).

There is some evidence that a short interview can be reliable, although there is bound to be some loss of information (Miller & Salter 1984). The list of threatening experiences is based on the fact that most threatening events were found in 12 categories of life events (severe illness to subject, severe illness or death of close relative, marital separation, unemployment, etc.) (Brugha *et al.* 1985). Events in these categories accounted for 92% of the marked or moderately threatening events in the full interview. On this basis a much shorter interview was derived in which the respondent is only asked about events in these 12 categories (Brugha *et al.* 1985). The instrument demonstrated a significant difference between depressed patients and controls, but the difference was less pronounced than would be expected with experience using the full instrument (Brugha & Conroy 1985). The disadvantage with this instrument is that it has only been derived for a particular population – it may not be used in other populations without checking in which categories the majority of severe events occur.

### Distorted recall

One reason that self-administered questionnaires may be inaccurate is the influence of current mood state on recall. Depressed subjects may examine their recent life experience in order to find a reason for the development of their illness. This 'effort after meaning' may lead to a spuriously high rate of events being recorded for the weeks prior to illness onset, providing an apparent relationship between negative life events and depression.

Experimental manipulation of mood in college students can mimic this effect; depressed mood state was associated with more negative life events and fewer social supports being reported (Cohen *et al.* 1988). Strict definition of events and careful interviewing can overcome this tendency for 'effort after meaning', and the Munich group were able to demonstrate similar and satisfactory results for discharged depressed and schizophrenic patients whether or not they still had significant psychiatric symptoms (Wittchen *et al.* 1989).

There is nothing that a self-administered questionnaire can do about this potential artefact. The research interviewer, on the other hand, uses probe questions, reminders and strictly defined events to ensure that both ·experimental and comparison groups recall events in an identical fashion. The LEDS requires training to become familiar with the detailed criteria for each event. For example, being off work has to last four weeks or more to be included as an event affecting the respondent; if it is the breadwinner in the respondent's household who is off work, the minimum time is eight weeks.

## Basic life events results in depression and schizophrenia

The first LEDS study compared 50 schizophrenic patients at relapse with 325 normal subjects, assessing life events over the preceding three months (Brown & Birley 1968). During the three weeks immediately prior to the relapse 60% of the schizophrenic patients had experienced an event compared to 20% of the controls. The latter figure was similar to the 'usual' rate over the previous weeks (Table 10.2), indicating the close association between experience of event and relapse of the schizophrenia. This increase was recorded for all types of events; thus relatively minor events, such as promotion or an uncomplicated house move, were associated with the relapse of schizophrenia.

The next major study concerned depression; for this purpose 114 inpatients and outpatients attending the Maudsley Hospital and 37 women in the community with recent onset of depression were compared with 382 normal women in the community (Brown & Harris 1978a). Life events were elicited for a full 12 months prior to the onset of the depression, or before the interview

Table 10.2 Percentage with at least one event in the four 3-week periods before onset (schizophrenic patients, $n = 50$) and interview (general population, $n = 325$)

|  | 3-week periods before onset/interview | | | |
|---|---|---|---|---|
|  | Furthest 4th* | 3rd* | 2nd* | 1st[†] |
| *Independent events* |  |  |  |  |
| Schizophrenic patients | 14 | 8 | 14 | 46 |
| General population | 15 | 15 | 14 | 14 |
| *Possibly independent events* |  |  |  |  |
| Schizophrenic patients | 16 | 10 | 6 | 22 |
| General population | 6 | 5 | 5 | 5 |
| *All events* |  |  |  |  |
| Schizophrenic patients | 30 | 18 | 20 | 60 |
| General population | 21 | 20 | 18 | 19 |

* No differences are significant.

[†] $P < 0.001$ in all three groups.

in the case of healthy comparison women. The results were again clear. During the 38 weeks prior to the onset of depression (or date of interview) 61% of depressed patients (68% of depressed women in the community) had experienced a *severe* event compared to 20% of controls ($P < 0.001$). The difference between depressed subjects and controls held for the three weeks immediately prior to onset but did *not* hold for all events, or those of mild/no threat; it was only events with a severe threat which were more common among the depressed group.

## Life events and illness onset – the direction of causation

Once it has been established that events and illness onset are significantly associated, it is necessary to establish the direction of causality between them. This is done by examining the temporal relationship of events and illness onset and by excluding any events that might result from the illness rather than cause it. (The latter task includes checking that the apparent statistical relationship between events and illness onset is not an artefact due to biased measurement.)

### Temporal relationship

It is not sufficiently appreciated that the life events research method is only really applicable for illnesses that have a clear dateable onset. Only under these circumstances can the researcher be sure events *prior* to onset are being considered in the aetiology of the illness. Some physical illnesses are ideal in this respect as the onset of pain leading to appendectomy (Creed 1981) or indicating myocardial infarction (Connolly 1976) can usually be established within a few hours. The onset or relapse of schizophrenia can be ascertained with reasonable certainty (Brown & Birley 1968, Day *et al.* 1987). The onset of depression in the community is more difficult, so Brown & Harris (1978a) spent considerable time with their respondents checking the dates of onset and events using diaries and anchor dates such as Christmas and bank holidays to establish exact dating of each. In this way it could be ascertained whether a relevant event preceded or followed the onset of illness. Such checking is, of course, impossible with a self-administered questionnaire.

In order to determine whether life events precede or follow the onset of an illness, the latter must be accurately established (Craufurd *et al.* 1990, Sclare & Creed 1990). Too often in life events research the date of being seen at a clinic, for example for back pain (Leavitt *et al.* 1979), or the date of admission, for example for mania (Kennedy *et al.* 1983, Ambelas 1987), is taken as the point of onset, when the illness may have been present for some days or weeks prior to the hospital attendance. In each case the researcher runs the risk of including events such as 'being off work' or 'having difficulties in close relationships', which occurred *after* the back pain or mania commenced. It would be quite fallacious to attribute the illness to such events.

### Independence of events and illness

In addition to the concern about correct timing of events and illness onset, there remains the possibility that events occurring shortly before the illness were due to subtle changes resulting from the developing illness. This problem is overcome by including only events which can definitely be regarded as independent of the developing illness. Thus loss of job through factory closure represents an event that is clearly independent of a developing schizophrenic episode, whereas loss of job in other circumstances might represent declining performance due to insidious illness onset (Brown & Birley 1968). In the study previously mentioned the proportion of schizophrenic patients and controls who had experienced an independent event during the three weeks prior to onset were 46% and 14%, respectively (Table 10.2). This indicated that the significant result mentioned above was not simply due to events which might have resulted from the developing schizophrenia. The proportions in the depression study who had experienced an independent event were 50%, 57% and 16% respectively for hospital patients, depressed women in the community and comparison subjects.

A self-administered questionnaire has, of

course, no way of subdividing events into independent and possibly independent categories. In fact, some questionnaires include both a large number of potentially illness-related events, for example 'experiencing difficulties at work', and also a number of actual symptoms, for example 'change in sleeping and eating habits' (Holmes & Rahe 1967).

Consideration of those life events independent of a developing illness is a necessary step in indicating the true relationship between life event experience and illness onset. It does *not* imply that independent life events are the only ones associated with onset of illness – marital separation, for example, is not an independent event but may be associated with the onset of depression (Miller *et al.* 1986).

### Dose–response relationships

Cooke (1986) has argued, like Susser (1973), that a linear relationship between dose (events) and response (e.g. depression) is persuasive of a causal relationship. Cooke quotes two community studies which support this hypothesis (Miller & Ingham 1979, Cooke 1981). Such studies assessed the number of depressive symptoms and found an association between symptom score and number of recent threatening situations.

This is a complicated issue because two different questions are being examined. The cross-sectional studies quoted by Cook inevitably included some subjects with established depression, in whom life events occurring *after* the onset of the depression were included. In these subjects the events probably exacerbate the pre-existing depression; so more events are found in those with most symptoms. On the other hand, Brown and colleagues have primarily been concerned with events prior to the onset of depression and pose a different question – do a greater number of events increase the chances of depression occurring (Brown & Harris 1989e)? To examine this issue in depth requires consideration of how life events are scored.

All life event scoring systems accept that the experience of bereavement is different from that of a routine job change. The Schedule of Recent Experience (SRE) used the concept of 'life change units': death of spouse scored 100 whereas a job change was awarded 36 (Holmes & Rahe 1967). Although there was widespread agreement about the scores awarded to particular events, this approach failed to take account of the meaning of an event to a particular individual. This is unlikely to affect death of spouse, which is always severely threatening. However, the circumstances surrounding job change may vary greatly; a routine change which represents promotion is quite different from the change to a job which carries less status and pay. The SRE would score both as 36. Similarly theft of a car may be a relatively trivial event for someone who has adequate insurance and generous financial resources, but it could be devastating for an individual who depends on the car to get to work yet has no insurance and no possibility of replacing the car. The threat is further increased if the individual has recently moved and depended on the car to keep in touch with family and friends.

An additional problem, relevant to the dose–response argument, relates to scoring. Simply adding up life change scores may produce extraordinary results, as the following example demonstrates. Brown & Harris (1978b) calculated that a young man who had recently been awarded a scholarship at Oxford could gain a total score of 79 life change units (end of formal schooling = 26, outstanding personal achievements = 28, a vacation = 13, Christmas = 12). This score of 79 would be greater than that for a man whose wife has left him (65).

A more sophisticated approach gives each life event a rating of threat or unpleasantness, according to the individual's biographical and current situation. In addition, events may be classified according to certain dimensions: desirable/undesirable, controllable/uncontrollable, entry/exit (from the person's social sphere), loss/non-loss.

The threat scales of the LEDS (Brown & Harris 1978a) and Paykel & Mangen (1980) are similar. The LEDS uses a four-point scale of threat or unpleasantness, and this rating is applied to both immediate and longer-term threat. For example, involvement in an accident may carry high threat (grade 1) in the short term, but if there are no lasting consequences at the end of the week the threat rating may have dropped to low level (grade 4) in the long term. By contrast, diagnosis of cancer in a spouse will carry high threat both at the time of discovery and one week later; it is such severely threatening events which are involved in the aetiology of depression. Work with the LEDS has shown that the experience of a single severely threatening life event (or analogous ongoing chronic difficulty) is sufficient to provoke depression and at first sight this is contrary to the dose–response argument. (A marked chronic difficulty is like a severe event, but represents an ongoing problem rather than a discrete change. Examples are marital or financial problems and these are associated with onset of depression in the same way as events.)

Does the experience of more than one event increase the chance of depression? This issue of additivity of events has been discussed in detail by Brown & Harris (1986, 1989a) and Miller & Ingham (1985b). All these authors agree that several minor events do not add up to exert the same effect as a severely threatening event, as in the example from the SRE quoted above. However, there is some evidence that two severe events are more than likely than a single severe event to cause depression. Of the total Camberwell sample studied by Brown & Harris (1978a) (114 hospital patients, 37 onset cases in the community and 382 normals), 35 women had experienced two or more severe events and 80% of those had become depressed. Of the 135 women who had experienced a single severe event, 50% became depressed; so it did appear that two severe events may be more stressful than a single one.

Brown & Harris studied the severity question by examining the time between onset of depression and admission to hospital for the inpatients. Of those women who had a dateable worsening of their depressive symptoms during this time, 47% had experienced a severe independent event immediately prior to the exacerbation. This compared with 16% of the women who had not had such a 'change point' in their depression during this time.

The dose–response effect is therefore seen most clearly in those studies which correlate severity of life events with number of depressive symptoms, rather than the number of severe events prior to onset. However, the effect is seen in the Brown & Harris model in terms of vulnerability factors, which will be discussed below. The more vulnerability factors that were present, the more likely depression was to occur if the woman was exposed to a severe event.

## Rate of events or binary method

This consideration of the life event scoring methods would not be complete without mentioning the various methods of scoring life events. Some reports quote the rate of events (per 100 subjects) for each group, others use the number of subjects who have experienced a particular type of event in a particular time period. These two methods were compared by Surtees & Duffy (1989) using data collected by the LEDS on a total of 1029 women in surveys at Edinburgh, Camberwell and Islington. The binary expression (severe life events present or absent) explained a slightly smaller proportion of the variance than the rate method, suggesting that the latter was the preferable measure. The authors did accept, though, that examining the effect of a specific type of event (e.g. loss events, exit events or events related to an ongoing difficulty) requires the binary method of analysis.

Brown & Harris provide a possible theoretical objection to the rate method (Brown & Harris 1989g). Half of the depressed women included in their Islington survey had experienced more than one severe event prior to onset, and would therefore be scored as having a higher rate of events. The events, however, were sometimes related. Examples included the starting of an affair (17 weeks before onset of depression) and ending it (immediately before onset); diagnosis of cancer in a relative (many weeks before onset) and death (immediately before onset). These pairs of events actually reflect a single ongoing process that affect particular women. Brown & Harris feel that it is inappropriate to allow these additional events to inflate the overall rate of severe events because they are really links in a single causal chain, and a conservative measure should be used to test the link between events and illness onset.

## Theoretical construct

This section concerning a theoretical construct linking life events and onset of disorder will be divided into two parts. First, the type of events linked to onset of depression and schizophrenia will be considered. Second, a theoretical model, including vulnerability factors, will be described.

### *Specific relationship between life events and disorder*

#### COMPARISON OF DEPRESSION AND SCHIZOPHRENIA

We have already noted that events of all magnitudes were related to the onset of schizophrenia, but only severely threatening events were associated with the onset of depression: 16% of schizophrenic patients experienced a severely threatening event in the 12 weeks before relapse, compared to 44% of depressed patients (Brown & Harris 1978c). Leff & Vaughn (1980), on the other hand, did not find any difference between depression and schizophrenia in terms of the proportion who experienced an undesirable event. At first sight this may appear to contradict the Brown & Harris finding but there are two important differences between the studies. The Brown & Harris study included all events, including serious arguments and disruption of close ties, which were excluded by the restricted analysis of Leff & Vaughn to independent events. Secondly, the latter study required that the patient be living with a relative, whereas this would not be the case for the Brown & Harris subjects.

The second difference between events in depression and schizophrenia relates to timing. The excess of events in schizophrenia was confined to the three weeks immediately prior to the relapse; in depression the difference was observed as far back as nine months prior to onset. This finding was similar in the Leff & Vaughn (1980) study just mentioned.

The relative importance of the time between events and onset of illness has been studied using a concept of brought forward time. This mathematical calculation makes an assumption that the episode of schizophrenia or depression would have occurred sooner or later anyway, but the episode is brought forward by the experience of a life event. The calculation employs a difference between the ill population and normal controls. It is very similar to the epidemiological concept of relative risk.

The brought forward time for schizophrenia was a mere ten weeks. This is a short time and has led to the conclusion that an episode of schizophrenia was imminent and the experience of a life event brought this forward only a short period in time. In depression the brought forward time was nearly two years, leading Brown & Harris to conclude that the experience of a severe life event is in some way formative rather than simply a trigger, i.e. the episode of depression might not have occurred but for the experience of a severe life event. Brown & Harris (1978a) calculated the brought forward time for other studies – in Paykel's depression study (Paykel *et al.* 1969) it was 2.7 years for exit events, and for Parkes' study of bereavement it was 2.5 years (Parkes 1964).

#### SEVERE EVENTS AND DEPRESSION

Further work by the Bedford College Group has explored the particular types of severe life events that are associated with the onset of depression. Three aspects of severe life events have been associated with onset of depression:

1 Events occurring in the context of prior commitment (C event). An event occurring in the area of a woman's particular commitment, for example, to marriage, to children, to work, was particularly likely to cause depression.

2 Events concerning role conflict (R event). Some women had a conflict about their role, for example, full-time work versus time spent with their children. An event concerning such role conflict was particularly linked to the onset of depression. Such R events were often closely related to an ongoing difficulty.

3 Severe events arising from an ongoing difficulty (D event). Examples of ongoing difficulties would

be: (i) a husband's disability following a stroke, or (ii) a severe marital problem. The respective D events would be a further stroke, or actual marital separation. Such events were among the most severe events in the threat ratings and often led to profound hopelessness. Thus any hope that the woman's husband might recover from the first stroke, or that the marriage might improve, were dashed by the subsequent event.

In the prospective Islington study, 37% of women with a severe C or D event became depressed, compared to 8% of those with other severe events (Brown & Harris 1989d).

## Vulnerability

Paykel (1978) has clearly demonstrated that most people who experience a severe life event do not develop depression. Using data from his own research he noted that 25% of depressed patients had experienced an exit event during the previous six months compared to 5% of healthy controls. He extrapolated these figures in a theoretical way to 10 000 subjects in the general population. If 2% of subjects become depressed during a six-month period then 200 new depressives can be compared with the 9800 non-depressed subjects. Since 25% of the former have experienced an exit event this will have occurred in 50 subjects. In addition, 5% of the 9800 non-depressed subjects will have experienced an exit event = 490 exit events which are not followed by depression. Thus of 540 exit events only 50 of these (9%) will lead to the subject becoming depressed. Thus factors other than life event experience must be involved in the aetiology of depression.

The original Camberwell study of Brown & Harris (1978a) did much to identify the vulnerability factors involved in an inner city urban population. The women were rated in terms of the closeness of their key relationships, and those without a close confiding relationship were more likely to develop depression if they also experienced a severely threatening life event. Ten per cent of the women who had a close confiding relationship with their husband or cohabitee and who had *also* experienced a severe event or major difficulty developed depression, compared to 41%

of women who had no such confiding relationship and experienced a severe event or major difficulty.

Three other factors were related in a similar fashion. Women who had lost their mother before the age of 11 years, those who were unemployed and those who had three or more children under 14 years old living at home were all more vulnerable to develop depression if they experienced a severe event. When all of these factors are taken together the results were additive. Although the numbers were small, all the women with the four vulnerability factors (absence of a confiding relationship, loss of mother when young, unemployment and young children at home) *and* who had experienced a severe event or difficulty developed depression: the more vulnerability factors that were present the more likely depression was to be recorded (Brown & Harris 1978d). In this way the dose–response relationship was upheld.

The assessment of vulnerability factors has been challenged on the basis that they are not truly independent of the threat rating given to events; an event might have been rated as severe partly because of the woman's unsupported status – without a confiding relationship (Tennant *et al.* 1981a). However, vulnerability has also been examined in a prospective way to examine whether factors assessed at the first interview relate to development of depression at follow-up.

The large Islington study of the Bedford College Group (Brown *et al.* 1987) assessed 400 women in the community on two occasions one year apart. Of those who experienced a severe event during this time one-fifth developed depression. These women, compared to the remaining four-fifths, were more likely to have experienced an event involving personal loss, and/or a particular commitment (C event, see above), *and* to have been without a close confiding relationship at the first interview. The importance of the last was confirmed prospectively: those who could not recruit emotional support at the time of a severe event were at greatest risk of developing depression.

An additional variable recorded at the first interview was also predictive of later depression – low self-esteem (Brown *et al.* 1986a). This could have been an indicator of pre-existing depression, rather than a true vulnerability factor

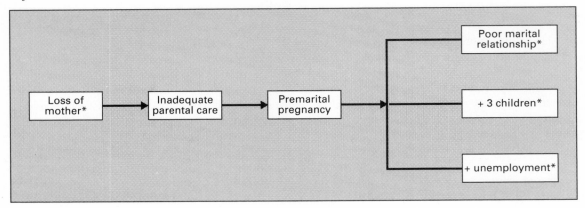

**Fig. 10.1** 'Conveyor belt' demonstrating the development of vulnerability factors for depression(*).

(Brown *et al.* 1986b, Miller *et al.* 1989). Two studies examined this possibility using multiple regression; both demonstrated that even after variance attributed to pre-existing depression was accounted for there was an additional effect attributable to low self-esteem.

In the Edinburgh study (Miller *et al.* 1989) stressful life events, in the absence of low self-esteem, led to anxiety and minor, but not major, depression. Major depression occurred when stressful life events interacted with prior low self-esteem. The low self-esteem appeared to have resulted from a prior life event, one involving severe stress within a close relationship (rows and arguments with someone close to the subject). Thus major depression was best predicted by a two-stage model: the experience of an event which led to low self-esteem followed by a stressful event which interacted with the low self-esteem.

These findings from the Edinburgh study are compatible with the model developed by the Bedford College Group to link the various vulnerability factors to subsequent depression (Bifulco *et al.* 1987, Harris *et al.* 1987). Loss of mother before the age of 15 years was not in itself linked to later depression; it was the lack of adequate parental care thereafter. Those who experienced such inadequate care were at greater risk of both a premarital pregnancy and an unsatisfactory 'marital' relationship. In this context young children at home and no employment outside the home were common sequelae, rendering the woman vulnerable to depression if she experienced a severe event. Brown & Harris have referred to this as a 'conveyor belt' (Fig. 10.1), on which working class women were much more likely to become trapped than middle class women (Harris & Brown 1986). The latter might escape if they did not become tied to an unsatisfactory 'marital' relationship at the point of a premarital pregnancy.

Further work has considered the role of low self-esteem in the vulnerability model (Brown *et al.* 1990a,b,d). However, this is a difficult task because low self-esteem is one of several factors which predict depression, and predict R and D events, and is itself closely related to current depressive symptoms: women with clinical depression are four times more likely than normal women to have low self-esteem; those with subclinical depression twice as likely.

Thus it was necessary for Brown and colleagues to exclude women with definite depression at first interview and perform multivariate analyses to establish the role of negative self-esteem *vis-à-vis* that explained by chronic subclinical depression. It was found that negative self-esteem and chronic subclinical depression were associated with the experience of inadequate parenting as a child, and negative elements in current relationships (i.e. lack of a confiding relationship and overt problems in interaction with husband and children).

In the Islington study 303 women who were not depressed at first interview were interviewed one year later. Of the 32 who became depressed during the follow-up year, 29 had experienced a severe event prior to the onset of depression. (A further 101 women had experienced a severe event without becoming depressed, in line with Paykel's theoretical calculation mentioned above.) The majority (78%) of those who became depressed had both negative elements in close relationships *and* negative self-esteem/chronic subclinical symptoms assessed at the first interview, and it turned out that the relatively small group of women with these two vulnerability factors (23% of the 303) were responsible for 75% of those who became depressed.

A series of multivariate analyses indicated that negative self-esteem, chronic subclinical symptoms and R and D events were contributing to the subsequent depression and an interactive model explained the most variance. Early inadequate parenting was associated with negative elements in close relationships and negative self-esteem, but not to the occurrence of D and R events.

## LIFE EVENTS AND RECOVERY FROM DEPRESSION

Several small studies have indicated that recovery from depression may be associated with events which 'neutralize' the adverse effects of previous severe life events (e.g. starting a new close relationship neutralizes the adverse effect of the previous broken one) (Tennant *et al.* 1981b, Parker *et al.* 1985). Two other studies concerned patients attending the GP with depression, where a positive or neutralizing event and good social support were associated with recovery over a six-month period (Davies *et al.* 1983, Parker *et al.* 1986). Among psychiatric outpatients continued relationship difficulties and/or further threatening events prevent recovery (Paykel & Tanner 1976).

Two community studies have allowed further examination of recovery from depression independent of treatment; the numbers involved were necessarily small (Miller *et al.* 1987, Brown *et al.* 1988). In the Islington study 26 women suffering from chronic depression at the first interview had

recovered by the second interview (Brown *et al.* 1988). Compared with women who continued to be depressed, recovery was associated with reduction in chronic difficulties and the experience of 'fresh start' events. The latter usually occurred in the context of considerable hardship, which was relieved by such changes as rehousing or the start of a new relationship.

Positive self-esteem and lack of negative self-esteem (the two were measured separately) have also been associated with recovery from chronic depression (Brown *et al.* 1990b). These patterns of self-esteem also predicted 'difficulty-reduction' and 'fresh start' events, indicating once again a link between background factors, psychological state and the later occurrence of events. It was inevitable that self-esteem had to be measured while the woman was depressed, but severity of depressed mood did not relate to improvement as the initial mean PSE scores of the recovered and non-recovered groups were similar (24 and 22 respectively).

The Islington results were very similar to those of the Edinburgh study (Miller *et al.* 1987), where remission of chronic illness was associated with good self-esteem, severe events not involving relationship stress and neutralizing events/reduction of difficulties. The Edinburgh study also examined factors associated with onset of transient illness as opposed to longer illness. The latter was associated with widowed, separated or divorced status and stressful life events involving uncertainty of outcome, for example, heart attack of spouse, threats of redundancy or stormy uncertain relationships with boyfriends. By contrast, onset of transient illness was associated with no previous consultation for nerves, and with life events restricted to health problems and more minor problems, such as burglaries (i.e. *not* involving uncertainty, relationship problems, deaths, exits or financial problems).

Miller and colleagues postulate that there are two patterns of illness. Chronic illness develops, they suggest, when severe relationship stress (of uncertain outcome) affects a divorced, separated or widowed woman, who has poor social support and poor self-esteem. Transient illness (less than 13 weeks) occurs in those with no previous psychiatric complaints who experience less severe stresses.

The Edinburgh study found that neither absence of a confidant nor separation before age 11 were predictive of recovery, and social class and employment status were not predictive once the other variables had been entered into the discriminant analysis. These findings are reminiscent of the Islington study, in which early inadequate parenting was linked to negative elements in core relationships and low self-esteem, but not of itself to those severe (D and R) events associated with the onset of depression. Such results emphasize two steps in the development of vulnerability to depression: distant historical ones and more recent psychological and environmental ones.

## Life events results in different populations

### Schizophrenia

Replication of the original LEDS research in schizophrenia has been patchy. The original study was concerned with schizophrenic relapse; there has been no adequate study which distinguishes first episode from relapse, or which has used a narrow definition of schizophrenia. The largest study, concerned mostly with first episodes, used a modified version of the LEDS and was performed at nine centres around the world (Day *et al.* 1987). The study included 386 patients with an ICD-9 diagnosis of schizophrenia, paranoid state or schizophreniform reactive psychosis.

The results were essentially similar to the original study. At six centres there were significantly more events experienced in the three weeks immediately prior to onset of schizophrenia than in the previous weeks; the proportions were similar to those in the original Camberwell study. At the remaining three centres the numbers were too small for statistical analysis – at two of these the trends were very much in the expected direction. The results were confirmed even when 'independent' events were analysed separately.

Unfortunately, there were no community controls, and there were differences in method between the centres. The study was limited to patients with a clear datable onset of psychosis (it had to be datable to within one week) and an onset within six months. Such inclusion criteria have clear advantages for a study which needs to ensure exact dating of events and onset, but may have biased the study towards patients with schizophreniform reactive psychosis. This diagnosis may be more likely than DSM-III schizophrenia to be preceded by threatening life events (Chung *et al.* 1986). However, the overall results are impressively similar to those of the original Camberwell study (Brown & Birley 1968).

One further study confirmed life events immediately prior to onset only in first episodes of schizophrenia, and not relapses (Al Khani *et al.* 1986).

A larger American study (Dohrenwend *et al.* 1987) included 66 cases of 'schizophrenic disorder'; once again schizophreniform disorder, brief reactive psychosis, schizoaffective psychosis and atypical psychosis were included. Patients in these groups had experienced a higher rate of events, but only those which may have been influenced by the subject or by insidious onset of illness: divorce, imprisonment, marital infidelity/separation, cessation of work, broken friendship. The pattern was similar for first onset or relapse of schizophrenia, but there was no build-up of events over the three weeks immediately preceding onset/relapse.

A small prospective study of schizophrenic patients in aftercare demonstrated a significantly greater number of events in the three months prior to relapse compared to similar times in the absence of relapse (Malla *et al.* 1990). This study, like that of Brown & Birley, was concerned with the timing of relapse, that is a triggering effect, not a causal one. It will be recalled that the short brought forward time indicates that the relapse was likely to occur soon anyway. It is very likely that in schizophrenia only a small proportion of overall variance is accounted for by life events. Future studies need to include biological variables as well as psychosocial ones (Day 1989). One study has suggested that the experience of a life event increases psychophysiological arousal – an effect which is further exacerbated by the presence of a critical relative (Tarrier & Lader 1979).

More studies of this type are required to integrate biological and social factors in schizophrenia.

## Depression

In contrast to the studies in schizophrenia, there have been numerous replications of the life events results in depression. In ten population studies using the LEDS (Brown & Harris 1989b) the original results have been repeated, and the total results indicated that 84% of 312 onset cases of depression in the community had experienced a severe event or marked difficulty in the previous 38 weeks compared to 32% of 1745 non-cases in the community.

There have been 11 studies of depressed patients under psychiatric care using an acceptable methodology (Brown & Harris 1989c). The results are essentially similar, with 45−70% of patients (compared to 10−25% of controls) having experienced an event variously described as severely threatening, undesirable, major role loss, exit, uncontrollable.

## Comparison of depression and schizophrenia

It has already been noted that schizophrenic relapse was preceded by life events of all grades of threat whereas depression was associated with severely threatening events (Brown & Birley 1968, Brown & Harris 1978a). Jacobs *et al.* (1974) also found that patients with depression, compared to those with schizophrenia, had experienced more undesirable events and more events categorized as 'exits' (from the social field). Of the 59 events, only two occurred significantly more frequently among the depressives: serious arguments with non-resident family members, and serious arguments with fiancé, girlfriend or boyfriend. These would correspond to the most frequent type of severe events in the Brown & Harris work.

A similar finding has been reported in the American study (Dohrenwend *et al.* 1987): 'independent fateful events', such as serious physical illness/death of a close relative, involvement in a disaster, infertility, redundancy, were significantly more frequent in depressed patients than either schizophrenic patients or healthy controls.

A somewhat different finding was reported by Leff & Vaughn (1980). They found that whereas relapse of schizophrenia was associated with *either* high Expressed Emotion *or* an independent life event, depression was associated with a *combination* of an undesirable event and a critical relative. The latter would have considerable similarity with the combination of a severe event in the presence of a non-confiding relationship in the Brown & Harris work.

## Epidemiology of life events

There has been relatively little work investigating the epidemiology of life events. There are two competing views: one suggests that events occur on a random or quasi-random basis in the community, the other suggests that certain environmental and personal factors determine the life event exposure. All the evidence supports the latter. Fergusson & Horwood (1987) recognized that marital and financial problems, employment changes and illness in the family are determined by systematic social, demographic and personal factors and inquired whether the same was true for formal life event scores. In a prospective study they found that 30% of the variance in reported life events exposure could be attributed to a common factor, which was highest among women from socially disadvantaged backgrounds and among women with high neuroticism score. These variables made largely independent contributions to the variability of life event exposure over a five-year period.

Miller *et al.* (1986) also assessed the distribution of life events according to social status. They analysed the life events occurring to 576 women in Edinburgh over a six-month period and found an overall event rate of 166 per 100 women per six months, which was remarkably close to the rates of 159.7 and 150 found in other surveys (Brown & Harris 1978a, Surtees & Ingham 1980). Compared to middle class women, working class women experienced more independent events, more severely threatening events and more serious health problems.

Brown & Harris (1978a) also found a higher rate of severe events in working class compared to middle class women, but the difference was only found in one category of severe events, household events, those affecting family members and the household as a whole*. The difference did not hold for health and other severe events, although working class women did suffer significantly more chronic difficulties in both health and household categories.

Vulnerability factors (early loss of mother, no confidant, young children at home and unemployment) were also significantly more common in working class women and it was a combination of the excess of severe household events, marked chronic difficulties, and vulnerability factors that accounted for the class difference in incidence of depression.

In the Edinburgh study (Miller *et al.* 1986) increasing age was associated with a decreasing total number of events (especially work and marital events), but an increasing number of independent health problems. Overall, older women did not differ significantly from younger women in terms of the number of severely threatening events they experienced. In Camberwell a similar pattern was found, with the overall rate of events dropping by more than 50% from the women in the age range 18–35 years and without children, to the group aged 36–65 years without children at home (Brown & Harris 1989f). There was no relationship between age and rate of severe events, indicating the fallacy of measuring event rates without reference to threat (e.g. Goldberg & Comstock 1980).

A further comparison, using the same instrument, has been made between two very different communities – an inner city area, Camberwell, and the rural islands of the Outer Hebrides (Brown & Prudo 1981). Severe events in both Camberwell and Outer Hebrides constituted approximately 15% of all events, but there was a difference in the proportion of women who had experienced a severe life event: 31% of

Camberwell women had experienced a severe event in the last year, compared to 21% of women in the Hebrides. The difference was only found in household and sociosexual events, such as broken close relationships, burglaries and marked financial problems. Other types of events, including illnesses and deaths, were similarly prevalent in the two communities.

Vulnerability factors were also studied in the Outer Hebrides and compared with those in Camberwell (Prudo *et al.* 1981). Two were identical in the two locations (lack of a confiding relationship, three or more children at home), but the others were different; lack of regular churchgoing and not living in a croft were the additional factors in the Hebrides. Churchgoing and living in a croft indicated integration into the local community – lack of integration made depression more likely.

In view of these findings that life events are not distributed randomly throughout the population, but are to some extent determined by social grouping, it is not too surprising that the tendency to experience life events has a familial component (McGuffin *et al.* 1988). These authors investigated the relative contributions of genetic influences and life events in the aetiology of depression, assuming these to be mutually exclusive aetiological agents. They studied two groups of patients, those with a life event/difficulty prior to onset and those without, expecting only the latter to have an increased risk of depression among first-degree relatives. This was not the case – both risk of depression and risk of life event experience were increased among relatives, indicating that both biological and environmental aetiological factors occur simultaneously (Dolan *et al.* 1985). There is a dearth of *research in depression where concomitant life events and biological measurements have been studied simultaneously*; it is likely that genetic factors will increase further our understanding of vulnerability. Brown *et al.* suggest that they are likely to explain some of the variance not accounted for by the very comprehensive psychosocial model (Brown *et al.* 1990b). It may be that the inadequate parenting–lack of confiding relationship model has a biological element.

* Examples of household events were: husband's loss of a job, son in trouble with the police, husband being imprisoned, son killed, woman stopping work to look after disabled son, eviction, step-daughter's overdose, an unwanted abortion because of extreme housing difficulties.

## LIFE EVENTS AND PERSONALITY

The intriguing result of Fergusson & Horwood (1987), mentioned above, correlating tendency to report high life events exposure to neuroticism may have several explanations. First, since the authors did not use a reliable interview method, the results might simply indicate that neuroticism determines a reporting style with the life events questionnaire. Alternatively, however, certain personality types are more likely to be involved in, or create social environments in which there is a greater chance of life event exposure. A third possibility is the reciprocal relationship of personality and life event exposure so that distant or recent event exposure (e.g. loss of mother when young or lack of a confiding relationship) might modify 'personality' in terms of neuroticism or self-esteem.

One study (Sievewright 1987) concurrently assessed personality *disorder* and life events in patients presenting with anxiety and depressive disorders. Disordered personality was not associated with total number of events or stressful events, but the single category, sociopathic personality, was associated with an increased number of undesirable and self-generated events.

It remains an open question whether personality factors bring about the event, the depression or both. In the Islington study, the independence categories of events experienced by depressed and non-depressed women were largely similar, except for events involving an argument, breaking off contact or other 'love' event (Brown & Harris 1989h). These events, which are most likely to be related to personality, were more common in the depressed group, but the balance of evidence suggested that personality may be linked to the likelihood of experiencing an event and possibly vulnerability, rather than to the onset of depression itself. This is a complicated area and further prospective research is needed.

## Life events and other conditions

No other condition has been studied as extensively as depression; the main results for conditions other than depression and schizophrenia will be considered briefly in this section.

### Anxiety

In order to compare anxiety and depression, Finlay-Jones & Brown (1981) studied life events in patients presenting to their GPs. Similar sized groups of patients with anxiety, depression and mixed symptoms were studied and in each group practically all the subjects had experienced a severe event in the preceding year compared to only one-third of comparison subjects. However, the nature of the severe events differed; loss events preceded depression (such as loss of a valued person through death or separation or loss of the respondent's physical health), whereas danger events preceded anxiety. The latter involved some kind of future threat to the subject, such as being told that a bodily symptom might be cancer, or by being involved in an affair, where the consequences of discovery will be disastrous to the subject.

One other study characterized the events preceding depression as those involving threat and choice of action, whereas those preceding anxiety involved threat, uncertainty of outcome but not involving loss (Miller & Ingham 1985a).

Faravelli & Pallanti (1989) also found that severe events were more common in subjects before the onset of DSM-III panic disorder or agoraphobia with panic attacks than in control subjects (6% versus 35%); the difference remained significant when only independent events were considered. However, this study found loss not danger events were involved, perhaps reflecting the similarity of panic disorder patients to depressives, rather than to the 'pure' anxiety seen in the general practice setting of Finlay-Jones & Brown.

### Mania

Results concerning mania are conflicting. Although several studies appear to have shown a link between life events and the onset of mania, most have not used an interview method of assessment or determined the exact date of onset (Sclare & Creed 1990). Only three studies used an interview method which allowed independent events to be assessed; one found a significant relationship between severe events and the onset of mania (Kennedy *et al.* 1983) and two did not (Chung *et al.* 1986, Sclare & Creed 1990). However, the Kennedy study examined life events before admission, not onset of symptoms, and there appears to be a considerable delay between onset of first manic symptom and admission (Winokur *et al.* 1969, Sclare & Creed 1990). During this time events may well be related to the illness, especially as the most common events involve work and close relationship difficulties, which might arise with early hypomanic irritability.

An interesting example of the study of a single life event is relevant here. Aronson & Shukla (1987) noted that 14% of lithium clinic attenders relapsed when exposed to the catastrophic effects of a hurricane, whereas 86% remained well. Those authors suggested that there is a subgroup of affective disorder patients who are liable to relapse into mania when exposed to environmental stress.

### Self-poisoning patients

It has long been recognized that deliberate self-harm is preceded by adverse life events; the interest lies in comparing these patients with those included in other life events studies. Paykel *et al.* (1975) reported twice as many events in the six months prior to a suicide attempt than for a comparable time before onset of depression. Farmer & Creed (1989) also found an increased rate of severe events for the three-week period prior to self-poisoning, and throughout the preceding year. The excess involved events that were not independent, commonly broken relationships and contact with police/court appearance.

This study demonstrated a link between total number of severe events and extrapunitive hostility, indicating the importance of underlying personality in this group of patients. Once again, however, the personality dimension was measured when the subject was depressed; the extrapunitive-

ness might have reflected both the tendency to experience events and to become irritable and hostile when depressed. This finding does accord with the observation that women who had lost their mother when young had an increased tendency to show suicidal plans or acts when depressed (Brown *et al.* 1985). Depression was thought to bring out hostile and attention-seeking behaviours in such women – an association between past experience, current 'personality', and predominant symptom-pattern when depressed.

The Farmer & Creed study (1989) compared two groups of deliberate self-poisoning patients: those with a depressive illness and those without. The pattern of life events was similar but the depressed subjects had experienced significantly more chronic difficulties over several months prior to the self-poisoning. It may have been the additional stress of a severe life event together with an ongoing difficulty that was related to the self-harm – it will be recalled that difficulty related events are particularly potent in causing hopelessness. Similarly, Slater & Depue (1981) demonstrated that a high incidence of further exit events *after* the onset of depression was associated with parasuicide in depressed patients.

### Conclusion

This review of life events research in relation to psychiatric illness has been confined to studies using a reliable measure. The research concerning life events and the onset of depression largely fulfilled the criteria set out at the beginning of the chapter concerning aetiology. The results for other conditions are relatively limited. Further work requires more detailed consideration of vulnerability factors (including personality and biochemical indicators), as it is the *interaction* between life events and vulnerability factors which has been the clue to aetiology in depression.

### References

Al Khani M.A.F., Bebbington P.E., Watson J.P. & House F. (1986) Life events and schizophrenia: a Saudi Arabian study. *British Journal of Psychiatry* 148, 12–22.
Ambelas A. (1987) Life events and mania – a special

relationship? *British Journal of Psychiatry* 150, 235–240.

Aronson T.A. & Shukla S. (1987) Life events and relapse in bipolar disorder: the impact of a catastrophic event. *Acta Psychiatrica Scandinavica* 75, 571–576.

Bifulco A.T., Brown G.W. & Harris T.O. (1987) Childhood loss of parent, lack of adequate parental care and adult depression: a replication. *Journal of Affective Disorders* 12, 115–128.

Brown G.W. (1989) Life events and measurements. In Brown G.W. & Harris T.O. (eds) *Life Events and Illness*, pp. 3–45. Guilford Press, New York.

Brown G.W., Adler Z. & Bifulco A. (1988) Life events, difficulties and recovery from chronic depression. *British Journal of Psychiatry* 152, 487–498.

Brown G.W., Andrews B., Harris T. *et al.* (1986a) Social support, self-esteem and depression. *Psychological Medicine* 16, 813–832.

Brown G.W., Andrews B., Bifulco A. & Veiel H. (1990a) Self-esteem and depression. 1. Measurement issues and prediction of onset. *Social Psychiatry and Psychiatric Epidemiology* 25, 200–209.

Brown G.W., Bifulco A. & Andrews B. (1990b) Self-esteem and depression. 111. Aetiological issues. *Social Psychiatry and Psychiatric Epidemiology* 25, 200–209.

Brown G.W., Bifulco A. & Andrews B. (1990c) Self-esteem and depression. IV. Effect on cause and recovery. *Social Psychiatry and Psychiatric Epidemiology* 25, 244–249.

Brown G.W., Bifulco A. & Harris T.O. (1987) Life events, vulnerability and onset of depression – some refinements. *British Journal of Psychiatry* 150, 30–42.

Brown G.W., Bifulco A.T., Harris T.O. & Bridge L. (1986b) Life stress, chronic subclinical symptoms and vulnerability to clinical depression. *Journal of Affective Disorders* 11, 1–20.

Brown G.W., Bifulco A., Veiel H. & Andrews B. (1990d) Self-esteem and depression. 11. Social correlates of self-esteem. *Social Psychiatry and Psychiatric Epidemiology* 25, 200–209.

Brown G.W. & Birley J.L.T. (1968) Crises and life changes and the onset of schizophrenia. *Journal of Health and Social Behaviour* 9, 203–214.

Brown G.W., Craig T.K. & Harris T.O. (1985) Depression: disease or distress? Some epidemiological considerations. *British Journal of Psychiatry* 147, 612–622.

Brown G.W. & Harris T.O. (1978a) *Social Origins of Depression: A Study of Psychiatric Disorder in Women*. Tavistock, London.

Brown G.W. & Harris T.O. (1978b) *Social Origins of Depression: A Study of Psychiatric Disorder in Women*, p. 107. Tavistock, London.

Brown G.W. & Harris T.O. (1978c) *Social Origins of Depression: A Study of Psychiatric Disorder in Women*, p. 125. Tavistock, London.

Brown G.W. & Harris T.O. (1978d) *Social Origins of Depression: A Study of Psychiatric Disorder in Women*, p. 181. Tavistock, London.

Brown G.W. & Harris T.O. (1982) Fall-off in the reporting of life events. *Social Psychiatry* 17, 23–28.

Brown G.W. & Harris T.O. (1986) Establishing causal links: the Bedford College studies of depression. In Katschnig H. (ed.) *Life Events and Psychiatric Disorders: Controversial Issues*, pp. 107–187. Cambridge University Press, Cambridge.

Brown G.W. & Harris T.O. (eds) (1989a) *Life Events and Illness*, pp. 71–81. Guilford Press, New York.

Brown G.W. & Harris T.O. (eds) (1989b) *Life Events and Illness*, p. 55. Guilford Press, New York.

Brown G.W. & Harris T.O. (eds) (1989c) *Life Events and Illness*, p. 56. Guilford Press, New York.

Brown G.W. & Harris T.O. (eds) (1989d) *Life Events and Illness*, p. 67. Guilford Press, New York.

Brown G.W. & Harris T.O. (eds) (1989e) *Life Events and Illness*, pp. 81–82. Guilford Press, New York.

Brown G.W. & Harris T.O. (eds) (1989f) *Life Events and Illness*, p. 336. Guilford Press, New York.

Brown G.W. & Harris T.O. (eds) (1989g) *Life Events and Illness*, p. 397. Guilford Press, New York.

Brown G.W. & Harris T.O. (eds) (1989h) *Life Events and Illness*, pp. 393–396. Guilford Press, New York.

Brown G.W., Harris T.O. & Peto. (1973) Life events and psychiatric disorder: 2. Nature of causal link. *Psychological Medicine* 3, 159–176.

Brown G.W. & Prudo R. (1981) Psychiatric disorder in a rural and an urban population: 1. Aetiology of depression. *Psychological Medicine* 11, 581–599.

Brugha T., Bebington P., Tennant C. & Hurry J. (1985) The list of threatening experiences: a subset of 12 life event categories with considerable long-term contextual threat. *Psychological Medicine* 15, 189–194.

Brugha T. & Conroy R. (1985) Categories of depression: reported life events in a controlled design. *British Journal of Psychiatry* 147, 641–646.

Chung R.K., Langeluddecke P. & Tennant C. (1986) Threatening life events in the onset of schizophrenia, schizophreniform psychosis and hypomania. *British Journal of Psychiatry* 148, 680–685.

Cleary P.J. (1980) A checklist for life event research. *Journal of Psychosomatic Research* 24, 199–207.

Cohen L.H., Towbes L.C. & Flocco R. (1988) Effects of induced mood on self-reported life events and perceived and received social support. *Journal of Person and Social Psychology* 55, 669–674.

Cohen S. & Wills T.A. (1985) Stress, social support and the buffering hypothesis. *Psychological Bulletin* 98, 310–357.

Connolly J. (1976) Life events before myocardial infarction. *Journal of Human Stress* 2, 3–17.

Cooke D.J. (1981) Life events and syndromes of depression in the general population. *Social Psychiatry* 16, 181–186.

Cooke D.J. (1986) Inferring causality in life event research. *Stress Medicine* 2, 141–152.

Craufurd D.I.O., Creed F. & Jayson M.D. (1990) Life

events and psychological disturbance in patients with low-back pain. *Spine* 15, 490–494.

Creed F. (1981) Life events and appendicectomy. *Lancet* i, 1381–1385.

Creed F. (1985) Life events and physical illness. *Journal of Psychosomatic Research* 29, 113–123.

Davies M.H., Rose S. & Cross K.W. (1983) Life events, social interaction and psychiatric symptoms in general practice: a pilot study. *Psychological Medicine* 13, 159–163.

Day R. (1989) Schizophrenia. In Brown G.W. & Harris T.O. (eds) *Life Events and Illness*, pp. 113–137. Guilford Press, New York.

Day R., Nielsen H., Korten A. *et al.* (1987) Stressful life events preceding the acute onset of schizophrenia: a cross-national study from the World Health Organization. *Culture, Medicine and Psychiatry* 11, 1–123.

Dohrenwend B.P., Levav I., Shrout P.E. *et al.* (1987) Life stress and psychopathology: process on research begun with Barbara Snell Dohrenwend. *American Journal of Community Psychology* 15, 677–715.

Dolan R.J., Calloway S.P., Fonagy P., De Souza F.V.A. & Wakeling A. (1985) Life events, depression and hypothalamic-pituitary-adrenal axis function. *British Journal of Psychiatry* 147, 429–433.

Faravelli C. & Pallanti S. (1989) Recent life events and panic disorder. *American Journal of Psychiatry* 146, 622–626.

Farmer R. & Creed F. (1989) Life events and hostility in self-poisoning. *British Journal of Psychiatry* 154, 390–395.

Fergusson D.M. & Horwood L.J. (1987) Vulnerability to life events exposure. *Psychological Medicine* 17, 739–749.

Finlay-Jones R.A. & Brown G.W. (1981) Types of stressful life event and the onset of anxiety and depressive disorders. *Psychological Medicine* 11, 803–815.

Goldberg E.L. & Comstock G.W. (1980) Epidemiology of life events: frequency in general populations. *American Journal of Epidemiology* 111, 736–752.

Harris T.O. & Brown G.W. (1989c) The LEDS findings in the context of other research: an overview. In Brown G.W. & Harris T.O. (eds) *Life Events and Illness*, pp. 385–437. Guilford Press, New York.

Harris T.O., Brown G.W. & Bifulco A.T. (1987) Loss of parent in childhood and adult psychiatric disorder: the role of social class position and premarital pregnancy. *Psychological Medicine* 17, 163–184.

Holmes T.H. & Rahe R.H. (1967) The social readjustment rating Scale. *Journal of Psychosomatic Research* 11, 213–218.

Hudgens R.W., Robins E. & Delong W.B. (1970) The reporting of recent stress in the lives of psychiatric patients, non-patients and their partners. *British Journal of Psychiatry* 117, 635–643.

Jacobs S., Prusoff B. & Paykel G. (1974) Recent life events in schizophrenia and depression. *Psychological Medicine* 4, 444–453.

Jenkins C.D., Hurst M.W. & Rose R.M. (1979) Life changes: do people really remember? *Archives of General Psychiatry* 36, 379–384.

Johnson J.H. & Sarason I.G. (1978) Life stress, depression and anxiety: internal-external control as a moderator variable. *Journal of Psychosomatic Research* 22, 205–208.

Kennedy S., Thompson R., Stancer H.C. *et al.* (1983) Life events precipitating mania. *British Journal of Psychiatry* 142, 398–403.

Klein D.N. & Rubovits D.R. (1987) Reliability of subjects' reports on stressful life events inventories – longitudinal studies. *Journal of Behavioural Medicine* 10, 501–512.

Leavitt F., Garron D.C. & Bieliauskas A. (1979) Stressing life events and the experience of low back pain. *Journal of Psychosomatic Research* 23, 49–55.

Leff J. & Vaughn C. (1980) The interaction of life events and relatives' expressed emotion in schizophrenia and depressive neurosis. *British Journal of Psychiatry* 136, 146–53.

McGuffin P., Katz R. & Bebbington P. (1988) The Camberwell Collaborative study. III. Depression and adversity in the relatives of depressed probands. *British Journal of Psychiatry* 152, 775–782.

Maes S., Vingerhoets A. & Van Heck G. (1987) The study of stress and disease: some developments and requirements. *Social Science Medicine* 25, 567–578.

Malla A.K., Cortese L., Shaw T.S. & Ginsberg B. (1990) Life events and relapse in schizophrenia. *Social Psychiatry and Psychiatric Epidemiology* 25, 221–224.

Miller P.Mc., Dean C., Ingham J.G., Kreitman N.B., Sashidharan S.P. & Surtees P.G. (1986) The epidemiology of life events and long-term difficulties, with some reflections on the concept of independence. *British Journal of Psychiatry* 148, 686–696.

Miller P.McC. & Ingham J.G. (1979) Reflections on the life-event-to-illness link with some preliminary findings. In Sarason I.G. & Spielberger C.D. (eds) *Stress and Anxiety* vol. 6. Wiley, New York.

Miller P.Mc. & Ingham J.G. (1985a) Dimensions of experience and symptomatology. *Journal of Psychosomatic Research* 29, 475–488.

Miller P.Mc. & Ingham J.G. (1985b) Are life events that cause each other additive in their effects? *Social Psychiatry.* 20, 31–41.

Miller P.Mc., Ingham J.G., Kreitman N.B. *et al.* (1987) Life events and other factors implicated in onset and in remission of psychiatric illness in women. *Journal of Affective Disorders* 12, 73–88.

Miller P.Mc., Kreitman N.B., Ingham J.G. & Sashideran S.P. (1989) Self esteem, life stress and psychiatric disorder. *Journal of Affective Disorders* 17, 65–75.

Miller P.McC. & Salter D.P. (1984) Is there a short-cut? *Acta Psychiatrica Scandinavica* 70, 417–427.

Neilson E., Brown G.W. & Marmot M. (1989) Myocardial infarction. In Brown G.W. & Harris T.O. (eds) *Life Events and Illness*, pp. 313–343. Guilford Press, New York.

Parker G., Holmes S. & Manicavasagar V. (1986) Depression in general practice attenders. 'Caseness', natural history and predictors of outcome. *Journal of Affective Disorders* 10, 27–35.

Parker G., Tennant C. & Blignault I. (1985) Predicting improvement in patients with non-endogenous depression. *British Journal of Psychiatry* 146, 132–139.

Parkes C.M. (1964) Recent bereavement as a cause of mental illness. *British Journal of Psychiatry* 110, 198–204.

Paykel E.S. (1978) Contribution of life events to causation of psychiatric illness. *Psychological Medicine* 8, 245–253.

Paykel E.S. (1983) Methodological aspects of life events research. *Journal of Psychosomatic Research* 27, 341–352.

Paykel E.S. & Mangen S.P. (1980) *Interview for Recent Life Events*. St George's Hospital Medical School, London.

Paykel E.S., Myers J.K., Dienelt M.N. *et al.* (1969) Life events and depression: a controlled study. *Archives of General Psychiatry* 21, 753–760.

Paykel E.S., Prusoff B.A. & Myers J.K. (1975) Suicide attempts and recent life events: a controlled comparison. *Archives of General Psychiatry* 32, 327–333.

Paykel E.S. & Tanner J. (1976) Life events, depressive relapse and maintenance treatment. *Psychological Medicine* 6, 481–485.

Prudo R., Brown G.W., Harris T. & Dowland J. (1981) Psychiatric disorder in a rural and an urban population: 2. Sensitivity to loss. *Psychological Medicine* 11, 601–616.

Schmid I., Scharfetter C. & Binder J. (1981) Lebensereignisse in Abhangigkeit von soziodemographischen Variablen. *Social Psychiatry* 16, 63–68.

Sclare P. & Creed F. (1990) Life events and the onset of mania. *British Journal of Psychiatry* 156, 508–514.

Sievewright N. (1987) Relationship between life events and personality in psychiatric disorder. *Stress Medicine* 3, 164–168.

Slater J. & Depue R.A. (1981) The contribution of environment, events and social support to serious suicide attempts in primary depressive disorder. *Journal of Abnormal Psychology* 90, 275–285.

Sobell L.C., Toneatto T., Sobbell M.B., Schuller R. & Maxwell M. (1990) A procedure for reducing errors in reports of life events. *Journal of Psychosomatic Research* 34, 163–170.

Steele G.P., Henderson S. & Duncan-Jones P. (1980) The reliability of reporting adverse experience. *Psychological Medicine* 10, 301–306.

Surtees P.G. & Duffy J.G. (1989) Binary and rate measures of life events experience: their association with illness onset in Edinburgh and London community survey. *Journal of Affective Disorders* 16, 139–150.

Surtees P.G. & Ingham J.G. (1980) Life stress and depressive outcome application of a dissipation model to life events. *Social Psychiatry* 15, 21–31.

Susser M. (1973) *Causal Thinking in Health Sciences*. Oxford University Press, New York.

Tarrier N. & Lader M.H. (1979) Bodily reactions to people and events in schizophrenics. *Archives of General Psychiatry* 36, 311–315.

Tennant C., Bebbington P. & Hurry J. (1981a) The role of life events in depressive illness: is there a substantial causal relation? *Psychological Medicine* 11, 379–389.

Tennant C., Bebbington P. & Hurry J. (1981b) The short-term outcome of neurotic disorders in the community: the relation of remission to clinical factors and to 'neutralizing' life events. *British Journal of Psychiatry* 139, 213–220.

Winokur G., Clayton P.J. & Reich T. (1969) *Manic Depressive Illness*. CV Mosby, St Louis, Missouri.

Wittchen H.-U., Essau C.A., Hecht H., Teder W. & Pfister H. (1989) Reliability of life event assessments: test-retest reliability and fall-off effects of the Munich Interview for the assessment of life events and conditions. *Journal of Affective Disorders* 16, 77–92.

# Chapter 11
## Social Factors and Alcohol Abuse

BETSY THOM

### 'Our favourite drug'

In most industrialized countries today alcohol is an integral part of the religious and secular life of the community. Not only do most people drink, but, in what has been called the 'post-war drinking binges' of 1950–75, alcohol consumption rose in many societies (Smart 1989).

Because alcohol is 'our favourite drug' (Royal College of Psychiatrists 1986), legally available and widely used, there is no clear dividing line between non-harmful alcohol *use* and alcohol *abuse*; alcohol abuse, alcoholism, alcohol dependence or problem drinking are all 'labels', the product of some form of assessment procedure, which, despite attempts to achieve definitional clarity, can mean different things to different people. Behind the 'labels' lie numerous causal theories for alcohol abuse, drawing most prominently on biomedical, psychological and sociological theories, and producing varying explanations for alcoholism which may be seen as a disease, a state of dependence, a learned behaviour disorder or an effect of the social and cultural setting in which drinking occurs. Alongside such 'scientific' and professional explanations, we still find the centuries old perceptions of alcoholism as a moral weakness or a sin or a form of criminal deviance. (See Robinson (1976) and Heather & Robertson (1985) for a discussion of these concepts.)

Current thinking most commonly urges the need for a multidisciplinary and multifactorial approach which recognizes the interrelationship between the physical, psychological and social dimensions of alcohol abuse. Genetic vulnerability, the development of physiological tolerance and dependence, and the individual's personality and perceived needs should be seen in conjunction with the social context (Royal College of Psychiatrists 1986).

In this chapter, however, the focus is on the social factors in alcohol abuse and we can only acknowledge the importance of the biomedical and psychological approaches. Even so, the task of examining the social aspects remains immense. Some consideration must be given to the structure of the society in which we live, the opportunities it affords for drinking, the restrictions it imposes, the beliefs and attitudes towards alcohol it sustains, the ways in which the boundaries between use and abuse are defined. The influence of major social categories such as gender or ethnicity, warrants examination, as does the influence of social groups and networks to which individuals belong – the family, occupational groups, peers and friendship networks. It is important also to examine the effects of change in the social context; the fact that the individual passes through different life stages, enters or leaves different social settings, possibly with ensuing changes in drinking habits. Finally, we must take account of an individual's interpretation of the social situation, the significance bestowed on events, and the effort to make sense of the world.

### Alcohol use

#### National patterns of consumption

Fluctuations in the total quantity of alcohol consumed by a nation have occurred regularly throughout history. In the UK, for instance, consumption decreased steadily throughout the first half of this century until the end of World War II when it began to rise again, almost doubling between 1950 and 1976 before the decline set in once more (Royal College of Psychiatrists 1986). Similar fluctuations in per capita consumption of alcohol have been reported from other countries (Romelsjo 1987, Hilton 1988, Rahkonan & Ahlstrom 1989). Many reasons may contribute to the rise or fall in national consumption rates: the fruitfulness of the harvest, the economic health of the society, political motivation to manipulate the supply of alcohol, the power of the alcohol industry, the attitudes of the populace towards alcohol use and the influence of advertising and the media are only some of the economic and social forces which help to shape the pattern of alcohol consumption.

The decline in the UK rate of consumption earlier this century was undoubtedly influenced by the onset of World War I, the economic depression of the 1930s and the controls imposed by government to curb the availability of alcohol. The subsequent rise in consumption was at least partly due to increased consumer spending, a drop in the real price of alcohol and a more relaxed attitude towards the use of alcohol in everyday life (Royal College of Psychiatrists 1986).

Of course, individuals vary enormously in the amounts they consume – some drink nothing at all while others drink very heavily, some drink only on special occasions, others like a drink most days, and individuals, like nations, change their drinking habits, consume more or less, depending perhaps on the company they keep or on how much they earn. Fluctuations in the total quantity of alcohol consumed by a nation are a reflection of changes in individuals' drinking habits and patterns throughout the society; generally speaking, when consumption rises, it is not just because heavy drinkers are drinking more but because everyone tends to do so.

## Group variations in consumption

Within the broad national picture, the consumption patterns of groups of people also vary. Belonging to a particular religion or religious sect (Adlaf & Smart 1985, Cochrane & Bal 1990), to a particular ethnic or cultural group (Pittman & Snyder 1962, Leland 1984, Babor 1986, Herd 1987), or to an immigrant population (Heok

1987) is likely to bring different pressures to drink or abstain from drink, different beliefs and attitudes towards the appropriate use of alcohol and different expectations of drinking behaviour and rituals.

One of the best-known examples is the well-documented difference in rates of drinking pathologies between American Irish (who have a high rate) and American Jews (who have a low rate). Bales (1962) has attempted to provide an explanation by comparing the historical and cultural backgrounds of the two groups. Bales describes the widespread utilitarian use of alcohol in traditional Irish culture, as a medicine, as a substitute for food (often in short supply in the homeland), as a reward to children, as a means of releasing sexual and aggressive tensions generated by the structure of Irish family life with its strict sexual mores and tightly controlled economic relations. Equally important are the symbolic uses of alcohol. Much of Irish drinking is convivial, having social rather than religious meaning, a manifestation of solidarity with kinship or friendship groups, an expression of hospitality and also of hostility towards opponents. By comparison, the use of alcohol in orthodox Jewish culture is woven into a network of sacred beliefs and activities expressed in religious and secular rituals and internalized at a very early age. In this context, stable attitudes towards drinking are formed and incorporated into powerful religious sentiments which are constantly renewed through the ceremonial aspects of group life and thus help to maintain sobriety. Other analyses have added to Bales' explanation by suggesting that the status of Jews as a minority group has influenced Jewish drinking habits in that minorities fear the reaction of powerful majorities to behaviour which is regarded as unacceptable (Snyder 1962).

The influence of changing social factors on the drinking habits of a particular group are well illustrated in the case of women's drinking which, it has been argued, has been increasing over the past 30 years (Fillmore 1984, Goddard & Ikin 1988). Women's alcohol consumption is, of course, subject to the same factors which influence supply and demand for the whole society: price, availability, restrictions on access and so on.

However, there are additional factors which have strongly affected women's drinking habits over the centuries and which do not apply to men. Perhaps the most important of these are the attitudes and values concerning acceptable use of alcohol by women, attitudes which, traditionally, have been strongly linked to expectations of women's roles in the family and to perceptions of 'appropriate' feminine behaviour. Unwritten codes of behaviour have generally served to restrict women's use of alcohol, at least in public, and have entailed informal sanctions – shame or embarrassment – on those who transgressed (Camberwell Council on Alcoholism 1980). Not so long ago, it was common for public houses to refuse women entry to the public bar; 'ladies' were confined to the saloon bar and pints of beer, if served at all, were likely to be offered in two half-pint glasses. Over the second half of this century, attitudes changed; many public houses rejected their 'male' image and, along with the alcohol industry, began to woo the female consumer. Advertising was aimed directly at women, the desirability of alcohol use conjured up in lavish portrayals of beautiful women drinking in sophisticated, glamorous and romantic settings. The new sales outlets, supermarkets, grocery stores and wine bars were unstigmatizing and particularly acceptable to women.

The power of the sales drive directed at women is obviously not the sole reason either for changing attitudes towards women's drinking or towards their rising rates of consumption. In many ways the alcohol industry was responding to changes already taking place in women's roles in society. Women were becoming more economically active with more money of their own to spend and greater independence and power to spend it as they chose. Many areas of life which had been restricted or closed to women were being challenged, including the male preserve of the public bar! Nowhere have the changes been more marked than among younger women, and it is perhaps in the behaviour and attitudes of younger women that the influence of social change becomes most visible. Studies in Britain reported less difference between the drinking habits of young women and young men than between the sexes in older age groups. Girls, for example, were taking their turn to buy rounds of drinks (Dorn 1983). A survey of women's drinking in England and Wales found that young women (under 25 years) were more likely than older women to believe that sex differences in drinking expectations were not general among their age group (Breeze 1985). A narrowing in the gap between the genders' views on alcohol use has also been reported from other countries, including Finland where the increase in drinking was most apparent among girls (Rahkonen & Ahlstrom 1989) and where differences in the frequency of intoxication between young men and women diminished in the 1980s.

There are, then, a wide range of social factors which influence whether people drink alcohol at all, how much they drink and how they behave when drinking. But whatever the individual variations in drinking habits, in most societies alcohol use is 'normal', commonplace behaviour and before we can talk about abuse we must define what is meant by the term.

## Use and abuse – the boundaries

Tolerance of the use of alcohol and the boundaries between what society regards as acceptable or unacceptable use have changed over time, from culture to culture and between different groups in society. The degree of tolerance afforded to any individual may depend on factors such as sex, age, social status or on the occasion when drinking takes place. The young man who becomes intoxicated at a friend's birthday party will arouse little comment; if he decides to drive home, he may well be criticized by others for his abuse of alcohol.

While there are many unwritten rules about what constitutes appropriate uses of alcohol and appropriate drinking behaviour, the widespread acceptance of alcohol use as a normal, everyday occurrence makes it all the more difficult to define what is meant by 'abuse'.

### How much is too much?

There are no formal rules or regulations beyond such minimal legislation as the legal age of drinking; medical guidelines are open to interpretation and debate and professional definitions of abuse, or harmful drinking, are often not accepted by the layman. The conscientious GP who advises a male patient to reduce his drinking to the recommended 10–11 pints per week may well be ignored because the patient regards his 15 pints as very moderate when compared to the amounts consumed by his companions.

The difficulty of deciding on the dividing line between use and abuse is not helped by the fact that professional guidelines and definitions also change depending on current knowledge and assessment of risk.

The criteria used in research and surveys are equally volatile. One author listed the variability between seven studies in their measures of the minimum amount of drinks needed to qualify as a 'heavy drinker'; the amounts were: five drinks once in the last year plus 45 drinks in 30 days; one and a half pints of beer every day; got drunk four times in the last year; three and a half pints of beer once a week; one pint of beer twice a week; five drinks once a month; one drink five days out of seven (Knupfer 1987).

Then there is the question of how important it is to assess abuse according to the quantity of alcohol consumed or according to the physiological, psychological and social damage it incurs. Is heavy drinking in itself an abuse of alcohol even if the drinker appears to suffer no harm and others do not complain of adverse effects on their lives?

Examining the problem of how to define alcohol abuse so that the definition might be of some practical use to the worried individual or the concerned professional, the Royal College of Psychiatrists took the stance that 'a person has a drink problem if his or her drinking is, or soon will be, causing him or her any sort of harm or causing harm to any other person' (Royal College of Psychiatrists 1986). This definition is not so far from the much earlier definition of 'alcoholism' proposed by Jellinek – 'any use of alcoholic beverages that causes any damage to the individual or society or both' (Jellinek 1960). However, despite Jellinek's careful distinction between 'alcoholism' in the broad sense and 'alcoholics' who suffered from a form of alcoholism which could be considered a disease, the terms 'alcohol-ism' and 'alcoholic' both became linked to the disease concept and, in the popular view, to heavy, seriously damaging consumption.

The move towards use of the terms 'problem drinker' and alcohol-related problems avoids the pitfalls of equating alcohol abuse with heavy consumption or with the concepts of 'alcoholism', 'addiction' or 'dependency' which tend to focus attention on the heavy drinker with severe alcohol-related difficulties. The terms 'problem drinker' and 'problematic drinking' encompass both the heavy or dependent drinker and the moderate or light drinker who, nevertheless, is experiencing problems or is at risk of doing so (Heather & Robertson 1985).

### How many problems make a 'problem drinker'?

All the same, difficulties of measurement still arise in trying to assess alcohol abuse by the existence of alcohol-related problems. Do we accept the drinker's assessment (or a relative's or employer's) or do we try to find some 'objective' way of measuring whether the drinking is harmful? How many problems must an individual report to be considered 'a problem drinker'? One American researcher acknowledged the difficulty of deciding where the boundary lay between problematical and non-problematical use of alcohol. He reported that in a recent survey he had included 13 items about alcohol dependence:

> If the respondents said yes to three or more of these items, I counted them as problem drinkers. To be more precise, I counted them as having 'problematic drinking' at a moderate level of severity. According to this method of estimation, 5.7 million men and 2.5 million women were problem drinkers. But if I had used a stricter definition of problem drinking, requiring respondents to say yes to four or more items, the estimates would have been lowered to 3.7 million men and 1.5 million women. On the other hand, if I had used two or more items as the criterion, the estimates would have been raised to 8.8 million men and 4.2 million women. (Hilton 1989)

Thus, in a sense, where the line is drawn between

alcohol use and alcohol abuse is itself determined by social forces: the interaction between current knowledge about the effects of alcohol, attitudes towards its use, who is defining the boundaries and for what purpose.

This is not to deny that there are very real physiological reactions and changes which clearly indicate that alcohol has been misused (Royal College of Psychiatrists 1986). However, the development of symptoms is not always easily detected and to wait for the possible appearance of clear evidence of harm misses many individuals whose drinking is causing problems both to themselves and others.

### Consumption and harm

We return, now, to the question of the relevance of per capita consumption of alcohol as a factor in the level of alcohol abuse in society.

The relationship between the scale of alcohol-related problems and the average consumption of alcohol in a country was first observed by a French mathematician and demographer, Ledermann, in the 1950s (Ledermann 1956). Although his theories have been refined and extended in subsequent years (Duffy 1986), there is still a general consensus, based on an accumulation of evidence from many countries, that, in a given population, changes in average consumption over time will lead to predictable changes in the same direction in the scale of alcohol-related harm. (e.g. Bruun *et al.* 1975, Royal College of Psychiatrists 1986).

At the national level, indices of alcohol-related problems such as convictions for drunkenness or drunk driving, deaths from alcoholic cirrhosis of the liver or hospital admissions for alcohol dependence provide some indication of the extent of alcohol abuse in the society (or less broadly within a subgroup of the population). Taken singly, fluctuations in any one indicator may be accounted for in numerous ways – changes in police procedures, in diagnostic knowledge and skills, or in medical technology, in official recording or in the willingness of individuals to seek help for their problems. Taken together, however, such indices are generally accepted as a reliable gauge of the scale of harm attributable to alcohol consumption.

The review by Kendell *et al.* (1983) of trends in Scotland provides one specific example. Between 1978 and 1982, when there was a reduction of 11% in alcohol consumption, first admissions to hospital for alcohol dependence also fell (by 19%), convictions for drunkenness (by 16%) and for drunk driving (by 7%); mortality from liver cirrhosis fell by 4%. Similar associations have been recorded in Sweden (Nordstrom 1987), in Canada (Smart & Mann 1987), in Poland (Wald & Moskalewicz 1984), in the USA (Hilton 1988) and in many other countries.

The association between consumption and harm also holds true when we consider subgroups in the population. Returning to the earlier example of women's rising consumption of alcohol, we find that in England and Wales the indices of harmful drinking rose during the 1960s and 1970s. In 1967 female offences for drunkenness were 5.8% of the total; by 1976 they were 8.0% of all offences. Convictions for drinking and driving rose from 1.1% of all offences in 1968 to 3.1% in 1977. Between 1964 and 1975, the number of males diagnosed as alcoholics doubled but the number of females trebled, thus lowering the ratio of men to women alcoholics in mental hospitals from 4:1 to 2.7:1. (Camberwell Council on Alcoholism 1980).

It has been estimated that, in the UK, alcohol-related problems cost the country over £160 million in 1983. The estimate took account of costs to industry from sickness and unemployment, the cost of lost days in housework among economically inactive women, working years lost through premature death, the cost to the National Health Service, and the cost of criminal activity including material damage, road accidents or fire (McDonnell & Maynard 1985). Such estimates are unable to take account of the sum of individual damage to health and well-being, the social and psychological damage and the misery suffered not only by the drinker but by family and other associates.

## Alcohol abuse and government intervention

Government policy, directly and indirectly, influences both the availability of alcohol and the demand for alcohol. The formation of policy with the explicit aim of reducing alcohol consumption depends on whether on not alcohol consumption has been defined as a social problem which warrants, and is susceptible to, intervention at a national level. By defining alcohol consumption as a problem, it becomes an object of public attention and responsibility permitting the development of appropriate agencies and agents to address the problem (Gusfield 1982). Over the centuries, aspects of alcohol use have been defined as a social problem demanding legislative action. Higgs (1984), for instance, recounts how in England 'Acts of 1495 and 1504 had empowered justices to suppress alehouses in their neighbourhoods which diverted people from the martial art of archery', and an act of 1552 'enforced the licensing of alehouses by justices in order to prevent "the intolerable hurts and troubles to the commonwealth of the realm daily increasing."' Gutzke (1984) examines the nineteenth century Edwardian campaign against maternal drinking which linked drinking by working class women to infant mortality rates and racial degeneration and resulted in legislation to prohibit children under 14 from licensed premises.

The general acceptance in the latter half of this century of the consumption–harm theory has led to consideration of a wide range of national control policies as a means of restricting per capita consumption and thereby reducing the level of alcohol-related problems. Measures have included taxation and legislation as well as education and publicity campaigns.

It is not always easy to assess the effect of social intervention on alcohol consumption and harm, particularly in the case of attempts to change behaviour through promoting education and awareness. Health educators face a complex task in trying to target and monitor educational efforts, and although health education programmers have been shown to increase knowledge about alcohol, their effect on deeply held attitudes is less clear. Nor is there any good evidence that drinking behaviour is altered either by increased awareness of alcohol or by a change in attitudes (Royal College of Psychiatrists 1986).

Evidence for the effectiveness of government intervention is stronger when we look at efforts to manipulate the availability of alcohol through legislation and taxation. Even so, it is still difficult to know whether any one form of control strategy alone will achieve the desired effect. Governments often implement more than one change at a time, and it is rarely possible to conduct any satisfactory investigation of the part played by concurrent social and economic trends which may also influence peoples' drinking habits and their experience of alcohol-related problems.

### Availability and harm – some examples

There are a considerable number of studies where an association has been found between government intervention – either the imposition of control measures or changes in legislation – and a corresponding change in the level of consumption and alcohol-related harm in a target population.

The effectiveness of *price* as a regulator of alcohol consumption has been demonstrated in many countries and over different periods of time. The report from the Royal College of Psychiatrists (1986) summarizes price responsiveness in England over the centuries, recording, for instance, that beer consumption in England dropped sharply when duty was tripled in 1690 and again when the price of malt rose in 1791; consumption of beer rose again with rising national prosperity and a reduction in duty in 1880. Price controls introduced in the second half of the eighteenth century helped to reduce the notorious abuse of gin. In recent times, a drop in the real price of alcohol has been one of the factors associated with rising consumption since the 1950s.

Other studies have indicated how levels of consumption and harm may respond to changes in the laws regarding the legal age of drinking. For example, concern over the incidence of road crashes among 16–20 year olds in New York led to a decision to raise the *minimum legal age* for purchasing alcoholic beverages from 18 to 19 years. Surveys were conducted the month before legislation became effective, and one year and three years after legislation. It was found that, prior to the change, 18 year olds' purchasing patterns had been much the same as for 19–20 year olds. Following legislation, there was a decrease in reported alcohol purchasing by that age group and the decrease was maintained in the longer term. Purchasing by other age groups did not change significantly over this period. The short-term decreases in alcohol consumption were found to coincide with decreases in reported drinking and driving, alcohol-related crashes and alcohol-related traffic convictions (Williams & Lillis 1988). The opposite effect was found when the drinking age was lowered in three Australian States; there was an increase in male juvenile crime by as much as 20–25% in two of the three states (Smith & Burvill 1987).

Restricting or expanding *sales outlets* is another way in which government action may influence the level of alcohol abuse in society. In 1978 the State laws in North Carolina were changed to allow distilled spirits to be sold by the individual drink for the first time since Prohibition. Between 1973 and 1982 there was an increase of between 6% and 7.4% in total distilled spirits sold in areas where liquor-by-the-drink was implemented. No comparable change was found for a comparison group of areas where the law remained unchanged. The observed increases occurred immediately after the effective date of legislation and persisted throughout the four years of the study (Holder & Blose 1987).

The association between consumption and legislative action is, however, rarely as clear-cut as the above examples suggest and other social and economic forces can operate to produce unpredictable results. There are, for instance, occasions when increasing the availability or decreasing the price of alcohol has not resulted in increased levels of consumption and harm (Duffy & Plant 1986, Davies 1988, Mulford & Fitzgerald 1988).

A clear instance of an unexpected outcome of policy comes from Sweden. Between 1920 and 1955, Sweden operated a rationing system which gave citizens over the age of 20 (with the exception of married women) an allowance of between one and four litres of spirits per month, the amount depending on marital and social status and social stability. The price of spirits during this period was low. With the abolition of rationing in 1955, the price of spirits rose; but for heavy drinkers, the price was now less than they had had to pay during rationing to obtain alcohol extra to their allowance from black market sources or at restaurant prices. Thus, while alcohol was more expensive for moderate and light drinkers, it was cheaper for those who drank heavily; their level of consumption rose with an attendant sharp rise in male mortality from liver cirrhosis (Nordstrom 1987).

Clearly, caution is required in using national trends and patterns of alcohol consumption as a predictor of levels of alcohol abuse or in interpreting the possible effects of government intervention on trends in consumption and harm. Nevertheless, in the broadest sense, the structure of society – the economy, political activity and regulatory institutions – and the general beliefs and attitudes towards alcohol use held by a society, provide the framework within which patterns of consumption and harm evolve. However, in seeking to explain the existence of variations in alcohol use and abuse among particular groups or, even more so, differences between individuals, we must delve more closely into the particular context of people's lives, the social groups and social networks to which they belong.

## Social groups and social networks

In the course of everyday activities, most people are involved with a variety of groups and social networks, some of them close-knit such as the family, others more diffuse such as university colleagues working in the same discipline or old school friends. These 'reference groups' impart to the members codes of beliefs and behaviour, the 'rules' of the group, which are learned by new members and sustained through remaining in contact or engaging in activity with others (Becker *et al.* 1972, Becker 1973).

General attitudes towards drug use may be conveyed along with other values, and existing members of the group may act as 'role models', providing examples of expected patterns of drug-using behaviour. Membership of a variety of groups or networks is likely to expose the individual to conflicting values and expectations concerning drug use but most people have little difficulty in adapting their behaviour to suit the social context and not all reference groups exert an equal influence over the individual's attitudes and behaviour. However, the importance of alcohol use as a symbol of group cohesion and belonging may lead the individual consciously or subconsciously to adopt drinking habits and drinking styles which are ultimately harmful. The most obvious and extreme example is the 'skid row' drinker. The deviant, criminal, or alienated drinker who finds a new network of social relationships on skid row adopts the drinking 'culture' of the new group and finds an alternative form of social organization and social values built around the safe procuring and consuming of alcohol (Rubington 1962, Archard 1975).

In more general terms, when considering alcohol use and the development of problematical drinking behaviour, three groups are of particular importance, the family, the peer group and the occupational group to which the individual belongs.

### Family and peer group

Families play an important role in conveying attitudes towards alcohol use to the young child (Casswell *et al.* 1985), and although outside influences, particularly the media, are also influential (Jahoda *et al.* 1980, Casswell *et al.* 1988), direct experience of alcohol and alcohol users is largely confined to the home until a child reaches adolescence when peer influence enters the picture (Kandel & Andrews 1987, Wilks & Callan 1988, Wilks *et al.* 1989). The mechanisms by which parents and peers influence drinking behaviour are not necessarily exactly the same (O'Connor 1978, Biddle *et al.* 1980, Bank *et al.* 1985, Kandel & Andrews 1987, Wilks *et al.* 1989), nor is the process necessarily the same for boys and girls. One study, for example, found that among other sex differences, the strongest predictors of alcohol use by adolescent girls

were their perceptions of best friend's drinking and their best friend's normative standards; the strongest predictors of alcohol use for boys were their perceptions of parental drinking and actual consumption by fathers (Wilks *et al.* 1989). Drinking habits and beliefs about alcohol are then, to some extent, 'handed down' through the family and peer group as part of the normal process of socialization into group life.

In considering the influence of family and peers on drinking behaviour an important question is whether heavy drinking in youth is likely to continue into adulthood or result in problematical drinking later in life. Alcohol consumption and the experience of alcohol-related problems have been found to vary by age in both cross-sectional and longitudinal research studies (Fillmore 1987, Hauge & Irgens-Jensen 1987). The general pattern to emerge from the findings of these studies is that, as people get older, the incidence of heavy drinking and alcohol-related problems decreases; chronicity of alcohol problems is highest in middle age; and age, irrespective of alcohol consumption or drinking pattern, influences the nature of negative consequences of alcohol. Hauge & Irgens-Jensen (1987), for example, comment that:

> acting out behaviour seems to be more common among young people, while experiencing health problems and social reactions on the part of family and peers because of the respondent's own drinking seems to be rather more common amongst older people.

Some studies suggest that heavy drinking in youth does increase the risk of alcohol abuse later in life. Evidence from a UK longitudinal study found that those young people who drank most and more frequently at 16 years of age were most likely at 23 to report heavy alcohol consumption (Ghodsian & Power 1987). Fillmore (1975), in a 20-year follow-up study of students in 27 American colleges, concluded that if a respondent drank in youth *and* reported alcohol problems it was likely that that person would report problems 20 years later.

Other studies lend support to Blane's (1979) view that 'frequent heavy drinking is a self limiting condition'. Donovan *et al.* (1983) reported that male and female college students classified as problem drinkers while adolescents in 1972–73, tended to be non-problem drinkers as young adults in 1979. Plant *et al.* (1985) found that drinking habits among a sample of Scottish school children aged 15–16 years were only a poor predictor of drinking in young adulthood, even among those who reported heavy drinking in the school survey.

Predictors other than the amount of alcohol consumed may, however, be more useful indicators of later problem drinking. Plant *et al.* (1985) found that for females the experience of alcohol-related problems in 1979–80 predicted problem drinking in 1983. A diverse range of specific risk factors in adolescence has been suggested, for example, binge drinking (Fillmore 1975), early personality problems (Donovan *et al.* 1983, Cox 1985), drinking in public houses at an early age (Plant *et al.* 1985), prolonged unemployment in adolescence (Power & Estaugh 1990). However, research evidence is not strong enough to distinguish with any certainty specific indicators or groups of risk factors which associate adolescent drinking with problem drinking in adulthood.

More important, perhaps, is the conclusion reached by Fillmore (1975) that 'problems which tend to characterise young problem drinkers are not necessarily those which serve as good predictive tools for later problems'. As illustration, she notes the well-established association between drinking by young men and driving offences, accidents and belligerent behaviour; she notes that in her study these associations did not predict later problem drinking unless they were accompanied in youth by at least infrequent intoxication and symptomatic drinking.

In other words, we need to distinguish whether there are particular sets or groups of risk factors which can more accurately predict which young drinkers are likely to abuse alcohol in later years while acknowledging that the majority of young people mature out of heavy drinking as they become involved in jobs, marriages and other interests.

One particular risk factor to receive considerable attention has been the influence of a childhood spent in a family with a history of problem drinking.

## ALCOHOLIC FAMILIES

The expanding literature on genetic factors in alcoholism and the increasing probability that some people may inherit greater genetic vulnerability than others to the effects of alcohol (Adityanjee & Murray 1991) has not diminished the importance of investigating environmental and social contextual factors which influence whether persons 'at risk' will, in fact, drink problematically.

The possibility discussed above, that attitudes and behaviour patterns are transmitted between generations, does not mean that children will inevitably use alcohol in ways, or quantities, similar to their parents or develop alcohol-related problems if brought up in homes with a problem-drinking parent (Harburg *et al.* 1990). Studies of 'resilience' have indicated a number of personality factors and environmental contexts which may be protective or help to counter the experience of being brought up in an 'alcoholic' family (Woodside 1988). However, the ill-effects of a childhood spent in a family where one or both parents have an alcohol problem have been well documented in many countries (Woodside 1988, Orford & Velleman 1990) and, despite conflicting findings in the research, the offspring of families with a history of drinking problems are still generally considered to be at risk of becoming problematical drinkers in adulthood. The mechanisms through which the transmission of inter-generational alcohol problems takes place remain, unfortunately, obscure (Orford & Velleman 1990). Explanations incorporate a variety of hypotheses; for instance that the risk is greater in a family context where there is a heavy drinking parent, especially a same-sex parent; where there is stress in the family and the disruption of family rituals; or where the child witnesses excessive drinking in the home. Research by Orford & Velleman (1990) examining these explanations concluded that 'the offspring of parents with drinking problems are probably at somewhat increased risk from drinking excessively in adulthood . . . However, each of the studies mentioned finds only a minority of offspring to be particularly at risk.' That being the case, the authors support investigation of the mediating variables which might explain why some offspring develop problems while others do not. From their own work, they suggest that where two parents are problem drinkers or where excessive drinking occurs often in the home, offspring may experience a greater degree of 'non-specific family disharmony' and that 'discord or disharmony at home, rather than alcohol-specific effects themselves, may be the factor that confers vulnerability'.

## Employment and unemployment

Employment, like the family, is a central part of most people's lives. Professions and workplaces transmit attitudes and values, encourage or discourage modes of behaviour, influence feelings of self-esteem and identity and the formation of social networks in much the same way as does the family (Plant 1979). The use of alcohol plays a prominent part in the working lives of many people and is often woven closely into the accepted 'culture' of occupations and work institutions, be it the business executive entertaining clients or the army recruit proving his affinity with his peers.

### OCCUPATIONAL RISKS

Indications that employment in particular professions or occupational groups carries an increased risk of developing drinking problems can be found in detailed studies of occupational groups with high rates of alcoholism, data from treatment agencies which show that people in some occupations are more likely than others to seek help for alcohol problems, and high rates of mortality from liver cirrhosis in certain occupations (Plant 1979). Typically, occupations such as the armed forces, the medical profession, occupations associated with the food and drink industry and with entertainment come high on the list (Plant 1979, Slattery *et al.* 1986).

It may be, of course, that people who are predisposed to drink excessively are attracted to particular occupations rather than that the work structure and situation encourage heavy drinking. This possibility was considered by Plant (1979) in a study of Scottish male manual workers, one sample of men being employed in the drink trade in brewing and distilling, the 'high risk' group, and the second sample, the control group, being employed in industries which were not considered as 'high risk'. The findings of the study lent some support to the theory that among the new recruits, the drink industry was more likely than the control industries to attract heavy drinkers; however, recruits joining the drinks industry were not more likely than controls to report alcohol-related problems. A year after joining the brewing and distilling trade, occupation was found to have had a significant impact on the men's drinking habits and on their experience of alcohol-related problems. Some men had left the industry specifically to reduce pressures to drink. The three-year follow-up confirmed that 'current job status was closely related not only to the general level of alcohol consumption but also to the level of alcohol-related problems and to a range of perceptions of drinking levels and alcohol-related harm amongst one's workmates'.

From a review of the literature on alcohol and occupation, Plant (1979) proposed a number of factors common to occupational groups at high risk of developing alcohol problems. They were:
1 Availability of alcohol.
2 Social pressure to drink.
3 Separation from normal social or sexual relationships.
4 Freedom from supervision.
5 Very high or very low income.
6 Collusion by colleagues.
7 Strains, stresses, and hazards.
8 Preselection of 'high-risk' people.

The way in which occupational activity integrates with other spheres of life may also influence when and how an individual drinks. A good example is provided by a study of offshore oil rig workers in Scotland. While on duty, the men were strictly forbidden to drink alcohol, but approximately 30% of the 213 men studied had drunk amounts above the safe limits recommended by the Royal College of Psychiatrists (1986) during the week preceding their duty spell. The authors of the study comment that:

> ... many of these men are drawn from a background where heavy drinking is the norm, are being introduced into a shift system which completely disrupts normal social life, are being paid very high wages immediately prior to having a fortnight of idleness in which to spend them – all circumstances which must exacerbate drinking. (Aiken & McCance 1982)

While being in certain occupations may carry an increased risk of developing harmful drinking practices, becoming unemployed or being long-term unemployed brings its own stresses which, it has been argued, are likely to result in heavier alcohol consumption.

THE RISKS OF BECOMING UNEMPLOYED

Studies of the psychological reactions to unemployment indicate that there are a number of different stages and phases through which the individual typically passes and which involve changes in mood, in sense of identity and self-esteem, in level of purposeful activity and, of course, in economic status and social integration. (Research on phases in unemployment is summarized in Winton *et al.* 1986.)

Since susceptibility to the stresses and frustrations of unemployment is highly individual, variations in drinking behaviour in the stages leading up to and following unemployment are to be expected. Reduced financial circumstances, for instance, may lead to cutting down expenditure on alcohol; on the other hand, redundancy money and unaccustomed leisure could result in heavier drinking, at least in the short term. Reactions to changes in social circumstances are also likely to be influenced by the individual's age, social class, marital status or sex (Layne & Whitehead 1985, Whitehead & Layne 1987, Whitehead *et al.* 1987, Lee *et al.* 1990, Power & Estaugh 1990). The young unemployed male is, perhaps, more likely to spend his redundancy money on drinking than the older married man with a family to support. Research studies have produced confusing and contradictory findings on the effect of unemploy-

ment on alcohol consumption, so much so that Crawford *et al.* (1987) in a review of the literature concluded that 'unemployment either affects alcohol use and abuse or it does not'. Despite such a doubtful summation, there is considerable evidence that the unemployed are more at risk of developing hazardous drinking practices than are the employed (Crawford *et al.* 1987, Lee *et al.* 1990). To take one example, comparing the drinking habits of fully employed and unemployed males in three areas of Britain, Crawford *et al.* (1987) found that in the week prior to interview, the unemployed had consumed significantly greater amounts of alcohol during their heaviest drinking day, and reported longer drinking periods and faster consumption rates; they were also more likely to report a range of adverse consequences from drinking over the preceding two years.

As with employment and unemployment, the social and psychological consequences of change in other areas of life may also affect drinking habits. The 'empty nest syndrome', for example, feelings of role loss when children leave home, has been one of the factors thought to account for the onset of heavy drinking in middle-aged women (references in Camberwell Council on Alcoholism 1980). On the other hand, changing circumstances such as in place of residence or in job, getting married, or breakdown in health have been found to initiate remission from excessive drinking (Smart 1976). It is important, then, to consider the relationship between the development of drinking patterns and changing social circumstances.

### Alcohol abuse and change in social networks

The notion of 'career' has been used to describe ways in which drinking patterns evolve and change over time (Plant 1979, Edwards 1984). Edwards (1984) sketches the course of a typical drinking career, in as far as that exists, as follows: as a child, the individual is totally abstinent or drinks only on special occasions or under family supervision and control; then follows a period of adolescent transitions in the course of which the young person enters fully into the drinking role;

this is succeeded by several decades of mature adult drinking before consumption is reduced as retirement age approaches. Variations in the basic career pathway arise from cultural and social differences and a drinking career may include periods of deviant or problematical drinking with the individual moving in and out of deviant drinking more than once in the course of a lifetime.

If, as prior discussion suggests, the use and abuse of alcohol is linked in some way to an individual's social situation, then, as social circumstances and social networks change, so we might expect the drinking career to be affected with some social situations resulting in the onset of deviant drinking patterns.

One way in which researchers have attempted to examine and account for changes in alcohol consumption and the experience of alcohol problems is by studying 'life events'. Events such as marriage, the birth of a child, sudden illness, divorce, unemployment, changes in job or in place of residence, retirement, etc., signal a transition from one social situation or social status to another and bring changes in roles or role expectations which are often accompanied by fundamental psychological and social change, in self-perception perhaps, or in self-esteem, in social standing or in financial status. An extensive 'life events' literature has demonstrated the importance of such events in the aetiology of a wide range of physical and psychiatric disorders (Brown & Harris 1989) and, theoretically, it seems reasonable to suppose that life events might also trigger changes in a drinking career with stressful events leading to heavier drinking.

Unfortunately, the association between life events and the onset of problem drinking is not at all clear (reviewed in Allan & Cooke 1985, O'Doherty & Davies 1987). Morrisey & Schuckit (1978) and Cooke & Allan (1984), for instance, found no association between life events and the onset of women's problem drinking. On the other hand, Gorman & Peters' (1990) study of men and women supported the view that stressful events may, in part, lead to heavier drinking.

It is not surprising that the link between stressful events and onset of problem drinking is difficult to establish. For one thing, people try to

make sense of the world they live in and of their own behaviour; the way in which an event is interpreted and the meaning bestowed on situations is likely to influence the degree to which stress is experienced and the kind of action taken by individuals. For another, most of the research on life events and alcohol use is retrospective; excessive drinkers, especially women, may cite stressful events as a reasonable explanation for behaviour which society condemns (Dahlgren & Myrhed 1977). Then there is the problem of timing onset of an event and onset of change in drinking habits (Gorman 1987). These are only some of the theoretical and methodological problems which beset the literature on life events and alcohol abuse and make it difficult to establish the connection between social change and the onset of change in drinking patterns. However, the evidence from research on age and changing patterns of alcohol consumption cited earlier and on the part played by life events in spontaneous remission from alcoholism (Smart 1976), is more encouraging of the basic contention that the individual's drinking career is intricately linked with other careers, as spouse, employee, parent, etc., and that change in social roles and social circumstances is likely to influence drinking habits.

## Social factors and the response to alcohol abuse

Societies and social groups respond in very different ways to the problems of alcohol misuse. Even if we limit ourselves to a discussion of organized responses in western industrialized countries, we encounter a vast array of different approaches and organizational structures each embedded in its own particular social and political context.

The struggle to implement control measures in England provides a good example. Proposals put forward in 1834 to reduce problems of drunkenness by introducing a rational licensing policy were laughed out of Parliament and the Select Committee which had attempted their introduction was dubbed the 'Drunken Committee' (Longmate 1982). However, the growing power of the Temperance Movement kept the question of alcohol control on the political agenda throughout the century and inspired the Liberal Government's 1908 Major Licensing Bill which again attempted to impose extremely strict controls on alcohol availability. This bill was rejected by the House of Lords on the grounds that it was not in the interests of the ordinary working man. A few years later, with the outbreak of war in 1914 and concern over the effects of drunkenness on the war effort, far stricter licensing restrictions were imposed and implemented without protest. As one historian of the family points out, 'What concern for the drunkard's family had failed to achieve in a century of agitation, anxiety about delay in turning out the means to kill fellow human beings accomplished overnight' (Longmate 1982). Fed by the wide acceptance of consumption-harm theories in the latter half of this century, discussion of control methods and questions of public health have again gathered momentum, although not without controversy (Anderson 1989, Baggott 1990). Powerful commercial interests, the demands of pressure groups concerned with alcohol misuse, the weight of medical opinion, increasing research activity producing 'scientific' evidence of alcohol-related harm and the need for sensitivity to public opinion are only some of the social pressures which have contributed to the development of UK alcohol policy in recent years.

Historically, other countries have adopted quite different approaches to the imposition of control measures, from the minimal legislation enforced in some of the wine-producing countries such as Spain or Italy – where for trade purposes quality control has been of greater importance than the control of consumption – to much stricter measures in the Scandinavian countries (Davies & Walsh 1983).

Differences in the structure and nature of alcohol treatment services provide further examples of how social forces shape policy formation and outcome. The surgical approach to chronic alcoholism – sterilization – was noted as the major response in Germany in 1936 where existing facilities for the treatment of alcoholism had largely been destroyed and local clinics were marked out as centres of 'subversive activity' (Baumohl & Room 1987). In England (as elsewhere in Europe and America) the institutional

response to alcohol treatment has its roots in the nineteenth century with the development of inebriate asylums or reformatories for the control and treatment of habitual drunkards. Although manifestly a failure (the asylums ceased to exist around 1915), the institutional response was strongly supported both by the Temperance Movement and by the medical profession and survived as the dominant British response to treatment until the 1970s. The movement over the last 20 years towards community-based agencies, notably councils on alcoholism, alcohol advisory services and community alcohol teams, is a result of many trends from changing perceptions of the problem to the necessity of coping with new client groups with different needs, to changing sources of funding for services, and the input of new ideas from greater numbers of psychologists and social workers entering the expanding world of alcohol treatment (Heather & Robertson 1985, Collins 1990).

At quite another level, the successful implementation of treatment policy depends on a host of social and cultural factors operating at the point of service delivery. For instance, a decentralized system of service management and funding may result in variable provision in different regions depending on local perceptions of needs and priorities, local pressure groups, cultural traditions in the area and so on. The uneven development of alcohol treatment units in different health authority regions in England and Wales is one example (Baggott 1990).

A further consideration is the sociocultural factors which influence access to treatment or people's willingness to use the services provided, and the symptoms they present when they do attend. As Babor & Mendelson (1986) comment, 'Modes of treatment may differ in their appropriateness for various population groups. Treatment personnel may respond differently to patients by using ethnic stereotypes to assign treatments. Patients may respond differently to personnel who do not belong to the same cultural group.' In recent years, much discussion has centred on ways of adapting services to make them more acceptable to women or to ethnic minorities, more attractive to young people or more relevant to homeless drinkers or other 'special populations'.

One illustration comes from experiments to incorporate traditional healing approaches within the provision of alcohol services for American Indian populations. Until they came into contact with Europeans, American Indians had virtually no access to alcohol. Without culturally established patterns of alcohol use or cultural controls on drinking behaviour, the introduction of alcohol into traditional Indian societies had devastating effects. According to Hall (1986), three environmental hypotheses may account for the relatively high level of alcohol abuse found in Indian populations today. First, Indian societies, which had developed highly structured ways of handling social problems, were exposed to alcohol at a time when they faced many other direct and indirect threats and when it was difficult to integrate the new drug in a positive fashion into Indian social life. As a result, alcohol became a symbol of Indian subjugation to the extent that Indian drinking patterns have been called 'the world's oldest ongoing protest movement'. A second hypothesis draws on social modelling concepts – one generation learning the habits of another – to account for current patterns of abuse. Thirdly, alcohol abuse among Indians has been linked to continuing adverse socioeconomic conditions: poverty, unemployment and low access to social status and positions of power. While traditional healing practices were not called on in the past as a response to alcoholism, the recent revival of native traditions has led to an interest in using traditional rituals and healing methods alongside modern approaches to alcohol treatment. Adapted alcohol treatment programmes have successfully provided, or encouraged the use of, a sweat lodge, a therapeutic ritual common to the cultural heritage of American Indians; some programmes also used a traditional medicine man or the Native American Church alongside contemporary approaches such as family therapy, behaviourist techniques or Alcoholics Anonymous (Hall 1986).

Finally, the nature and scale of alcohol consumption and alcohol-related problems, and the development of prevention and treatment policies are subject to changing socioeconomic trends at international level. While the aim of national policy may be to reduce consumption and harm, the level of domestic consumption depends on the interaction of international supply and demand and the development of international trade, which may conflict with or act as a constraint on the implementation of preventive health policy (Powell 1989). International marketing strategies and the alcohol industry's quest for new markets have been shown to destabilize traditional drinking habits and result in forms of abuse which communities are unprepared to face. For example, in developing countries, the diffusion of European-style drinks has added to rather than substituted for traditional brews and increasing tourism has had a major impact on the availability and use of alcohol, in some cases incurring considerable hidden economic and social costs (McBride & Mosher 1985). Within the European Community, harmonization policies, aiming to remove barriers to trade and promote price competition across the Community, have been criticized as conflicting with UK public health objectives to reduce alcohol consumption and the level of alcohol abuse (Maynard & O'Brien 1982, Braine 1990).

International trade processes may seem very remote from the everyday work of the clinician trying to help an individual with drinking problems. They are, nevertheless, part of the complex interplay between societal and individual factors which determine both the problem and the response to the problem. The above examples are merely illustrative of a very wide range of factors which influence the perceptions and behaviour of the state, professionals, the public and those who require help for drinking problems.

## Conclusion

Over the past century, causal explanations for alcohol abuse have changed from seeing the problem as a moral or legal concern – the appropriate response being control and punishment by incarceration in jail or, in England, in the workhouse – to regarding it as a medical or public health concern demanding a prevention-treatment response.

More recently biomedical explanations and

responses, embodied in the 'disease' concept of alcoholism, have been tempered and broadened by social-psychological and sociological theory, with a shift of emphasis from 'person-centred' to 'situation-centred' explanations for problem drinking.

Current professional thinking now offers a complex model of causation which views any individual's drinking as a movable point located on a continuum from low-risk to high-risk drinking and which links biomedical, psychological and social factors in explaining movement in any direction along the continuum. The point at which alcohol abuse occurs on the continuum is the outcome of a definitional process taking place both at the level of society as a whole, for instance in defining 'safe limits', and at the level of each individual where the 'label' is generally the result of interaction between the drinker, family or associates, and medical professionals.

The focus of this chapter has been to illustrate how alcohol consumption and alcohol abuse are responsive to social change in the widest sense. Drinking habits may change along with the availability of alcohol in society or general attitudes towards the appropriate use of alcohol. Changes in the reference groups more immediately meaningful to individual life-styles – the family, peer group or occupational group – or changes in the particular circumstances of any person's life – in their financial status perhaps, their marriage or state of health – may also affect drinking patterns.

It is not possible to describe exactly the mechanisms and processes which influence levels of alcohol consumption and the nature of drinking habits, nor to provide precise details of which social factors or groups of factors will accurately predict alcohol abuse. Nevertheless, an emphasis on alcohol consumption and alcohol abuse as social phenomena puts at our disposal a wider range of concepts and theories than has hitherto been available both for understanding and for responding to drinking problems. Since alcohol abuse is no longer confined to an abnormal minority of drinkers but is a risk run by everyone who drinks, finding an appropriate response demands consideration of a wide range of measures which address the problems not only at the

individual level but nationally and internationally at the level of society as a whole.

## References

Adityanjee & Murray R.M. (1991) The role of genetic predisposition in alcoholism. In Glass I.B. (ed.) *International Handbook of Addiction Behaviour*. Routledge, London.

Adlaf E.M. & Smart R.G. (1985) Drug use and religious affiliation, feelings and behaviour. *British Journal of Addiction* 80, 163–171.

Aiken G.J. & McCance C. (1982) Alcohol consumption in offshore oil rig workers. *British Journal of Addiction* 77, 305–310.

Allan C.A. & Cooke D.J. (1985) Stressful life events and alcohol misuse in women: a critical review. *Journal of Studies on Alcohol* 46, 147–152.

Anderson D. (ed.) (1989) *Drinking to Your Health. The Allegations and the Evidence*. The Social Affairs Unit, London.

Archard P. (1975) *The Bottle Won't Leave You. A Study of Homeless Alcoholics and their Guardians*. Alcoholics Recovery Project, London.

Babor T.F. (ed.) (1986) Alcohol and culture: comparative perspectives from Europe and America. *Annals of the New York Academy of Sciences* 472.

Babor T.F. & Mendelson J.H. (1986) Ethnic/religious differences in the manifestation and treatment of alcoholism. In Babor T.F. (ed.) *Alcohol and Culture: Comparative Perspectives from Europe and America*, pp. 46–59. The New York Academy of Sciences, New York.

Baggott R. (1990) *Alcohol, Politics and Social Policy*. Gower Publishing Company, Aldershot.

Bales R.F. (1962) Attitudes toward drinking in the Irish culture. In Pittman D.J. & Snyder C.R. (eds) *Society, Culture, and Drinking Patterns*. John Wiley, Chichester.

Bank B.D., Biddle B.J., Anderson D.S. *et al.* (1985) Comparative research on the social determinants of adolescent drinking. *Social Psychology Quarterly* 48, 164–177.

Baumohl J. & Room R. (1987) Inebriety, doctors, and the State. Alcoholism treatment institutions before 1940. In Galanter M. (ed.) *Recent Developments in Alcoholism*, vol. 5, New York, Plenum.

Becker H.S. (1973) *Outsiders: Studies in the Sociology of Deviance*, pp. 41–58. Free Press, New York.

Becker H.S. *et al.* (1972) *Boys in White: Student Culture in Medical School*. Brown, Chicago.

Biddle B.J., Bank B.D. & Marlin M.M. (1980) Social determinants of adolescent drinking: what they think, what they do and what I think and do. *Journal of Studies on Alcohol* 41, 215–241.

Blane H.T. (1979) Middle aged alcoholics and young drinkers. In Blane H.T. & Chafetz M.E. (eds) *Youth, Alcohol and Social Policy*. Plenum, New York.

Braine Rt Hon Sir B. (1990) A British perspective on alcohol problems in relation to European Community policy. *British Journal of Addiction* 85, 677–681.

Breeze E. (1985) *Women and Drinking*. HMSO, London.

Brown G.W. & Harris T. (eds) (1989) *Life Events and Illness*. Guilford Press, New York.

Bruun K., Lumio M. & Makela K. *et al.* (1975) *Alcohol Control Policies in Public Health Perspective*. Finnish Foundation for Alcohol Studies, Helsinki.

Camberwell Council on Alcoholism (1980) *Women and Alcohol*. Tavistock, London.

Casswell S., Brasch P., Gilmore L. & Silva P. (1985) Children's attitudes to alcohol and awareness of alcohol-related problems. *British Journal of Addiction* 80, 191–194.

Casswell S., Gilmore L.L., Silva P. & Brasch P. (1988) What children know about alcohol and how they know it. *British Journal of Addiction* 83, 223–227.

Cochrane R. & Bal S. (1990) The drinking habits of Sikh, Hindu, Muslim and white men in the West Midlands: a community survey. *British Journal of Addiction* 85, 759–769.

Collins S. (ed.) (1990) *Alcohol, Social Work and Helping*. Tavistock/Routledge, London.

Cooke D.J. & Allan C.A. (1984) Stressful life events and alcohol abuse in women: a general population study. *British Journal of Addiction* 79, 425–430.

Cox M.N. (1985) Personality correlates of substance abuse. In Galizio M. & Maisto S.A. (eds) *Determinants of Substance Abuse. Biological, Psychosocial and Environmental Factors*. Plenum, New York.

Crawford A., Plant M.A., Kreitman N. & Latcham R.W. (1987) Unemployment and drinking behaviour: some data from a general population survey of alcohol use. *British Journal of Addiction* 82, 1007–1016.

Dahlgren L. & Myrhed M. (1977) Female alcoholics. *Acta Psychiatrica Scandinavica* 56, 39–49.

Davies P. (1988) The Licensing (Scotland) Act 1976. *British Journal of Addiction* 83, 129–130.

Davies P. & Walsh D. (1983) *Alcohol Problems and Alcohol Control in Europe*. Croom Helm, London.

Donovan J.E., Jessor R. & Jessor L. (1983) Problem drinking in adolescence and young adulthood: a follow-up study. *Journal of Studies on Alcohol* 44, 109–137.

Dorn N. (1983) *Alcohol Use and the State*. Croom Helm, London.

Duffy J.C. (1986) The distribution of alcohol consumption – 30 years on. *British Journal of Addiction* 81, 735–741 (and three comments on J.C. Duffy's paper pp. 743–748).

Duffy J.C. & Plant M. (1986) Scotland's liquor licensing: an assessment. *British Medical Journal* 292, 36–39.

Edwards G. (1984) Drinking in longitudinal perspective: career and natural history. *British Journal of Addiction* 79, 175–183.

Fillmore K.M. (1975) Relationships between specific drinking problems in early adulthood and middle age. *Journal of Studies on Alcohol* 36, 882–917.

Fillmore K.M. (1984) 'When angels fall': women's drinking as cultural preoccupation and in reality. In Wilsnack S.C. & Beckman L.J. (eds) *Alcohol Problems in Women*. Guilford Press, New York.

Fillmore K.M. (1987) Prevalence, incidence and chronicity of drinking patterns and problems among men as a function of age: a longitudinal and cohort analysis. *British Journal of Addiction* 82, 77–83.

Ghodsian M. & Power C. (1987) Alcohol consumption between the ages of 16 and 23 in Britain: a longitudinal study. *British Journal of Addiction* 82, 175–180.

Goddard E. & Ikin C. (1988) *Drinking in England and Wales in 1987*. HMSO, London.

Gorman D.M. (1987) Measuring onset of 'caseness' in studies of stressful life events and alcohol abuse. *British Journal of Addiction* 82, 1017–1020.

Gorman D.M. & Peters T.J. (1990) Types of life events and the onset of alcohol dependence. *British Journal of Addiction* 85, 71–79.

Gusfield J.R. (1982) Deviance in the Welfare State: the alcoholism profession and the entitlements of stigma. *Research in Social Problems and Public Policy* 2, 1–20.

Gutzke D.W. (1984) The cry of the children: the Edwardian medical campaign against maternal drinking. *British Journal of Addiction* 79, 71–84.

Hall R.L. (1986) Alcohol treatment in American Indian populations: an indigenous treatment modality compared with traditional approaches. In Babor T.F. (ed.) *Alcohol and Culture: Comparative Perspectives from Europe and America*. New York Academy of Sciences, New York.

Harburg E., Gleiberman L., Franceisco W., Schork A. & Weissfeld L. (1990) Familial transmission of alcohol use. III. Impact of imitation/non-imitation of parent alcohol use (1960) on the sensible/problem drinking of their offspring (1977). *British Journal of Addiction* 85, 1141–1155.

Hauge R. & Irgens-Jensen O. (1987) Age, alcohol consumption and the experiencing of negative consequences. *British Journal of Addiction* 82, 1101–1124.

Heather N. & Robertson I. (1985) *Problem Drinking. The New Approach*. Penguin, Harmondsworth.

Heok K.E. (1987) Drinking in Chinese culture: old stereotypes re-examined. *British Journal of Addiction* 82, 224–225.

Herd D. (1987) Rethinking black drinking. *British Journal of Addiction* 82, 219–223.

Higgs E.J. (1984) Research into the history of alcohol use and control in England and Wales: the available sources in the Public Record Office. *British Journal of Addiction* 79, 41–47.

Hilton M.E. (1988) Trends in US drinking patterns: further evidence from the past 20 years. *British Journal of Addiction* 83, 269–279.

Hilton M.E. (1989) How many alcoholics are there in the United States. *British Journal of Addiction* 84, 459–460.

Holder H.D. & Blose J.O. (1987) Impact of changes in distilled spirits availability on apparent consumption: a time series analysis of liquor-by-the-drink. *British Journal of Addiction* 82, 623–631.

Jahoda G., Davies J.B. & Tagg S. (1980) Parents' alcohol consumption and children's knowledge of drinks and usage patterns. *British Journal of Addiction* 75, 297–303.

Jellinek E.M. (1960) *The Disease Concept of Alcoholism.* Hillhouse Press, Newhaven.

Kandel D.B. & Andrews K. (1987) Processes of adolescent socialisation by parents and peers. *International Journal of the Addictions* 22, 319–342.

Kendell R.E. de Roumanie M. & Ritson E.B. (1983) Effects of economic changes on Scottish drinking habits 1978–82. *British Journal of Addiction* 78, 365–379.

Knupfer G. (1987) New directions for survey research in the study of alcoholic beverage consumption. *British Journal of Addiction* 82, 583–585.

Layne N. & Whitehead P.C. (1985) Employment, marital status and alcohol consumption of young Canadian drinkers. *Journal of Studies on Alcohol* 46, 538–540.

Ledermann S. (1956) *Alcool, Alcoolisme, Alcoolisation.* Presses Universitaires de France, Paris.

Lee A., Crombie I.K., Smith W.C.S. & Tunstall-Pedoe H.D. (1990) Alcohol consumption and unemployment among men: the Scottish Heart Health Study. *British Journal of Addiction* 85, 1165–1170.

Leland J. (1984) Alcohol use and abuse in ethnic minority women. In Wilsnack S.C. & Beckman L.J. (eds) *Alcohol Problems in Women.* Guilford Press, New York.

Longmate N. (1982) Alcohol and the family in history. In Orford J. & Harwin J. (eds) *Alcohol and the Family.* Croom Helm, London.

McBride R. & Mosher F. (1985) Public health implications of the international alcohol industry: issues raised by a World Health Organisation project. *British Journal of Addiction* 80, 141–147.

McDonnell R. & Maynard A. (1985) The costs of alcohol misuse. *British Journal of Addiction* 80, 27–35.

Maynard A. & O'Brien B. (1982) Harmonisation policies in the European Community and alcohol abuse. *British Journal of Addiction* 77, 235–244.

Morrisey E.R. & Schuckit M.A. (1978) Stressful life events and alcohol problems among women seen at a detoxification centre. *Journal of Studies on Alcohol* 38, 1559–1576.

Mulford H.A. & Fitzgerald J.L. (1988) Per capita alcohol sales, heavy drinker prevalence and alcohol problems in Iowa for 1958–1985. *British Journal of Addiction* 83, 265–268.

Nordstrom T. (1987) The abolition of the Swedish alcohol rationing system: effects on consumption distribution and cirrhosis mortality. *British Journal of Addiction* 82, 633–641.

O'Connor J. (1978) *The Young Drinkers: A Cross National Study of Social and Cultural Influences.* Tavistock, London.

O'Doherty F. & Davies J.B. (1987) Life events and addiction: a critical review. *British Journal of Addiction* 82, 127–137.

Orford J. & Velleman R. (1990) Offspring of parents with drinking problems: drinking and drug-taking as young adults. *British Journal of Addiction* 85, 779–794.

Pittman D.J. & Snyder C.R. (eds) (1962) *Society, Culture and Drinking Patterns.* John Wiley, Chichester.

Plant M.A. (1979) *Drinking Careers, Occupations, Drinking Habits and Drinking Problems.* Tavistock, London.

Plant M.A., Peck D.F. & Samuel E. (1985) *Alcohol, Drugs and School Leavers.* Tavistock, London.

Powell M. (1989) The health policy implications of international trade and alcohol and tobacco products. *British Journal of Addiction* 84, 1151–1162.

Power C. & Estaugh V. (1990) Employment and drinking in early adulthood: a longitudinal perspective. *British Journal of Addiction* 85, 487–494.

Rahkonan O. & Ahlstrom S. (1989) Trends in drinking habits among Finnish youth from 1973–1987. *British Journal of Addiction* 84, 1075–1083.

Robinson D. (1976) *From Drinking to Alcoholism: A Sociological Commentary.* John Wiley, Chichester.

Romelsjo A. (1987) Decline in alcohol-related in-patient care and mortality in Stockholm County. *British Journal of Addiction* 82, 653–663.

Royal College of Psychiatrists (1986) *Alcohol our Favourite Drug.* Tavistock, London.

Rubington E. (1962) 'Failure' as a heavy drinker: the case of the chronic-drunkenness offender on skid row. In Pittman D.J. & Snyder C.R. (eds) *Society, Culture, and Drinking Patterns.* John Wiley, Chichester.

Slattery M., Alderson M.R. & Bryant J.S. (1986) The occupational risks of alcoholism. *International Journal of the Addictions* 21, 929–936.

Smart R.G. (1976) Spontaneous recovery in alcoholics: a review and analysis of the available research. *Drug and Alcohol Dependence* 1, 277–285.

Smart R.G. (1989) Is the post war drinking binge ending? Cross-national trends in per capita alcohol consumption. *British Journal of Addiction* 84, 743–748.

Smart R.G. & Mann R.E. (1987) Large decreases in alcohol-related problems following a slight reduction in alcohol consumption in Ontario 1975–1983. *British Journal of Addiction* 82, 285–291.

Smith I. & Burvill P.W. (1987) Effect on juvenile crime of lowering the drinking age in three Australian states. *British Journal of Addiction* 82, 181–188.

Snyder C.R. (1962) Culture and Jewish sobriety: the ingroup–outgroup factor. In Pittman D.J. & Snyder C.R. (eds) *Society, Culture, and Drinking Patterns.* John Wiley, Chichester.

Wald I. & Moskalewicz J. (1984) Alcohol policy in a crisis situation. *British Journal of Addiction* 79, 331–335.

Whitehead P.C. & Layne N. (1987) Young female Canadian drinkers: employment, marital status and heavy drinking. *British Journal of Addiction* 82, 169–174.

Wilks J. & Callan V.J. (1988) Expectations about appropriate drinking contexts: comparisons of parents, adolescents and best friends. *British Journal of Addiction* 83, 1055–1062.

Wilks J., Callan V.J. & Austin D.A. (1989) Parent peer and personal determinants of adolescent drinking. *British Journal of Addiction* 84, 619–630.

Williams T.P. & Lillis R.P. (1988) Long-term changes in reported alcohol purchasing and consumption following an increase in New York State's purchase age to 19.

*British Journal of Addiction* 83, 209–217.

Winton M., Heather N. & Robertson I. (1986) Effects of unemployment on drinking behaviour: a review of the relevant evidence. *International Journal of Addictions* 21, 1261–1283.

Woodside M. (1988) Research on children of aicoholics: past and future. *British Journal of Addiction* 83, 785–792.

# Chapter 12
## Drug Use, Drug Problems and Drug Addiction: Social Influences and Social Responses

### JOHN STRANG & MICHAEL GOSSOP

### Introduction

The abuse of drugs creates many social problems within society. Over the past 20 years or so there have been many changes in how these problems have been perceived in the UK as well as changes in the nature and delivery of responses. These include a decrease in emphasis upon individual psychiatric disorders and psychopathology and an increased awareness of the importance of social factors upon the initiation of drug use, upon the development of drug problems, upon the course of such problems and upon their short-term and long-term outcome − both with and without treatment. In this chapter an examination is undertaken of the social influences and social responses which may influence drug use, drug problems and drug addiction.

### Drug use, drug problems and drug addiction − terminology

Two terms have been widely used which relate to the condition under consideration: 'problem drug taking' and 'drug dependence'. It is the more sociologically orientated terms which have become more widely used recently with consideration of the 'problem drinker' (Advisory Committee on Alcoholism (Kessel Report) 1978) and 'problem drug taker' (Advisory Council on the Misuse of Drugs 1982). The problem drug taker is defined as 'any person who experiences social, psychological, physical or legal problems related to intoxication and/or regular excessive consumption and/or dependence as a consequence of his/her own use of drugs or other chemical substances...'. Over the same time period, much work has been done to define more precisely the concept of dependence. Much of this work has

been done in the field of alcohol (Edwards & Gross 1976, Stockwell *et al.* 1979), but only more recently and less extensively in the opiate field (Phillips *et al.* 1986, Sutherland *et al.* 1986). It is often mistakenly presumed that the terms 'problem drug taking' and 'drug dependence' and linked areas of understanding merely reflect a medical or sociological terminology for the same phenomenon; however, on closer study it becomes evident that there may be value in considering them as largely independent dimensions (insofar as each of them might legitimately be considered as a single dimension). Thus consideration of two individual drug takers might find one scoring highly on problems but low on dependence, whilst the loading was reversed for the other.

In an attempt to identify a limited set of terms and concepts around which consensus might gradually form, the World Health Organization (WHO) put forward proposals for more specific terms for the various phenomena under study (Edwards *et al.* 1981):

1 Unsanctioned use: use of a drug that is not approved by a society, or a group within that society. When the term is used, it should be made clear who is responsible for the disapproval. The term implies that we accept disapproval as a fact in its own right without having to determine or justify the basis of that disapproval.

2 Hazardous use: use of a drug that will probably lead to harmful consequences for the user − either to dysfunction or to harm. This concept is similar to the idea of risky behaviour. For instance, smoking 20 cigarettes each day may not be accompanied by any present or actual harm but we know it to be hazardous.

3 Dysfunctional use: use of a drug that is leading to impaired psychological or social functioning (e.g. loss of job or marital problems).

4 Harmful use: use of a drug that is known to have caused tissue damage or mental illness in the particular person.

Edwards *et al.* also take up the increasing dissatisfaction with the apparent dichotomy between physical dependence and psychological/psychic dependence. They propose use of the term 'neuroadaptation' which covers the changes associated with physical and psychological withdrawal phenomena and also with the development of tolerance. Thus neuroadaptation covers the cellular, metabolic and behavioural adaptations that occur in response to drug use. The term may also be extended to the concept of reciprocal neuroadaptation to discover the phenomenon previously described as cross-tolerance.

The proposed definition for 'dependence' is based on the prior work from Edwards and his colleagues (e.g. Edwards & Gross 1976) and is viewed as 'a syndrome manifested by a behavioural pattern in which the use of a given psychoactive drug, or class of drug, is given a much higher priority than other behaviours that once had higher value'. Dependence is considered as a clustering of cognitive, behavioural and physiological phenomena. Methods of assessment should consider the following:

1 Subjective awareness of compulsion to use a drug or drugs, usually during attempts to stop or moderate drug use.
2 A desire to stop drug use in the face of continued use.
3 A relatively stereotyped drug-taking habit (i.e. a narrowing of the repertoire of the drug-taking behaviour).
4 Evidence of neuroadaptation (tolerance and withdrawal symptoms).
5 Use of the drug to relieve or avoid withdrawal symptoms.
6 The salience of drug-seeking behaviour relative to other important priorities.
7 Rapid reinstatement of the syndrome after a period of abstinence.

Finally the WHO memorandum proposes a model for the initiation, continuation and discontinuation of drug and alcohol use (see Edwards *et al.* 1981). A first set of stimuli bears on the individual and the initial drug-taking behaviour. This then leads to a range of consequences which act as deterrents or reinforcers of further drug seeking or drug use. These events are then modulated by various other learning processes which must be considered. Drug-seeking behaviour and drug use will also be subject to influence by factors leading to cessation of drug taking on a permanent or temporary basis. Finally the model may be used for consideration of the restarting of drug taking after a period of cessation, with attendant factors influencing the nature of that reinstatement.

In recent years shorthand terms have been developed in the drug field which describe the different significance of the drug use to the individual. Thus drug use might be seen as experimental, recreational or compulsive/dependent. Whilst it may well be the case that these terms do not describe discrete entities, the terminology may nevertheless be of value to aid communication between researchers and workers (and certainly seems to have meaning to drug takers themselves).

Experimental drug use is often prompted by curiosity about the nature of the drug effect. It is typically a peer group activity. Of those who have become experimental users of a particular drug, some will refrain from any further use whilst others will continue to take the drug in order to obtain a known effect (typically perceived as positive at this stage) and these users might be described as recreational users. From amongst these drug users, a proportion will develop dependence and/or other problems: this may be accompanied by a tolerance of damage to personal or family well-being and as the use of the drug becomes a more exclusive pursuit and activity it may no longer be associated primarily with the pursuit of positive effects but may be taken primarily for the abolition of negative physical or psychological effects: at this stage the drug user might be regarded as a compulsive or dependent user (Yates 1985).

## Epidemiology

The majority of the commonly abused drugs are subject to legal restrictions. Consequently the people who use them tend by definition to be law-breakers and this immediately raises a number of difficulties in attempting to reach valid estimates of prevalence. Various measures do exist. Attempts have been made to estimate the prevalence of various types of drug taking through self-report surveys or by using official notification figures. Other approaches have attempted to gauge trends rather than actual numbers and have used other sorts of measures. These include various morbidity and mortality data such as drug-related deaths, hepatitis B statistics, non-fatal drug emergencies and law enforcement data.

In the UK the Home Office reports two indirect indicators of drug trends. The first relates to the number of 'addicts' and the other presents data on the numbers of people who have been cautioned or convicted of drugs offences (for description see Edwards 1982, Mott 1992). All medical practitioners in the UK have a statutory duty to notify the Home Office of anyone who is addicted to heroin, cocaine or one of a list of other notifiable drugs. This Home Office Addicts Index has been criticized on a number of grounds. It undoubtedly underestimates the actual number of addicts since many addicts will not present to medical agencies (Hartnoll *et al.* 1985). Also there is good evidence that many medical practitioners do not in fact make notifications as required (e.g. see Strang & Shah 1985). However, it probably does bear some relationship to national trends, and shows that the number of addicts has steadily increased since 1968 and that this increase appears to have accelerated since 1980. The suggestion of a rising trend is supported by the drugs offences indicators.

There are no routine national surveys of drug use in Britain. However, a number of independent surveys have been carried out. In his review of the available UK surveys Plant (1990) suggested that these show that a large and probably increasing minority of young adults (between 10% and 30%) have used an illegal drug at some time or other. It is also clear that there are marked regional variations. These apply both to the prevalence of drug use and to the type of drugs used. Most surveys indicate that the majority of those people who have used illegal drugs have done so on relatively few occasions and that the

overwhelming majority of 'drug users' were not regular users, and they had not used heroin or injected drugs. In a follow-up study of more than a thousand young people in Scotland, Plant *et al.* (1984) found that 15% of the males and 11% of the females had used an illegal drug at the start of the survey (at this point subjects were aged 15–16 years) and that this increased to 37% and 32% respectively by the end (aged 19–20 years). This study also found a strong link between drug use and unemployment.

In a series of surveys from Wolverhamptom, UK, Wright & Pearl (1986, 1990) reported on the changes in knowledge about drugs and extent of use of different drugs amongst fourth year pupils in secondary schools during the mid 1960s and mid 1980s. Over the 20-year period the proportion of pupils who knew somebody taking drugs had more than doubled from 15% to 31%, and over the same period the proportion who had been offered drugs rose from 5% to 19%.

Further UK data are available in a survey of substance use by Swadi (1988) based on self-report questionnaires from 3333 school children aged between 11 and 16 in London. Swadi found that 20% of these school children had used solvents or illegal drugs on at least one occasion, with rates of 13% in the 11 year olds, rising to 26% in the 16 year olds. More than 10% also used alcohol at least once a week. Regular use of solvents or other illicit drugs was markedly less but was still much higher than had previously been reported in the UK, with figures rising to 16% of 16 year olds. Heroin use was reported by 1.7% of the group and 2% reported use of cocaine. (Swadi also records his failure to obtain data from 13% of school children who were truanters who might well represent a particularly high risk population.)

In the USA national high school surveys on patterns of drug use have been conducted annually since 1975, and a national household survey of drug use since 1972. These provide estimates of drug-using trends. Based on information from these surveys, the lifetime prevalence of cannabis use among adolescents increased steadily during the 1970s, from 14% in 1972 to 31% in 1979. During the 1980s this trend has stabilized and has shown signs of decline. Among high school students for instance, the percentage of people smoking cannabis in the past month declined from 37% in 1979 to 29% in 1982 (Spiegler & Harford 1987). The use of most illicit drugs showed a similar trend during this time, though the use of stimulant drugs differed from the overall pattern by showing an increase during the 1980s, especially for the use of cocaine by adults aged 26 years or older (US Institute of Medicine 1990).

The 1988 US national survey was the first to collect information on items that are part of the ICD-10 and DSM-III-R criteria for drug dependence and abuse. The data on each individual in the survey were classified to yield categories of clear, probable, possible, and unlikely need for treatment. On the basis of these calculations, out of an estimated 14.5 million people (about 7.3% of the population aged 12 years or older) who used any illicit drug at least once in the month prior to the survey, 1.5 million could be regarded as having a clear need for treatment at the time of the survey, that is, they showed more than the minimum clinical diagnostic criteria for dependence. Another 3.1 million people were seen as having a probable need for treatment. These combined groups of 'problematic drug takers' make up 4.6 million people; this figure represents one-third of the current month drug takers, and about 2.3% of the population aged 12 years or older.

In the USA, as in the UK, for almost all categories of drug taking, especially for heavy use, the proportion of males tends to be higher than that for females. Interestingly, there is a marked racial effect in the USA with regard to heroin use which is two to three times more prevalent among blacks and Hispanic groups – an effect that appears absent or even reversed in the UK with drugs such as heroin.

## Special studies

### *The Vietnam study*

In their NIDA Monograph and a series of papers, Robins and her colleagues describe the extraordinary story of heroin use by US army personnel during and after the Vietnam War (Robins *et al.*

1974, 1975). Robins looked at two samples. One sample comprised 500 army-enlisted men drawn randomly from those returning home from Vietnam during September 1971. Forty-three per cent had used an opiate while in Vietnam, and nearly half of these men had used opiates on at least a weekly basis for six months or longer. A fifth of this general sample of Vietnam veterans were of the view that they had been addicted to heroin while in Vietnam. The sample were followed up on their return home, and when interviewed eight to ten months later, only 10% had used opiates since their return to the USA, and only 1% were of the view that they had been addicted since their return. The other sample studied by Robins was a group of 500 'drug positive' men (soldiers known to be or to have been drug users). Three-quarters of these men had been addicted to opiates whilst in Vietnam, but on interview 8–12 months after return to the USA, only a third had used any opiates since Vietnam and only 7% of the sample believed that they had been addicted since their return.

A number of points are vividly demonstrated by the Robins papers which need to be borne in mind in separate considerations of the significance of drug use to the individual and to society. If the circumstances are right (or to be more precise, if the circumstances are wrong) the extent of use of prohibited drugs such as heroin can be remarkably high – levels of heroin use of nearly 50% of the population far exceed the levels which legitimately cause such concern in society today. Whilst the level of use seen in Vietnam would be unlikely to be found in most ordinary circumstances, it would be naive to presume that the problems of heroin use and heroin addiction were somehow restricted only to a minority with some unspecified addiction-prone qualities. Winick (1980) has described how the extent of drug use within a society may be determined by three factors: the availability of the drug, the degree of social proscription, and the extent of conflict or stress. In Vietnam, heroin was not only readily available but was of high purity and at low cost relative to surplus income. As the use of heroin by smoking and injecting became more widespread amongst American soldiers, so the extent of moral censorship or social proscription against personal use of such drugs became much less. The extent to which role strain might have existed for American soldiers in Vietnam may appear self-evident, but there is further evidence to support Winick's hypothesis: the concept of role strain is not just an index of the stressful nature of the situation – it also requires a sense of dissonance between one's aspirations and the circumstances in which one finds oneself. Surprisingly the levels of heroin addiction were higher amongst those men who had volunteered for service in Vietnam than in those who had been drafted, and Winick suggests that this might be the result of the greater level of inner dissonance amongst those who had volunteered to serve than amongst those who had been drafted. The drafted men may be similarly stressed at the circumstances but would not experience the same degree of dissonance (Winick 1980).

The findings from Vietnam also provide interesting information on the non-dependent use of heroin. Many users did not become dependent during their use of heroin. More specific study of this area has been undertaken in different settings by Zinberg (1984), who describes the patterns of use and social structure of groups of heroin users who abide by strict internal rules (e.g. avoidance of dose escalation, avoidance of use on consecutive days, preservation of outside interests and friendship networks, etc.) which Zinberg put foward as factors which were protective against the development of the more typical dependent pattern of heroin use.

A third area in which the Vietnam studies may provide us with insight is with regard to the reversability of the heroin-using and heroin-addicted status. Virtually all non-dependent heroin users and the vast majority of heroin addicts in Vietnam did not use heroin after they had returned to the USA. This geographical move will obviously have been associated with changes in the areas described above by Winick (i.e. reversal of the availability, social proscription and role strain), and whilst this is an example of a considerable piece of engineering of the social environment, it nevertheless stands as a clear demonstration of the evident reversibility of the heroin-using and heroin-addicted conditions.

## Addict doctors

Medical practitioners represent a group with higher than average rates of alcohol and other drug addictions. When we consider specifically the raised levels of opiate addiction (Stimson *et al.* 1984), it seems unlikely that this reflects any pre-addiction characteristics of the population as there are different rates of addiction seen within the different subspecialties (e.g. higher levels in general practice and anaesthetics) where the opportunities for initially undetected diversion of supplies are greater. Certain forms of medical practice offer considerable access to the drugs (e.g. consider the GP collecting stocks of controlled drugs for transport in his doctor's bag during home visits); the degree of social proscription may be less for doctors who have seen the extensive analgesic use of morphine and heroin without the instant emergence of addiction, so that some of the protective taboos which apply to most of society may be eroded. Finally, the motivations behind the decisions to enter medicine may not sit comfortably with much of the reality of clinical practice for many practitioners so that considerable dissonance and role strain is generated. Study of the natural history of addiction in doctors also provides an opportunity to look at how outcome may be influenced. The treatment of addicted doctors is notable for the extent to which it contains infringements of civil liberties to a greater extent than would normally be entertained (e.g. supervised administration of opiate antagonists; random call-up for physical examination and/or supervised urine specimens; compulsory attendance at support groups; alerting systems 'for family and colleagues so as to identify and abort relapses at an early stage; etc.) as described by Crowley and colleagues (Anker & Crowley 1982, Crowley 1984). These appear to be widely accepted by both the individual and the system, and may go some way to explain the good recovery rates.

## UK studies of neighbourhoods

One of the earlier studies of illicit drug use in a UK neighbourhood was undertaken in Crawley New Town during the late 1960s. In an elegant series of studies, de Alarcon & Rathod documented the 'epidemic' of heroin use amongst local residents and the gradual consolidation of this epidemic. From an initial base of two separate heroin addicts, 50 confirmed users and 48 probable users were identified (de Alarcon & Rathod 1968). They explored the mode of transmission and identified that this was not via dealer networks but was as a result of peer influence (de Alarcon 1969). They described three phases of the epidemic: an initial stage during which a small number of individuals had come into contact with heroin whilst living elsewhere; a subsequent phase during which these users returned to Crawley and formed a nucleus of local heroin users; and a third stage during which the size of the drug-using population grew from this nucleus to the larger initiative drug-using group. From this information base, the authors were then able to examine the impact of different public health interventions, as with the control of the methylamphetamine epidemic (de Alarcon 1972).

The Cambridge studies involved a similar approach, although greater reliance was placed on tracing through the social network of users themselves emanating from an initial four heroin users. During the years of study, the variations in use of various drugs, including heroin, cocaine, methylamphetamine and methadone, were studied (Kosviner *et al.* 1968, Zacune *et al.* 1969, Hawkes 1976). A particular finding from these studies was that of the intermittent users of these drugs: at any one time more than half of the study group were using opiates on a less than daily basis. Evidence was also presented which indicated that the extent of use of opiates appeared to reduce over time.

Plant undertook an extensive study using a social network method amongst drug users in Cheltenham. He interviewed 200 drug users between 1970 and 1972. All of the drug users had used cannabis, three-quarters had used hallucinogens and half had used amphetamines; 30 of these 200 drug users had injected drugs on at least one occasion, but only three of them injected regularly. Plant found that levels of physical morbidity or material harm as a consequence of this drug use seemed to be low, although one in eight of the drug takers had consulted a doctor at some time in connection with their drug use. Higher levels of associated problems were seen with injectors than non-injectors (Plant 1973, 1975).

Studies in North London have been undertaken by Hartnoll and colleagues (Hartnoll *et al.* 1985, Drug Indicators Project 1989). They explored the extent to which different numerator techniques may be used directly or indirectly as the basis for estimating the extent of opioid dependence in a community, and they proposed use of indirect methods including use of routine public health, morbidity and mortality data, surveys of local agencies and detached fieldwork as sources of information (Hartnoll *et al.* 1985). Subsequent work from the same group looked at factors promoting and interfering with the process of help seeking (Drug Indicators Project 1989).

Drug use in the Wirral was studied by Parker *et al.* (1987, 1988). They showed the rapid and extensive spread of heroin use over the course of a year or two in a community of variable social deprivation and in which extensive heroin use was previously unknown.

Pearson and colleagues showed considerable variation in the extent of use in different local communities across the north of England, including variation in the distribution networks, the balance between amphetamines and heroin, and the prevailing popularities of different routes of administration (Pearson *et al.* 1986, 1987a). In particular, the strong association between the extent of spread of heroin use and the existing levels of unemployment and other indices of socioeconomic disadvantage was noted (Pearson 1987b). Parker *et al.* (1987) had similarly noted such an association and had also observed the spread of the effect of such disadvantage to adjacent townships whose association with the disadvantage was only geographical.

## The social and psychological context of drug use

Three major parameters operate to determine drug effects. Zinberg (1984) referred to these as drug, set and setting. The pharmacological factors are the most clearly understood and would include dose level and frequency and route of administration. Set (that is, beliefs or expectations about drug effects) also has a powerful influence, especially when the drug is one with which the individual has had considerable prior experience. Finally, the setting in which the drug is taken (e.g. alone or in the company of others, in a hospital or in a recreational setting) will also influence the way in which the individual responds to it.

The impact of expectancy has often been studied in placebo studies, and has been clearly shown in what Marlatt & Rohsenow (1980) refer to as the 'balanced placebo design'. These studies used alcohol rather than any of the illicit drugs but they have direct relevance to the abuse of drugs. One study investigated the link between alcohol and aggression (Lang *et al.* 1975). The subjects were a group of male, heavy drinkers. They were given either vodka and tonic (to a blood alcohol level of 0.10%), or tonic only, under one of two conditions − expect alcohol and expect no alcohol. They were then asked to carry out a motor coordination test and half of the subjects were strongly criticized for their poor performance. The subjects who *believed* that they had consumed alcohol responded more aggressively to this criticism than the others who believed that they had received no alcohol, and among those who believed that they had drunk alcohol there was no difference in aggression between the alcohol and the placebo groups. In their review of this and other studies, Marlatt & Rohsenow (1980) conclude that expectancy effects may be more important than pharmacological/physiological factors in determining various interperson and social behaviours as well as in determining craving for an actual consumption of alcohol. This expectation effect has been shown to be an important determinant of the severity of the heroin withdrawal syndrome (Phillips *et al.* 1987), and the provision of accurate and reassuring information has been found to reduce withdrawal discomfort (Green & Gossop 1988).

A classic paper on the way in which the social context influences cannabis use was published by Becker in 1953. The paper shows how cannabis smoking may be understood as a behaviour which is the result of social experiences during which the person acquires a conception of the meaning of cannabis use including perceptions and judgements of other people, objects and events which make the activity possible and desirable. The novice cannabis smoker typically does not experience any marked positive or euphoric effect the first time that they smoke the drug. Indeed, they may even experience the effects as physically unpleasant. They must learn correct techniques of inhalation, and during this time they are 'coached' by experienced users both in technique and in perceptions and attitudes towards the experience and its meaning. There is nothing unique about cannabis in this respect. The same principles would apply to a drug such as heroin. Many (or even most) first-time heroin users are physically sick when they take the drug; novices also require an initial period during which they learn correct techniques and appropriate interpretations of effects (Gossop 1987).

## Drug careers or the natural history of addiction?

These two perspectives on an individual and his or her drug use relate to fundamentally different models of understanding of the phenomenon. The concept of a drug-using career has been developed extensively from the interactionist studies of Everett Hughes and colleagues at the Chicago School of Sociology. Life itself might be considered as a career during which the individual enters and leaves various activities. Thus prostitution or drug use may be considered as an 'occupation' within a deviant career. The Hughes model involves consideration of external influences on the drug taking (contingency) and the position of choice over behaviour (voluntarism). In the UK Young (1973) has considered drug use as part of a deviant career and has put forward his 'deviancy amplification theory' in which society's own reaction to the initial deviant act acts as a potent reinforcer of the very behaviour which society is seeking to reduce. Various studies do indeed provide evidence of individuals moving in and out of drug use during a 'career' which has been described by Parker *et al.* (1988) as the 'incidence' and 'outcidence' of the behaviour which between them dictate the prevalence.

A different perspective is obtained from study of the literature on the natural history of addiction. At one level, workers from various backgrounds have referred to 'epidemics' with the linked presumption of greater risk of 'infection' in the disadvantaged or vulnerable. Thus sociologists (e.g. Parker *et al.* 1988) and epidemiologists (e.g. Hunt & Chambers 1976) have found these terms to be a useful metaphor. But are there circumstances in which the term refers to concept rather than mere metaphor? Certainly the writings of Winick (1962) and Vaillant (1973) consider the natural history of the condition in a more literal sense, although the condition under study still seems elusively imprecise. More recently Edwards (1984) has described a tighter concept of natural history as being 'the sequential development of designated biological processes within the individual'. This approach allows for a longer-term perspective, for different degrees of involvement with the drug at different points in time and certainly represents a more tangible concept for consideration and debate. The two concepts may not be mutually exclusive, but confusion between the two serves only to obscure one's vision.

### The impacts of new drugs and new technologies

From time to time new drugs are discovered or, more usually, old drugs are adapted to produce related products with a new profile of effects. Thus whilst the development of cocaine in the mid nineteenth century and the development of LSD in the mid twentieth century represent genuinely new drugs, the more recent 'new drugs' such as Ecstasy (3,4-methylenedioxy methamphetamine, MDMA) is in fact old-fashioned amphetamine which has undergone refinement in the hands of a blackmarket biochemist to produce an amphetamine with LSD-like properties. Developments in technology and new methods of use can also bring about changes in patterns of drug taking. Thus the discovery around 1980 in the UK that heroin could be inhaled as it sublimated off the surface of heated tin foil undoubtedly contributed to the explosion of heroin use at that time. Likewise during the 1980s, awareness grew in the USA that cocaine could be taken by freebasing, and subsequently by smoking it as crack

so as to produce a markedly greater initial effect – as if injecting but without the attendant risks of needle and syringe.

The issue to be considered is not just the new substance or the new equipment: it is the new relationship which develops between man and drug. The substance may even remain the same, but changes in the technology can upset a balance which may have prevailed for up to centuries. Recent examples include the extensive problems now being identified in South American urban and rural settings with the increasingly widespread smoking of pasta and basuco (contaminated precursors in the production of blackmarket cocaine) despite centuries of unremarkable chewing of the coca leaf from earlier generations. In another part of the world a similar disturbance of the balance is only now being recognized with the emergence of a major indigenous heroin problem in countries which have become producer countries for the new blackmarket in heroin. During the 1980s the North West Frontier of Pakistan has been one of the major producer regions for blackmarket heroin for export around the world and, despite a long history of culturally bound smoking of the opium poppy, the refined product (heroin) is decimating the young male population with current estimates that there are in excess of one million young men who have recently become addicted to heroin in Pakistan (Gossop 1989).

The adoption of new drugs and new technologies may not be haphazard. Frequently the drug serves some adaptive function – not merely through the social function of shared drug use, but possibly also at the pharmacological level. It is said that the Viking warriors who invaded the English shores would deliberately take quantities of hallucinogenic mushrooms prior to battle to give them a greater fighting spirit (indeed these warriors were called berserkers, from which the word berserk is derived). More recently it has been suggested that the choice of barbiturates (often with alcohol) as a drug of use by punks represents the selection of a drug whose pharmacological effects are well suited to nihilism and anarchy, and Burr (1984) has recently provided an anthropological perspective on how this choice of drug may be linked to the punk ideology of despair.

## Treatment – determinants of outcome

In a consideration of treatment outcome it must be recognized that the actual treatment procedures are only one set of variables that affect any changes that might occur. Outcome is also affected by demographic and psychological subject characteristics, and by a range of social and environmental factors.

The majority of studies of demographic factors affecting response to methadone maintenance treatments have found that older patients are more likely to remain in treatment and are more likely to perform better during treatment in terms of reduced illicit drug use, improved health status, etc. (McLellan 1983). The patients' background has also been found to have an impact upon their response to treatment. In a study of more than 17 000 patients in methadone programmes, Gearing & Schweitzer (1974) found that those individuals with skilled or semi-skilled employment histories were more likely to respond well to treatment both in terms of reduced drug use and in employment. Similarly in a study of an alcohol treatment programme, Moos et al. (1990) found that both life context factors and sociodemographic characteristics were predictive of treatment outcome. This observation would apply equally to outcome among drug abusers where many of the factors that are most strongly associated with relapse are related to social and environmental events and circumstances (Bradley et al. 1989).

In the massive treatment outcome perspective study (TOPS) conducted in the USA with more than 10 000 drug abuse patients, it was found that the most important factors relating to post-treatment heroin use were the severity of drug use and drug-related problems at treatment entry, and the time spent in treatment (Hubbard et al. 1984, 1989). This time in treatment effect is one which has been found in many other studies. De Leon & Jainchill (1982) noted that time in treatment has been found to be an important determinant of good outcome among opiate addicts in therapeutic communities such as Phoenix House. A similar result was reported by Gossop et al. (1990) in their study of predictors of outcome among a group of opiate addicts being treated in a London inpatient drug-dependence unit. This sort of 'time in treatment' effect should be interpreted with some caution, since time spent in treatment is itself a complex variable which is affected by many client, treatment and non-treatment conditions.

None the less, the weight of evidence from many studies of different treatment modalities in different countries increasingly points to the fact that treatments for drug dependence can have an important effect upon outcome. In their prospective follow-up study of a group of opiate addicts after treatment, Gossop et al. (1989) found that six months after leaving treatment 45% of the sample were abstinent from opiates and living in the community. Longer-term follow-up studies have also shown that the numbers of addicts who are able to remain abstinent after treatment are much higher than was once thought. Hubbard et al. (1984) found abstinence rates at one year of between 40% and 50% for such drugs as heroin and cocaine; these reductions were evident at three- to five-year follow-up after a specific treatment episode. The authors of the TOPS report concluded that drug-dependence treatment programmes can be effective in reducing drug abuse and also that such treatment can have an impact upon other drug-related behaviours such as criminality. Indeed, on this latter point the authors note that 'while drug abuse treatment has been shown to be a good return on investment simply in terms of crime reduction, the returns may be substantially greater' (than those actually demonstrated by their data).

However, it remains true that such studies do not demonstrate *direct* effects of treatment on post-treatment behaviours. Treatment programmes have no direct control of behaviour after clients leave treatment. Instead the treatment interventions may influence post-treatment behaviour indirectly through changes in psychological states and behaviour during treatment. Treatment may have a number of positive influences on short-term outcome, but both short-term and long-term outcomes are powerfully affected by the patients' personal and environmental circumstances.

## Community-based treatment and other initiatives

During the last few years of the 1980s a debate began involving the competing goals and strategies of personal and public health. The advent of HIV has brought attention to the drug field which is borne not out of concern for the individual drug taker but stems from anxieties that sexually active injecting drug users might form what is now being referred to as a 'bridgehead' into the wider general public. Often the goals and methods will be compatible or identical across consideration of personal health and public health, but there remain areas in which planners and clinicians are bitterly divided with a damaging effect on the services – not pulling together but falling apart. Thus in the USA there is still bitter argument as to whether needle and syringe exchange schemes should be established (or whether over-the-counter sales should be permitted) as in the UK, Australia, and much of Europe and the rest of the world: by 1991, the arguments did not seem any further advanced than when the debate began in earnest a full five years previously, but the positions have certainly become more entrenched (see Stimson *et al.* 1990, Power *et al.* 1991, Stimson *et al.* 1992). Another area of active debate concerns the role that might be played by different prescribing strategies. Within the UK context, where more than 100 needle exchange schemes have already been established (Lart & Stimson 1990) and where over-the-counter sales of needles and syringes by pharmacists are already fairly widespread (Glanz *et al.* 1989), it is the prescribing debate which is attracting most attention – even though the debate as presently framed is only applied to consideration of opiate users.

The 1980s have seen the widespread establishment of community drug teams in the UK – along the lines of community mental health teams, community elderly teams and community alcohol teams (see Stockwell & Clement 1987). Some description has been made of the context and work of community drug teams (Strang 1989, 1991, Strang *et al.* 1992), but there has been surprisingly little critical study of the process or outcome of this new method of organizing drug treatment services. In the seven years following the establishment of the first community drug team (1983–90), 75 community drug teams have been established in England alone (MacGregor *et al.* 1991), with some Regions in the country now sporting at least one community drug team in every District Health Authority or town. In common with other community mental health initiatives, the staffing is typically multidisciplinary, and has a strong community outlook. Effort is directed towards recruitment of generic input (e.g. from GPs and generic social workers); however, the extent of successful recruitment has been disappointing (see Bell *et al.* 1990), such that many community drug teams now appear to be abandoning the higher-level goal of consultancy work (as described by Shaw *et al.* 1978, Spratley 1987) with a shift of emphasis away from enabling the contribution of others towards the more direct provision of services (Strang 1991). The goal of greater generic input (e.g. from GPs) remains the long-term objective, but rapid change of attitudes and behaviour is unlikely to occur in the broad mass of these generic care-providers, and the advent of HIV does not allow the luxury of an exclusive investment in a long-term training strategy.

Various other approaches have been used to work with drug users whilst they remain in the social setting in which their drug problems have developed. Perhaps the most well established have been the residential drug free rehabilitation houses. These have traditionally been described as falling into three categories – concept-based therapeutic communities, Christian houses and community-based hostels. They receive referrals from various sources – an analysis in 1980 for the Advisory Council on the Misuse of Drugs (ACMD 1982) found that 29% of referrals came from courts, prison or probation; 28% self-referral; 26% from non-specialist services and non-statutory agencies; and 17% from drug clinics and GPs.

### *Rehabilitation houses/therapeutic communities*

Concept-based therapeutic communities form the largest section of residential houses (e.g. Phoenix

House). They are derived from the original Synanon in California in 1958, and despite the subsequent demise of Synanon itself, the therapeutic community movement has established itself as a worldwide network of aftercare and recovery. Typically such houses are staffed by a mixture of professionally trained personnel working alongside former addicts who have usually graduated from the treatment programme. Mahon (1973) has described the structure of the Concept House as rigidly hierarchical – an element which is an essential part of the therapeutic community and relates to the strict work ethic. Initially the new resident absolves themselves of all responsibility which is taken over by the community; but gradually the resident assumes responsibility for self, for an extended network of residents, and gradually to the wider community. This is often extended to include voluntary work outside the house as well as occupying a quasi-staff position within the community. Recent developments in the UK have included the creation of half-way houses and bridging accommodation for graduates from therapeutic communities so as to ease the passage back into the general community. As with virtually all drug treatment programmes, therapeutic communities are dogged with the problem of early self-discharge: a study by Ogborne & Melotte (1977) reported that a third left within the first month, and only a third stayed for more than six months in a treatment programme intended to last at least a year. Length of stay correlated positively with subsequent drug-free status.

Christian houses form a smaller body within UK rehabilitation houses. Two clear subcategories appear to exist – one relates to houses in which the Christian faith is part of the motivation of the staff but in which faith is not a prerequisite for entry by a resident; whereas with the other group the profound Christian faith is seen as essential to recovery, and hence the commitment to Christianity on the part of the resident is deemed essential.

Community houses represent the smallest group within this section and appear to be least well defined. Theoretically the emphasis is placed on reintegration back into the community during this period of recovery, with early encouragement to develop links with the local community. Typically these houses contain a less rigid structure with less reliance on confrontational and group psychotherapeutic techniques.

During the last decade there has been a minor revolution within the therapeutic community movement in the UK, with active questioning of the previous central position of confrontational techniques. The result has been a widespread evolution of these programmes so as to be more adaptable to the characteristics of the individual resident (for description of these changes see Toon & Lynch 1992). This internal review of methods and objectives has been further applied since the advent of HIV, with incorporation of harm-minimization education and a more adaptable programme (Cooke *et al.* 1990).

During the mid and late 1980s, the UK has seen a considerable growth in treatment programmes based on the 'Minnesota Model' – residential/inpatient programmes of a shorter duration (about two months) in which the style of work is based strongly on the 12 Step programmes of Alcoholics Anonymous and Narcotics Anonymous (for a description of this work see Wells 1987a, 1987b, 1992, Cook 1988a,b).

### Day centres

Twenty years ago day centres formed a significant part of the London treatment response (for a description see Chapple & Gray 1968). A seemingly never-ending stream of problems plagued day centres with conflict about whether they allowed injecting on the premises, violence, and other questions relating to the purpose and 'ownership' of these centres. By 1980 the only remaining drug day centre was the Lifeline Project in Manchester: it is interesting to note that this had been one of the few day centres to adopt a 'no drugs on the premises' policy and to decide not to open a 'fixing room' in which addicts could inject drugs (as was present in several other Day Centres – see Dorn & South 1985). Thus Yates (1981) describes the style of work at the Lifeline Day Centre as 'encouraging the individual to take responsibility for his attitudes and actions in order to understand the possibility of, and need for, personal change'. Staff at Lifeline placed responsibility on the individual (irrespective of addict status) and hence countered the position commonly adopted of powerless/victim/inadequate role – thus challenging many of the stereotypes of both society and the drug-takers themselves.

During the mid/late 1980s a new creature has risen from the ashes of the old day centre. Several day centres have recently been established with more specific briefs and hence serving a more clearly defined subsection of the drug-taking population. All are within their first few years of work and none has yet published any information on their work or impact, but the emphasis includes a more clear focus on practical change including retraining, re-employment and the development of personal skills. Clearly the reborn day centre has turned away from the original role as a drop-in for dropouts.

### Street agencies

The collapse/closing of day centres in the mid 1970s provoked an existential crisis on the part of many voluntary agencies. Dorn & South (1985) describe the clashes between staff and clients over ownership and direction of the projects. The result was the move by most projects to being 'street agencies' who provided points of contact for drug-users at which they might obtain advice and counselling, and referral to other agencies. In their analysis of these evolutions, Dorn & South describe four overlapping forces:

1 Changing drug systems and cultures (reduced availability of prescribed injectable drugs); the spread of intravenous barbiturate use with associated chaos and danger, etc.
2 Worsening housing and employment prospects.
3 Changes in the nature of social work (professionalization; the drift to more analytical and psychotherapeutic work, etc).
4 Financial insecurity of the agencies.

Over the years that followed, many street agencies introduced an appointment system and thus lost the on-the-street or drop-in nature of their contact. Nevertheless the groundwork had been done for the next step in the evolution during the late 1980s with the development of out-reach programmes and the creation of needle exchange schemes.

### Injecting equipment exchange schemes

The first UK needle exchange scheme was opened in 1987 and more than a dozen schemes were set up as part of a Department of Health initiative (see description by Stimson *et al.* 1988a, 1990). In the three years that followed more than 100 exchange schemes have been established across the UK (Lart & Stimson 1990) – some freestanding, some linked to pre-existing non-statutory drug agencies; and some linked to NHS drug treatment centres. Thus an estimated two million needles and syringes were distributed in the UK during 1989, mostly in exchange for used needles and syringes (Donoghoe 1991); in addition to this a further estimated two million needles and syringes were sold over the counter by community pharmacists, usually without any facility for disposal of used needles and syringes (Glanz *et al.* 1989). Exchange schemes were originally set up by the junkiebonden in Amsterdam during the early 1980s in response to a concern about hepatitis B, and thus represented an early example of addict self-help organization (see Nelles 1990) and also an example of harm-minimization strategies which acknowledged the likelihood of continued injecting by a proportion of drug-users (see Buning 1990, Stimson 1992). Such schemes have been successful in making contact with drug-users who were otherwise not currently in contact with drug treatment services. Although 75% were opiate users, 17% reported that amphetamine was their main drug – a population not normally seen in drug treatment centres (Stimson *et al.* 1988a). A third were currently in treatment, a third had previously been in treatment, and the remaining third had never previously had any treatment contact. Unfortunately exchange schemes seem dogged by similar high drop-out rates from continued contact, so that one-third of clients attended only once and less than half attended for more than two visits (Stimson *et al.* 1988b). Disappointingly, exchange schemes do not seem to be used particularly by young drug-users or -injectors earlier in their injecting career, so that there is typically a lag of several years before first attendance, with an average age of 26.8 years, and an average of 7.7 years since first injection (Stimson *et al.* 1988c). Moderately high levels of needle sharing were reported by clients on entry into exchange schemes (34% having shared in the last month), and when reinterviewed three months later this figure had reduced, but not greatly, to 27% who had shared in the last month (Stimson *et al.* 1989). Twenty-one per cent of clients reported that they continued to share at least as frequently as prior to their first attendance.

### The problem of relapse

Relapse may be regarded as one of the most central clinical problems in the addictions. Even for the heavily dependent drug-taker it is relatively easy to stop taking drugs; it is very difficult to remain drug free. The early studies of Hunt and his colleagues demonstrated nearly identical patterns of relapse in groups of heroin addicts, alcoholics and cigarette smokers (Hunt *et al.* 1971). This finding has been repeatedly confirmed and it has been suggested that there may be common patterns of relapse for the various addictive behaviours (Cummings *et al.* 1980).

In a prospective study of relapse among heroin addicts after treatment, Gossop *et al.* (1989) found that the critical period for relapse was immediately after leaving treatment. A large proportion of their subjects used opiates within a matter of only days or a few weeks of leaving an intensive inpatient treatment programme. Forty-two per cent of the sample had used heroin at least once within one week of leaving treatment, and at six-week follow-up 71% had lapsed. This finding would appear to confirm the most pessimistic views about the prognosis of heroin addicts. However, these apparently depressing findings must be seen in the broader context of subsequent events. It is clear from the results cited by Gossop *et al.* (1989) that the initial lapse to opiate use did not herald a full-blown relapse to an addictive pattern of use. There was a clear 'recovery-after-lapse' effect during the six-month follow-up period which showed increasing numbers of subjects moving towards abstinence. By the six-month point, 45% of the sample were abstinent from opiates (as confirmed by urine analysis) and were living in the community.

The research that has been conducted into the process and correlates of relapse has been accompanied by the development of a clinical framework for relapse prevention. A good deal of the impetus behind this treatment approach has been provided by Alan Marlatt and his colleagues. Relapse Prevention is a self-management programme which combines behavioural skill training, cognitive interventions, and life-style change procedures. It is designed to help support the maintenance stage of change, and its goal is to teach individuals who are trying to change their behaviour now to anticipate and cope with the problems that will increase their risk of relapse (Marlatt & Gordon 1985).

The two central pillars of the Relapse Prevention approach are the identification of high-risk situations and the development and strengthening of coping strategies. The Relapse Prevention approach regards the individual's likelihood of avoiding relapse as being determined largely by these two factors. In Litman's (1986) model of survival the chances of avoiding relapse are seen as depending upon an interaction between:

1 Situations perceived to be dangerous for the individual in that they may precipitate relapse.
2 The coping strategies available within the individual's repertoire to deal with these situations.
3 The perceived effectiveness of these coping behaviours.
4 The individual's self-perception and self-esteem and the degree of learned helplessness with which they view their situation.

Among the high-risk situations which are a common problem for ex-addicts attempting to maintain their abstinence from heroin are negative mood states (such as sadness, boredom and anxiety), external events and cognitive factors (Bradley *et al.* 1989). Several studies have indicated that interpersonal factors may play an important role in relapse (e.g. Marlatt & George 1984). There are also strong risks attached to being exposed to drug-related cues and the role of these in producing craving or urges to use drugs has been emphasized by Stallard *et al.* (1987). In an investigation of the factors associated with relapse during outpatient detoxification treatment Unnithan *et al.* (1992) found that as many as 79% of their sample had met other drug-users in the week prior to interview and 62% had actually been offered drugs. The attrition rates among addicts during outpatient detoxification are high with less than 20% successfully completing treatment (Gossop *et al.* 1986), and the frequency with which they are exposed to such high-risk situations could easily be understood to greatly increase the risks of relapse among addicts at this vulnerable stage of change.

In Relapse Prevention treatments an important first task for the client is to develop an understanding of the way in which internal and external cues may create a high-risk situation. Clients may be encouraged to keep regular diaries detailing their use of drugs, the extent to which they have encountered possible precipitants of relapse, and a summary of their response. The therapist may assist in conducting a behavioural analysis of these situations and teach the client how to conduct such a behavioural analysis themselves. Structured problem-solving techniques are employed alongside rehearsal/role play. The client is warned of the dangers of the way in which covert planning may lead to relapse, and of apparently irrelevant decisions which may 'by chance' lead the client to happen to find himself outside his old drug dealer's house. The client must learn to spot early warning signals for these potential relapse situations.

On occasions when the client begins craving, he must learn to accept that this feeling can be tolerated and that it will dissipate. Marlatt somewhat poetically refers to this technique as 'urge-surfing'; the client is encouraged to allow the feeling to wash over and beyond him. On occasions when a lapse occurs and drugs are taken, then the client must resume control, realizing that drug use or abstinence is not an on/off behaviour, and thus avoid an undampened oscillation of perceived control which Marlatt terms the 'Abstinence Violation Effect'.

Thus, specific intervention strategies should be considered which would include extinction (or re-duction) or the conditioned stimulus-conditioned response link, the correction of identified physical or psychological handicaps, or relapse rehearsal to develop alternative coping strategies. These should be supplemented by global self-control strategies such as the learning of new 'positive addictions' and consideration of strategies for stimulus control and stimulus avoidance.

Annis (1986) has presented a relapse prevention model based on social learning approaches and, in particular, self-efficacy theory. This self-efficacy model sees the effectiveness of treatment as exerting its influence by enhancing the client's own efficacy expectations (defined as a judgement that one has the ability to execute a certain behaviour pattern). The expectations of the individual about their own self-efficacy are seen as having an impact upon the initiation, generalization and maintenance of coping behaviours, and the strength of the efficacy expectations will determine how long the coping behaviours will be maintained under stress. Self-efficacy theory provides a strong statement of the cognitive perspective in that it predicts that treatment is effective only insofar as it increases the client's own expectations of what they can themselves achieve and maintain.

## The malleability of behaviour and natural recovery

A substantial body of evidence now exists to illustrate the malleability of drug-taking behaviour amongst those who continue to use drugs. In a study from the early 1970s, Hawks reports on the follow-up of a cohort of opiate addicts in an English provincial town and reports that at three-year follow-up many had reduced the frequency of their injecting even though they continued to use (Hawkes 1976). More recently Strang *et al.* (1987) have described evidence for moderation of the drug habit in 55 ongoing drug-users (part of a two-year follow-up sample) – 45% had reduced dose substantially, whilst 42% had reduced frequency of injecting, even though they continued to use drugs. Likewise Ghodse *et al.* (1987) have reported on the apparently spontaneous reductions in the extent of needle sharing amongst opiate addicts attending a London drug treatment centre over the period during which there was the first extensive public HIV information campaign. Evidence is now available from studies of needle exchange schemes which show that at least some drug injectors are able to move away from particularly high-risk behaviours – for example, labelling their own personal syringe, using clean syringes, restricting the number of their needle-sharing partners, etc. (see Stimson *et al.* 1988c, 1990). Indeed this form of work is now termed 'harm minimization' and is becoming a major theme within the broader drug treatment strategy (Stimson 1992). In the same vein, US data on the promotion of bleach as an agent for cleaning needles and syringes (the teach and bleach campaign) shows reported use of bleach to have increased from 5% to 50% in San Francisco (Newmeyer 1988). Power *et al.* (1988) reports that in his sample of London drug addicts, the fear of HIV and its consequences was identified most commonly as the issue prompting the recently observed changes away from injecting. In New York, Jackson & Rotkiewicz (1987) reported on their findings that HIV outreach work also appeared to be effective in diverting drug-users into treatment programmes, even though the overt strategy was one of harm minimization during continued use.

Little attention has been paid to apparently spontaneous or natural patterns of recovery. Reference is occasionally made to Winick's early description of the 'maturing out' process in which recovery was seen as a spontaneous result of age and length of addiction (Winick 1962). Subsequent analyses have seen fit to consider the factors (including age and length of addiction) which might influence the timing of this seemingly spontaneous recovery. Anglin *et al.* (1986) report on their large-scale follow-up study and note that natural recovery appears to be influenced by addiction-related or contextual factors (e.g. property crime and drug dealing) which may retard the rate of any natural recovery. Stimson & Oppenheimer (1982) report on their London study of heroin addicts recruited from treatment centres in 1968. Over the course of a decade 35% became stably drug free, but had travelled down

many different pathways to reach this status. Attributions from the subjects themselves included the achievement of employment, new friends and the giving up of former addict friends; and for many a geographical move had been central. Wille (1981) looked at data from the same cohort and identified two basic patterns of recovery – a planned, internally motivated, voluntary way of becoming abstinent; and a separate, external-enforced way (both of which had been successful with different individuals). Specific study of spontaneous recovery from heroin addiction was undertaken by Schasre (1966) who reported on findings from 40 subjects who identified the following key factors – negative experiences with peers, pressure from partner/spouse, increased awareness of the stigma of addiction, geographical move, the disappearance of the regular drug dealer. Waldolf & Biernacki have undertaken a series of studies of natural recovery amongst San Francisco heroin addicts, and in their review of the literature (Waldorf & Biernacki 1979) they propose that the process of natural recovery concerns change in a person's identity, with the replacement of the addict identity by some more ordinary identity. In this regard it is interesting to consider the intermediate state between these identities that might be achieved by successful recruitment into methadone maintenance programmes which Preble & Miller described as the 'inter-world' (Preble & Miller 1977). This may perhaps link with Biernacki's later proposal (1983) that for the entrenched addict it may be necessary to provide this new identity in order to facilitate natural recovery (i.e. in contrast to relying on some pre-existing perceived role set). Likewise Jorquez (1983) suggests that recovery involves two concurrent processes – extrication from the social ties and dependencies of the drug world, and accommodation to the new ordinary life-style.

## Manipulating the environment

Change is undoubtedly achievable: certain key studies provide evidence of the feasibility of changes in drug status, whilst at the same time being tantalizingly imprecise about the factors which have led to the change observed. Thus the Vietnam veteran studies described above (Robins *et al.* 1974, 1975) stand as a vivid illustration of the malleability of heroin-taking behaviour and heroin addiction, with figures of less than 10% using opiates and less than 1% being addicted in the year after their return to the USA. But what were the actual factors associated with this extraordinary follow-up data? The problem is that the return from Vietnam to the USA contains so many possible causal factors that it is so difficult to disentangle the various influences: but the study demonstrates the power of these forces if only they can be harnessed. More parochially, a series of studies by Oppenheimer and her colleagues have studied three cohorts of London drug addicts recruited from each of a drug treatment centre (outpatient), a drug-free residential therapeutic community, and a short-stay crisis intervention centre (Oppenheimer *et al.* 1988, 1990). Here again there is evidence of surprisingly high levels of substantial change in drug taking, with follow-up data three to five years later finding that 59% had not used opiates for at least a year, and that 75% had not used any opiates at all during the month prior to interview. Their study straddled the period of time during which HIV/AIDS reached public awareness and may have contributed to the extensive change observed, but once again the study provides evidence of the extent to which change is achievable if the relevant forces can be brought to bear.

Recently more attention has been paid to factors which may be associated with treatment outcome which exist within the community. Hawkins (1983) has recently reviewed this area and suggests that 'community' may be seen in five ways:

1 A geographical environment defined by the sociodemographic characteristics of residence.

2 A set of organizations which an individual may encounter.

3 A culture, set of expectations and beliefs localized in a geographical setting.

4 A neighbourhood in which people carry out their daily routine and with which they may identify.

5 The people with whom an individual interacts in the routines of daily living.

Each of these community perspectives leads to different areas of enquiry with different possible intervention strategies.

### Manipulating the home environment

Azrin and colleagues (Hunt & Azrin 1973, Azrin 1976, Azrin *et al.* 1982) have studied various community reinforcement strategies in the treatment of recovering alcoholics (although the data have yet to be replicated with subjects dependent on other drugs). Their approach is based on principles of operant reinforcement and involves the systematic rearrangement of existing community reinforcers such as job, family, social and recreational opportunities. These are rearranged in such a way that further drinking results in time out from these reinforcers. The model is further developed by the incorporation of a buddy system, a telephone report-in system, an early warning relapse notification system, and group counselling (Azrin 1976); and in a later study by an additional component built around self-administration of disulfiram (Antabuse) (Azrin *et al.* 1982). The authors report on the strikingly better progress of alcoholics assigned to the community reinforcement programme, with the study group spending only 2% of their time drinking compared with 55% for the control group, and with similar differences in outcome measures of employment, time with families and time out of institutions. The effects were also remarkably durable, and were in large part maintained at this level of magnitude for the two-year follow-up period.

Certain cities have set up re-employment programmes, such as those attached to methadone maintenance programmes in the USA (see Gearing 1974). Certainly there is a continuing practice of discrimination against addicts and ex-addicts seeking employment, and Hawkins (1983) expresses concern that the structure of methadone maintenance programmes seems unlikely to support improved functioning in the community following treatment, whilst allowing the discrimination against this group by other organizations to continue. It is not surprising, then, to discover that many former heroin addicts in methadone maintenance programmes live in neither the addict world nor the straight world but in a detached 'inter-world'.

## Studies of the neighbourhood and its influence

Hughes and colleagues (1971) found surprisingly little community awareness of drug dealing and drug use. Hughes concludes that neighbourhoods are not sufficiently integrated to serve as reliable influences either for or against drug use, and that any such influences are more likely to be found at the peer group rather than neighbourhood level.

Study of the social network of drug-users may be expected to be a more productive line of enquiry. As yet, this area has been minimally studied as a possible area for intervention, although the current enthusiasm for detached social work and for outreach work represent possible avenues into this field of enquiry and intervention. Hawkins & Fraser (1981) found strong correlations between frequency of opiate use and the degree of engagement in drug-using networks (and also the degree of disengagement from non-using networks). This included the number of contacts from work, school or other organizations, and the authors concluded that many such opiate addicts entering treatment were now in social relationships in which the drug use and criminal behaviour were valued positively by their peers who saw little reward associated with more socially acceptable activities. In an extension of this study they looked at the post-treatment progress of former heroin addicts leaving a residential treatment programme; here again Hawkins & Fraser found that high levels of continued contact with drug-users was associated with higher levels of relapse back to heroin use (Hawkins & Fraser 1981). The evidence from these authors accords with the findings from the naturalistic studies described above (e.g. Waldorf & Biernacki 1979) – that social network support from key individuals appears to be influential on both drug use and subsequent recovery, and there may be considerable scope for adaptation of the immediate social environment of addicts during and after treatment.

## Legal constraints and coercion

It goes against the instincts of many drug workers to look at the potentially beneficial influence of coercion. However, the data would certainly suggest that this is an area requiring more serious consideration. For example, Vaillant (1974) has explored the necessary intimate partnership between law and medicine, and has also provided data on the apparently successful use of coercion within the treatment programme (Vaillant 1974). The treatment histories and incarcerations of 100 heroin addicts were studied: only 10 out of 361 passages through treatment were followed by abstinence of one year's duration, whereas there was a successful drug-free interval of at least one year in the community after 24 of the 34 prison sentences (in this study prison sentence was followed by a year of strict parole with a requirement of employment, abstinence from opiates and regular reporting to parole officer). Inadvertently the criminal justice system appeared to have stumbled across a powerful therapeutic intervention, but here again the challenge is to tease out the components which are responsible for the different course or outcome.

Subsequent work from California has explored the beneficial results of civil commitment (Anglin & McGlothlin 1984). In a series of studies, the Los Angeles group has gathered extensive data on the time-related probabilities of different outcomes of addicts in methadone treatment programmes, on the one hand, and in Civil Addict Programmes (CAP) – a compulsory treatment approach provided under the auspices of the Department of Correction. Their results indicate that both civil commitment and methadone maintenance are effective in reducing drug use, drug dealing, acquisitive crime (i.e. crime to raise funds for drug use), and arrests; and that there is also some evidence (albeit less striking) for improvement in employment situation and assumption of family responsibilities. The benefit appears to be related positively to the length of time in active treatment, which also seems to result in longer duration of benefit. For the majority of these subjects methadone maintenance was available within the CAP. Anglin & McGlothlin (1984) conclude that it is the behavioural elements of the CAP which have been instrumental in bringing about these results. First, there is a clear behavioural goal of abstinence (apart from prescribed methadone); secondly there was tight monitoring of behaviour by parole officers (supplemented by urine testing) which typically revealed relapse at an early stage; and thirdly the return to addictive opiate use resulted in immediate reincarceration. The incarceration periods included educational and vocational training as well as specific drug counselling, and were followed up by supervision by parole officers who ensured further educational and vocational assistance.

## Conclusion

There is clear evidence that social and environmental factors influence the extent of drug use both within the community and within the individual. Furthermore, the time-course and nature of continued drug use within individuals and within groups appears susceptible to influence in ways that produce strikingly different outcome data in different studies. However, as yet, efforts to tease out the active factors in bringing about these different outcome data have been disappointingly imprecise: certainly one of the major areas of continued research must be in the area of factors influencing the natural history or career of drug use at the individual and group level, until such time as the essential therapeutic components can be isolated and subsequently administered in a deliberate and controlled approach. There will then exist the task of identifying different matchings of individuals and treatments so as to ensure maximum compatibility and acceptability of different approaches (see Glaser 1980, Glaser & Skinner 1981). As yet our interventions remain more of a blunderbuss approach. The study of drug use and addiction in its social context offers a suitable laboratory for the development of tomorrow's preventive and treatment techniques.

## References

Advisory Committee on Alcoholism (Kessel Report) (1978) *The Pattern and Range of Services for Problem Drinkers.* HMSO, London.

Advisory Council on the Misuse of Drugs (1982) *Treatment and Rehabilitation Report.* HMSO, London.

Anglin M.D., Brecht M.L. & Woodward J.A. (1986) An empirical study of maturing out: conditional factors. *International Journal of the Addictions* 21, 233–246.

Anglin M.D. & McGlothlin W.H. (1984) Outcome of narcotics addict treatment in California. In Tims F. & Ruchman N. (eds) *Drug Abuse Treatment Evaluation: Strategies, Progress and Prospects.* NIDA Research Monograph Series. US Government Printing Office, Washington DC.

Anker A.L. & Crowley T. (1982) Use of contingency contracting in speciality clinics for cocaine abuse. In Harris L.S. (ed.) *Problems of Drug Dependence 1981.* NIDA Research Monograph 41, pp. 452–459. NIDA, Washington DC.

Annis H.M. (1986) A relapse prevention model for treatment of alcoholics. In Miller W.R. & Heather N. (eds) *Treating Addictive Behaviors*, pp. 407–433. Plenum Press, New York.

Azrin N.H. (1976) Improvements in the community-reinforcement approach to alcoholism. *Behaviour Research and Therapy* 14, 339–348.

Azrin N.H., Sisson R.W., Meyers R. & Godley M. (1982) Alcoholism treatment by disulfiram and community reinforcement therapy. *Journal of Behavior Therapy and Experimental Psychiatry* 13, 105–112.

Becker H.S. (1953) Becoming a marihuana user. *American Journal of Sociology* 59, 235–242.

Bell G., Cohen J. & Cremona A. (1990) How willing are general practitioners to manage narcotic misuse? *Health Trends* 22, 56–57.

Biernacki P. (1983) *Pathways from Heroin Addiction: Recovery without Treatment.* Temple University Press, Philadelphia.

Bradley B., Phillips G., Green L. & Gossop M. (1989) Circumstances surrounding the initial lapse to opiate use following detoxification. *British Journal of Psychiatry* 154, 354–359.

Buning E. (1990) The role of harm-reduction programmes in curbing the spread of HIV by drug injectors. In Strang J. & Stimson G. (eds) *AIDS and Drug Misuse: The Challenge for Policy and Practice in the 1990s.* Routledge, London.

Burr A. (1984) The ideologies of despair: a symbolic interpretation of punks and skinheads' usage of barbiturates. *Social Science and Medicine* 19, 929–938.

Chapple P. & Gray G. (1968) One year's work at a centre for the treatment of addicted patients. *Lancet* i, 908–911.

Cook C. (1988a) The Minnesota model in the management of drug and alcohol dependency: miracle or myth? Part 1. The philosophy and the programme. *British Journal of Addiction* 83, 625–634.

Cook C. (1988b) The Minnesota Model in the management of drug and alcohol dependency: miracle, method or myth? Part 2. Evidence and conclusion. *British Journal of Addiction* 83, 735–748.

Cooke L., Barrett A. & Tomlinson D. (1990) HIV positivity and health in the therapeutic community. In Strang J. & Stimson G. (eds) *AIDS and Drug Misuse: The Challenge for Policy and Practice in the 1990s*. Routledge, London.

Crowley T. (1984) Contingency contracting treatment of drug-abusing physicians, nurses and dentists: behavioural intervention techniques in drug abuse treatments. *NIDA Research Monograph* 46, 68–83.

Cummings C., Gordon J.R. & Marlatt G.A. (1980) Relapse: prevention and prediction. In Miller W.R. (ed.) *The Addictive Behaviors*, pp. 291–321. Pergamon Press, New York.

de Alarcon R. (1969) The spread of heroin abuse in a community. *Bulletin on Narcotics* 21, 17–22.

de Alarcon R. (1972) An epidemiological evaluation of a public health measure aimed at reducing the availability of methylamphetamine. *Psychological Medicine* 2, 293–300.

de Alarcon R. & Rathod N.H. (1968) Prevalence and early detection of heroin abuse. *British Medical Journal* 2, 549–553.

de Leon G. & Jainchill N. (1982) Male and female drug abusers: social and psychological status two years after treatment in a therapeutic community. *American Journal of Drug and Alcohol Abuse* 8, 465–497.

Donoghoe M.C. (1991) Syringe exchange: has it worked? *Druglink* January/February, 8–11.

Dorn N. & South N. (1985) *Helping Drug Users*. Gower, Aldershot.

Drug Indicators Project (1989) *Report of Study on Help seeking*. Institute for the Study of Drug Dependence, London.

Edwards G. (1982) *The Treatment of Drinking Problems – A Guide for the Helping Professions*. Grant MacIntyre, London.

Edwards G. (1984) Addiction: a challenge to society. *New Society* 25 October, 133–135.

Edwards G., Arif A. & Hodgson R. (1981) Nomenclature and classification of drug and alcohol related problems: a shortened version of a WHO memorandum. *British Journal of Addiction* 77, 287–306.

Edwards G. & Gross M.M. (1976) Alcohol dependence: provisional description of a clinical syndrome. *British Medical Journal* 1, 1058–1061.

Gearing F.R. (1974) Methadone maintenance treatment five years later – where are they now? *American Journal of Public Health* 64, 44–50.

Gearing F.R. & Schweitzer M.D. (1974) An epidemiological evaluation of long-term methadone maintenance. *American Journal of Epidemiology* 100, 101–106.

Ghodse A.H., London M., Bewley T.H. & Baht A.V. (1987) In-patient treatment for drug abuse. *British Journal of Psychiatry* 151, 72–75.

Glanz A., Byrne C. & Jackson P. (1989) Role of community pharmacies in prevention of AIDS among injecting drug misusers: findings of a survey in England and Wales. *British Medical Journal* 299, 1076–1079.

Glaser F.B. (1980) Anyone got a match?: treatment research and the matching hypothesis. In Edwards G. & Grant M. (eds) *Alcohol Treatment in Transition*.

Glaser F.B. & Skinner H.A. (1981) Matching in the real world: a practical approach. In Gottheil E.A., McLellan A.T. & Donley K.A. (eds) *Matching Patient Needs and Treatment Methods in Alcoholism and Drug Abuse*. Charles C. Thomas, Springfield, Illinois.

Gossop M. (1987) What is the most effective way to treat opiate addiction. *British Journal of Hospital Medicine* 38, 161.

Gossop M. (1989) The detoxification of high dose heroin addicts in Pakistan. *Drug and Alcohol Dependence* 24, 143–150.

Gossop M., Green L., Phillips G. & Bradley B. (1989) Lapse, relapse and survival among opiate addicts after treatment: a prospective follow-up study. *British Journal of Psychiatry* 154, 348–353.

Gossop M., Green L., Phillips G. & Bradley B. (1990) Factors predicting outcome among opiate addicts after treatment. *British Journal of Clinical Psychology* 29, 209–216.

Gossop M., Johns A. & Green L. (1986) Opiate withdrawal: in-patient versus out-patient programmes and preferred versus random assignment to treatment. *British Medical Journal* 293, 103–104.

Green L. & Gossop M. (1988) The effects of information on the opiate withdrawal syndrome. *British Journal of Addiction* 83, 305–309.

Hartnoll R.L., Mitcheson M.C., Lewis R. & Bryer S. (1985) Estimating the prevalence of opioid dependence. *Lancet* i, 203–205.

Hawkes D. (1976) Heroin users in a provincial town and their follow-up over a three year period. In Edwards G., Russell M.A.H., Hawks D. & McCafferty M. (eds) *Drugs and Drug Dependence*. Saxon House, Farnborough, Hants.

Hawkins J.D. (1983) Community characteristics associated with treatment outcome. In Cooper J.R., Altman F., Brown B.S. & Czechowicz D. (eds) *Research on the Treatment of Narcotic Addiction: State of the Art*. National institute on Drug Abuse, Rockville, Maryland.

Hawkins J. & Fraser M.W. (1981) The Social Networks of Drug Abusers Before and After Treatment. Paper presented at the International Congress of Drugs and Alcohol, Jerusalem, Israel. Center for Social Welfare Research, University of Washington, Seattle.

Hubbard R.L., Marsden S.D., Rachal J.V. *et al.* (1989) *Drug Abuse Treatment: A National Study of Effectiveness*. University of North Carolina Press, Chapel Hill.

Hubbard R.L., Rachal J.V., Craddock S.G. & Cavanaugh E.R. (1984) Treatment outcome prospective study (TOPS): client characteristics and behaviors before, during and after treatment. In Tims F.M. & Ludford J.P. (eds) *Drug Abuse Treatment Evaluation: Strategies, Progress and Prospects*. National Institute on Drug Abuse, Rockville, Maryland.

Hughes P.H., Chappel J., Senay E. & Jaffe J. (1971) Developing in-patient services for community-based treatment of narcotic addiction. *Archives of General Psychiatry* 25, 278–283.

Hunt G.M. & Azrin N.H. (1973) A community-reinforcement approach to alcoholism. *Behavior Research and Therapy* 11, 91–104.

Hunt W.A., Barnett L.W. & Branch L.G. (1971) Relapse rates in addiction programmes. *Journal of Clinical Psychology* 27, 455–456.

Hunt L.G. & Chambers C.D. (1976) *The Heroin Epidemic: A Study of Heroin Use in the United States.* Spectrum Press, New York.

Jackson J. & Rotkiewicz L. (1987) A Coupon Programme. Paper presented at the Third International conference on AIDS, Washington, DC.

Jorquez J.S. (1983) The retirement phase of heroin using careers. *Journal of Drug Issues* 13, 343–365.

Kosviner A., Mitcheson M.C., Myers K. *et al.* (1968) Heroin use in a provincial town. *Lancet* i, 1189–1192.

Lang A.R., Goeckner D., Adesso V. & Marlatt G.A. (1975) The effects of alcohol on agression in male social drinkers. *Journal of Abnormal Psychology* 84, 508–518.

Lart R. & Stimson G. (1990) National survey of syringe exchange schemes in England. *British Journal of Addiction* 85, 1433–1444.

Litman G. (1986) Alcoholism survival: the prevention of relapse. In Miller W. & Heather N. (eds) *Treating Addictive Behaviours.* Plenum, New York.

MacGregor S., Ettore B., Croomber R., Crosier A. & Lodge H. (1991) *Drug Services in England and the Impact of the Central Funding Initiative.* ISDD Research Monograph 1. Institute for the Study of Drug Dependence, London.

McLellan A.T. (1983) Patient characteristics associated with outcome. In Cooper J.R., Altman F., Brown B.S. & Czenchowicz D. (eds) *Research on the Treatment of Narcotic Addiction: State of the Art.* National Institute on Drug Abuse, Rockville, Maryland.

Mahon T. (1973) Therapy or brain washing? *Drugs and Society* 2, (5), 7–10.

Marlatt G.A. & George W. (1984) Relapse prevention: introduction and overview of the model. *British Journal of Addiction* 79, 261–273.

Marlatt G. & Gordon J. (eds) (1985) *Relapse Prevention.* Guildford Press, New York.

Marlatt G.A. & Rohsenow, D.J. (1980) Cognitive processes in alcohol use: expectancy and the balanced placebo design. In Mello N.K. (ed.) *Advances in Substance Abuse: Behavioural and Biological Research.* JAI Press, Grennwich, Connecticut.

Moos R.H., Finney J.W. & Cronkite R.C. (1990) *Alcoholism Treatment: Context, Process and Outcome.* Oxford University Press, New York.

Mott J. (1992) The British Addict Notification System. In Strang J. & Gossop M. (eds) *Responding to Drug Abuse: The British System.* Oxford University Press, Oxford (in press).

Nelles W. (1990) Models of self-help for drug users with HIV/AIDS. In Strang J. & Stimson G. (eds) *AIDS and Drug Misuse: The Challenge for Policy and Practice in the 1990s.* Routledge, London.

Newmeyer, J.A. (1988) Why bleach? Development of a strategy to combat HIV contagion among San Franciscan drug users. In Battjes R.J. & Pickens R.W. (eds) *Needle Sharing Among Intravenous Drug Abusers: National and International Perspectives.* National Institute on Drug Abuse, Rockville, Maryland.

Ogborne A.C. & Melotte C. (1977) An evaluation of the therapeutic community for former drug users. *British Journal of Addiction* 72, 75–82.

Oppenheimer E., Sheehan M. & Taylor C. (1988) Letting the client speak: drug misusers and the process of help seeking. *British Journal of Addiction* 83, 635–648.

Oppenheimer E., Sheehan M. & Taylor C. (1990) What happens to drug misusers?: a medium-term follow-up of subjects new to treatment. *British Journal of Addiction* 85, 1255–1260.

Parker H., Bakx K. & Newcombe R. (1988) *Living with Heroin: The Impact of a Drugs 'Epidemic' on an English Community.* Open University Press, Milton Keynes.

Parker H., Newcombe R. & Bakx K. (1987) The new heroin users: prevalence and characteristics in Wirral, Merseyside. *British Journal of Addiction* 8, 147–157.

Pearson G. (1987a) *The New Heroin Users.* Basil Blackwell, Oxford.

Pearson G. (1987b) Heroin and unemployment. In Dorn N. & South N. (eds) *A Land Fit for Heroin: Drugs in Britain in the 1980s.* Macmillan, London.

Pearson G., Gilman M. & Mclver S. (1986) Young people and heroin: an examination of heroin use in the North of England. *Health Eduction Council Research Report No. 8.* Gower and Health Education Council, London.

Phillips G., Gossop M. & Bradley B. (1986) Influence of psychological factors on the opiate withdrawal syndrome. *British Journal of Psychiatry* 149, 235–238.

Phillips G.T., Gossop M., Edwards G., Sutherland G., Taylor C. & Strang J. (1987) The application of SODQ to the measurement of the severity of opiate dependence in a British sample. *British Journal of Addiction* 82, 691–699.

Plant M.A. (1973) The escalation theory reconsidered: drug takers in an English town. *British Journal of Addiction* 68, 305–313.

Plant M.A. (1975) Drug takers in an English town. *British Journal of Criminology* 15, 181–186.

Plant M.A. (1990) Epidemiology and drug misuse. In: Berridge V. (ed.) *Drug Research and Policy in Britain: A Review of the 1980s.* Avebury, Aldershot.

Plant M., Peck D. & Samuel E. (1984) *Alcohol, Drugs and School Leaves.* Tavistock, London.

Power R., Hartnoll R. & Daviaud E. (1988) Drug injecting, AIDS and risk behaviour: potential for change and intervention strategies. *British Journal of Addiction* 83, 649–654.

Power R., Stimson G. & Strang J. (1991) Drug prevention and HIV policy. *AIDS 1990* 4, (suppl), S263–S267.

Preble E. & Miller T. (1977) Methadone, wine and

welfare. In Weppner, R.S. (ed.) *Street Ethnography*. Sage, Beverley Hills, California.

Robins L.J., Davis D.H. & Goodwin D.W. (1974) Drug users in Vietnam: a follow-up on return to USA. *American Journal of Epidemiology* 99, 235–249.

Robins L.N., Helzer J.E. & Davis D.H. (1975) Narcotic use in South East Asia and afterwards. *Archives of General Psychiatry* 32, 955–961.

Schasre R. (1966) Cessation patterns among neophyte heroin users. *International Journal of the Addictions* 1, 23–32.

Shaw S., Cartwright A., Spratley T. & Harwin J. (1978) *Responding to Drinking Problems*. Croom Helm, London.

Spiegler D.L. & Harford T.C. (1987) Addictive behaviours among youth. In Nirenberg T.D. & Maislo S.A. (eds) *Developments in the Assessment and Treatment of Addictive Behaviours*. Ablex, Norwood, New Jersey.

Spratley T. (1987) Consultancy as part of community alcohol team (CAT) work. In Stockwell T. & Clement S. (eds) *Helping the Problem Drinker: New Initiatives in Community Care*. Croom Helm, London.

Stallard A., Heather N. & Johnson B. (1987) AIDS and intravenous drug use: what clinical psychology can offer. *Bulletin of the British Psychological Society* 40, 365–368.

Stimson G. (1992) Minimising harm from drug use. In Strang J. & Gossop M. (eds) *Responding to Drug Misuse: the British System*. Oxford University Press, Oxford (in press).

Stimson G.V., Alldritt L., Dolan K. & Donoghoe M. (1988a) Syringe exchange schemes for drug users in England and Scotland. *British Medical Journal* 296, 1717–1719.

Stimson G.V., Dolan K., Donoghoe M. & Alldritt L. (1988b) Syringe exchange: 1 *Druglink* May/June, 10–11.

Stimson G., Dolan K., Donoghoe M., Alldritt L. & Lart R. (1989) Syringe exchange 3: Can injectors change? *Druglink* January/February, 10–11.

Stimson G., Donoghoe M., Alldritt L. & Dolan K. (1988c) Syringe exchange 2: the clients. *Druglink* July/August, 8–9.

Stimson G., Donoghoe M., Lart R. & Dolan K. (1990) Distributing sterile needles and syringes to people who inject drugs: the syringe exchange experiment. In Strang J. & Stimson G. (eds) *AIDS and Drug Misuse: The Challenge for Policy and Practice in the 1990s*. Routledge, London.

Stimson G. & Oppenheimer E. (1982) *Heroin Addiction: Treatment and Control in Britain*. Tavistock, London.

Stimson G.V., Oppenheimer E. & Stimson C.A. (1984) Drug abuse in the medical profession: addict doctors and the Home Office. *British Journal of Addiction* 79, 395–402.

Stockwell T. & Clement S. (1987) *Helping the Problem Drinker: New Initiatives in Community Care*. Croom Helm, London.

Stockwell T., Hodgson R., Edwards G., Taylor C. & Rankin, H. (1979) The developments of a questionnaire to measure severity of alcohol dependence. *British Journal of Addiction* 74, 79–87.

Strang J. (1989) A model service: turning the generalist on to drugs. In MacGregor S. (ed.) *Drugs and British Society: Responses to a Social Problem in the 1980s*. Routledge, London.

Strang J. (1991) Service development and organisation: drugs. In Glass, Ilana B. (ed.) *The International Handbook of Addiction Behaviour*. Routledge, London.

Strang J., Heathcote S. & Watson P. (1987) Habit-moderation in injecting drug addicts. *Health Trends* 19, 16–18.

Strang J. & Shah A . (1985) Notification of addicts and the medical practitioner – an evaluation of the system. *British Journal of Psychiatry* 147, 195–198.

Strang J., Smith M. & Spurrell, S. (1992) The community drug team. *British Journal of Addiction* 87, 169–178.

Sutherland G., Edwards G., Taylor C., Phillips G., Gossop M. & Brady R. (1986) The measurement of opiate dependence. *British Journal of Addition* 81, 485–494.

Swadi H. (1988) Drug and substance use among 3333 London adolescents. *British Journal of Addiction* 83, 935–942.

Toon P. & Lynch R. (1992) Changes in therapeutic communities. In Strang J. & Gossop M. (eds) *Responding to Drug Misuse: The British System*. Oxford University Press, Oxford (in press).

Unnithan S., Gossop M. & Strang J. (1992) Factors associated with relapse among opiate addicts in an out-patient detoxification programme. *British Journal of Psychiatry* (in press).

US Institute of Medicine (1990) In Gerstein D.B. & Harwood H.-J. (eds) *Treating Drug Problems (vol. 1): A Study of the Evolution Effectiveness and Financing of Public and Private Drug Treatment Systems*. National Academy Press, Washington.

Vaillant G. (1973) A 20 year follow up of New York narcotic addicts. *Archives of General Psychiatry* 29, 237–241.

Vaillant G. (1974) The place of coercion in addiction treatment. In Bostrom H., Larsson T. & Ljungstedt N. (eds) *Drug Dependence: Treatment and Treatment Evaluation*. Almqvisd and Wiksell, Stockholm.

Waldorf D. & Biernacki P. (1979) Natural recovery from heroin addiction: a review of the literature. *Journal of Drug Issues* 9, 281–289.

Wells B. (1987a) NA and the Minnesota method in Britain. *Druglink* 2, (1), 8–9.

Wells, B. (1987b) Narcotics Anonymous: the phenomenal growth of an important resource. *British Journal of Addiction* 82, 1–2.

Wells, B. (1992) Narcotics Anonymous – growth of a

movement. In Strang J. & Gossop M. (eds) *Responding to Drug Misuse: The British System.* Oxford University Press, Oxford (in press).

Wille R. (1981) Ten-year follow-up of a representative sample of London heroin addicts. Clinic attendance, abstinence and morality. *British Journal of Addiction* 76, 259–266.

Winick C. (1962) Maturing out of narcotic addiction. *Bulletin of Narcotics* 142, 1–7.

Winick C. (1980) A theory of drug dependence based on role, access to, and attitudes towards drugs. In Lettieri D.J., Sayers M. & Pearson H.W. (eds) *Theories on Drug Abuse*, pp. 225–235. National Institute on Drug Abuse (NIDA), Washington.

Wright J.D. & Pearl L. (1986) Knowledge and experience of young people of drug abuse 1969–1984. *British Medical Journal* 292, 179–182.

Wright J.D. & Pearl L. (1990) Knowledge and experience of young people regarding drug abuse 1969–1989. *British Medical Journal* 300, 99–103.

Yates R. (1981) *Out from the Shadows – Lifeline Project.* NACRO (National Association for Care and Rehabilitation of Offenders), London.

Yates R. (1985) Addiction: an everyday disease. In Lishman, J. (ed.) *Approaches to Addiction.* Kogan-Page, London.

Young J. (1973) *The Drug Takers.* Paladin, London.

Zacune J., Mitheson M. & Malone, S. (1969) Heroin use in a provincial town – one year later. *International Journal of the Addictions* 4, 557–570.

Zinberg N. (1984) *Drug Set and Setting. The Basis for Controlled Intoxicant use.* Yale University Press, New Haven.

# Chapter 13
## Social Factors in Child Psychiatric Disorder

A.COX

### Introduction

There is increasing evidence about the nature and extent of continuities between psychiatric disorders in childhood and adult life (Rutter 1989a, Zeitlyn 1990). A wide range of social factors are associated with child psychiatric disorders and there is evidence that they may be influential, not only in the genesis and maintenance of disorders in childhood, but also their extension into adulthood (Rutter 1989a). Factors under consideration include characteristics of parents and care-givers, such as their mental state and personality and the quality of parents' marriages, the style of child rearing and the contexts in which it occurs, relationships between the child and other family members, family structure and aspects of family function, relationships with peers, school experience, and broader environmental circumstances such as housing and the impact of life events (Garmezy & Rutter 1985, Hersov 1985a, Rutter & Cox 1985, Wolkind & Rutter 1985a,b, Shaw & Emery 1988, Goodyer 1990a,b). The broad associations between these varied factors and child psychiatric disorders point to the need to comprehend the nature of the associations and the requirement to look for specificities linking particular factors and particular disorders. Links between specific social factors and specific diagnoses have not been easy to find and this is understandable given the multifactorial aetiology of most of the disorders (Reeves *et al.* 1987, Werry *et al.* 1987, Williams *et al.* 1990). Some reports have suggested that the broad groupings of factors such as life events, socioeconomic status, family structure and function and parental characteristics act in a non-specific fashion, but interact with each other so that the risk of disorder increases geometrically with the addition of successive adversities (Rutter & Quinton 1977, Cowen *et al.*

1990b). Furthermore, it has been pointed out that family disadvantage makes only a modest contribution to explaining the presence of child psychiatric disorders. One model proposes that life experience and family social and material conditions influence a non-specific vulnerability to disorder (Fergusson *et al.* 1990). However, several studies now find externalizing or conduct disorders in childhood associated with cumulative social adversity: internalizing or anxiety disorders with specific social adversities, especially depression and anxiety disorders in parents (Werry *et al.* 1987, Shaw & Emery 1988, Offord *et al.* 1989, Velez *et al.* 1989). In considering cumulative familial stressors Rutter (1978b) identified:

1 The father having an unskilled or semi-skilled job.
2 Overcrowding in the home or a large family size.
3 The mother suffering from depression or neurotic disorder.
4 The child ever having been in care.
5 The father having been convicted of any offence against the law.
6 Marital discord.

However, it can be argued that it is necessary to go beyond broad groups of social factors to an examination of more detailed processes if specificities are to be detected. Disentanglement of processes requires that social factors are considered alongside other factors, especially genetic factors and the characteristics of individual children (Rutter 1985b). These and broader cultural factors are not considered in detail here. In addition, a more discriminating approach is necessary to the broad range of social factors, including a recognition of their potential for protection from the development of disorder (Garmezy 1985, Rutter 1985a, 1987, Patterson *et al.* 1989, Rae-Grant *et al.* 1989). Risk factors are seen to predispose to poor outcomes; assets to good or adaptive outcomes; protective factors attenuate or remove the adverse consequences of risk factors (Patterson *et al.* 1989).

Although genetic factors will not be discussed fully, there is increasing evidence of their importance and the manner in which they may interact with social factors in the genesis of child psychiatric disorders. Indeed, the understanding of genetic factors is raising questions about the current categorization of child psychiatric disorders (Rutter *et al.* 1990a). A general model would propose that genetic factors interact with other personal child characteristics and predisposing influences in the environment, such as the impact of chronic environmental difficulties and provoking agents, in order to bring about child psychiatric disorder (Brown *et al.* 1986).

However, it is probably more important to consider social factors in respect to the maintenance of child psychiatric disorders rather than just to the genesis. Hence there needs to be a distinction between vulnerability in the individual and predisposing factors in the environment with regard to *both* provoking *and* maintenance factors. For example, a preschool child may have repeated episodes of physical illness leading to a lack of opportunities to develop confidence in interactions with peers, coupled with an overprotective parental approach. When school entry provokes anxiety in the child leading to school refusal, the disorder may be maintained by the parental response. A distinction is also necessary between the direct and indirect effect of factors so that in the example given the repeated childhood illnesses act in an indirect fashion through an influence on the child's experience and the parents' approach to the child.

## Social adversity

The high intercorrelation of the broad categories of social adversity also makes for difficulties in disentangling processes. For example, there is a very high correlation between maternal depression and discordant parental relationships, and both these factors are highly related to the pre- sence of child psychiatric disorder (Quinton & Rutter 1985a). It is thus necessary to be cautious in inferring causal relationships from the correlation of particular social adversities with disturbances in children's emotional and behavioural development.

In thinking about social factors, it is helpful to distinguish life events from chronic difficulties or adversities. Further distinctions separate out continuing difficulties of recent onset and 'daily hassles' (Goodyer 1990b). Most research in child psychiatry has been concerned with chronic difficulties, whether in relationships or circumstances; however, there has been a recent upsurge in interest in life events following the extensive work in this area for affective disorders in adult life (Brown *et al.* 1986, Goodyer 1990a,b). This interest has been further stimulated by the effects of specific disasters on children when aeroplanes have crashed or boats sunk (Garmezy & Rutter 1985, Pynoos *et al.* 1987, Yule 1989, Yule *et al.* 1990, Parry-Jones 1990) (see also Chapter 27). However, an earlier focus was on children's experience of separation from their parents (Bowlby 1951). There had been a tendency to consider this as a specific event with major long-term consequences, but it became apparent that separation needed to be related to its context and might be better conceptualized as the onset of a more extended experience which might or might not constitute a chronic difficulty (Rutter 1981b).

Before turning to particular categories of life event or chronic difficulty it is important to consider the developmental perspective and think further about the mechanisms through which social factors may bring about disorders. The effect of different social factors varies according to the developmental state of the child. The salient stage of the child's development may be determined by genetic or environmental factors. For example, the emergence of attachment behaviours during the second half of the first year of life is thought to be genetically determined and a prerequisite for the formation of specific attachment relationships (Bowlby 1982). Children who do not have the opportunity for stable and specific emotional attachments between six months and four years of age may have a characteristic personality development in which there is a lack of confiding relationships with peers and a lack of selectivity in choosing friends (Hodges & Tizard 1989b). On the other hand, whether and at what age school attendance is demanded by society varies from country to country so that an emotional disorder characterized by separation anxiety and school non-attendance may only become apparent when there is a societal demand that the child attends school. Again, although it is now recognized that major affective disorders occur in children before puberty, their prevalence is much lower than in adolescence and the sex ratio is more equal than in later life. These changes reflect developmental processes that are probably both biological and social, although their exact nature is not determined (Rutter 1986).

As already indicated, it is necessary that there is further disentangling of the manner in which social factors may bring about psychiatric disorders. Rutter has listed seven main ways in which earlier experiences may be linked with later psychiatric disorder (Rutter 1986). Although he was considering circumstances in which there might be a relatively long time-lag between the early experience and the later disorder, including links between childhood experiences and adult mental disorder, the proposed mechanisms are also relevant when the gap in time is much shorter. His phraseology has been adapted to take this into account:

1 They (the experiences) may lead to immediate disorder, with this disorder persisting for reasons that are largely independent of the initial causation or provocation.
2 They may lead to bodily changes, which in turn influence later functioning. The changes in the neuroendocrine system following acute physical stresses in infancy are one example.
3 They may lead directly to altered patterns of behaviour which although changed at the time of the event take the form of overt disorder some time later.
4 They may lead to changed family circumstances which then in turn predispose to later disorder.
5 They may operate through their action in altering sensitivities to stress or in modifying styles of coping, which then protect from or predispose

toward disorder in later life only in the presence of later stress events.
6 They may alter the individual's self-concept or attitudes or cognitive set, which in turn influence the response to later situations.
7 Finally, they may have an impact on later behaviour through effects on the selection of environments or on the opening up or closing down of opportunities (Rutter 1981a, 1983a).

It will be apparent from this list of processes that social experiences may often act indirectly but their recognition is important for the alleviation or prevention of disorders.

The central importance of child rearing and the quality of relationships both within and outside the family for the genesis, maintenance or prevention of child psychiatric disorders means that the interest in social factors extends beyond any presumed direct effect on child psychiatric disorders to the need to understand the way in which they influence parenting and relationships surrounding the child (Dunn 1986). For example, the nature of a child's relationships both within and outside the family, together with temperamental characteristics and intelligence, contribute to their resilience against the development of a disorder in the face of adversity (Garmezy 1985, Jenkins et al. 1989, Patterson et al. 1989, Cowen et al. 1990a,b, Jenkins & Smith 1990). Child rearing involves interactions between adults and children, and relationships between child and care-giver are a crucial component. Nevertheless, child rearing is about more than relationships and parent–child relationships are about more than child rearing (Hinde 1988). Parental interactions with the child have been conceived as the final common path for the influence of social factors (Belsky et al. 1989, Campbell 1990), but it has been cogently argued that non-genetic differences between siblings in psychopathology must reflect non-shared environmental influences; for example, not only differences in parent–child relationships, but also sibling and peer relationships (Dunn et al. 1990). Furthermore, the division of social factors into events and current difficulties in relationships or circumstances point to a wider range of processes mediating between social factors and disorders. For instance, separation from parents due to hospitalization, parental death or divorce all involve modifications to parent–child interaction and/or relationships, but such modifications do not fully describe the individual's experiences, nor how they are affected. Similarly, other traumatic or potentially traumatic events, and school, housing and area influences evidently include personal encounters but may also have effects by other means.

Rutter's list of processes mediating between social factors and child psychiatric disorder also emphasizes the need to distinguish chains of events or circumstances that alter risk for other risk factors or for the inception of disorder (Rutter 1989a), and circular processes that may sustain disturbance (Gorell Barnes 1985, Patterson 1982). For example, low socioeconomic status might increase the risk that a child lives in an area where there is an unsatisfactory school that in turn might increase the risk that the child fails educationally that in turn increases the risk that the child will develop a disorder of conduct (Wolkind & Rutter 1985b, Yule & Rutter 1985). On the other hand, low socioeconomic status increases the risk that a mother becomes depressed and that a coercive cycle develops between mother and child such that the child's non-compliant behaviour maintains the mother's hostile attitude towards the child; this hostile approach in turn sustaining the child's non-compliant behaviour (Patterson 1982, Cox *et al.* 1987).

## Life events

Stress is a confused concept and is used to apply equally to a form of stimulus (i.e. a stress or a response which may be a non-specific response of the body to any demand), a mental state (e.g. distress) and in a wider sense a state reached in response to a challenge (Rutter 1981a, Mitchell 1984). Stress is also used to refer to a strain, that is, either a stimulus requiring adaptation, or a response to challenge which exceeds the capacity of the organism to respond. In practice stress is commonly used for both stressors, i.e. certain challenges, and strain, i.e. human responses where there is overload. Not all life events are stressors and whether they are will depend not only on their

characteristics, but also the social context, how they are perceived, and previous experience (see also Chapter 10). Research in childhood in this field has suffered from many conceptual and methodological difficulties (Garmezy & Rutter 1985).

First, different forms of stressful experiences need to be discriminated. Studies of one-off disasters indicate that it is useful to disentangle discrete time-limited inherently unpleasant experiences not coming within the range of loss events or life changes that can be expected to occur in all people's lives at sometime. To these traumatic events there are a range of clearly described reactions which are thought by some to be distinctive manifestations of post-traumatic stress disorder (Garmezy & Rutter 1985, Pynoos *et al.* 1987, Yule 1989, 1991). As already indicated, persistently disturbed relationships and circumstances are also stressful but need to be considered separately. Garmezy & Rutter (1985) further distinguish losses associated with personal relationships, such as bereavements and rebuffs; life changes that alter the balance of family relationships, such as the birth of a younger sibling or hospitalization, and those that require social adaptation, such as starting school. Some would argue that the life changes listed all have inherent loss, or threat of loss of self-esteem or a relationship. Depressive feelings may be a consequence of either failure or loss of a relationship (Garmezy 1986).

Secondly there is evidence that for discrete, accumulated or repeated traumatic or undesirable experiences the outcome is influenced by personal and social antecedents and consequences, and whether they occur in the context of disturbed relationships or adverse social circumstances (Wolkind & Rutter 1985a, Garmezy & Rutter 1985, Rutter 1985b, Cicchetti & Schneider-Rosen 1986, Rutter 1987, Pianta & Castaldi 1989).

Thirdly the character or significance of experiences needs to be taken into account. In considering the unpleasantness or undesirability of experiences it is important to consider the meaning of the event. Stage of development and other characteristics of the child such as temperament, intelligence and physical state will influence how events are perceived and will need to be taken into account in measuring their quality (Goodyer 1990b). Although undesirability or unpleasantness of events has been linked particularly with 'exits' or losses (Rutter 1981a, Goodyer 1990b, Goodyer *et al.* 1985), there are undoubtedly events whose unpleasantness springs not just from a fear of loss of self-esteem or relationships or a threat to life. Controllability, responsibility, and whether the impact of the event is direct or indirect are also important in considering the effect of stressful events in children (Goodyer 1990b) as well as among adults (see Chapter 10). An inability to control may provoke a sense of helplessness. It has been suggested that this is particularly important in children who have much less control of their environment. The repeated experience of helplessness or even single major experiences of this type is thought to engender a persisting tendency to respond to stressful events with a sense of helplessness (Bowlby 1980, Seligman & Peterson 1986). This tendency is seen as a vulnerability with respect to the development of depression in adult life, and there is some evidence that children who lose their mother before the age of 11 are vulnerable to the development of depression as adults (Brown *et al.* 1986). Seligman & Peterson (1986) argue that the learned helplessness model is equally appropriate to the development of depression in childhood, but there is no direct evidence, and there are a number of other mechanisms that might be responsible for the continuity between childhood loss and depression in adult life other than a personal cognitive set arising from the loss. For example, it appears that the quality of care reported to have been experienced in childhood following the loss of the mother is of more importance both in contributing to a sense of helplessness in childhood and adult life, and also in predisposing to development of depression by other means (Brown *et al.* 1986). If this is so then the concurrent childhood consequences of an uncontrollable loss event may have more to do with consequences than the event itself (Dunn 1986).

With regard to responsibility, it is clear that objectively individuals may incur stressful events for which they are more or less responsible. A sense of responsibility for uncontrollable events forms part of the learned helplessness model of depression, and depressed children in comparison with controls have been shown to attribute bad events to themselves more often (Seligman & Peterson 1986). Young children may be particularly likely to infer that adverse events are their responsibility or have occurred because of some misdemeanour on their part (Wallerstein 1983, Hetherington 1983). Threat has also been found to be a relevant dimension and for adults it seems that perceived long-term threat is more likely to precipitate disorder than short-term threat (Brown & Harris 1978).

Two more recent studies of children have attempted to define life events and their characteristics more carefully (Goodyer *et al.* 1985, Goodyer 1990b). First, events were classified according to their undesirability, incorporating the notions of long-term threat and negative impact (Paykel 1983). Secondly only events that were independent or almost certainly independent of the disorder were included. In the first study there was found to be an increased frequency of moderate to severely undesirable life events in the 12 months before the onset of child psychiatric disorder. Mildly undesirable events were also associated where there was an onset of a conduct disorder but not an emotional disorder (Goodyer *et al.* 1985). This research was concerned with experiences such as accidents, illnesses, marriages, bereavements, family additions, house and social moves and natural disasters. The relative risk for developing emotional or conduct symptoms following an undesirable event was increased between three and six times (Goodyer *et al.* 1987). In a second related study analyses showed that recent events exert an influence independent of maternal adversity as assessed by poor confiding relations and the presence of maternal distress (Goodyer *et al.* 1988). However, other studies have suggested that life events contribute relatively modestly to explanatory models in the comparison with parental psychopathology (Berden *et al.* 1990, Jensen *et al.* 1990). In the Dutch study (Berden *et al.* 1990) which examined children aged 4–16 years over a 2-year period, the pre-event level of emotional and behavioural problems in the children was controlled for. Life event occurrences increased significantly with increasing age and were slightly, but significantly, more common amongst those of low socioeconomic status. Overall there was a significant relationship between the total score of negative life events in the 2-year period and changes in the level of emotional and behavioural problems in the children, but it was the preceding level of behavioural and emotional function that was most influential.

Although stressful events may precipitate child psychiatric disorder, certain repeated events, for at least some individuals, may have a steeling and strengthening affect. Indeed it is apparent that satisfactory development involves the successful response to challenges (Rutter 1981a).

It has already been indicated that various characteristics of the children themselves may influence the impact of events, for example, age or stage of development (Garmezy 1986). The sex of the child is also important so that in childhood males are more vulnerable than females to a wide variety of biological and psychosocial stress (Rutter 1985b, Werner 1985). Genetic factors and temperament may influence the extent or duration of the response to stressful events. A child's temperament is not just a matter of genetic constitution, and is influenced by parental perception and response (Dunn 1986). Temperament may influence not only the child's direct response but also the response to the parents' response to an event and the parents' response to them. This can be seen when an older child experiences the birth of a sibling (Dunn 1988). Intelligence is in general a protective factor but it is uncertain how it operates (Garmezy 1985, Werner 1985). It may be that a child of higher intelligence has more frequent experience of coping which contributes to self-esteem. The manner in which experiences are appraised may also be influenced by intelligence (Garmezy 1986).

The importance of the psychosocial context within which a child experiences stressful events emphasizes the interrelationship between events and chronic difficulties. First the presence of close supportive personal relationships is a protective factor for both discrete undesirable experiences and persistent adversities (Werner 1985, Cowen *et al.* 1990a,b). Commonly their absence constitutes a vulnerability factor. The morale of the group within which the child is or is living at the time of an event is also influential in determining outcome, whether in a positive or negative direction (Garmezy & Rutter 1985). This group might be a school class, a peer group or other family members. However, it is not just a question of morale in the sense of the extent to which members of the group are mutually supportive or take an optimistic attitude, but how individuals in the group react to the event themselves and to others' reactions to the events. For example, a mirror fell on a two-year-old child in a shop. The parents' anger with the shopkeeper and with delays in hospital and their blaming of each other constituted a crucial aspect of the context of the event. Indeed it could be argued that the whole character of the event was changed by virtue of the parental responses. Psychosocial context also includes the response of those with whom an individual child is in contact but who have not themselves been exposed to the event. Peers and other family members may respond to an exposed person by virtue of their knowledge that that person has had such an experience and/or as a reaction to the behaviour induced in the individual by the event. Such responses can sometimes set in chain a process which takes on its own momentum; in other words a circular process that sustains the disorder.

The manner in which children cope with adverse experiences has been much less studied than how disorders develop as a consequence, although stage of development, intelligence and/or attainment, temperament and the presence or absence of supportive relationships have all been found to be influential (Garmezy 1986, Patterson *et al.* 1989, Cowen *et al.* 1990a,b, Jenkins & Smith 1990). In broad terms coping may involve management of the environment or intrapsychic processes. More specifically there may be direct action to change threatening conditions, altered appraisal of experiences or regulation of the emotional response (Rutter 1981a). Children develop the ability to modulate their emotional response by the second year of life (Malatesta *et al.* 1989), although the ability to exhibit outwardly feelings that are contrary to those that are being experienced is probably not developed until five or six years of age (Malatesta *et al.* 1989). Cicchetti & Schneider-Rosen (1986) have reviewed the complex connections between competence, cognition and emotions during early development. Children are less able to take direct action on their environment and although less able to modulate their emotional response tend to have less persistent emotional responses to stressful events than adolescents and adults (Garmezy & Rutter 1985, Cicchetti & Schneider-Rosen 1986, Rutter 1986). Furthermore they may not appraise the full negative significance of adverse experiences, but they may view them in a fashion which is different from adults, so that the preschool child may already conclude that the absence of a parent constitutes abandonment. Somewhat older children may perceive parental rows as being their responsibility (Hetherington 1983, Wallerstein 1983). These considerations re-emphasize the importance of supportive relationships for children and there is now important evidence that they have a protective effect when a child is living with parents who have a disharmonious marriage (Jenkins & Smith 1990). Thus it is clear that life events and chronic adversity do affect children, the context being as important as reported among adults.

### Separation from parents

ATTACHMENT THEORY

Attachment theory (Bowlby 1982) has been very influential in an attempt to understand social and emotional development, including the significance for children of separation from parents. It has also stimulated a considerable quantity of research (Wolkind & Rutter 1985a, Hinde & Stevenson-Hinde 1988, Speltz *et al.* 1990). Essentially parents and younger children are thought to be genetically primed to respond to each other in ways that ensure the survival of defenceless young. In the latter part of the first year of life when children become mobile they display attachment behaviours that promote proximity to their care-giver, either by moving towards them themselves or by enlisting reponses in the care-giver that bring about proximity. The attachment behavioural system (Hinde 1982) which is thought to underlie this pattern of behaviours is seen to be 'turned on' in the presence of external threat. The manner in which parents and child respond to each other in these and other circumstances are seen to contribute to the formation of an attachment relationship. The 'biological' purpose of such earlier attachment relationships is to develop emotional security and social autonomy (Bowlby 1982). For a given child attachment relationships vary so that the quality of attachment to one parent is not necessarily the same as that with another (Lamb 1978, Main & Weston 1981). The influence of the relationships that develop is thought to extend beyond the infancy period. Modes of relating are thought to have 'continuity and coherence' (Sroufe & Fleeson 1988) through the development of 'working models' of relationships. These models have both cognitive and affective components and include an individual's expectations regarding intimacy and care from others (Belsky & Pensky 1988, Sroufe & Fleeson 1988, Speltz *et al.* 1990). Thus it is hypothesized that early interaction experiences guide 'interpersonal behaviour and the interpretation of social experience' through the development of working models — 'affectively-laden mental representations of relationships'. Although the models are conceived as relatively stable, they are modifiable (Belsky & Pensky 1988). However, it should be emphasized that the aspect of relationships encompassed by attachment concepts is only one facet of interpersonal relationships (Emde 1988).

There is now good evidence that assessments of the quality of attachment relationships with care-givers, usually mother's, around 12–24 months of age can predict the future social competence of the child, their approach to problem solving, and the affective quality of their interaction with others (Sroufe & Fleeson 1988, Speltz *et al.* 1990). Indeed they have been found to predict whether or not psychological disorders occur in boys up to five years later (Lewis *et al.* 1984, Grossmann 1988). The quality of attachment relationship has been classified in various ways: initially by children's responses to reunion with care-takers in the Ainsworth Strange Situation at one to two years of age (Ainsworth *et al.* 1978). However, instruments have now been constructed to make assessments of parent–child attachment later in childhood (Speltz *et al.* 1990) and retrospectively in adulthood (Grossmann *et al.* 1988, Dozier 1990).

## ATTACHMENT RELATIONSHIPS

The broad distinction is between a secure and an insecure attachment relationship. Insecure attachment is now subclassified into avoidant, ambivalent/resistant, controlling and disorganized-disoriented types (Speltz *et al.* 1990). A secure attachment relationship between mother and child is influenced by maternal responsiveness to the child during the first year of life (Crockenburg 1981, Ainsworth 1982, Sroufe 1985), and whether or not the mother is subject to environmental stress (Thompson *et al.* 1982) or depressed (Murray 1990) and by the quality of her marriage (Howes & Markman 1989). In general children with secure early attachment classification with respect to a care-giver have favourable social and emotional outcomes; insecure unfavourable (Grossmann 1988).

The proposal that the quality of early attachment relationships influences the development of working models of relationships which in turn affect the manner in which individuals interact with others at a later stage has already received support (Sroufe & Fleeson 1988). For example, there is evidence that children classified as having insecure attachment with their mothers at 18 months, some 2 or 3 years later respond differently to peers, and teachers respond differently to them (Sroufe & Fleeson 1988). However, the manner in which the children behave depends crucially on who it is they are interacting with. Thus the child who has been classified as having an earlier insecure attachment may interact harmoniously with another child classified as having an earlier secure attachment, though not with another child who has been insecurely attached. In this latter case the pattern exhibited is one of victimization, where one child system-

atically exploits, demeans or otherwise mistreats their partner (Troy & Sroufe 1987).

It must be re-emphasized that the attachment relationship only constitutes one aspect of parent–child relationships or indeed other relationships, and that there are many other aspects that are crucial for satisfactory child rearing, as for example the promotion of learning and self-control (Emde 1988). It should also be emphasized that it is not a question of presence or absence of attachment relationships or 'working models', but their quality. Attachment behaviours are exhibited by young children who are rejected or abused by their parents and by those who lack opportunities for developing persistent selective attachments. The extent and fashion in which they are shown will vary with stage of development, and the range and quality may not be adequately captured by the Ainsworth Strange Situation (Rutter 1988, Belsky & Pensky 1988, Sroufe & Fleeson 1988). It must also be recognized that separation from parents commonly involves far more than just separation. Thus there may be a difference in the quality of care during separation, or if the child is admitted to hospital they may be subjected to medical procedures (Wolkind & Rutter 1985a, Saylor *et al.* 1987).

## SEPARATION

The link between attachment theory and childhood experience of separation from care-givers is in the proposal that future quality of relationships is particularly vulnerable to disruption of early selective attachment. Between the ages of approximately six months and four years children show characteristic responses to brief separation from their parents, involving periods of up to one or two weeks (Bowlby 1973). For example, a typical pattern shown when young children enter hospital starts with 'protest', leads to 'despair' and then 'detachment' when the child appears less upset by a parental visit. On a reunion or return home the child may initially ignore or avoid the parents, become clingy or show anger towards them. These patterns are usually at a maximum when the child is about two years of age, but are least if the child stays in a familiar environment with familiar people. However, it seems that for weeks or even months after such an experience the child may resist being parted from the parent from whom they were separated. The parent–child relationships are more composite than a simple attachment relationship and it is the quality of the latter that determines the future interactions and feelings of being 'secure'.

## HOSPITALIZATION

Hospital admission is common as a cause of parent–child separation during early childhood so that a third of children admitted in the UK are admitted at least once, and 1 in 20 will have multiple admissions (Douglas 1975, Quinton & Rutter 1976). Preparing children for admission has been shown to reduce parental anxiety and, perhaps in consequence, children's distress (Wolfer & Visintainer 1975, Ferguson 1979). The way in which the child is handled in hospital is also important (Wolff 1973, Rutter 1979, Wolkind et al. 1982). Distress can be reduced by daily visits from parents (Illingworth & Holt 1935) and even more so if parents are admitted with their children. However, if parents are themselves very anxious during visits this may be unhelpful. The importance of parental anxieties is exemplified by the study which indicated that children admitted without their parents were more likely to be distressed if their parents considered that it was very important that they should be admitted with their children (Brain & MacKay 1968).

As an example of brief separation from parents, hospitalization emphasizes the need to take into account circumstances and relationships preceding a separation, the quality of experience during the separation, and circumstances and relationships following reunion in order to understand the connection between separation and the development of child psychiatric disorder (Wolkind & Rutter 1985a). The characteristics of the child will again be influential, so that, for example, Schaffer (1965) showed that children with an outgoing temperament continued to show developmental progress while they were in hospital in contrast to those who tended to withdraw into themselves. The child's own previous experience may help if they have had previous brief happy separations (Stacey et al. 1970) but previous unpleasant experiences may have the reverse effect. Repeated hospitalizations in the preschool period have been shown to be associated with an increased risk for later conduct disorder or delinquency (Douglas 1975, Quinton & Rutter 1976), and are also associated with other indices of adversity in children's circumstances. When these are taken into account an increased risk remains, which is more marked in discordant or disadvantaged families. Wolkind & Rutter (1985a) argue that this suggests that repeated hospitalization is not the direct cause of the higher rates of disorder.

For school-age children it seems that, if the effects of chronic illness are excluded, long-term consequences of hospitalization are infrequent (Werry 1979), and that short-term distress is related to premorbid psychological adjustment, and the number of physical stresses during admission (Saylor et al. 1987).

## BEREAVEMENT

An increased rate of psychological disturbance in children following the death of one parent has been found (Kanzler et al. 1990), symptoms being twice as common as in a control group a month after the event (Van Eerdewegh et al. 1982). Disturbance occurred in three-quarters of the children and ranged from depression to poor school performance and bed wetting. However, a severe depressive reaction of adult type was very uncommon. It appears that symptoms were unlikely to persist beyond a year unless there were other maintaining factors (Van Eerdewegh et al. 1982, Black & Urbanowitz 1987). Whether or not symptoms persisted is mediated by parental responses (Goodyer 1990a, Kanzler et al. 1990). Thus in the study by Black & Urbanowitz (1987) children over five that talked about the dead parent in the month following bereavement were less likely to have parents who were severely depressed or grieving and more likely to have a good psychological outcome a year later.

Grief reactions in young children tend to be milder and shorter than in adolescence (Rutter

1986). In general the likelihood that a child will develop psychiatric disorder is less following bereavement than it is following divorce. Longer-term outcome studies looking at the incidence of depression in women following the loss of a parent in childhood indicate that the loss of a mother is more significant than the loss of a father, that the age at which loss occurs may be important so that the maximum long-term effect is greater for those in middle childhood (age five to ten years), but that the long-term effects are substantially mediated by the quality and care that the child experiences following the loss (Brown *et al.* 1986, Garmezy 1986).

These long-term effects are more evident among working class families. If, as Brown *et al.* (1986) suggest, it is parental indifference and lack of control that mediate between childhood bereavement and adult disorder, then disorder during childhood is to be expected. Put together with the evidence for an impact on children during childhood they point to an increased risk for child psychiatric disorder amongst children who have been bereaved that is predominantly mediated by the emotional and physical circumstances antecedent and consequent on the loss of the parent (Rutter 1986). Pre-existing disorder is likely to be sustained.

LOSS OF A PARENT THROUGH DIVORCE

Parental divorce or separation is now the commonest reason why children are separated from a parent in childhood and some 30–40% of marriages in the UK end in divorce: in the USA the percentage is even higher (Block *et al.* 1988, Richards 1988). Although it may occur at a particular time from the point of view of the child's experience, divorce is not a time-limited event. It is often preceded by a long period of marital discord and unsupportive parenting of the children (Block *et al.* 1988), and may be followed by changes that have an additional significant impact on the quality of care experienced by the child. For example, there may be a marked reduction in financial resources, the remaining parent may be depressed, and there may be continuing tension over access between the separated parent and

the child (Wolkind & Rutter 1985a). Parental remarriage has further consequences for the home environment (Hetherington 1983).

A number of factors which increase the probability of divorce may also influence quality of care, and thus the likelihood that a child will develop psychiatric disorder even before the parents separate. These factors include young age of parental marriage, prenuptual conception, closely spaced conceptions after marriage and four or more children (Richards 1988). The importance of the finding that the quality of family relationships before the divorce is often unsatisfactory (Block *et al.* 1988) is that children exposed to persistent marital disharmony have an increased risk of disorder, especially if there is marital violence (Wallerstein 1983, Wolkind & Rutter 1985a, Johnston *et al.* 1987, Jenkins & Smith 1990). In the same prospective study Block and his co-workers showed that long before divorce occurred sons tended to be impulsive and undercontrolled compared with boys in families that remained intact (Block *et al.* 1986), emphasizing the significance of conditions antecedent to the divorce.

Within the family a good relationship between children and parents may be an asset, and the quality of relationships with siblings and grandparents may have a protective effect with regard to pre-existing and subsequent marital disharmony (Jenkins & Smith 1990).

Following divorce, disturbance in the children is particularly evident in the first two years (Wallerstein & Kelly 1980, Hetherington 1983). Although these problems may have their roots in the predivorce patterns (Block *et al.* 1988), following the marital break-up they may be compounded by alterations in the mental state of the custodial parent, depression and emotional lability being particularly common (Hetherington 1983). Outcomes with regard to child psychiatric disorder are significantly influenced by whether parents have been able to negotiate successfully about the care of the children before the divorce (Block *et al.* 1981, Johnston *et al.* 1987), when and whether remarriage of the custodial parent occurs, and the quality of the remarriage and style of parenting (Hetherington 1988).

The prospective study by Hetherington and her co-workers is illuminating for understanding outcomes for young children who were on average four years old at the outset of the study, but it should be noted that the families were middle class (Hetherington 1983, Hetherington *et al.* 1982, 1985). The study showed that following the parental separation a typical pattern amongst the young children was for there to be an increased rate of non-compliance with anxiously dependent demanding behaviour towards the custodial parent, the mother in this study. This pattern was much more common in boys and was likely to provoke an aversive response generating a potentially enduring coercive cycle. Non-compliance might also be manifested in the school environment, where a decline in school performance has been reported in children in the first two years after divorce (Wallerstein & Kelly 1980, Hetherington *et al.* 1982).

Pre-adolescent girls in the custody of their mothers showed no more problems than daughters in non-divorced families. If matters were handled satisfactorily by both home and school there was a decline in disturbance in children by two years following divorce. Where there was a less satisfactory outcome child coercion and ineffective parental control with poor supervision persisted. Remarriage was more likely to improve the position for boys than girls. An authoritative parenting style was associated with better outcomes, but if employed by step-parents worked better if it was gradually phased in. In the initial phase children's responses varied according to age, so that preschool children in addition to being clingy, felt responsible for the divorce and were irritable, tearful and aggressive. Children aged seven or eight were likely to be more pre-occupied with the father's departure and experience it as rejection. This group sometimes sought a replacement for their father through their mother's remarriage, but conflicts of loyality were more marked amongst those aged 9–12 years old who tended to take sides in the parental conflict and extend it into any attempted parental remarriage. Hetherington reports that remarriage when children were in the age range 9–14 was particularly difficult and carried an especially

poor prognosis for the adjustment of the child. As adolescence approached disturbance was more likely to be displayed in girls and this related either to the social precocity which girls in single-parent families manifested or to the conflicts that arose between girls and stepfathers, particularly if they joined the family when the daughter was at this stage of development.

In summary, conduct disorders in boys commonly emerge in the early phases following divorce and are likely to be sustained if they have been pre-existent, if there is a continuing interparental conflict and if the custodial parent's style of child rearing is not authoritative. Initial disturbance in girls is more likely to settle but problems may emerge later as they enter adolescence. Although parental remarriage may improve the mental state of the parent, this does not necessarily lead to an improvement in family relationships. It should however be emphasized that although many children may still feel distressed that their parents have separated at least 10 years after the divorce (Wallerstein 1984), emotional and behavioural disturbance is not shown by many, if not most, children (Wallerstein 1983, Amato & Edgar 1987).

### BIRTH OF A SIBLING

A series of studies have mapped the reactions of earlier-born young children to the birth of siblings (Dunn 1988). Although these studies do not indicate whether or not there were persistent psychiatric disorders in the earlier-born children, the research exemplifies ways in which relationships between mothers and children can be perturbed by events in such a way that longer-term disturbance might arise should other events impinge on the child or a negative cycle of interactions between parent and child persist. Most first-born children showed signs of disturbance alongside marked changes in their mothers. In the series of studies there was a decrease in maternal attention and play with the older child and an increase in punitive and restrictive behaviour. Responsibility for initiating communicative contact lay more with the first-born child than with the mother. There were big variations in the behaviour of the older children, who varied from being difficult and demanding or clingy and unhappy to withdrawing. However, half the children also showed positive changes in terms of their autonomy with increased independence for feeding, dressing and toileting.

A number of not necessarily mutually exclusive patterns are described. Those first borns who initially withdrew, a year later had mutually negative and hostile interactions with their sibling. The consequence of the birth of the sibling for family relationships was also influenced by pre-existing relationships between the mother and earlier-born child, so that first borns who had experienced high levels of play and joint attention with their mothers before the birth of the sibling showed more specific hostility to the newborn 14 months later, whereas those who had confrontative relationships with their mothers were particularly friendly to those siblings. In some cases the first born's hostility to the second born was proportionate to the mother's expressed affection to the second born, in others it related to differences in the mother's behaviour to the two children. When mothers prepared the older children for the arrival of the new child and continued to discuss them as a person with needs and feelings, it promoted friendly interaction between the siblings. Dunn (1988) points to the variety of processes involved and the varying character of mother–child and intersibling relationships. A study by Kreppner (1988) looked also at changes in fathers' behaviour during the first 8 or 9 months postnatally; when mothers were focusing more on the newborn children, the fathers interacted more with the first born.

TRAUMATIC EVENTS

There is now a wide range of information relating to children's responses to acute time-limited one-off traumatic events (Garmezy & Rutter 1985, Pynoos *et al.* 1987, Martini *et al.* 1990, Parry-Jones, 1990, Yule & Williams 1990, Yule *et al.* 1990, Yule 1991). These range from floods, cyclones, earthquakes and fires to plane crashes, shipwrecks, threat of a nuclear accident, radiation exposure and kidnapping. There are a number

of conclusions that can be drawn from the various studies. First the children can develop post-traumatic stress disorder in a form that is very similar to that found in adults, encompassing symptoms of increased fearful arousal, numbing and re-experiencing. For example, after the Lockerbie disaster when a plane crashed on the town 60% of a group of clinically referred children aged 3–14 years merited a diagnosis of post-traumatic stress disorder, symptoms being most severe in the 3–4 weeks following the crash. However, 56% of the children also showed altered mood and 24% eating difficulties (Parry-Jones 1990). Brett *et al.* (1988) suggest that additional features peculiar to children include re-experiencing through play, loss of recently acquired developmental skills and separation anxiety. Parry-Jones (1990) reports all these including the loss of acquired skills in 70%, especially amongst those under ten years. However, Garmezy & Rutter (1985) question whether the children's responses to such events are markedly different from emotional disorders not precipitated by severely traumatic experiences.

In some instances disorders following traumatic events appear to be exacerbations of pre-existing emotional and behavioural disorders (Garmezy & Rutter 1985, Martini *et al.* 1990, Parry-Jones 1990). In general the behavioural disturbance seems to be less intense than might have been expected, younger children showing fewer impairing symptoms than adolescents or adults. Disturbance is also more likely to persist in older children, the persistence of disturbance commonly paralleling that found in other family members. Where parents have interpersonal or mental health problems, or are experiencing stress for other reasons, then there is likely to be more disturbance in the children and it is more likely to persist. The extent to which children are directly exposed to the events is also important, so that at Lockerbie those children nearest the site of the crashed plane were most affected (Parry-Jones 1990). Those who lose family members, relatives and friends are also more likely to develop a disorder than those who lose material possessions. Although children were not killed in the kidnapping of 26 children reported by Terr (1979,

1981a,b, 1983), this was a particularly unpleasant experience and 4–5 years after the incident many of the children were still experiencing repetitive terror dreams, although they had declined in frequency, and most of the children were functioning adequately at school. Symptom severity was greatest amongst families with more chronic or recurrent problems springing from other sources. The report from this follow-up suggested that children were less likely than adults to have amnesia for events, psychic numbing or intrusive flashbacks. However, children who have witnessed a parental suicide have been shown to reiterate the event in play and behaviour, be preoccupied, experience mental intrusion of the event, and manifest affective disturbance and aggressive behaviour (Pynoos & Eth 1985). These examples again point to the importance of preceding relationships and experiences, context of the traumatic event and the contingent and subsequent responses of other people and the family.

### Circumstances and chronic difficulties

#### FAMILY STRUCTURE

Children from large families have delayed language development and lower verbal intelligence and reading attainment, although this association is less marked in higher social classes (Clausen 1966, Rutter & Madge 1976, Richman & Stevenson 1977, Fogelman 1985, Stevenson & Fredman 1990). The family environment is probably influential (Douglas *et al.* 1968, Rutter & Mittler 1972, Puckering & Rutter 1987, Richman & Stevenson 1977, Morisset *et al.* 1990), there being less opportunity for young children to interact with parents in larger families (Rutter & Cox 1985). Lower verbal intelligence and reading attainment are associated with child psychiatric disorders, particularly conduct disorders, but the reasons for the association are not entirely clear. There are probably both common underlying factors and mutual influences (Corbett 1985, Yule & Rutter 1985). Children from large families are in fact twice as likely to develop disorders of conduct and more likely to be delinquent (Rutter & Madge 1976, Rutter & Giller 1983), but this

association is most marked for boys, and indeed families containing mostly boys (Jones *et al.* 1980). There are various suggestions about the reasons for the association. Apart from the predisposing influence of educational retardation, other mechanisms include increased level of conflict in large families, and lower levels of parental disciplinary supervision (Rutter & Cox 1985). There is also the suggestion that amongst males antisocial behaviour may be spread by contagion (Robins *et al.* 1975) or by the way boys respond to each other to encourage antisocial behaviour (Jones *et al.* 1980). Although emotional disorders on their own may be somewhat more common amongst small families, it needs to be remembered that emotional disorder often co-occurs with conduct disorder.

With regard to ordinal position there seems to be a tendency for first-born children to have higher educational attainments (Rutter & Madge 1976) and for a last-born child to be more prone to school failure (Belmont *et al.* 1976). However, eldest children are somewhat more likely to develop emotional disorders (Rutter *et al.* 1970). Two main suggestions to account for this are that parents may be more anxious and controlling with their first-born children and that eldest children experience more sharply the change in family interactions and relationships following the birth of second and subsequent children (Rutter 1981b, Dunn 1988). A recent study suggests differences in maternal warmth as well as control may be important (Dunn *et al.* 1990).

Given that approaching half the children born in the UK will experience the divorce or separation of their parents (Richards 1988), many will spend at least part of their lives being reared by a single parent. Earlier discussion about parental separation and divorce and bereavements in families emphasizes that both the mode of onset and continuance of the single-parent state can vary very considerably. Indeed it is uncommon for children to stay in single-parent households throughout their childhood (Fogelman 1985). However, although the majority of children who are born illegitimate are living in two-parent families by the age of 11 (Lambert & Streather 1980), they are also more likely to be living in poorer socioeconomic circumstances and to have experienced admission to care (Rutter & Madge 1976).

The increased rate of educational, emotional, and behavioural difficulties in children who have been raised in one-parent families (Herzog & Sudia 1973, Ferri 1976, Lambert & Streather 1980, Hetherington *et al.* 1982) appears to have a number of explanations. Children from single-parent families or from families where there is a single parent following divorce or separation are overrepresented in clinical samples, while those whose parent is single following bereavement are not (Steinhausen *et al.* 1987). However, data from the Ontario Child Health Study indicated that the small but significant increased risk for psychiatric disorder, particularly conduct disorder and poor school performance, amongst children from one-parent families was not sustained when poverty was taken into account. Poverty and family dysfunction made the strongest independent contribution to the presence of disorder. Maternal education contributed most to school performance. Younger children of single parents and those in rural areas still had some increased risk of disorder, but the reason for single-parent status was not taken into account in this analysis (Monroe Blum *et al.* 1988). In contrast a UK study found that children born to single mothers were more neurotic and antisocial with poorer vocabulary scores even when income was taken into account (Wadsworth *et al.* 1985). It should be noted that the sample of children born to single parents will be different from a cross-sectional sample of children living with a single parent.

It needs to be emphasized that the overall increased rate for child disorder in single-parent families does not mean that being reared by a single parent is necessarily disadvantageous to children. This is apparent in the Lambert & Streather (1980) study where more social maladjustment was found amongst children who were living with a step-parent at 11 years of age and this may have reflected conflict in the reconstituted family. On the other hand single parents tend to be more socially isolated and experience more stressful life events, and these and the extent of support for the mothers can influence the quality of mother–child interaction (Weinraub & Wolf 1983).

Teenage mothers are more likely to be single parents, and if they marry or co-habit that relationship is more likely to break up than for women aged 20 years or more (McCluskey *et al.* 1983). Furthermore, they are more likely to develop depression while their children are young (Cox *et al.* 1987). However, it appears that if they receive a good extended family support the outcome when their children are three and a half years old may be no worse than for other mothers and children living in a similar area (Wolkind & Kruk 1985).

Parental death or mental illness in a parent may have a greater impact on the mental health of the same sex children (Rutter 1966, Quinton & Rutter 1985a, Wolkind & Rutter 1985a), but rearing by a single-parent mother or in a lesbian household does not increase the risk for homosexuality in boys (Biller 1971, Golombok *et al.* 1983, Huston 1983). The lack of a father may in the early years be associated with boys exhibiting less masculine behaviour and girls having more difficulty interacting with males (Huston 1983), but these tendencies do not amount to psychiatric disorder.

## PARENTAL CRIMINALITY

There is abundant evidence that parental criminality is associated with disorders of conduct and delinquency in children (Rutter & Giller 1983). The strength of the association increases if both parents have a criminal record, if they are recidivist and if their crime record extends into the period of child rearing (Robins *et al.* 1975, Osborn & West 1979). The presence of delinquency in sibs further increases the risk (West & Farrington 1973, Robins *et al.* 1975). There are many reasons for the association, but factors such as low social class and poverty, and selective surveillance and prosecution of those families with a criminal record do not provide adequate explanations (West & Farrington 1973, Robins *et al.* 1975, West 1982). For example, parental criminality has been linked to an increase in child psychiatric disorder and behavioural deviance in school amongst ten year olds – before prosecutions are undertaken (Rutter *et al.* 1975).

The association may be contributed to by personality abnormalities in parents such as excessive drinking or persistent aggression, modelling of deviant behaviour and child rearing that is neglectful, lacking in supervision or includes cruelty or hostility towards the children (McCord & McCord 1959, West & Farrington 1973, Robins *et al.* 1975, Rutter 1985b), but a genetic predesposition is considered to be at least a partial explanation (Dilalla & Gottesman 1989).

## PARENTAL MENTAL DISORDER

The link between parental psychiatric disorder and child psychiatric disorder has been documented in a wide range of studies, including studies of young children (Rutter *et al.* 1975). In general the form of a parent's mental disorder does not predict the nature of the disorder that may be manifest in one of their children during childhood. Although there is increasing evidence for a genetic contribution towards a wide range of disorders that may have their onset in childhood and adolescence, including childhood autism, schizophrenia, bipolar affective disorders, anti-social disorders and criminality (Rutter *et al.* 1990a), social mechanisms and gene–environment interactions play a significant role (Rutter 1989b). The association between parent and child disorder is a strong one; for example, when a mother is depressed the rates of disorder in children vary between one-third and two-thirds in a variety of studies (Cox 1988). The associations are strongest for personality disorder in parents (Rutter 1966, Quinton & Rutter 1985a) and somewhat greater for depression than schizophrenia (Rutter & Cox 1985).

Leaving aside the genetic contribution there have been a number of attempts to try to disentangle the nature of mechanisms involved. First, it has to be re-emphasized that the impact on the child may vary according to their sex, temperament and social development (Rutter 1989b). Secondly, there is the question whether any impact of parental mental disorder is due to exposure to specific parental symptoms or alterations

in parent–child interactions or child rearing. Thirdly, it may be asked whether the link between parent and child disorder is due to changes in family structure associated with parental disorder or to other correlated factors, either concurrently or in the parents' earlier experience (Cox 1988).

With regard to exposure to symptoms it needs to be remembered that many behaviours manifest by parents when they are mentally ill, such as irritability, crying or suicide attempts, are not necessarily specific to particular disorders (Cox 1988). Indeed most studies have been concerned with examining alterations in parenting rather than children's exposure to specific symptoms such as delusions or hopelessness, although Rutter's earlier study (Rutter 1966) pointed to the importance of the extent to which children are involved in symptoms for the risk of the development of disorder. A later study of children in families where a parent had had a mental illness indicated that direct involvement in parental symptoms was uncommon and suggested that parental mental disorder could be considered as one of a number of psychosocial adversities that in combination increased the risk for disorder in the children (Quinton & Rutter 1985a). The risk was thought to stem more from psychosocial disturbance in the families rather than the illness itself. In other words the effects were more through alterations in parent–child interaction than exposure to specific symptoms. Furthermore, exposure of the children to parental hostility was considered particularly important for the generation and maintenance of disorder, especially conduct disorder. Such hostility is not specific for specific parental disorders. There was a similar finding in the Waltham Forest study that followed up three-year-old children to the age of eight (Richman *et al.* 1982). Here it was again found that persistent hostility towards children was related to the persistence of child psychiatric disorders even when mothers had ceased to have psychiatric symptoms. In a prospective study persistence of maternal depression has been linked to both onset and maintenance of children's behavioural disorders (Egeland *et al.* 1990). Quinton & Rutter (1985a) emphasized that the mediation of effects through exposure to hostility does not rule out other mechanisms which may be different for different parental disorders or different child disorders. For example, Emery *et al.* (1982) found that child conduct disorder appeared to be accounted for by marital discord when parents had depression or personality disorder but not when they had schizophrenia. There is also evidence that points to parental discord being relevant for child conduct disorder as opposed to emotional disorder (Folstein *et al.* 1983, Quinton & Rutter 1985a).

These studies did not involve observation of parent–child interaction, although even in observation studies contrasts have often been between children whose parents have a specific psychiatric disorder and those whose parents have no disorder, as opposed to a comparison between different types of parental disorder (Cox 1988). This means that it is often difficult to establish what forms of parent–child interaction may be characteristic for a particular parental mental disorder. For example, it has been shown in a number of studies that depressed mothers are more negative towards their children, have less well-tuned responsiveness, use more instructions and commands and are more indecisive in comparison with control parents (Cox 1988). Apart from increased rates of child psychiatric disorder their offspring may show delays in development, particularly in the area of language, have temperamental difficulties, be more sensitive to emotional distress in others and manifest insecure attachment behaviour towards their parents (Radke-Yarrow *et al.* 1985, Cox 1988, Puckering 1989).

The complexity of the position for maternal depression is emphasized by the recognition that depressed mothers vary considerably in, for example, whether maternal depression is related to acute stress or arises in the context of more longstanding difficulties. Furthermore, the evidence of child disorder persisting when parental symptoms have remitted, suggests that patterns of parent–child relationship have been established which are sustained beyond a period of maternal illness (Pound *et al.* 1985, Cox 1988, Murray 1988).

These observations still leave open whether the child disorder is generated by other antecedent or concurrent factors than maternal depression. For example, there may be permanent or temporary changes in the family structure associated with parental mental disorder and this is evidently an additional risk factor for child disorder in some instances. The adverse effects of marital breakdown and/or the reception of children into foster or institutional care are well established (Wolkind & Rutter 1985a, Rutter *et al.* 1990b). Also there may be many factors in the backgrounds of parents with mental disorders, or in their current circumstances that may equally well account for the alterations in parent–child interaction and the increased rates of child psychiatric disorders. Indeed, recent studies (Cox *et al.* 1987, Murray 1990) suggest that in the case of maternal depression it is only in the presence of other vulnerability factors or chronic difficulties that there is disorder in the children. Predisposing factors in mothers include poor relationships with their own parents, unsatisfactory school experience, and birth of their first child before the age of 20 (Cox *et al.* 1987, Murray 1990). The most frequent and important current adversity is discordant relationships between parents, which occurs frequently with other parental mental disorders also, and is itself a major risk factor for child psychiatric disorder in children (Cox *et al.* 1987, Rutter 1989b, Murray 1990). It is interesting that there is increasing evidence for cross-generational continuities in poor quality parenting mediated by effects on the child's (future parents) personality development (Belsky & Pensky 1988, Caspi & Elder 1988, Belsky *et al.* 1989). It is therefore possible that adverse earlier experiences predispose to depression in adult life, a poor marriage *and* difficulties in the parent–child relationship. It has also been argued that while maternal depression and marital discord commonly coexist and sustain each other, the discord promotes conduct problems in the children while maternal depression leads to child depression (Downey & Coyne 1990).

The available data suggest that maternal depression alone, particularly if it is time limited, may not significantly increase the risk of child psychiatric disorder, but when it occurs in combination with factors in the mother that predispose to difficulties in the parent–child relationship, such as their own relationships with their own parents, current stresses or difficulties, or a discordant marital relationship, then the parental mental disorder has an impact that is additional to those other adversities working alone. However, there appear to be a number of different patterns. First there is preliminary evidence that depression in mothers during the first year of life may be particularly adverse for aspects of children's development other than language (D. Hay, 1989, personal communication). Later, expressive language development may be more likely to suffer (Cox 1988, Puckering 1989), and this is itself a risk factor for the development of behavioural disorder in children. Where there is associated marital difficulty or severe environmental stress then a cycle may develop in which the parent is less responsive, but also more irritable and negative towards the child who in turn coerces the parent to achieve their own ends (Radke-Yarrow *et al.* 1988, MacKinnon *et al.* 1990). A cycle of child non-compliance and parental hostility then leads to the maintenance of an oppositional or conduct disorder in the child. However, there is evidence for other patterns which may or may not coexist. For example, the depressed parent may have more difficulty in containing emotional distress in the child (Puckering 1989), increasing the likelihood that they will develop an emotional disorder. In other circumstances children will comfort their distressed parents so there may be a more or less persistent reversal of roles (Cox 1988, Engfer 1988, D. Hay, 1989, personal communication), and it has been suggested this may predispose to depression in adult life (Pound 1982), although the consequences for disorder in childhood are unknown.

It has already been indicated that the mechanisms operating may be different for different parental mental disorders, so that if a parent has a personality disorder the major effect may be through the child's exposure to hostile/aggressive behaviour (Quinton & Rutter 1985a), but there may be additional influences through the quality of discipline and supervision, and also influences through modelling (Rutter 1985b). In schizophrenia genetic influences may be more significant

and specifically it has been suggested that the quality of marriage is not such an important mediating factor in this case (Emery *et al.* 1982). Furthermore, alteration in parenting in schizophrenia had been reported less consistently (Melhuish *et al.* 1988). It may be either that the schizophrenic parent when ill is more likely to be out of the family, and/or that there is more likely to be a protective relationship with the unaffected parent in these circumstances than is the case when one of the parents has an affective disorder. Overall it is becoming apparent that although there may be deficiencies in child rearing such as poorly tuned responsiveness, or exposure of the child to persistently negative emotions, that may occur in a wide variety of parental mental disorders, there may be some specificities. In the case of parental depression this may relate to the failure to contain the child's emotional distress as evidenced by the higher rates of emotional distress in this group in comparison with children of parents who were institutionalized as children and failure to thrive children (C. Puckering, 1989, personal communication).

## INTERPARENTAL RELATIONSHIPS

The quality of the interparental relationship emerges as one of the most important factors associated with child psychiatric disorder in a wide range of studies (Wolkind & Rutter 1985a, Jenkins *et al.* 1989), often co-occurring with other major adversities such as parental mental disorder (Quinton & Rutter 1985a), or separation of parents. It is clear that overtly and markedly disharmonious families are particularly associated with conduct disorders and delinquency in children, particularly boys (Rutter & Giller 1983). However, clinical experience suggests that less readily detectable forms of dysfunction in interparental relationships may be of importance in the development of emotional disorders in children. Thus children's difficulties in separating from parents, as in school refusal, may occur when fathers are relatively disengaged from the family (Skynner 1974). Although Rutter has emphasized that marital discord is a weak risk factor in otherwise well-functioning families, and that it is the combination of adversities that is most damaging (Rutter 1978b), the different stresses potentiating each other (Rutter 1983b), it is likely that more specific connections between varieties of interparental relationship and different forms of child psychiatric disorder will become apparent as methods of assessment and measurement become more discriminating. Thus different mechanisms may operate for those aspects of child rearing that are concerned with children's cognitive and language development, their safety and physical health, their emotional development and socialization. For example, in the field of socialization parents' preoccupation with their negative interaction with each other may lead to a lack of supervision, or the parental disagreements may extend into approaches to discipline. Furthermore, parental discord may be diverted into hostility towards a specific child, increasing the possibility that child coercion of the parent will develop. Some support for these ideas comes from a study in families where a child had conduct problems and the parents had discordant marriages. These families were compared with controls. The children were aged between 5 and 13 years (Christensen & Margolin 1988). The parent's marital relationships were found to be weaker (more mutually negative) than other dyadic relationships in the family. The involvement of each parent with the target (symptomatic) child differed, so that fathers tended to be neutral, mothers involved in negative interaction with them. Parents' interaction with non-target children was more balanced. Conflict in the marital dyad tended to spread into other family interactions – containment of conflict being more effective in the control families.

In contrast, there may be circumstances where a poor marital relationship is associated with one parent becoming overinvolved with the child such that they share the parent's distress. One study of the development of parent–child relationships from birth (Engfer 1988) found some support for the compensatory hypothesis that mother–child relationships may sometimes 'make up' for deficits experienced in the marital relationship. There was even stronger evidence for a common factor in the mother's personality predicting quality of relationship with child and partner at three to four months after delivery.

A strong relationship between maternal responsivity or sensitivity and marital quality has been found in other studies (Cox *et al.* 1987, 1989). Although common factors in the mother's background are likely to be important in the explanations of this association, there are almost certainly effects of the marriage on the parent–child relationship as evidenced by the link between quality of marriage and parenting amongst mothers who have experienced institutional care in childhood (Quinton & Rutter 1985b). How good marital relationships can improve parent–child relationships is not clear, although Rutter (1988) points to anxiety reduction and reduced task demands, while acknowledging that the absence of discord is also significant.

A further issue concerns how children cope with parental quarrels. It has been found that psychological disturbance in children is associated with the frequency and severity of parents' quarrels; that children's level of intervention in those quarrels is related to the frequency and severity of quarrels and indeed that most children intervene to stop parents quarrelling and comfort them afterwards. Furthermore, there is a tendency for children's symptoms to be associated with the extent to which they intervene in the quarrels (Jenkins *et al.* 1989). The same study provides interesting evidence about factors protecting children living in disharmonious homes (Jenkins *et al.* 1989, Jenkins & Smith 1990). The authors distinguish protective factors that benefit children in the context of parental discord and those factors (sometimes called assets) that benefit children living with both good and bad parental marriages. Protective factors were a good relationship with someone outside the family, commonly a grandparent, a good sibling relationship and involvement in an activity for which the children received much positive recognition. Good parent–child relationships were assets.

The interparental relationships thus affect the child directly and indirectly. Modelling, altered atmosphere, arguments or support all produce some degree of effect on the child.

CHILD REARING

Child rearing or parenting is intimately related to its social context. First because the quality of parent or care-giver–child relationship influences the style of child rearing and its effectiveness, and secondly because parenting occurs in the context of a family system which is influenced by both internal and external forces (Quinton & Rutter 1985b, Hinde & Stevenson-Hinde 1988).

Much research and thinking has been concerned with parental discipline and one of the most influential formulations has been that of Maccoby & Martin (1983), characterizing it along two main dimensions of demanding/controlling–undemanding/low control and accepting/responsive–rejecting/unresponsive. It will be observed that the first dimension is concerned with control, the second with the quality of parent–child relationships. Authoritarian parenting is associated with firm limits but a lack of parental responsiveness and negotiation with their children, and there is evidence that this may lead to unhappy, socially withdrawn children who lack confidence (Baumrind 1967, Coopersmith 1967, Loeb *et al.* 1980). An indulgent, permissive approach with a lack of control but responsiveness to the child is associated with poor impulse control, increased aggression at home and a lack of self-reliance (Yarrow *et al.* 1968, Baumrind 1971, Olweus 1980a,b). Indifferent, uninvolved, neglecting parenting, that is both low on responsiveness and control, leads to low self-esteem in the child and an increased risk of involvement in antisocial and aggressive activities (Egeland & Sroufe 1981, Patterson 1982). The authoritative–reciprocal pattern which combines firm rules with child-centred responsiveness and negotiation has already been referred to as a style that is protective in the context of parental divorce and remarriage (Hetherington 1983), and there is other evidence that this is the approach that promotes mental health and protects against the development of child psychiatric disorder (Coopersmith 1967, Baumrind 1971, Comstock 1973).

In the consideration of parental discipline and control this two-dimensional formulation requires elaboration. Problems of discipline and control have been found to derive from interactions outside specific disciplinary confrontations (Quinton & Rutter 1985b). For example, the failure to prepare a child for care-giving may lead to a parent–child confrontation. This is not just a question of responsiveness but child-centredness. There is also the need to discriminate lack of control stemming from neglect and that deriving from ineffective attempts at control. Patterson & Dishion (1988) report the strong link between parents' irritable/explosive discipline and their children's antisocial behaviour. Related to this is the notion of inconsistent, unpredictable discipline that reflects parental moods or concerns rather than child behaviour (Caspi & Elder 1988). These features of parent–child interaction have been repeatedly documented as linked to aggressive antisocial child behaviour, but not all children who experience conflictful parent–child relationships develop behavioural problems. It is argued that it is necessary to take into account parent and child emotions and cognitions, as for example the extent to which the adult attributes control and power to the child who is perceived to misbehave intentionally (MacKinnon *et al.* 1990). These misperceptions are thought to be common in maltreating parents (Belsky 1980), who have also been found to be more negative, intrusive and controlling, and less responsive (Vondra *et al.* 1989). Maltreated children are at risk not only for behavioural disturbance but also delays in cognitive functioning and academic performance (Hill *et al.* 1989, Vondra *et al.* 1989).

However, the effects of discipline on socialization omit the consideration of other major aspects of child rearing, for example research on children's cognitive and language development indicates that the quality of parent's stimulation of their child is influential (Bradley & Caldwell 1976, Cantwell & Baker 1985, Melhuish *et al.* 1990b, Morisset *et al.* 1990). Relative delay in both general cognitive and language development are risk factors for child psychiatric disorder (Yule & Rutter 1985, Corbett 1985). Studies, already referred to, influenced by attachment theory that have used the Ainsworth Strange Situation assessment of attachment when the child is between one and two years of age, support the hypothesis that if a child is able to establish a secure emotional base with a parent they are protected against the onset of child psychiatric disorder and likely to be more confidently independent later in childhood (Lamb 1982, Ainsworth 1982, Grossmann 1988). Studies of adult psychiatric disorder suggest that the broader range of emotional disorders excluding manic-depressive psychoses and schizophrenia may be predisposed to by child rearing characterized by parental constraint, high anxiety and more particularly low affection (Parker 1983). Concurrent studies of young children (Baumrind 1967) also support the view that parents who are controlling with high expectations, but also warm and supportive, can be contrasted with those that are controlling but anxious and emotionally unsupportive. This latter pattern, which has been implicated in emotional disorders in childhood including school refusal (Hersov 1985b,c), can be characterized as overprotective and was examined in detail in a classical study by Levy (1943). This pointed the way in which a wide range of factors underlie the evolution of this pattern including the long-awaited child whose existence has been threatened by severe or repeated illness, born to mothers who lack the experience of warmth in their own childhood and whose marital partners are relatively emotionally uninvolved. There is some *empirical* support from a prospective study (Engfer 1988) for the postnatal development of a pattern of maternal anxious involvement with poor sensitivity alongside marital distress. When the children were 18 months old maternal overprotection was predicted by marital distress assessed 14 months earlier.

Although uninvolved fathers have been described in both emotional and conduct disorders, it will be seen that different outcomes may relate to both genetic and temperamental factors in the child, their sex, the presence or absence of developmental and physical disorders, whether paternal lack of involvement is associated with a discordant marriage, whether the mother's child rearing involves an authoritative approach to discipline and does or does not include satisfactory emotional support of the child.

Protective factors have been detected in a prospective study of a high-risk sample of children followed from birth to the age of eight (Egeland *et al.* 1990). Homes characterized by good levels of stimulation, predictability and organization were those in which children did not develop behavioural disorders. Furthermore, children who were anxiously attached to their mothers at 18 months and/or had preschool behaviour problems at $4\frac{1}{2}-5$ years, did not develop disorders or had lost them by 8 years if their family showed the protective factors.

In general it should be noted that the link between parenting and childhood externalizing disorders is better established than for internalizing disorders. This is exemplified by another study which originally assessed children aged three, then at school entry and at age nine. Leaving aside child factors, negative maternal control related to the persistence of conduct and oppositional disorders but not internalizing disorders. These latter disorders were associated with both prior and concurrent family stress (Campbell & Ewing 1990). This points to aetiological factors for internalizing disorders in the child, or factors in parenting which do not take the form of negative control but are influenced by stress in some other way.

There is now an increasing body of research linking parents' childhood experiences to the quality of their child rearing (Belsky 1984, Belsky & Pensky 1988, Caspi & Elder 1988, Belsky *et al.* 1989, Patterson & Dishion 1988). The medium of transmission is thought to be via the personality development of the parents, expecially the mothers (Caspi & Elder 1988). The parents 'working-models' of relationships are one concept employed (Belsky *et al.* 1989). Rutter (1989a) has outlined some of the continuities and discontinuities relevant to transmission of deviant parenting from one generation to the next. An important source of discontinuity is the quality of marital relationship established by an individual with adverse childhood experiences. Such adverse experiences increase the likelihood of making a poor marriage with consequent unsatisfactory parenting; but if a good marriage occurs it increases the chances of satisfactory parenting (Rutter 1988).

ADOPTION, FOSTERING AND DAY AND INSTITUTIONAL CARE

The increase in maternal employment has led to changing patterns in preschool day care which may nevertheless vary widely from child minding in a child's home to placement in a day nursery. While the overall quality of care was seen as important, an earlier review suggested that there was little evidence that the different modes of day care predisposed to the development of child psychiatric disorder, although it was suggested that independence and social assertiveness might develop earlier (Rutter 1981c). More recent research emphasizes the wide variations in interaction experience of children in different types of day care and also within each type (Melhuish *et al.* 1990a). The differences reflected in part variations in physical accommodation, group size and adult–child ratio. Cognitive development at 18 months of age was not influenced by the type of day care but children from socially advantaged homes did less well in language development than those cared for at home. It is not known whether this effect is of sufficient magnitude to constitute a risk factor for psychiatric disorder (Melhuish *et al.* 1990b).

Since Bowlby's studies 50 years ago (Bowlby 1946, 1951), there has been concern about the effects of institutional rearing on young children's later development (Rutter 1981b). More recent studies (Wolkind 1974, Roy 1983, Wolkind & Renton 1979, Hodges & Tizard 1989a,b) have confirmed the very high rates of disorder amongst children who have experienced institutional care. The quality of such care has undoubtedly improved in many instances so that earlier studies compounded institutional and poor quality care. Nevertheless, in a more recent study (Hodges & Tizard 1989a,b) it is evident that the children who spent at least the first two years of their lives in residential care were subject to multiple caretaking. In this study comparison was possible between those children who had experienced early institutional care and were later adopted and those returned to their own family. A few children remained in institutional care for much longer periods. Children adopted before four and a half years of age had much better outcomes for intellectual development than those restored to their families or adopted at a later age. At age eight both the adopted and restored children were showing higher rates of child psychiatric disorder than control children. Longer follow-up at age 16 found greater overall levels of disturbance amongst children restored to what were less than satisfactory families than those in which the adopted children were placed. Adopted children had higher levels of disturbance than controls but lower than the restored children, and it was less likely that their own disturbance took the form of conduct disorder. More importantly it appeared that there were characteristic differences in both the adopted and restored group of children in their capacity for peer relationships. A lack of confiding and close relationships with peers, while not constituting psychiatric disorder, is nevertheless a risk factor for disorder. Although Hodges & Tizard describe good quality relationships with parents amongst the adoptees at 16 years of age, it can be speculated that these may be perceived as inappropriately dependent and superficial at a later stage of development.

When the results of this study are combined with others it seems that if there has not been an opportunity for early secure, stable and specific attachments then later characteristic abnormalities in social development are apparent, including the failure to develop confiding, reciprocal relationships with peers. In Wolkind's study (1974) a pattern of superficial over-friendliness was largely confined to those admitted to the institution before the age of two, while antisocial behaviour was common amongst all the children regardless of their age of admission. Girls raised in foster-care or children's homes are more likely to become pregnant while in their teens and unmarried (Wolkind & Kruk 1985).

It will be seen that in many circumstances it is difficult to disentangle influences on the child prior to the admission to care, whether foster care or institution, and those deriving from their experience of care. Many studies have shown that children in foster care have an increased rate of emotional and behavioural difficulties and low levels of scholastic attainment (Wolkind & Rutter 1973, Rowe *et al.* 1984). Many children end up in foster care following family adversity and it is clear that much of the disturbance is the consequence of earlier family difficulties experienced before the placement (Hersov 1985a).

Behavioural and emotional disturbance are particularly common at the time of placement. Rushton *et al.* (1988) have mapped the pattern of disturbance over the first year after placement in 18 boys fostered following abuse and neglect. Disobedience, eating problems, poor concentration and bed wetting were very common at the outset but declined over the year. Emotional distress was of most concern after six months, while encopresis, difficulty making friends and a lack of expressed affection to the foster-mother persisted in a small proportion throughout the year. This catalogue of problems highlights the ease with which persistent disorder can be established if the child's behaviour generates inappropriate responses in the foster-parent. Thus it is easy to understand the high rate of fostering breakdown (Hersov 1985a).

## THE INFLUENCE OF SIBS AND PEERS

The significance and manner of influence of sibling and peer relationships on the initiation and maintenance of child psychological and psychiatric disorders have been relatively neglected. This is despite the fact that poor peer relationships are particularly highly correlated with significant child psychiatric disorder (Rutter *et al.* 1970, Hartup 1983, Kolko 1989). The quality of such relationships is also highly predictive of future or persistent disorder (Roff *et al.* 1972, Cowen *et al.* 1973), so that unpopularity at the age of seven predicts delinquency in the teenage years. Poor relationships with both peers and siblings predicted the persistence of disorders in children age ten followed up four years later (Cox 1976).

It is apparent that peer influences can work not only through modelling (Rutter 1985b), but the more direct effects of unpopularity, teasing and

bullying (Olweus 1980b, Patterson *et al.* 1989). Peer-rejected children tend to show more behaviour problems, including aggression and disruption. These disturbances have been shown to be less in six year olds if the children's mothers are warm and accepting of them (Patterson *et al.* 1989). Indeed the ability to make friends may follow from affectionate family relationships (Petit *et al.* 1988). Friendship difficulties occur more often in the year before the onset of emotional disorders than in controls (Goodyer *et al.* 1989), while children with disorders of conduct tend to lack the social skills that would make peer relationships more satisfactory (Kolko 1989).

The influence of sibling relationships will depend on the whole pattern of family relationships. The way in which the arrival of a second child can alter relationships between the mother and two children on the basis of existing relationships has already been discussed (Dunn 1988). A description has also been made of the manner in which there is modification of all the dyadic interactions involving both parents and both children (Kreppner 1988). The studies of the mother and two children suggest ways in which negative and conflictual patterns of interaction can develop which predispose to the development of child psychiatric disorder. A study of distressed families in which there was marital discord and child-conduct problems (Christensen & Margolin 1988) shows how conflict between siblings can spread to marital and parent–child conflict and vice versa. It was relatively uncontained spread of conflict that characterized the distressed rather than control families. This indicates ways in which child disorders can be predisposed to and sustained by intersibling conflict. Within the family, differences can be developed and accentuated in a fashion that may be particularly relevant for emotional disorders (Rutter 1985b).

## FAMILY RELATIONSHIPS

There have been very significant developments in the understanding of family systems and the network of family relationships (Gorell Barnes 1985, Hinde & Stevenson-Hinde 1988). Some progress has been made in attempts to characterize these relationships in a form that can be satisfactorily measured (Hinde & Stevenson-Hinde 1988). The work on the impact of high expressed emotion and communication deviance in families that has been done with adults in relationship to schizophrenia and major affective disorder has been replicated in adolescence (Asarnow *et al.* 1988), and there is a considerable body of research supporting the importance of the exposure of children to parental hostility in the maintenance of conduct disorders (Rutter 1985b, Quinton & Rutter 1985a). Rutter (1985b) argues that both weak family relationships and those characterized by discord contribute to disorders of conduct.

A wide variety of different patterns of family dysfunction are clinically described. Certain instruments have been developed to measure them. They include the Beavers–Timberlawn Family Ratings Scales (Beavers 1982), the Family Adaptation and Cohesion Scales (FACES; Olson 1986), and the card-sorting technique of David Reiss (Oliveri & Reiss 1982). The patterns include: disturbance in family communications, such as family members being unable to take turns or share a focus of attention; alterations in family structure, particularly the inadequate establishment of intergenerational boundaries; the reduced capacity to negotiate changes in the family lifecycle, for example when children enter school; the pervasive influence of certain family beliefs affecting the perceived meaning of others' actions and experiences; and impaired capacities of the family to problem solve (Gorell Barnes 1985, Minuchin 1988).

### Circumstances

#### SCHOOLING

It had previously been thought that school influences on the development of child psychiatric disorders were relatively minimal in comparison with those emanating from the family, but several studies (Wolkind & Rutter 1985b, Maughan 1988) have demonstrated systematic links between aspects of schools as social organizations and children's behaviour and attainments.

Wolkind & Rutter (1985b) identified three major aspects of schools: the composition of the student body, the qualities of the school as a social organization and the efficiency of classroom management techniques.

It seems that children's behaviour and attainments are worse if many children in the school have poor behaviour and attainment. Favourable school qualities are: high expectations for work and behaviour, good models of behaviour provided by teachers, a respect for children in their achievements with opportunities for them to be involved in the school as an organization, clear disciplinary rules with an emphasis on encouragement of good behaviour and sparing use of punishment, pleasant working conditions and good teacher–child relationships and a supportive, coherent structure for teachers. Overall there need to be established goals, values and norms that are known to both pupils and staff. Classroom management techniques also contribute: a minimum of non-teaching activity by the teacher in lesson time (e.g. setting-up), class-orientated instruction, plentiful use of praise with disciplinary actions kept as low as possible, prompt beginning and ending of lessons, and clear feedback to children on how they are doing. Thus the role of school as an institution with clearly defined and available tasks and expectations can work out to the child's advantage.

#### SOCIOECONOMIC CIRCUMSTANCES

Although rates of childhood psychiatric disorders are higher in families of low socioeconomic status, the association is less strong than in adults and less strong than the association between disorder and family discord. The link is somewhat stronger for delinquency and disorders of conduct, but parental occupation is still less important than other family characteristics (Wolkind & Rutter 1985b). However, high socioeconomic status may have a protective effect with regard to adversity, as for example against the deleterious effect of severe perinatal stress on IQ (Werner 1985). The meaning of social class is complex and may reflect aspects as diverse as differences in material resources or living conditions, and attitudes to education. Earlier reference was made to six major psychosocial factors that are considered adversities that can contribute to conduct disorder in children. One of these was the father being in an unskilled or semi-skilled job.

The higher rates of child psychiatric disorder in urban, particularly inner city areas, points to further factors that may predispose to disorder or protect (Richman 1985, Wolkind & Rutter 1985b). The nature of the factors associated with child psychiatric disorders tends to be similar in different areas and differences seem to be largely attributable to the higher rates of adversities known to be associated with child psychiatric disorders, for example, parental mental health, interparental relationships, quality of housing, schooling. The reasons for the differences in the levels of family adversities are not entirely clear. One possibility is that there is less social cohesion and thus social support for parents in child rearing. Secondly, flats and high-rise buildings are associated with greater rates of disorder in pre-school children. This may be partly because of increased risks for maternal depression in these circumstances (Richman 1977, Brown & Harris 1978). Thirdly, it may be that people feel less sense of control over their environment in large cities (Wolkind & Rutter 1985b). Maternal depression and disorder in preschool children in an inner city area were found to be associated with the level of environmental threat assessed by knowledge or experience of violence (Cox *et al.* 1987). Coleman (1985) has shown that certain features of housing estate design are associated with antisocial behaviour by young males and there is little doubt that this contributes to the sense of threat experienced by mothers with young children. These design features, which essentially promote the unimpeded and unsupervised movement of young adolescents, also contribute to difficulty in supervision of young children.

## Summary

There is a very wide range of social factors that may be influential either directly or indirectly in the development or maintenance of child psychiatric disorders. In many instances the influence

can be understood to be working through the quality of relationships between parent and child or the quality of child rearing, but this is very far from entirely the case as the evidence from research with peer relationships and schools demonstrates. However, again it seems to be the quality of relationships that is important, and this is re-emphasized by the research indicating the protective influence that good relationships may have in preventing disorders amongst those exposed to a variety of adversities, ranging from specific disasters, to living with parents who do not get on well together.

## References

Ainsworth M. (1982) Attachment: retrospect and prospect. In Parkes C.M. & Stevenson-Hinde J. (eds) *The Place of Attachment in Human Behaviour*, pp. 3–30. Tavistock, London.

Ainsworth M.D.S., Blehar M.C., Waters E. & Wall S. (1978) *Patterns of Attachment: A Psychological Study of the Strange Situation.* Erlbaum, Hillsdale, New Jersey.

Amato P. & Edgar D. (1987) *Children in Australian Families. The Growth of Competence.* Prentice-Hall, Sydney.

Asarnow J.R., Goldstein M.J. & Ben-meir S. (1988) Parental communication deviance in childhood onset schizophrenia spectrum and depressive disorders. *Journal of Child Psychology and Psychiatry* 29, 825–838.

Baumrind D. (1967) Child care practices anteceding three patterns of pre-school behaviour. *Genetic Psychology Monographs* 75, 423–488.

Baumrind D. (1971) Current patterns of parental authority. *Developmental Psychology Monographs* 4, (1. Pt. 2).

Beavers W. (1982) Healthy, mid-range and severely dysfunctional families. In Walsh F. (ed.) *Normal Family Process.* Guilford, New York.

Belmont L., Sein S.A. & Wittes J.L. (1976) Birth order, family size and school failure. *Developmental Medicine and Child Neurology* 18, 421–430.

Belsky J. (1980) Child maltreatment. *American Psychologist* 35, 320–335.

Belsky J. (1984) Determinants of parenting: a process model. *Child Development* 55, 83–96.

Belsky J. & Pensky E. (1988) Developmental history, personality and family relationships: towards an emergent family system. In Hinde R. & Stevenson-Hinde J. (eds) *Relationships within Families: Mutual Influences*, pp. 193–217. Oxford University Press, Oxford.

Belsky J., Youngblade L. & Pensky E. (1989) Child-rearing history, marital quality, and maternal affect: intergenerational transition in a low risk sample. *Develop-*

ment and Psychopathology 1, 291–304.

Berden G.F.M.G., Altaus M. & Verhulst F.C. (1990) Major life events and changes in behavioural functioning in children. *Journal of Child Psychology and Psychiatry* 31, 949–959.

Biller H.P. (1971) *Father, Child and Sex Role: Paternal Determinants of Personality Development.* Heath, Lexington.

Black D. & Urbanowitz M.A. (1987) Family intervention with bereaved children. *Journal of Child Psychology and Psychiatry* 28, 467–476.

Block J.H., Block J. & Gjerde F. (1986) The personality of children prior to divorce. *Child Development* 57, 827–840.

Block J., Block J.H. & Gjerde P. (1988) Parental functioning and home environment in families of divorce: prospective and concurrent analyses. *Journal of the American Academy of Child and Adolescent Psychiatry* 27, 207–213.

Block J.H., Block J. & Morrison A. (1981) Parental agreement-disagreement and child-rearing orientations and gender-related personality correlates in children. *Child Development* 52, 965–974.

Bowlby J. (1946) *Forty-fourth Juvenile Thieves; Their Characters and Home-life.* Bailliere, Tyndal and Cox, London.

Bowlby J. (1951) *Maternal Care and Mental Health.* WHO, Geneva.

Bowlby J. (1973) *Attachment and Loss,* vol. 2: *Separation, Anxiety and Anger.* Hogarth, London.

Bowlby J. (1980) *Attachment and Loss,* vol. 3: *Anxiety and Depression.* Hogarth, London.

Bowlby J. (1982) *Attachment and Loss,* vol. I: *Attachment,* 2nd edn. Hogarth, London.

Bradley R.H. & Caldwell B.M. (1976) The relation of infants' home environment to mental test performance at fifty-four months: a follow-up study. *Child Development* 47, 1172–1174.

Brain D.J. & MacKay I. (1968) Controlled study of mothers and children in hospital. *British Medical Journal* 1, 278–280.

Brett E.A., Spitzer R.C. & Williams J.B.W. (1988) DSM-III-R criteria for post-traumatic stress disorder. *American Journal of Psychiatry* 145, 1232–1236.

Brown G. & Harris T. (1978) *Social Origins of Depression.* Tavistock, London.

Brown G.W., Harris T.O. & Bifulco A. (1986) Long-term effects of early loss of parent. In Rutter M., Izard C.E. & Read P.B. (eds) *Depression in Young People: Developmental and Clinical Perspectives,* pp. 251–296. Guilford, New York.

Campbell S.B. (1990) *Behaviour Problems in Pre-school Children: Clinical and Developmental Issues.* Guilford, New York.

Campbell S.B. & Ewing L.J. (1990) Follow up of hard-to-manage pre-schoolers: adjustment at age 9 and predictors of continuing symptoms. *Journal of Child Psychology and Psychiatry* 31, 871–889.

Cantwell D. & Baker L. (1985) Speech and language: development and disorders. In Rutter M. & Hersov L. (eds) *Child and Adolescent Psychiatry: Modern Approaches,* pp. 526–544. Blackwell Scientific Publications, Oxford.

Caspi A. & Elder G.H. (1988) Emergent family patterns: intergenerational construction of problem behaviour and relationships. In Hinde R. & Stevenson-Hinde J. (eds) *Relationships within Families: Mutual Influences,* pp. 218–240. Oxford University Press, Oxford.

Christensen A. & Margolin G. (1988) Conflict and alliance in distressed and non-distressed families. In Hinde R. & Stevenson-Hinde J. (eds) *Relationships within Families. Mutual Influences,* pp. 263–282. Oxford University Press, Oxford.

Cicchetti D. & Schneider-Rosen K. (1986) An organisational approach to childhood depression. In Rutter M., Izard C.E. & Read P.B. (eds) *Depression in Young People: Clinical Perspectives,* pp. 71–134. Guilford, New York.

Clausen J.A. (1966) Family structure, socialisation and personality. In Hoffman L.W. & Hoffman M. (eds) *Review of Child Development Research,* vol. 2, pp. 1–53. Russell Sage, New York.

Coleman A. (1985) *Utopia on Trial: Vision and Reality in Planned Housing.* Hilary Shipman, London.

Comstock M.L.C. (1973) Effects of perceived parental behaviour on self-esteem and adjustment. *Dissertation Abstracts* 34, 465b.

Coopersmith S. (1967) *The Antecedents of Self-esteem.* Freeman, San Francisco.

Corbett J. (1985) Mental retardation: psychiatric aspects. In Rutter M. & Hersov L. (eds) *Child & Adolescent Psychiatry: Modern Approaches,* pp. 661–678. Blackwell, Oxford.

Cowen E.L., Pederson A., Babigian H., Izzo L.D. & Trost M.A. (1973) Long term follow-up of early detected vulnerable children. *Journal of Consulting in Clinical Psychology* 41, 438–446.

Cowen E.L., Pedro-Carroll J.L. & Alpert-Gillis L.J. (1990a) Relationships between support and adjustments among children of divorce. *Journal of Child Psychology and Psychiatry* 31, 727–735.

Cowen E.L., Wyman P.A., Work W.C. & Parker G.R. (1990b) The Rochester child resilience project: overview and summary of first year findings. *Development and Psychopathology* 2, 193–212.

Cox A. (1976) The association between emotional disorders in childhood and neuroses in adult life. In Van Praag H.M. (ed.) *Research in Neurosis,* pp. 40–58. Bohn, Scheltema and Holkema, Utrecht.

Cox A.D. (1988) Maternal depression and impact on children's development. *Archives of Disease and Childhood* 63, 90–95.

Cox A.D., Puckering C., Pound A. & Mills M. (1987) The impact of maternal depression in young children. *Journal of Child Psychology and Psychiatry* 28, 917–928.

Cox M.J., Tresch Owen M., Lewis J.M. & Henderson B.K.

(1989) Marriage, adult adjustment and early parenting. *Child Development* 6, 1015–1024.

Crockenberg S. (1981) Infant irritability, mother responsiveness and social support influences on the security of mother–infant attachment. *Child Development* 52, 857–865.

Dilalla L.F. & Gottesman I. (1989) Heterogeneity of causes for delinquency and criminality: life-span perspectives. *Development and Psychopathology* 1, 339–349.

Douglas J.W.B. (1975) Early hospital admissions and later disturbances of behaviour and learning. *Developmental Medicine and Child Neurology* 17, 456–480.

Douglas J.W.B., Ross J.M. & Simpson H.R. (1968) *All Our Future: A Longitudinal Study of Secondary Education*. Peter Davies, London.

Downey G. & Coyne J. (1990) Children of depressed parents: an integrative review. *Psychological Bulletin* 108, 50–76.

Dozier M. (1990) Attachment organisation and treatment use for adults with serious psychopathological disorders. *Development and Psychopathology* 2, 47–60.

Dunn J. (1986) Stress, development and family interaction. In Rutter M., Izard C.E. & Read P.B. (eds) *Depression in Young People: Clinical and Developmental Perspectives*, pp. 479–489. Guilford, New York.

Dunn J. (1988) Connections between relationships: implications of research on mothers and siblings. In Hinde R. & Stevenson-Hinde J. (eds) *Relationships within Families: Mutual Influences*, pp. 168–180. Oxford University Press, Oxford.

Dunn J., Stocker C. & Plomin R. (1990) Non-shared experiences within the family: correlates of behavioural problems in middle childhood. *Development and Psychopathology* 2, 113–126.

Egeland B., Kalkoske E.M., Gottesman N. & Erickson M.F. (1990) Pre-school behavioural problems: stability and factors accounting for change. *Journal of Child Psychology and Psychiatry* 31, 891–909.

Egeland B.R. & Sroufe L.A. (1981) Developmental sequelae of maltreatment in infancy. In Rizley R. & Cicchetti D. (eds) *Developmental Perspectives in Child Maltreatment (New Directions for Child Development No. 11)*. Jossey Bass, San Francisco.

Emde M.D. (1988) The effect of relationships on relationships: a developmental approach to clinical intervention. In Hinde R. & Stevenson-Hinde J. (eds) *Relationships within Families: Mutual Influences*, pp. 354–364. Oxford University Press, Oxford.

Emery R.E., Weintraub S. & Neale J.M. (1982) Effects of marital discord on the school behaviour of children of schizophrenic, affectively disordered and normal parents. *Journal of Abnormal Child Psychology* 10, 215–228.

Engfer A. (1988) The inter-relatedness of marriage and the mother–child relationship. In Hinde R. & Stevenson-Hinde J. (eds) *Relationships within Families: Mutual Influences*, pp. 104–118. Oxford University Press, Oxford.

Ferguson B.F. (1979) Preparing young children for hospitalisation. *Paediatrics* 64, 656–664.

Fergusson D.M., Horwood L.J. & Lawton J.M. (1990) Vulnerability to childhood problems and family social background. *Journal of Child Psychology and Psychiatry*, 31, 1145–1160.

Ferri E. (1976) *Growing Up in a One-parent Family*. National Foundation for Educational Research, Slough.

Fogelman K. (1985) Exploiting longitudinal data: examples from the National Child Development Study. In Nicol A.R. (ed.) *Longitudinal Studies in Child Psychology and Psychiatry*, pp. 241–261. Wiley, Chichester.

Folstein S.E., Franz M.L., Jensen B.A., Chase G.A. & Folstein M.F. (1983) Conduct disorder and affective disorder amongst the offspring of patients with Huntington's disease. *Psychology Medicine* 13, 45–52.

Garmezy N. (1985) Stress-resistant children: the search for protective factors. In Stevenson J. (ed.) *Aspects of Current Child Psychiatry Research*, pp. 213–233. (Journal of Child Psychology and Psychiatry (Book Supplement No. 4).) Pergamon, Oxford.

Garmezy N. (1986) Developmental aspects of children's response to separation and loss. In Rutter M., Izard C.E. & Read P.B. (eds) *Depression in Young People: Developmental and Clinical Perspectives*, pp. 297–233. Guilford, New York.

Garmezy N. & Rutter M. (1985) Acute reactions to stress. In Rutter M. & Hersov L. (eds) *Child & Adolescent Psychiatry: Modern Approaches*, pp. 152–176. Blackwell Scientific Publications, Oxford.

Golombok S., Spencer A. & Rutter M. (1983) Children in lesbian and single-parent households: psychosexual and psychiatric appraisal. *Journal of Child Psychology and Psychiatry* 24, 551–572.

Goodyer I. (1990a) Family relationships, life events and childhood psychopathology. *Journal of Child Psychology and Psychiatry* 31, 161–192.

Goodyer I. (1990b) Life events and psychiatric disorder. *Journal of Child Psychology and Psychiatry* 31, 839–848.

Goodyer I.M., Kolvin I. & Gatzanis S. (1985) Recent undesirable life events and psychiatric disorder in childhood and adolescence. *British Journal of Psychiatry* 147, 517–523.

Goodyer I.M., Kolvin I. & Gatzanis S. (1987) The impact of recent life events and psychiatric disorders of childhood and adolescence. *British Journal of Psychiatry* 151, 179–185.

Goodyer I.M., Wright C. & Altham P.M.E. (1988) Maternal adversity and recent stressful life events in anxious and depressed children. *Journal of Child Psychology and Psychiatry* 29, 651–667.

Goodyer I., Wright C. & Altham P.M.E. (1989) Recent friendships in anxious and depressed school-age children *Psychological Medicine* 19, 165–174.

Gorell Barnes G. (1985) Systems theory and family theory. In Rutter M. & Hersov L. (eds) *Child and Adolescent Psychiatry Modern Approaches*, pp. 216–229. Blackwell Scientific Publications, Oxford.

Grossmann K.E. (1988) Longitudinal and systemic approaches in the study of biological high- and low-risk groups. In Rutter M. (ed.) *Studies of Psychosocial Risk: The Power of Longitudinal Data*, pp. 138–157. Cambridge University Press, Cambridge.

Grossmann K., Fremmer-Bombik E., Rudolf J. & Grossmann J. (1988) Maternal attachment representations as related to patterns of infant–mother attachment and maternal care during the first year. In Hinde R. & Stevenson-Hinde J. (eds) *Relationships within Families: Mutual Influences*, pp. 241–260. Oxford University Press, Oxford.

Hartup W.W. (1983) Peer relationships. In Hetherington E.M. (ed.) *Socialisation, Personality, and Social Development*, vol. 4, *Handbook of Child Psychology*, 4th edn, pp. 103–196. Wiley, New York.

Hersov L. (1985a) Adoption & fostering. In Rutter M. & Hersov L. (eds) *Child & Adolescent Psychiatry: Modern Approaches*, pp. 101–117. Blackwell Scientific Publications, Oxford.

Hersov L. (1985b) Emotional disorders. In Rutter M. & Hersov L. (eds) *Child and Adolescent Psychiatry: Modern Approaches*, pp. 368–381. Blackwell Scientific Publications, Oxford.

Hersov L. (1985c) School refusal. In Rutter M. & Hersov L. (eds) *Child and Adolescent Psychiatry: Modern Approaches*, pp. 382–399. Blackwell Scientific Publications, Oxford.

Herzog E. & Sudia C.E. (1973) Children and fatherless families. In Caldwell B.M. & Ricciuti H.N. (eds) *Review of Child Development Research*, vol. 3, pp. 141–232. University of Chicago Press, Chicago.

Hetherington E.M. (1983) Parents, children and siblings: six years after divorce. In Hinde R.A. & Stevenson-Hinde J. (eds) *Relationships within Families: Mutual Influences*. Oxford University Press, Oxford.

Hetherington E.M. (1988) Parents, children and siblings: six years after divorce. In Hinde R.A. & Stevenson-Hinde J. (eds) *Relationships within Families: Mutual Influences*, pp. 311–331. Oxford University Press, Oxford.

Hetherington E.M., Cox M. & Cox R. (1982) Effects of divorce on parents and children. In Lamb M.E. (ed.) *Non-traditional Families: Parenting and Child Development*, pp. 233–288. Erlbaum, Hillsdale, New Jersey.

Hetherington E.M., Cox M. & Cox R. (1985) Long-term effects of divorce and remarriage on the adjustment of children. *Journal of the American Academy of Child and Adolescent Psychiatry* 24, 518–530.

Hill S., Bleichfeld B., Brunstetter R.D., Hebert J.G. & Steckler S. (1989) Cognitive and physiological responsiveness of abused children. *Journal of the American Academy of Child and Adolescent Psychiatry* 28, 219–224.

Hinde J. (1982) Attachment: some conceptual and biological issues. In Parkes C.M. & Stevenson-Hinde J. (eds) *The Place of Attachment in Human Behaviour*, pp. 60–76. Basic Books, New York.

Hinde R. (1988) Introduction. In Hinde R. & Stevenson-Hinde J. (eds) *Relationships Within Families: Mutual Influences*, pp. 1–4. Oxford University Press, Oxford.

Hinde R. & Stevenson-Hinde J. (eds) (1988) *Relationships Within Families: Mutual Influences*. Oxford University Press, Oxford.

Hodges J. & Tizard B. (1989a) IQ and behavioural adjustment of ex-institutional adolescents. *Journal of Child Psychology and Psychiatry* 30, 53–75.

Hodges J. & Tizard B. (1989b) Social and family relationships of ex-institutional adolescents. *Journal of Child Psychology and Psychiatry* 30, 77–97.

Howes P. & Markman H.J. (1989) Marital quality and child functioning: a longitudinal investigation. *Child Development* 6, 1044–1051.

Huston A.C. (1983) Sex-typing. In Hetherington E.M. (ed.) *Socialisation, Personality and Social Development*, vol. 4, *Handbook of Child Psychology*, 4th edn, pp. 387–467. Wiley, New York.

Illingworth R.S. & Holt K.S. (1955) Children in hospital: some observations on their reactions with special reference to daily visiting. *Lancet* ii, 1257–1262.

Jenkins J.M. & Smith M.A. (1990) Factors protecting children living in disharmonious homes: maternal reports. *Journal of the American Academy of Child & Adolescent Psychiatry* 29, 60–69.

Jenkins J.M., Smith M.A. & Graham P.J. (1989) Coping with parental quarrels. *Journal of the American Academy of Child and Adolescent Psychiatry* 28, 182–189.

Jensen P.S., Bloedau L., Degroot J., Ussery T. & Davis H. (1990) Children at risk: I. Risk factors and symptomatology. *Journal of the American Academy of Child and Adolescent Psychiatry* 29, 51–59.

Johnston J.R., Gonzalez R. & Campbell L.E.G. (1987) Ongoing-post-divorce conflict and child disturbance. *Journal of Abnormal Child Psychology* 15, 493–509.

Jones M.B., Offord D.R. & Abrams N. (1980) Brothers, sisters and antisocial behaviour. *British Journal of Psychiatry* 136, 139–145.

Kanzler E.M., Shaffer D. Wasserman G. & Davies M. (1990) Early childhood bereavement. *Journal of the American Academy of Child and Adolescent Psychiatry* 29, 513–520.

Kolko D.J. (1989) Conduct disorder. In Hersen M. (ed.) *Innovations in Child Behaviour Therapy*, pp. 243–269. Springer, New York.

Kreppner K. (1988) Changes in dyadic relationships within a family after the arrival of a second child. In Hinde R. & Stevenson-Hinde J. (eds) *Relationships Within Families: Mutual Influences*, pp. 143–167. Oxford University Press, Oxford.

Lamb M.E. (1978) Qualitative aspects of mother– and father–infant attachments. *Infant Behaviour and Development* 1, 265–275.

Lamb M.E. (1982) Paternal influences on early socio-emotional development. *Journal of Child Psychology and Psychiatry* 23, 185–190.

Lambert L. & Streather J. (1980) *Children in Changing Families: A Study of Adoption and Illegitimacy*.

Macmillan, London.

Levy D.M. (1943) *Maternal Over-protection*. Columbia University Press, New York.

Lewis M., Feiring C., McGuffog C. & Jaskir J. (1984) Predicting psychopathology in six year olds from early social relations. *Child Development* 55, 123–136.

Loeb R.C., Horst L. & Horton P.J. (1980) Family interaction patterns associated with self-esteem in pre-adolescent girls and boys. *Merrill-Palmer Quarterly* 26, 203–217.

McCluskey K.A., Killarney J. & Papini D.R. (1983) Adolescent pregnancy and parenthood: implications for development. In Callaghan E.J. & McCluskey K.A. (eds) *Life-span Developmental Psychology: Non-normative Life Events*, pp. 69–113. Academic, New York.

Maccoby E.E. & Martin J.A. (1983) Socialisation in the context of the family: parent–child interaction. In Hetherington E.A. (ed.) *Socialisation, Personality and Social Development*, vol. IV, *Handbook of Child Psychology*, 4th edn, pp. 1–101. Wiley, New York.

McCord W. & McCord J. (1959) *Origins of Crime*. Columbia University Press, New York.

MacKinnon C.E., Lamb M.E., Belsky J. & Baum C. (1990) An affective-cognitive model of mother–child aggression. *Development and Psychopathology* 2, 1–13.

Main M. & Weston D. (1981) The quality of the toddler's relationship to mother and father. *Child Development* 52, 932–940.

Malatesta C.Z., Culver C., Tesman J.R. & Shephard B. (1989) The development of emotions expression during the first two years of life. *Monographs of the Society for Research in Child Development* 54, nos 1–2.

Martini D.R., Ryan C., Nakayama D. & Ramenofsky M. (1990) Psychiatric sequelae of traumatic injury: the Pittsburgh regatta accident. *Journal of the American Academy of Child and Adolescent Psychiatry* 29, 70–75.

Maughan B (1988) School experiences as risk/protective factors. In Rutter M. (ed.) *Studies of Psychosocial Risk: The Power of Longitudinal Data*, pp. 200–220. Cambridge University Press, Cambridge.

Melhuish E.C., Gamble C. & Kumar R. (1988) Maternal mental illness and the mother–infant relationship. In Kumar R. & Brockington I. (eds) *Motherhood and Mental Illness, 2: Causes and Consequences*, pp. 191–211. Wright, London.

Melhuish E.C., Mooney A., Martin S. & Lloyd E. (1990a) Type of child care at eighteen months – I. Differences in interactional experience. *Journal of Child Psychology and Psychiatry* 31, 849–859.

Melhuish E.C., Lloyd E., Martin S. & Mooney A. (1990b) Type of child care at eighteen months – II. Relations with cognitive language development. *Journal of Child Psychology and Psychiatry* 31, 861–870.

Minuchin P. (1988) Relationships within the family: a systems perspective on development. In Hinde R. & Stevenson-Hinde J. (eds) *Relationships Within Families: Mutual Influences*, pp. 7–26. Oxford University Press, Oxford.

Mitchell R.G. (1984) Childhood stress – future research strategies. In Butler M.R. & Corner B.D. (eds) *Stress and Disability in Childhood: The Long-term Problems*, pp. 113–118. Wright, Bristol.

Monroe Blum H., Boyle M.R. & Offord R. (1988) Single-parent families: child psychiatric disorder and school performance. *Journal of the American Academy of Child and Adolescent Psychiatry* 27, 214–219.

Morrisset C.E., Barnard K.E., Greenberg M.T., Booth C.L. & Spieker S.J. (1990) Environmental influences on early language development: the context of social risk. *Development and Psychopathology* 2, 127–149.

Murray L. (1988) Effects of postnatal depression on infant development: direct studies of early mother–infant interactions. In Kumar R. & Brockington I. (eds) *Motherhood and Mental Illness, 2: Causes and Consequences*, pp. 159–190. Wright, London.

Murray L. (1990) Regulation of contact between young infants and their mothers. Paper delivered at the World Association of Infant Psychiatry and Allied Disciplines Conference: The Effect of Relationships on Relationships, 9–10 November 1990, London.

Offord D.R., Boyle M.H. & Racine Y. (1989) Ontario child health study: correlates of disorder. *Journal of the American Academy of Child and Adolescent Psychiatry* 28, 856–860.

Oliveri M. & Reiss D. (1982) Family styles of construing the social environment: a perspective on variation among non-clinical families. In Walsh F. (ed.) *Normal Family Process*. Guilford, New York.

Olson D. (1986) Circumplex Model VII validation studies and FACES III. *Family Process* 25, 337–351.

Olweus D. (1980a) Familial and temperamental determinants of aggressive behaviour in adolescent boys: a causal analysis. *Developmental Psychology* 16, 644–665.

Olweus D. (1980b) Bullying among schoolboys. In Barnes R. (ed.) *Children and Violence*. Academic Literature, Stockholm.

Osborn S.G. & West D.J. (1979) Conviction records of fathers and sons compared. *British Journal of Criminology* 19, 120–133.

Parker G. (1983) *Parental Overprotection: A Risk Factor in Psychosexual Development*. Grune & Stratton, New York.

Parry-Jones W. (1990) The Lockerbie Disaster. Paper presented at the Annual Residential Conference of the Child and Adolescent Psychiatry Section of the Royal College of Psychiatrists, Glasgow, September 1990.

Patterson C.J., Cohn D.A. & Kao B.T. (1989) Maternal warmth as a protective factor against risks associated with peer rejection among children. *Development and Psychopathology* 1, 21–38.

Patterson G.R. (1982) *Coercive Family Process*. Castalia, Eugene, Oregon.

Patterson G.R. & Dishion T.J. (1988) Multi level family process models: traits, interactions and relationships. In Hinde R.A. & Stevenson-Hinde J. (eds) *Relationships within Families: Mutual Influences*, pp. 283–310.

Oxford University Press, Oxford.

Paykel E.S. (1983) Methodological aspects of life events research. *Journal of Psychosomatic Research* 29, 341–352.

Petit S.G., Dodge K.A. & Brown M.M. (1988) Early family experience and social competence. *Child Development* 59, 107–120.

Pianta R.C. & Castaldi J. (1989) Stability of internalising symptoms from kindergarten to first grade and factors related to instability. *Development in Psychopathology* 1, 305–316.

Pound A. (1982) Attachment and depression. In Parkes C.M. & Stevenson-Hinde J. (eds) *The Place of Attachment in Human Behaviour*, pp. 118–130. Basic Books, New York.

Pound A., Cox A., Puckering C. & Mills M. (1985) The impact of maternal depression on young children. In Stevenson J.E. (ed.) *Recent Research in Developmental Psychopathology*, pp. 3–10. Pergamon, Oxford.

Puckering C. (1989) Maternal depression. *Journal of Child Psychology and Psychiatry* 30, 807–817.

Puckering C. & Rutter M. (1987) Environmental influences on language development. In Yule W. & Rutter M. (eds) *Language Development and Disorders*, pp. 103–128. Blackwell Scientific, Oxford.

Pynoos R. & Eth S. (1985) Developmental perspective on psychic trauma in children. In Figley C. (ed.) *Trauma and its Wake*. Brunner-Mazel, New York.

Pynoos R.S., Frederick C., Nader K. *et al.* (1987) Life threat and post-traumatic stress in school-age children. *Archives of General Psychiatry* 47, 1057–1063.

Quinton D. & Rutter M. (1976) Early hospital admissions and later disturbances of behaviour: an attempted replication of Douglas's findings. *Developmental Medicine and Child Neurology* 18, 447–457.

Quinton D. & Rutter M. (1985a) Family pathology and child psychiatric disorder: a four-year prospective study. In Nicol A.R. (ed.) *Longitudinal Studies in Child Psychology and Psychiatry*. Wiley, Chichester.

Quinton D. & Rutter M. (1985b) Parenting behaviour of mothers raised 'in care'. In Nichol A.R. (ed.) *Longitudinal Studies in Child Psychology and Psychiatry*, pp. 157–201. Wiley, Chichester.

Radke-Yarrow M., Cummings E.S., Kuczynski L. & Chapman M. (1985) Patterns of attachment in two- and three-year olds in normal families and families with parental depression. *Child Development* 56, 884–893.

Radke-Yarrow M., Richter S.J. & Wilson W.E. (1988) Child development in a network of relationships. In Hinde R. & Stevenson-Hinde J. (eds) *Relationships Within Families: Mutual Influences*, pp. 48–67. Oxford University Press, Oxford.

Rae-Grant N., Thomas B.H., Offord D. & Boyle M. (1989) Risk, protective factors and the prevalence of behavioural and emotional disorders in children and adolescents. *Journal of the American Academy of Child and Adolescent Psychiatry* 28, 262–268.

Reeves J.C., Werry J.S. & Zametkin A. (1987) Attention deficit, conduct, oppositional and anxiety disorders in children. II. Clinical characteristics. *Journal of the American Academy of Child and Adolescent Psychiatry* 27, 144–155.

Richards M.P.M. (1988) Parental divorce and children. In Burrows G. (ed.) *Handbook of Studies in Child Psychiatry*. Elsevier, Amsterdam.

Richman N. (1977) Behaviour problems in pre-school children: family and social factors. *British Journal of Psychiatry* 131, 525–527.

Richman N. (1985) Disorders in pre-school children. In Rutter M. & Hersov L. (eds) *Child and Adolescent Psychiatry: Modern Approaches*, pp. 336–350. Blackwell Scientific Publications, Oxford.

Richman N. & Stevenson J. (1977) Language delay in three year olds: family and social factors. *Acta Paediatrica Belgica* 32, 213.

Richman N., Stevenson J. & Graham P.A. (1982) *Preschool to School: A Behavioural Study*. Academic, London.

Robins L.N., West P.A. & Herjanic B.L. (1975) Arrests and delinquency in two generations: a study of black urban families and their children. *Journal of Child Psychology and Psychiatry* 16, 125–140.

Roff M., Sells S.B. & Golden M.M. (1972) *Social Adjustment and Personality Development*. University of Minnesota Press, Minneapolis.

Rowe J., Cain H., Hundleby M. & Keane A. (1984) *Long-term Foster Care: Child Care Policy and Practice*. Batsford, London.

Roy P. (1983) Is Continuity Enough? Substitute Care and Socialisation. Paper presented at the Spring Scientific Meeting: Child and Adolescent Psychiatry Specialist Section of the Royal College of Psychiatrists, London, March 1983.

Rushton A., Treseder J. & Quinton D. (1988) New parents for older children. *BAAF Discussion Series* 10.

Rutter M. (1966) Children of sick parents: an environmental and psychiatric study. *Institute of Psychiatry Maudsley Monographs No. 16*. Oxford University Press, London.

Rutter M. (1978a) Family, area and school differences in the genesis of conduct disorders. In Hersov L. & Shaffer D. (eds) *Aggression and Anti-social Disbehaviour in Childhood and Adolescence*, pp. 95–114. Pergamon, Oxford.

Rutter M. (1978b) Early sources of security and competence. In Bruner J.S. & Garton A. (eds) *Human Growth and Development*, pp. 33–61. Oxford University Press, London.

Rutter M. (1979) Protective factors in children's response to stress and disadvantage. In Kent M.W. & Rolfe J.E. (eds) *Primary Prevention of Psychopathology. Social Competence in Children*, vol. 3. Hanover Press, University of New England, Arundale, AL.

Rutter M. (1981a) Stress, coping and development: some

issues and some questions. *Journal of Child Psychology and Psychiatry* 22, 323–356.

Rutter M. (1981b) *Maternal Deprivation Re-assessed*, 2nd edn. Penguin, Harmondsworth.

Rutter M. (1981c) Social/emotional consequences of day-care for pre-school children. *American Journal of Orthopsychiatry*. 51, 4–28.

Rutter M. (1983a) Continuities and discontinuities in socio-emotional development: empirical and conceptual perspectives. In Emde R. & Harmon R. (eds) *Continuities and Discontinuities in Development*, pp. 41–68. Plenum, New York.

Rutter M. (1983b) Statistical and personal interactions: facets and perspectives. In Magnusson D. & Allen V. (eds) *Human Development: An Interactional Perspective*, pp. 295–317. Academic, New York.

Rutter M. (1985a) Resilience in the face of adversity. *British Journal of Psychiatry* 147, 598–611.

Rutter M. (1985b) Family and school influences: meanings, mechanisms, and implications. In Nicol A.R. (ed.) *Longitudinal Studies in Child Psychology and Psychiatry*, pp. 357–403. Wiley, Chichester.

Rutter M. (1986) The developmental psychopathology of depression: issues and perspectives. In Rutter M., Izard C.E. & Read P.B. (eds) *Depression in Young People: Clinical and Developmental Perspectives*. Guilford, New York.

Rutter M. (1987) Psychosocial resilience and protective mechanisms. *American Journal of Orthopsychiatry* 57, 316–331.

Rutter M. (1988) Functions and consequences of relationships: some psychopathological considerations. In Hinde R. & Stevenson-Hinde J. (eds) *Relationships Within Families: Mutual Influences*, pp. 332–353. Oxford University Press, Oxford.

Rutter M. (1989a) Pathways from childhood to adult life. *Journal of Child Psychology and Psychiatry* 30, 23–51.

Rutter M. (1989b) Psychiatric disorder in parents as a risk factor for children. In Shaffer D., Phillips I. & Enzer N.B. (eds) *Prevention and Mental Disorders, Alcohol and Other Drug Use in Children and Adolescents. OSAP Prevention Monograph* 2, pp. 157–189. Office for Substance Abuse Prevention, US Dept of Health and Human Services, Rockville, Maryland.

Rutter M. & Cox A. (1985) Other family influences. In Rutter M. & Hersov L. (eds) *Child & Adolescent Psychiatry: Modern Approaches*, pp. 58–81. Blackwell, Oxford.

Rutter M. & Giller H. (1983) *Juvenile Delinquency: trends and perspectives*. Guilford, New York.

Rutter M., Macdonald H., Le Couteur A., Harrington R., Bolton P. & Bailey A. (1990a) Genetic factors in child psychiatric disorders – II. Empirical findings. *Journal of Child Psychology and Psychiatry* 31, 39–83.

Rutter M. & Madge N. (1976) *Cycles of Disadvantage: A Review of Research*. Heinemann, London.

Rutter M. & Mittler P. (1972) Environmental influences in language development. In Rutter M. & Martin J.A.M. (eds) *The Child with Delayed Speech, Clinics in Developmental Medicine*, no. 43, pp. 52–67. Heinemann/Spastics International Medical Publications, London.

Rutter M. & Quinton D. (1977) Psychiatric disorder-ecological factors and concepts of causation. In McGurk H. (ed.) *Ecological Factors in Human Development*, pp. 173–187. North-Holland, New York.

Rutter M., Quinton D. & Hill J. (1990b) Adult outcome of institution reared children: males and females compared. In Robins L. & Rutter M. (eds) *Straight & Deviant Pathways from Childhood to Adulthood*, pp. 135–157. Cambridge University Press, Cambridge.

Rutter M., Tizard J. & Whitmore K. (1970) *Education, Health and Behaviour*. Longman, London.

Rutter M., Yule B., Quinton D., Rowlands O., Yule W. & Berger M. (1975) Attainment & adjustment in two geographical areas. III: Some factors accounting for area differences. *British Journal of Psychiatry* 126, 520–583.

Saylor C.F., Pallmeyer T.P., Finch A.J., Eason L., Trieber F. & Folger C. (1987) Predictors of psychological distress in hospitalised pediatric patients. *Journal of the American Academy of Child and Adolescent Psychiatry* 26, 232–236.

Schaffer H.R. (1965) Changes in developmental quotient under two conditions of maternal separation. *British Journal of Social and Clinical Psychology* 4, 39–46.

Seligman M.E.P. & Peterson C. (1986) A learned helplessness perspective on childhood depression: theory and research. In Rutter M., Izard C.E. & Read P.B. (eds) *Depression in Young People: Developmental and Clinical Perspectives*, pp. 223–249. Guilford, New York.

Shaw D. & Emery R. (1988) Chronic family adversity and school age children's adjustment. *Journal of the American Academy of Child and Adolescent Psychiatry* 27, 200–206.

Skynner R. (1974) School phobia: a reappraisal. *British Journal of Medical Psychology* 47, 1–16.

Speltz M., Greenberg M.T. & Deklyen M. (1990) Attachment in pre-schoolers with disruptive behaviour: a comparison of clinic-referred and non-problem children. *Development and Psychopathology* 230, 1–46.

Sroufe L.A. (1985) Attachment classification from the perspective of infant–care-giver relationships and infant-temperament. *Child Development* 56, 1–14.

Sroufe A.L. & Fleeson J. (1988) The coherence of family relationships. In Hinde R. & Stevenson-Hinde J. (eds) *Relationships Within Families: Mutual Influences*, pp. 27–47. Oxford University Press, Oxford.

Stacey M., Dearden R., Pill R. & Robinson D. (1970) *Hospitals, Children and Their Families: The Report of a Pilot Study*. Routledge and Kegan, Paul, London.

Steinhausen H.C., Von Aster S. & Gobel D. (1987) Family composition and child psychiatric disorder. *Journal of the American Academy of Child and Adolescent Psychiatry* 26, 242–247.

Stevenson J. & Fredman G. (1990) The social environmental correlates of reading ability. *Journal of Child Psychology and Psychiatry* 31, 681–698.

Terr L.C. (1979) Children of Chowchilla: a study of psychic trauma. *Psychoanalytic Study of the Child* 34, 552–623.

Terr L.C. (1981a) Psychic trauma in children: observations following the Chowchilla school-bus kidnapping. *American Journal of Psychiatry* 138, 14–19.

Terr L.C. (1981b) Forbidden games: post-traumatic children's play. *Journal of the American Academy of Child Psychiatry* 20, 741–760.

Terr L.C. (1983) Chowchilla revisited: the effects of psychic trauma four years after a school-bus kidnapping. *American Journal of Psychiatry* 140, 1543–1550.

Thompson R.A., Lamb M.E. & Estes D. (1982) Stability of infant–mother attachment and its relationship to change in life circumstances in an unselected middle-class sample. *Child Development* 53, 144–148.

Troy M. & Sroufe L.A. (1987) Victimization among pre-schoolers: the role of attachment relationship history. *Journal of the American Academy of Child Psychiatry* 26, 166–172.

Van Eerdewegh M., Bieri M.D., Parrilla R.H. & Clayton P.J. (1982) The bereaved child. *British Journal of Psychiatry* 140, 23–29.

Velez C.N., Johnson J. & Cohen P. (1989) A longitudinal analysis of selected risk factors for childhood psychopathology. *Journal of the American Academy of Child and Adolescent Psychiatry* 28, 861–864.

Vondra J., Burnett D. & Cicchetti D. (1989) Perceived and actual competence among maltreated and comparison children. *Development and Psychopathology* 1, 237–255.

Wadsworth J., Burnell I., Taylor B. & Bartlett T. (1985) The influence of family type on children's behaviour and development at five years. *Journal of Child Psychology and Psychiatry* 26, 245–254.

Wallerstein J. (1983) Children of divorce: stress and developmental tasks. In Garmezy N. & Rutter M. (eds) *Stress Coping and Development*, pp. 265–302. McGraw-Hill, New York.

Wallerstein J.S. (1984) Parent–child relations following divorce. In Anthony J. & Chiland C. (eds) *Clinical Parenthood*, vol. 8. *The Year Book of the International Association of Child & Adolescent Psychiatry*. Wiley, New York.

Wallerstein J.S. & Kelly J. (1980) *Surviving the Break-up: How Children and Parents Cope with a Divorce*. Basic Books, New York.

Weinraub M. & Wolf B.M. (1983) Effects of stress and social supports on mother–child interactions in single- and two-parent families. *Child Development* 54, 1297–1311.

Werner E.E. (1985) Stress and protective factors in children's lives. In Nicol A.R. (ed.) *Longitudinal Studies in Child Psychology in Psychiatry: Practical Lessons from Research Experience*, pp. 335–355. Wiley, Chichester.

Werry J.S. (1979) Psychosomatic disorders, psychological symptoms and hospitalisation. In Quay H.C. & Werry J.S. (eds) *Psychopathological Disorders in Childhood*, 2nd edn, pp. 134–184. Wiley, New York.

Werry J.S., Reeves J.C. & Elkind G.S. (1987) Attention deficit, conduct, oppositional and anxiety disorders in children. I. A review of research on differentiating characteristics. *Journal of the American Academy of Child and Adolescent Psychiatry* 26, 133–143.

West D.J. (1982) *Delinquency: Its Roots, Careers and Prospects*. Heinemann, London.

West D.J. & Farrington D.P. (1973) *Who Becomes Delinquent?* Heinemann, London.

Williams S., Anderson J., McGee R. & Silva P.A. (1990) Risk factors for behavioural and emotional disorders in pre-adolescent children. *Journal of the American Academy of Child and Adolescent Psychiatry* 29, 413–419.

Wolfer J.A. & Visintainer M.A. (1975) Pre-hospital psychological preparation for tonsillectomy patients: effects on children's and parents' adjustment. *Paediatrics* 64, 646–655.

Wolff S. (1973) *Children under Stress*. Penguin, Harmondsworth, Middlesex.

Wolkind S.N. (1974) Sex differences in the aetiology of antisocial disorders in children in long-term residential care. *British Journal of Psychiatry* 125, 125–130.

Wolkind S. & Kruk S. (1985) From child to parent: early separation and the adaptation to motherhood. In Nicol A.R. (ed.) *Longitudinal Studies in Child Psychology and Psychiatry*, pp. 53–74. Wiley, Chichester.

Wolkind S.N. & Renton G. (1979) Psychiatric disorders in children in long-term residential care: a follow up study, *British Journal of Psychiatry* 135, 129–135.

Wolkind S.N. & Rutter M. (1973) Children who have been 'In-care' – an epidemiological study. *Journal of Child Psychology and Psychiatry* 14, 97–105.

Wolkind S. & Rutter M. (1985a) Separation, loss and family relationships. In Rutter M. & Hersov L. (eds) *Child & Adolescent Psychiatry: Modern Approaches*, pp. 34–57. Blackwell Scientific Publications, Oxford.

Wolkind S. & Rutter M. (1985b) Socio-cultural factors. In Rutter M. & Hersov L. (eds) *Child & Adolescent Psychiatry: Modern Approaches*, pp. 82–100. Blackwell Scientific Publications, Oxford.

Wolkind S., Vyas I. & Harris R. (1982) Families and children–child psychiatric contributions in the general hospital. In Creed F. & Pfeffer S.M. (eds) *Medicine and Psychiatry: A Practical Approach*, pp. 213–228. Pitman, London.

Yarrow M.R., Campbell J.D. & Burton R.V. (1968) *Child Rearing: An Enquiry into Research and Methods*. Jossey-Bass, San Francisco.

Yule W. (1989) The effects of disasters on children. *Association for Child Psychology and Psychiatry Newsletter* 11, 3–6.

Yule W. (1991) Children in shipping disasters. *Journal of the Royal Society of Medicine* 84, 12–15.

Yule W. & Rutter M. (1985) Reading and other learning difficulties. In Rutter M. & Hersov L. (eds) *Child and Adolescent Psychiatry: Modern Approaches*, pp. 444–464. Blackwell Scientific Publications, Oxford.

Yule W., Udwin O. & Murdoch K. (1990) The 'Jupiter' sinking: effects on children's fears, depression and anxiety. *Journal of Child Psychology and Psychiatry* 31, 1051–1061.

Yule W. & Williams R.N. (1990) Post-traumatic stress reactions in children. *Journal of Traumatic Stress* 3, 279–295.

Zeitlyn H. (1990) Current interests in child–adult psychopathological continuities. *Journal of Child Psychology and Psychiatry* 31, 671–679.

# Chapter 14
## Social Psychiatry of Adolescence

PETER HILL

Adolescence is itself a social construct. Some societies do not recognize it as a stage of development and those that do have only done so in comparatively recent times, arguably since about 1900 (Aries 1962). In western societies it is a biopsychosocial concept within which the early physical changes of puberty usher in a phase of rapid development in physical, psychological and social terms, the developmental processes of each domain interweaving with and influencing the others.

It is impossible to divorce the social psychiatry of adolescence from the social psychiatry of childhood. Similar conceptual models for the genesis and maintenance of psychiatric disorder can be applied to both developmental epochs of immaturity: prepubertal childhood and postpubertal adolescence. A number of the studies providing supportive evidence for these models as they are applied to children have included young, school-age adolescents as well as prepubertal children. When social factors are considered, the broad framework of an interacting field and historical sequence of risk factors, protective factors, individual vulnerabilities and assets, and the division between precipitating and maintaining influences, are widely accepted. Similarly, the concept that social influences can form causal chains, the links of which combine to provide more than the arithmetical sum of their separate impacts, is increasingly rehearsed (a particularly elegant instance of how such a model can illuminate links between childhood and adult life is provided by Rutter (1989)). For such reasons at least, no assessment of the social psychiatry of adolescence can neglect social antecedents in childhood; they will mitigate, amplify or resonate with social factors impinging during adolescence. This chapter must therefore be read in conjunction with the preceding chapter by Cox.

### Development in adolescence

Adolescence itself can be defined from three perspectives: physical, chronological and developmental. The statement above that it is a biopsychosocial concept requires some justification.

For instance, it can be argued that adolescence starts at puberty and ends with physical maturity. Yet the psychological and social aspects of adolescence do not merely follow physical development as evidenced by instances of precocious puberty in childhood. Although such children display all the physical characteristics of puberty before the age of eight or nine, they remain children psychologically. In no way are they adolescent in their interests or other aspects of psychological development. Conversely, teenagers with delayed puberty will, depending on the cause, usually participate in a range of typical adolescent activities. Puberty appears to be a somewhat subsidiary issue.

Nevertheless, the usual convention is that adolescence commences with the observable changes of puberty (Tanner stage II) so that there is a biological marker as the conventional entry threshold. Since there is a wide individual variation in the age of onset of puberty and a very substantial difference (about two years) in the mean age of onset between the sexes, it becomes impossible to characterize the onset of adolescence precisely in age terms. Nor is it any easier to define the end of adolescence in age terms for the same reasons. For instance girls stop growing about two years before boys. Society does not consistently recognize this and prescribes, for instance, the same ages for social responsibility for both boys and girls except where it actually grants responsibility earlier to boys – as in the fact that boys can join the armed forces one year earlier than girls.

In accordance with the definition of adolescence afforded by the Oxford English Dictionary it is a period of development between what is obviously childhood and what might be regarded as adulthood. However, serious problems arise with the latter threshold if adulthood is held to be full developmental maturity in all modalities, since physical maturation, psychological maturation

**Table 14.1** Indices of psychosocial maturity

*Emotional*
Tolerance of frustration and ability to postpone gratification
Capacity to control impulses
Even-temperedeness and serenity; minimal resentment
Acceptance of ambivalence
Minimal dependency needs
Ability to give and receive affection without fear of losing one's own integrity
Ability to enjoy without guilt

*Social*
Ability to be alone
Self-determination
Capacity for measured assertion
Material independence
High priority for human relationships
Gradation of intensity in human relationships
Capacity for graded judgements about others (without polarization)
Accurate empathy and perception of needs of others
Consolidated personal identity actively derived from own experience
Freedom from pretence

*Intellectual*
Capacity for abstract thought and hypothetical planning
Ability to detach logic from immediate experience
Increasing generality and diminishing specificity in reasoning
Breadth of perspective indicating 'wisdom'

*Spiritual and moral*
Rational and consistent personal standards
Consciousness of own mortality without panic
Awareness of one's own capacity for initiative and choice
Ability to weigh personal and wider social priorities
Capacity for continued adaptation

and recognition of social maturity (by, say, an age of majority) do not coincide, even in a single given society. For instance, there is no single age at which full civic responsibility is granted in the UK, although many thresholds of responsibility are crossed at the eighteenth birthday. When maturity is considered in psychosocial terms, it is hard to see how this can be achieved by most 18 or 21 year olds (see Table 14.1), particularly as adult life is increasingly seen as a period of continuing development.

There is thus a choice and a dilemma. It is convenient to mirror social legislation and assign an age range to adolescence. This has advantages for administrative purposes and economy of thought. The administrative aspects will tie in with social provisions such as schooling or psychiatric inpatient units which tend to operate age limits. Alternatively, the developmental processes which are particularly linked with transition between childhood and maturity could be identified as markers for adolescence, which then becomes a developmental rather than a chronological concept. If the developmental option is selected, an acknowledgement needs to be made that this is likely to encompass a wider age range with no obvious upper limit and possibly an extension into a lower age than 13 for some children in special circumstances. For instance, children who lose one or both parents can be catapulted into a premature assumption of adult responsibilities which accelerates their social development (Wallerstein & Kelly 1980). Without being explicit as to which model is employed, any discussion of adolescent psychiatry will be ambiguous as to its axioms.

Whilst acknowledging this, many would accept a hybrid yet practical notion of adolescence as starting with the pubertal development of externally recognizable secondary sexual characteristics (where this is not precocious in age terms) and ending at some point around the ages of 18 or 21. This is a compromise; selecting as the end-point the major thresholds of civic adulthood rather than maturity. The focus of development is upon changes and advances made in a five- to eight-year epoch which includes certain physical changes such as the development of sexual interest and capability, and social transitions such as that from school to work. By such a convention the limits become biosocially, not merely biologically, defined. The social component is crucial.

The point that adolescence is largely a social construct is underscored by the way in which most authorities on human development point to task-mastery as a core concept in powering psychological development during adolescence (the adolescent process). The idea is that the physical changes imposed on the individual by puberty, the social demands imposed by social expectations, prohibitions and requirements, and the new abilities in language and cognition which emerge during the teenage years combine to create tasks and problems which the individual adolescent must master, resolve, adjust to or otherwise cope with in order to minimize personal distress or hardship. In meeting such challenges and discovering their solutions, new skills are forged or insights are acquired which result in psychological growth.

For instance, for an adolescent girl, the changes in body shape and the growth of breasts which accompany puberty will alter the responses of those around her. She has to accommodate to obvious sexual interest shown by boys, possibly the diminution of physical affection shown to her by her father, and generally becomes aware of herself as a sexual being. Such an identity carries with it new social rules about, for instance, allowing a little sexual play with boys but not, in early adolescence, full sexual activity. As there is considerable ambiguity and variation between social groups as to what such rules actually state, the girl has herself to resolve the problem as to how to negotiate emergent sexuality, balancing curiosity and pleasure (or a lack of it) with risks of sexually transmitted disease or pregnancy. To do so, she must make her own decisions and state her own views. She can follow those of others or decide her own. In doing so she defines her social position and adds to her own repertoire of insights, responses and principles. In the terms of Piaget, her schemata must accommodate, she must develop new understandings of the world in order to make sense of it and newly valid responses to cope with it. The alternative is denial and avoidance of growth or regression, a flight from it.

**Table 14.2** Developmental tasks of adolescence

*Tasks set by biological maturation*
Accommodating to accelerated linear growth and the way in which this alters how one is perceived by others
Accommodating to changes in body shape and secondary sexual characteristics and the way these alter the reactions of others
Coping with libido and fertility without precipitating pregnancy
Managing powerful emotions such as crushes and falling in love
Accepting own personal appearance and level of attractiveness

*Tasks set by drive for independence*
Increasing autonomy from parents in various areas (money, social support, leisure, dress)
Developing individual moral standards
Self-sufficiency in dealing with practical and emotional difficulties
Balancing need for acceptance by peer group with need to retain links with parents
Active exploration of personal identity as opposed to passive acceptance of family of origin's view

*Tasks set by general social expectations*
Leaving school and starting work
Taking or not taking public exams, making a career choice
Acquiring new skills or liberties by passing age thresholds (driving, legal sex, drinking alcohol)
Having conventional heterosexual relationships
Managing opportunities for risk and excitement
Preserving satisfactory status in peer group by own efforts

Not all tasks are set by biological change. In accordance with general social expectations, adolescents leave school between the ages of 16 and 19. They have no choice in the matter (apart from progressing to higher education) and move in one bound from an environment where they are surrounded by other teenagers of the same age into a world of work, peopled by individuals of varying ages who come from different family backgrounds and will not share the same values or leisure pursuits as the family members or school friends who have hitherto formed the social milieu of the adolescent. Within this new social environment, values have to be defended or assumed, ways of relating to adults who are not relatives and have none of the authority of teachers or parents have to be learned, and work habits substituted for study habits. Again, there are new skills to be learned and new insights gained. The individual, by doing so, gains in complexity and develops.

A sample list of the various tasks set by adolescence is exhibited in Table 14.2. Some of these are at a different level than those mentioned above. For instance, the individual adolescent has to master a range of tasks while preserving a coherent sense of identity and without becoming overwhelmed; a personal sense of continuity and consistency is maintained in healthy development. Bearing in mind the number of tasks, it is a little surprising at first sight that most adolescents manage a transition through adolescence without excessive or handicapping stress. The answer seems likely to be that they concentrate on certain issues at certain times rather than trying to progress on a broad front. This is the central theme of Coleman's focal theory of adolescent development for which there is a certain amount of empirical support (Coleman 1980), not that this is a field in which tight hypotheses are plentiful. A task-mastery model is more descriptive than predictive and is difficult to cast in falsifiable terms. Nevertheless, it provides a useful unifying approach for conceptualizing adolescent development and there are no serious current contenders as models for adolescent psychological development.

## Minor psychological disturbance in adolescence

A task-mastery model helps to understand and explain psychological development in adolescence but is not at all a complete explanation. Adolescents have pasts, families and personalities and their psychological development will inevitably be influenced by many of the factors that influenced childhood development. For example, an institutional upbringing in infancy can affect psychological development in childhood (Tizard & Hodges 1978) and still have an effect in adolescence (Hodges & Tizard 1989a,b). In this particular instance, the effect will be mediated by, among other things, family relationships and attitudes during both childhood and adolescence. There is a large element of continuity between childhood and adolescence which partly reflects continuity of

social situations, partly the impact of the child's personality which will contain continuous as well as discontinuous elements. Some of these are reflections of experiences and learning within the family, school and peer group. On the other hand, the developmental tasks of adolescence are self-evidently relatively specific for adolescence in western culture, and the number of them posed within the developmental epoch is comparatively large compared with the eight or so years of middle childhood. Identifying the tasks involved means that it is possible to be specific about adolescent development and examine to what extent psychological disturbance in adolescence might be considered linked to the process of adolescence itself, in terms of the type of tasks and the rate at which they present.

Psychological disturbance here is intended to be revealed by symptoms or behavioural abnormalities which are not handicapping or associated with significant suffering and do not represent major mental illness. It is meant to refer to a state which is less severe than that indicated by the term psychiatric disorder and which is strikingly more common among adolescents than children.

This question of adolescent psychopathology short of disorder is addressed by the various studies into so-called adolescent turmoil, particularly the Isle of Wight follow-up (Rutter *et al.* 1976). There seems little dissent from the assertion that many adolescents experience mood fluctuations, social sensitivity, hypochondriacal concerns, exhibit minor social withdrawal or irritability, even that a substantial minority toy with ideas of suicide, but that these symptoms and behaviours are not associated with impaired social functioning and are not sufficiently severe to be cause of substantial suffering. The number of adolescents with any of such symptoms is unknown, but cross-sectional studies suggest it is at last half (Rutter *et al.* 1976, Kandel & Davies 1982, Schoenbach *et al.* 1982, Ostrov *et al.* 1989).

A common assumption is that these symptoms are related to hormonal changes, but the evidence is that the effect of these is very small (see Hill 1993) and it seems probable that such symptoms mainly stem from adolescents' perceptions of the responses of others, an essentially social phenomenon. Elkind (1967) makes the point that self-centred behaviour and social sensitivity derive from incompletely developed formal operational thought so that the adolescent's new-found capacity for thinking about thinking means that he or she confuses his thoughts with the thoughts attributed to others. Doubts about self are, he or she assumes, shared by others. Similarly, concerns about developing body shape, particularly among girls, can be linked to inappropriate but not morbid preoccupations about fatness (Nylander 1971, Bowden *et al.* 1989) and how it is judged by others. Depressive swings which are commoner in girls have been thought to stem from the behaviour of teachers in their criticisms of teenage girls' school work (Dweck *et al.* 1978), and concerns about personal identity related to an interaction between family environment and task presentation (Adams & Adams 1989). It has been argued that the common disagreements and mild degrees of alienation between parents and adolescents are most likely to be the result of living within the same household rather than adolescence *per se* (Rutter 1979). In other words there are good grounds for thinking that a number of minor psychological symptoms are related predominantly to interpersonal issues and developmental challenges rather than organic processes.

## Psychiatric disorder in adolescence

The considerable continuity between childhood and adolescence is not only true for psychosocial development and its deviations but for psychiatric disorder too. According to the age of the adolescents studied, up to one-half of those with psychiatric disorder will display a disorder that is a continuation of psychiatric disorder first manifest in childhood (see Hill 1989). This will obviously be the more the case, the younger the adolescent group in question.

It is evident from epidemiological studies (e.g. Rutter *et al.* 1976, Offord *et al.* 1987) that there are no psychiatric disorders which occur or first appear only in adolescence as defined by the teenage years; nor are there any which are absolutely confined to that epoch when it is defined in age terms as is necessary for epidemiological enquiry. In general terms there is a spectrum of conditions ranging from those predominantly arising in, and typical of childhood to those conventionally regarded as adult disorders. Early adolescence will contain a predominance of the former, late adolescence the latter. There might therefore be two components to adolescent psychiatry. First, the requirement to assess the pathoplastic effect of adolescence on the presentation of disorder. This assumes that adolescence is important because it may affect such features as mode of presentation of disorder or, conversely, the presentation of treatments so that they are appropriate for a teenage population. Secondly, there is the possibility that although an age definition of adolescence does not illuminate disorders specific to adolescence, a developmental approach could do so by identifying certain disorders as perversions or distortions of adolescent developmental process.

### Pathoplastic effects of adolescence

For psychiatric conditions occurring in adolescence, it might be expected that their presentation or prognosis would be altered by the fact that they are present in an adolescent person. In this respect the presentation of, for example, depression is different in several ways from childhood or adult life. Depressed adolescents are more likely than depressed adults to display separation anxiety, complain of pain, overeat, act antisocially and abscond from home (see review in Hill 1989). On the other hand they are more likely than children to commit suicide or commit other acts of deliberate self-harm. The most probable explanation for such differences is that they are distributed on a continuum of maturity from childhood to adulthood since, to take one instance, suicide rates for adolescence are intermediate between those for childhood and adult life (Hawton 1986). This approach obscures certain gender differences so that depression in young adolescent boys is more likely to be associated with antisocial behaviour than is the case with girls, yet depression is relatively commoner among girls in adolescence, becoming more so with advancing age. A more discriminating picture emerges when gender and age are considered separately within adolescence. These trends: for depressed adolescent boys to be relatively more antisocial and for depressed girls to be relatively compliant, reflect the ordinary range of gender differences of feelings and actions in normal adolescents (Ostrov *et al.* 1989).

The pathoplastic effect of adolescence may reflect the adolescents' social situation rather than global maturational state. The surge in incidence of antisocial acts which occurs in the middle teens reflects, in part, less parental supervision and, for boys at any rate, may subsequently be lessened by the resumption of accountability to other household members with the formation of more enduring relationships with girlfriends and wives in the late teens (Osborn & West 1980). It may be impossible to separate the two factors of maturation and social situation. For instance, the common irritability shown by adolescents in dealings with their parents may be a function of chafing at parental restrictions as the adolescent prepares to leave the family home or a way of negotiating release from an erstwhile dependent relationship – fighting one's way out as a developmental process (Haley 1980). On the other hand, it may be a consequence of independent-minded people, adolescents and their parents, sharing a common household within which shared living arrangements mean that compromises are necessary (though granted only grudgingly). Similarly, as teenagers leave school and enter work, they appear to experience an increase in psychological well-being as indicated by a fall in their scores on the General Health Questionnaire. There is evidence that this is related both to a release from the pressures of public examinations – essentially a social factor specific to adolescence – and general developmental factors, since a decline in scores continues for years after the examination period (Cairns *et al.* 1991).

### Disorders specifically related to adolescent developmental process

An alternative way of considering whether there might be specifically adolescent psychiatric disorders is to relate the developmental processes which are specific to adolescence to known psychiatric conditions. This will exclude some conditions which not uncommonly first present in adolescence but are not obviously linked to developmental processes. These include schizophrenia, manic-depressive disorder or obsessive-compulsive disorder, all of which can first occur at any stage of life, though there is a tendency for first manifestation to be in the teenage years. For a disorder to be specifically an adolescent psychiatric disorder it should be:

1 First apparent most commonly in adolescence, rather than earlier or later, and

2 Capable of being related aetiologically to developmental processes peculiar to adolescence.

The case of anorexia nervosa being specifically linked to the adolescent developmental process is probably the strongest (see also Chapter 16). Most formulations stress that the condition is a biopsychosocial one and that pubertal changes interact with social and family expectations. The modal age of onset is 17 (Crisp 1980), cases occurring before puberty are rare (Jacobs & Isaacs 1986, Lask & Bryant-Waugh 1990), as are those arising for the first time in later life. When cases outside the usual age range have been described, there is frequently a comment by the authors that the condition seemed linked to premature or unresolved psychosocial developmental demands of the type experienced by adolescents. Several explanatory models or aetiological mechanisms for anorexia nervosa have been described, and are detailed below.

*1 Self-starvation as a reaction to erroneous perception of body shape with the possibility of entering a vicious spiral as starvation increases the magnitude of the perceptual error* (Crisp & Kalucy 1974, Russell *et al.* 1975)

It is generally found that a large proportion of mid-adolescent girls in the general population (of the order of 70%) judge themselves to be fatter then they would like and that this seems to be based in part upon a perceptual error (see e.g. Bowden *et al.* 1989). The origins of such a misperception may be biological, but in view of large differences in the inception rate of anorexia nervosa between cultures, concern about it seems likely to be fuelled by cultural standards for physical attractiveness conveyed by mass media and commercial interests such as slimming magazines which both exploit and intensify the concern, thus both reflecting and intensifying current social values. Exceptional sensitivity to the perceptions of others is a common feature of adolescence and may derive from the mechanism suggested by Elkind (1967) wherein, as a consequence of early formal operational thought, the girl has difficulty separating her own judgements of herself from those attributed by her to others. Self-starvation intensifies distortion in self-perception; the thinner the girl gets, the more she is prone to overestimate her own size. She will intensify calorie restriction and maintain a vicious spiral because she values her thinness.

## 2 Self-starvation as a means to obtain control over body shape and therefore personal destiny, a sense of power otherwise unavailable (Bruch 1974)

Developing autonomy as a component of the individuation process in adolescence requires the adolescent to possess adequate self-esteem and a sense of personal competence. Bruch describes a number of ways in which girls with anorexia nervosa feel inadequate to the task and experience a feeling of powerlessness. This may be accentuated by the essentially passive experience of the pubertal changes imposed upon young adolescents. The discovery that they can exert some control over themselves by changing the shape of their bodies enables a sense of control over one's destiny to be recovered.

## 3 Self-starvation as a means whereby the maturational demands of adolescence can be postponed or avoided by physiological regression into a prepubertal state (Crisp 1980)

This is a particularly well-developed theory derived from extensive experience with patients who have severe, chronic anorexia nervosa. The social expectations of adulthood which begin to be communicated and experienced in adolescence may alarm the young teenager with low self-esteem

and a compliant habit, who feels unprepared for autonomy, responsibility, sexuality and meeting the demands of others for self-reliance. Self-starvation in ordinary, common teenage dieting brings welcome feelings of control and confidence which cause dieting to be prolonged so that the weight threshold for initiating puberty (about 48 kg) is crossed in reverse, menstruation ceases and further pubertal development is halted. The girl is now effectively prepubertal in physiological terms and has negotiated for herself a biological and psychosocial regression, thus retreating from and avoiding further adolescent challenges.

## 4 Self-starvation as a device for diverting interparental conflict by imposing the need to unite in caring for a sick child (Minuchin et al. 1978)

The impact of a daughter, intent upon self-starvation to illogical lengths and pursuing a diet with heedless obstinacy, provokes parents to abandon marital disputes and reunite in parenting tasks which were becoming less demanding as their daughter became more independent of care-giving. The argument that this is most likely to occur in adolescence hinges upon the individuation process of adolescence and the consequent changes in role for parents in relation to the daughter, especially if she is the youngest child whose departure from the family will result in an empty nest and a necessity for the parents to revert to a two-person household. The parents may themselves feel apprehensive or ambivalent about this and may even convey this indirectly to their daughter. Marital discord can supervene as they renegotiate their relationship with each other. Having a 'sick' daughter restores the feeling of pre-individuation security and continuity which was otherwise threatened by parental disputes. The daughter experiences a calmer household.

These theories postulate mechanisms which are not mutually exclusive and in clinical practice appear to have differing heuristic power in different cases, or at different times in the same case, or to combine simultaneously. Mechanism (1) may act as an initiating factor, but mechanism (2) may maintain self-starvation, for instance. Nor is there convincing evidence that any one theory explains all cases. For instance, not all patients will show over-estimation of their own fatness (see Bowden *et al.* 1989) and both closeness and disruption may be seen in the families of a series of patients (e.g. Heron & Leheup 1984).

The argument that anorexia nervosa is linked to social adolescent developmental process rests partly on its modal age of onset and the fact that onset is rare before puberty and uncommon after the teenage years. It also derives from the logical link between the misperception of self as fat which reaches a peak at about the age of 17 and is largely a female phenomenon, as is anorexia nervosa. Theories (2) and (3) above would most easily be cast as maintaining factors, which would supervene after self-starvation had been initiated as a means to slim in response to the combined pressure of wider cultural influence which favours thinness or as a reaction to teasing about puppy fat (Crisp 1980). The girl discovers that her dieting produces desirable gains in other areas of life and these become the principle motive to continue. Given a certain degree of obsessional determination and drive, starvation is maintained in the face of hunger and a biologically determined preoccupation with food which is an innate reaction to starvation. The moral attitudes adopted (fat is bad) and the single-minded concern with control develop as a consequence of this struggle against hunger and preoccupation with food. The physical aspects such as amenorrhoea, lanugo hair, tolerance of cold and bradycardia are physical consequences of starvation, in part a form of semi-hibernation.

Although there is a little evidence that genetic influences play an aetiological role, it is unclear how. In the absence of an identifiable organic basis for the vast majority of cases, some influence on personality seems likely. The fact that dieting to lose weight is common and anorexia nervosa uncommon implies that either personality, peer group or family variables represent vulnerabilities for the eventual development of the condition. Estimating premorbid personality is difficult since starvation and the struggle against appetite alters personality, but there is a consensus that girls who

develop anorexia nervosa are unusually quiet, compliant, industrious, and orderly (see e.g. Heron & Leheup 1984). Little is known about peer group variables though a proportion of girls report teasing centred on fatness in their childhood or early teens (Crisp 1980). Clinical studies of families containg adolescents with anorexia nervosa suggest that family functioning is distorted (Minuchin *et al.* 1978, Yager 1982), and this can be demonstrated by formalizing observations using, for instance, Benjamin's Structural Analysis of Social Behaviour (Humphrey 1987). It has not yet been established to what extent this is cause or consequence. Nevertheless, the evidence for social impact upon aetiology is overwhelming, the physical signs (and much of the typical mental state) being essentially the consequence of starvation rather than primary factors. What seems likely is the interaction between cultural values or habits (such as slimming) and developmental processes in girls with vulnerable personalities or, just possibly, vulnerable families.

The other group of disorders which might relate specifically to adolescent development is the constellation of anxieties around the perceptions of self by others. The categories of social phobia and dysmorphophobia are somewhat heterogeneous but share the common feature of an inappropriate and morbidly anxious concern about being judged adversely by other people. Both are virtually unknown in middle childhood and are most likely to become apparent in the middle to late teens. Mild apprehension about the judgements of others as to one's worth and a preoccupation with appearance as the teenager adjusts to pubertal changes in their body are common in ordinary teenagers. As mentioned above, fleeting ideas of self-reference and hypochondriacal concerns are not uncommon mild psychological disturbances in this developmental epoch. The importance of the views of others is arguably an extension of three elements. First, the hypothesis of Elkind: that developing formal operational thought causes a faulty attribution of the adolescent's own preoccupations to an 'audience' thought to share the teenager's own judgements about their own appearance. Secondly, the role of advertising and fashion in emphasizing the social importance of appearance and establishing standards of physical attractiveness, dress, speech and behaviour for a teenage market. Thirdly, the developmental move from reliance upon parental guidance on standards to the acquisition of individual personal standards, a process which amplifies the importance of peer group opinions as the teenager sifts through a repertoire of alternative possibilities to parental standards. Satisfactory involvement in peer group activities requires adequate social skills and popularity is enhanced by physical attractiveness (see Hartup 1983). Not surprisingly, demeanour and appearance are major fulcra in all this. Furthermore, adolescents who are themselves anxious about the acceptability of their own attractiveness and competence in these areas will use mechanisms of projection and externalization in order to avoid psychological discomfort; they will persecute and tease those less attractive than themselves. Given the tendency for adolescents to gather in age-related groups, such defences can exacerbate pathology in other adolescents; social unease is infectious.

## The sources of social influence on psychiatric disorder

There is some advantage in considering continuous and discontinuous sources separately for the sake of clarity, though the distinction is somewhat academic; a continuous stressor such as marital discord also makes a discontinuous event such as a parent leaving the family home more likely. Some apparent life events such as parental divorce may be better conceptualized as continuous processes or indeed stand as proxies for previous chronic marital discord (Wallerstein & Kelly 1974).

Those continuous sources to be considered would arise within family, school, work and peer group. Only family influences have been conceptualized or explored in any detail in adolescence, though a few findings about school, work and peer group influences deserve note.

### *Family life*

Task-mastery models of human development are not restricted in their usefulness to adolescence. For instance, Solomon (1973) has proposed such a model for the development of the family unit, though his suggestion might well be considered more a description of the development of parental skills than of the whole family unit since he emphasizes challenges set by child rearing. There is an epigenetic notion underlying such an approach which has some plausibility: parents must have dealt with earlier tasks of establishing a family (such as separating themselves from their families of origin) and with earlier tasks of child rearing (such as facilitating both attachment and separation in the child's infancy) before they can satisfactorily assist their adolescent offspring's individuation from their family. When applied to the tasks of parenting adolescents, a list of parenting tasks can be created which is, to a large extent, the obverse of developmental tasks facing individual adolescents. That is to say that parents should support the adolescent in the mastery of their own developmental tasks by:

1 Providing a sense of continuous yet developing identity throughout the physical changes of puberty.

2 Providing realistic feedback on personal style and posture without damaging self-esteem, and allowing reasonable experimentation.

3 Providing adequate information and guidance about the world outside the family home and the school.

4 Demonstrating and teaching social skills such as self-presentation and negotiation.

5 Adjusting but not abandoning family structure of authority, exerting limit setting and discipline especially with respect to aggressive and sexual behaviour within the home without compromising the appropriate development of autonomy.

6 Reinforcing sexual boundaries within the family system to contain sex within the parental marriage, separate from the activities of sexually experimenting offspring.

7 Letting go so that the peer group can establish standards of behaviour and risk taking beyond the supervision of parents.

8 Being prepared to rescue disasters caused by adolescent misjudgement.

9 Enabling their children to leave the family home free of guilt or rancour.

Such standards of parenting are not easy to establish or maintain. The fundamental requirement is that parents sustain their child-rearing practices whilst attuning them to the fact that their child is becoming an adult. Both parents need to agree about the developmental needs of their child and this is not easy when the teenager selects one or other parent with whom to deal with when confiding or negotiating new limits of supervision (as they may often do; see Monck 1991). Parents may be out of tune with his or her developmental status; a situation commoner in families containing a psychiatrically disordered adolescent (Fischer 1980). Furthermore, it needs to be appreciated that, for many adolescents, their teenage years will coincide with their parents' middle age and their tackling of adolescent developmental tasks will be paralleled by their parents' preoccupations with mid-life challenges. Fathers are prone to question themselves about their own careers or work achievements and assess how well these represent the fulfilment of ideals they possessed when they themselves entered work in mid or late adolescence. Mothers may have sacrificed paid vocation for the sake of child rearing and sought satisfaction in and through their children who are now soon to leave the family home. A mother may consider returning to work but find her ambition compromised by her husband's expectations that she continue as the homemaker he has grown accustomed to. Both parents are likely to be past their conventional physical prime and compare themselves and each other critically with adolescents in and around the home. Such factors can easily compromise the extent to which parents carry out their duties to their children. The extent to which this occurs seems, on clinical grounds, to underpin a number of the common intrafamilial resentments which form a large proportion of referrals to psychiatric services.

A distinction can be drawn between conditions arising for the first time in adolescence and those which occur in adolescence but began in childhood. The latter are chronic child psychiatric problems about which a fair amount is known but the former have been comparatively poorly studied so that a degree of clinical speculation is appropriate. For instance, an interlocking of parental behaviour and adolescent reaction can often be observed in teenagers who are apparently grumpy and truculent to the degree which prompts psychiatric referral. One particular model for this has been described by Hill (1989) as the 'strop cycle' and proposes a vicious spiral of wavering self-confidence and parental criticism. This implies a degree of alienation of parents from adolescents which is by no means usual among normal adolescents (see e.g. Offer & Offer 1975, Ghodsian & Lambert 1978). The perception by teenagers of their parents as being unfair, incomprehending and intolerant is often assumed to be normal by mental health professionals, yet this is not likely to be so (Offer *et al.* 1981) unless the teenager is psychiatrically disordered (Hartlage *et al.* 1984).

How significant family issues are in the aetiology of disorder arising for the first time in adolescence can be called into question. Rutter *et al.* (1976) showed that, for psychiatric disorder arising in adolescence, family factors such as poor parental marriage and parental psychiatric disorder were less powerful associations than for disorder arising in childhood; roughly 20% of cases compared with approximately 30%. The effect of duration of influence was not tightly controlled but the assertion seems plausible.

What of an interaction between family and genetic, neurological, school or peer group factors? There is no direct answer, though Kashani *et al.* (1987) argue that on the basis of data derived from a community study using structured interviews and formal assessment instruments with adolescents and parents, adolescent psychiatric cases demonstrated a close interaction of parenting behaviour, personality and psychopathology. Family rapport was the most commonly expressed concern (out of 8 available possibilities including e.g. peer acceptability and self-concept) by all adolescents, cases and non-cases. For the adolescents judged to be psychiatric cases (28 out of a total sample of 150), family rapport was a concern in 79% compared with 51% of non-cases. Naturally such a study cannot separate cause from effect but it implies that it is necessary to take family relationships into consideration in clinical practice. Certainly clinicians think so; in an opinion study rating psychosocial stressors in adolescence, family factors occupied 22 out of 30 of the most severe ratings, virtually all the others being varieties of sexual abuse (Plapp *et al.* 1987). The extremes of family breakdown might be thought to be abuse and divorce. Most instances of intrafamilial abuse presenting in adolescence represent the disclosure or identification of abusive patterns which have begun in childhood, there are no studies of the effect of abuse which has been confined to adolescence (though it is known to occur) and there is little to suggest that adolescence has more than a pathoplastic effect on any psychiatric disorder with which abuse is associated. The situation with respect to divorce is a little different and suggests that parental divorce has a rather different effect upon adolescents compared with children. In a comprehensive follow-up study, Wallerstein (Wallerstein & Kelly 1974, 1980, Wallerstein 1985) showed that for those who were teenagers at the time of their parents' divorce, substantial psychopathology resulted. At five-year follow-up, one-third were considered to show moderate to severe clinical depression. This needs to be set against the finding that some showed an 'impressive developmental spurt' displaying a positive response to apparent adversity and becoming mature, compassionate and altruistic with respect to their parents. One implication is that divorce can act as a particularly severe developmental challenge which can be mastered positively with consequent gains. At ten-year follow-up, painful feelings about their parents' divorce were still common among young adults who experienced parental divorce in their teens, and for over 80% the divorce seemed to the interviewer to still hold a central position in their psychological functioning. Half of these young adults asserted that it was a continuing major influence upon their lives. No hard ratings of psychiatric disorder were specified at ten-year follow-up, but one-third of the women were particularly fearful of personal betrayal, had continuing problems maintaining sexual relationships and were inclined to drift in terms of occupation, elements which hint at personality disorder.

### School factors

Early studies on the association of schools and referral rates to psychiatric services suggested that different schools displayed different rates of referral to clinics which could not be completely explained by the catchment areas from which they drew their pupils (see e.g. Gath *et al.* 1977). The original and significant study by Rutter and his colleagues (1979) carried out in 12 London secondary (age 11–16+) schools was able to standardize for differences in intake policy which might account for such school differences, and although it did not examine psychiatric referral rates or psychiatric disorder directly, assessed variables exhibited by pupils (delinquency, truancy and bad behaviour) which might stand as proxies for mental health problems. In short, schools were shown to have an independent effect on such variables. Differences between schools in exerting such effects were stable and could not be completely explained by differences in intake or catchment area. The outcome variables: academic attainment, attendance, behaviour and delinquency, tended to covary so that 'good' schools were generally better than 'bad' schools on all measures. The impact, for good or ill, of the school was through its effect as a social institution. Physical factors such as the size of the school or the age of its buildings were unimportant, as were broad administrative differences such as whether schools were coeducational or not or whether their pastoral care was organized on a year or house system. What was significant included such factors as teachers' expectations and disciplinary style, teachers' own behaviour in demonstrating standards, use of feedback to pupils, formalization of pupil responsibilities, and the consistency of school values. The detail need not be spelled out here since what was under study was not psychiatric disorder, yet schools were demonstrated to influence pupil behaviour. Some of the mechanisms elucidated suggest strongly that they are a potential source of social influence upon the genesis and maintenance of psychiatric disorder in adolescence even though recent work suggests that the size of the effect may be smaller and less stable than previously thought (see Reynolds & Cuttance 1991).

One suggested mechanism whereby a particular school variable, namely teacher feedback, might influence psychiatric morbidity is provided by Dweck's studies (Dweck & Bush 1976, Dweck *et al.* 1978). Although teachers were generally more critical of adolescent boys than girls, this was expressed more diffusely to boys but girls were criticized for their intellectual shortcomings. Encouragement, conversely, was more specific for boys and diffuse for girls. This, coupled with the finding that girls were more likely than boys to blame their academic failure on their own shortcomings and were more likely to give up rather than try harder, provides an instance of how social and individual factors might combine to yield a vulnerability factor (learned helplessness) which could conceivably contribute to the increased rate of depression among adolescent girls compared with boys.

## Peer group

It has long been recognized that good peer relations are a powerful positive prognostic factor for psychiatric disorder in both childhood and adolescence. Adversities within the peer group could be loosely considered to be group-syntonic, as might operate in the aetiology of socialized conduct disorder, or group-dystonic as in rejection and victimization of which mobbing (being bullied by a large group) would be an instance. In the study of social pathology such as delinquency, the impact of the peer group in fostering criminal activity has long been recognized – most juvenile delinquency and nearly all first crime is carried out in the company of others (see Rutter & Giller 1983). Similar arguments and observations apply to the initiation and maintenance of drug abuse, but in both delinquency and drug abuse a strong interaction between peer group and family factors has been documented (Rutter & Giller 1983, Hawkins *et al.* 1984). This seems likely to be the case for adolescent deliberate self-harm, too (Hawton 1986). Group dystonic influences might reasonably be thought to be associated with more severe psychopathology, as has been argued for volatile substance abuse (see Hill 1989), though this assertion is supported only by clinical experience. Similar findings might be expected to apply to psychiatric pathology but the area is relatively unexplored. An exception is the study of Goodyer *et al.* (1991) which demonstrated an adverse effect of poor peer relations on outcome of depression in late child-

hood and early adolescence though whether these were cause or consequence could not be elucidated. Poor peer relationships may be a result of psychiatric disorder or an indicator of poor personality development but isolated clinical instances of adolescents being driven to suicide by peer group rejection, depression following the loss of a close friend or of dysmorphophobia apparently secondary to teasing are common enough to warrant further scientific enquiry of this source of social influence.

It is important to note that neither the adolescent peer group nor the way it impinges on social relationships should be conceptualized as homogeneous, whether by age or sex. For instance, in a study of late adolescent girls with high scores on a screening instrument for depression, Monck (1991) found differing patterns of confiding according to age. Throughout the age range 15–19 inclusive, these girls were much more likely to confide in their mothers and girlfriends than in boys. Only among the 19 year olds did the practice of confiding in a boyfriend rather than in a girlfriend or mother begin to become noticeable as a practice.

## Work

As with adults, there is an indication that unemployment has a deleterious effect on adolescent mental health (see also Chapter 21). Employment prospects are a common source of anxiety among adolescents (Porteous 1985). Studies of school leavers show a higher rate of minor psychiatric morbidity among the unemployed compared with employed (e.g. Stafford *et al.* 1980) and longitudinal approaches implicate unemployment as a causal factor rather than a consequence of earlier morbidity (Banks & Jackson 1982, Donovan *et al.* 1986). The authors of the latter study suggest the lack of general peer contact (not the lack of a confiding relationship) as an implicated variable.

## Life events

Events are discontinuous influences but some can, of course, indicate chronic, continuous processes, as remarked above with respect to divorce. Adolescents probably experience a high rate of events compared with young adults, certainly this was true of the 15–20-year-old girls studied by Monck & Dobbs (1985). Their study demonstrated the considerable problems of method in ascertaining life events experienced by an adolescent population. Parental report is inadequate as a source for any but severe events and the discrepancy between informant and parent increases with age. They argue strongly that checklist approaches are likely to be inadequate for use with adolescents. Goodyer *et al.* (1986), using an interview ultimately based on Coddington's scale, were unable to show any effect of age (over or under age 12) on the association of life events with psychiatric disorder in a clinic sample of children and young adolescents so that it may be reasonable to assume that the findings described by Cox (see Chapter 13) would hold for young teenagers.

In an interview study of a community sample of late teenage girls in London, Monck and her colleagues (E. Monck, personal communication 1991) were able to demonstrate an increased rate of recent life events in those girls who were diagnosed depressed at interview. However, this finding had no separate predictive power in identifying depressed girls when ratings of maternal depression, quality of relationship between mother and her husband/partner, and the quality of relationship between mother and daughter were taken into account. The conceptual difficulties associated with this area of research are highlighted by the fact that some life events were shared between mother and daughter (and might thus influence maternal mental state) and the possible mutual contamination of various measures of marital relationship, maternal mental state and life events.

That some life events have a direct impact on adolescent mental health is illustrated by the studies of teenage survivors of disasters. In spite of earlier scepticism, the clinical evidence that horrifying experiences which are beyond the usual can produce in school-age children the constellation of symptoms known as post-traumatic stress disorder (PTSD) is now very strong indeed (Pynoos 1990) (see also Chapter 27). Indeed, there are grounds for thinking that, among adolescent girls, it is the most likely pattern of psychological mor-

bidity after such an experience (Anthony 1986). Whereas some adolescents respond to disasters with a depressive reaction, the constellation of fear- and anxiety-centred features characteristic of PTSD is the most striking and frequent response. Yule *et al.* (1990), in their study of the effect of a maritime diaster on mid-adolescent girls, argue that, on the basis of what is known about the origins of fears and the components of PTSD, the most plausible mechanism linking the disaster event and the persisting psychological reaction is one of conditioned fear.

## Conclusion

This brief account, intentionally selective for adolescence and for major psychiatric (rather than social) pathology, can only draw upon a sparse scientific literature compared with what is available in studies of adults and younger children. Nevertheless, there are sufficient indicators that social factors are important, even crucial elements in the precipitation and perpetuation of much psychiatric disorder in adolescence. To quantify the magnitude of their impact would be artificial; they interact with constitutional variables and with each other in complex, transactional, systemic modes.

## References

Adams G. & Adams C. (1989) Developmental issues. In Hsu G. & Hersen M. (eds) *Recent Developments in Adolescent Psychiatry*, chap. 2. John Wiley, New York.

Anthony E.J. (ed.) (1986) Special section: children's reactions to severe stress. *Journal of the American Academy of Child Psychiatry* 25, 299–392.

Aries P. (1962) *Centuries of Childhood*. Jonathan Cape, London.

Banks M. & Jackson P. (1982) Unemployment and risk of minor psychiatric disorder in young people: cross-sectional and longitudinal evidence. *Psychological Medicine* 12, 789–798.

Bowden P., Touyz S., Rodriguez P., Hensley R. & Beumont P. (1989) Distorting patient or distorting instrument? Body shape disturbance in patients with anorexia nervosa and bulimia. *British Journal of Psychiatry* 155, 196–201.

Bruch H. (1974) *Eating Disorders*. Routledge and Kegan Paul, London.

Cairns E., McWhirter L., Barry R. & Duffy U. (1991) The development of psychological well-being in late adolescence. *Journal of Child Psychology and Psychiatry* 32, 635–643.

Coleman J. (1980) *The Nature of Adolescence*. Methuen, London.

Crisp A. (1980) *Anorexia Nervosa: Let Me Be*. Academic Press, London.

Crisp A. & Kalucy R. (1974) Aspects of the perceptual disorder in anorexia nervosa. *British Journal of Medical Psychology* 47, 349–361.

Donovan A., Oddy M., Pardoe R. & Ades A. (1986) Employment status and psychological well-being: a longitudinal study of 16-year-old school leavers. *Journal of Child Psychology and Psychiatry* 27, 65–76.

Dweck C.S. & Bush E. (1976) Sex differences in learned helplessness. I. Differential debilitation with peer and adult evaluators. *Developmental Psychology* 12, 147–156.

Dweck C.S., Davidson W., Nelson S. & Enna B. (1978) Sex differences in learned helplessness II. The contingencies of evaluative feedback in the classroom. III An experimental analysis. *Developmental Psychology* 14, 268–276.

Elkind D. (1967) Egocentrism in adolescence. *Child Development* 38, 1025–1034.

Fischer J. (1980) Reciprocity, agreement and family style in family systems with a disturbed and non-disturbed adolescent. *Journal of Youth and Adolescence* 9, 391–406.

Gath D., Cooper B., Gattoni F. & Rockett D. (1977) *Child Guidance and Delinquency in a London Borough*. Maudsley Monographs No. 24. Oxford University Press, London.

Ghodsian M. & Lambert L. (1978) Mum and Dad are not so bad: the views of sixteen-year-olds on how they get on with their parents. *Journal of the Association of Educational Psychologists* 4, 27–33.

Goodyer I., Germany E., Gowrusankur J. & Altham P. (1991) Social influences on the course of anxious and depressive disorders in school-age children. *British Journal of Psychiatry* 158, 676–684.

Goodyer I., Kolvin I. & Gatzanis S. (1986) Do age and sex influence the association between recent life events and psychiatric disorders in children and adolescents? – A controlled enquiry. *Journal of Child Psychology and Psychiatry* 27, 681–687.

Haley J. (1980) *Leaving Home*. McGraw-Hill, New York.

Hartlage S., Howard K. & Ostrov E. (1984) The mental health professional and the normal adolescent. In Offer D., Ostrov E. & Howard K. (eds) *Patterns of Adolescent Self-Image*. Jossey Bass, San Francisco.

Hartup W. (1983) Peer relations. In Mussen P. (ed.) *Handbook of Child Psychology: IV. Socialization, Personality and Social Development*. Wiley, New York.

Hawkins J.D., Lishner D. & Catalano R. (1984) Childhood predictors and the prevention of adolescent substance abuse. In Jones C.L. & Battjes R.J. (eds) *Etiology of Drug Abuse: Implications for Prevention*. NIDA Research Monograph 56. National Institute on Drug Abuse, Rockville, Maryland.

Hawton K. (1986) *Suicide and Attempted Suicide among Children and Adolescents*. Sage, London.

Heron J. & Leheup R. (1984) Happy families? *British Journal of Psychiatry* 145, 136–138.

Hill P. (1989) *Adolescent Psychiatry*. Churchill Livingstone, Edinburgh.

Hill P. (1993) Recent advances in selected aspects of adolescent development. *Journal of Child Psychology and Psychiatry* 34 (in press).

Hodges J. & Tizard B. (1989a) IQ and behavioural adjustment of ex-institutional adolescents. *Journal of Child Psychology and Psychiatry* 30, 53–75.

Hodges J. & Tizard B. (1989b) Social and family relationships of ex-institutional adolescents. *Journal of Child Psychology and Psychiatry* 30, 77–97.

Humphrey L.L. (1987) Comparison of bulimic-anorexic and nondistressed families using structural analysis of social behaviour. *Journal of the American Academy of Child Psychiatry* 26, 248–255.

Jacobs B. & Isaacs S. (1986) Pre-pubertal anorexia nervosa: a retrospective controlled study. *Journal of Child Psychology and Psychiatry* 27, 237–250.

Kandel D. & Davies M. (1982) Epidemiology of depressive mood in adolescents. *Archives of General Psychiatry* 39, 1205–1212.

Kashani J., Hoeper E., Beck N. *et al.* (1987) Personality, psychiatric disorders and parental attitude among a community sample of adolescents. *Journal of the American Academy of Child and Adolescent Psychiatry* 26, 879–885.

Lask B. & Bryant-Waugh R. (1990) Childhood onset anorexia nervosa. In Meadow R. (ed.) *Recent Advances in Paediatrics VIII*, chap. 2. Churchill Livingstone, Edinburgh.

Minuchin S., Rosman B. & Baker L. (1978) *Psychosomatic Families*. Harvard University Press.

Monck E. (1991) Patterns of confiding relationships among adolescent girls. *Journal of Child Psychology and Psychiatry* 32, 333–345.

Monck E. & Dobbs R. (1985) Measuring life events in an adolescent population: methodologic issues and related findings. *Psychological Medicine* 15, 841–850.

Nylander I. (1971) The feeling of being fat and dieting in a school population. *Acta Sociomedica Scandinavica* 3, 17–26.

Offer D. & Offer J. (1975) *From Teenage to Young Manhood*. Basic Books, New York.

Offer D., Ostrov E. & Howard K. (1981) The mental health professional's concept of the normal adolescent. *Archives of General Psychiatry* 38, 149–152.

Offord D., Boyle M., Szatmari P. *et al.* (1987) Ontario child health study. II Six month prevalence of disorder and rates of service utilization. *Archives of General Psychiatry* 44, 832–836.

Osborn S. & West D. (1980) Do delinquents really reform? *Journal of Adolescence* 3, 99–114.

Ostrov E., Offer D. & Howard K. (1989) Gender differences in adolescent symptomatology: a normative study. *Journal of the American Acadamy of Child and Adolescent Psychiatry* 28, 394–398.

Plapp J., Rey J., Stewart G., Bashir M. & Richards I. (1987) Ratings of psychosocial stressors in adolescence using DSM-III axis IV criteria. *Journal of the American Academy of Child and Adolescent Psychiatry* 26, 80–86.

Porteous M. (1985) Developmental aspects of adolescent problem disclosure in England and Ireland. *Journal of Child Psychology and Psychiatry* 26, 465–478.

Pynoos R. (1990) Post-traumatic stress disorder in children and adolescents. In Garfinkel B., Carlson G. & Weller E. (eds) *Psychiatric Disorders in Children and Adolescents*. W. B. Saunders, Philadelphia.

Reynolds D. & Cuttance P. (eds) (1991) *School Effectiveness*. Cassell, London.

Russell G., Campbell P. & Slade P. (1975) Experimental studies on the nature of the psychological disorder in anorexia nervosa. *Psychoneuroendocrinology* 1, 45–56.

Rutter M. (1979) *Changing Youth in a Changing Society*. Nuffield Provincial Hospitals Trust, London.

Rutter M. (1989) Pathways from childhood to adult life. *Journal of Child Psychiatry and Psychology* 30, 23–51.

Rutter M. & Giller H. (1983) *Juvenile Delinquency: Trends and Perspectives*. Penguin, Harmondsworth.

Rutter M., Graham P., Chadwick O. & Yule W. (1976) Adolescent turmoil: fact or fiction. *Journal of Child Psychology and Psychiatry* 17, 35–56.

Rutter M., Maughan B., Mortimore P. & Ouston J. (1979) *Fifteen Thousand Hours: Secondary Schools and their Effects on Children*. Open Books, London.

Schoenbach V., Kaplan B., Grimson R. & Wagner E. (1982) Use of a symptom scale to study the prevalence of a depressive syndrome in young adolescents. *American Journal of Epidemiology* 116, 791–800.

Solomon M. (1973) A developmental, conceptual premise for family therapy. *Family Process* 12, 179–188.

Stafford E., Jackson P. & Banks M. (1980) Employment, work involvement and mental health in less qualified young people. *Journal of Occupational Psychology* 53, 291–304.

Tizard B. & Hodges J. (1978) The effect of early institutional rearing on the development of eight-year-old children. *Journal of Child Psychology and Psychiatry* 19, 99–118.

Wallerstein J. (1985) Children of divorce: preliminary report of a ten-year follow-up of older children and adolescents. *Journal of the American Academy of Child Psychiatry* 24, 545–553.

Wallerstein J. & Kelly J. B. (1974) The effects of parental divorce: the adolescent experience. In Anthony E.J. & Koupernik C. (eds) *The Child in his Family*. John Wiley, New York.

Wallerstein J. & Kelly J. B. (1980) *Surviving the Breakup*. Grant McIntyre, London.

Yager J. (1982) Family issues in the pathogenesis of anorexia nervosa. *Psychosomatic Medicine* 44, 43–60.

Yule W., Udwin O. & Murdoch K. (1990) The 'Jupiter' sinking: effects on children's fears, depression and anxiety. *Journal of Child Psychology and Psychiatry* 31, 1051–1061.

# Chapter 15
# Social Factors in Forensic Psychiatry

PHILIP JOSEPH

## Introduction

Forensic psychiatry is concerned in its broadest sense with the interaction between law and psychiatry, a vast area demonstrated by the recent publication in the UK of the first major textbook on the subject comprising 141 contributors and 150 chapters (Bluglass & Bowden 1990).

The modern forensic psychiatrist is no longer confined to issues of insanity and criminal responsibility, but has helped broaden the legitimate concerns to include amongst others civil litigation, the psychiatry of disasters, and victimology. Nevertheless this chapter will revert to the traditional focus of the forensic psychiatrist, namely the mentally disordered offender, a victim of a cycle of social disadvantage causing, perpetuating and resulting in his or her position as a social 'outsider'.

The first part of the chapter examines social factors implicated in the development of criminal behaviour. The perspective is criminological, drawing primarily on the work of Farrington. Are these factors of relevance to the development of mental disorder? The work of Robins from the USA looking at childhood precursors of adult antisocial behaviour is of particular relevance. A consideration will then be given to some theories which seek to account for the development of criminal behaviour.

The second part of the chapter seeks to establish whether there is an association between mental disorder and criminal behaviour. This topic has generated a vast body of research by criminologists, psychologists and psychiatrists in the USA and UK, and an attempt will be made to draw some general conclusions from often contradictory findings.

Social considerations falling under the rubric of the criminalization of the mentally ill are dealt with in the third part of the chapter. Has the closure of psychiatric hospital beds under the policy of deinstitutionalization led to the translocation of the mentally ill in prison? It is difficult to carry out methodologically sound research in this area and a comparison of statistics from hospital and prison populations can be misleading. Some research, mainly from the USA, will be reviewed to explore this proposition, but hard facts are difficult to disentangle from the polemic which is rife in this area. If the displaced hospital patients are not in prison, perhaps they are living on the streets. A brief review of the studies of the homeless mentally ill and their criminality will follow.

The fourth part of the chapter looks at the ways the mentally disordered offender can be diverted from the criminal justice system, thereby highlighting the balance which exists between factors which criminalize the mentally ill and those which medicalize criminal behaviour.

The final part of the chapter examines the settings available for the treatment of the mentally disordered offender, bearing in mind that imprisonment itself may exacerbate social disadvantage and mental disorder. In the light of recent prison disturbances, should alternatives to custody for mentally disordered offenders be sought whenever possible, or should existing medical facilities within prison be improved in order to provide humane treatment for those deemed unsuitable for admission to conventional hospital-based psychiatric services?

## Social factors and criminal behaviour

A substantial minority of individuals are convicted of a criminal offence during their lifetime. Farrington (1981) estimated prevalence figures based on 1977 conviction rates for non-motoring standard list offences in England and Wales of approximately 43% and 15% for men and women respectively. He commented: 'in the foreseeable future ... unconvicted males will be deviant in a statistical sense'.

It is difficult to identify specific social factors predicting such a widespread event, therefore it becomes necessary to concentrate on the more severe end of the offending spectrum. Farrington *et al.* (1986) have reviewed the different research strategies used in studying criminal behaviour. The three most common research designs are cross-sectional, longitudinal and experimental. Of these, longitudinal studies have been most successful in advancing knowledge of criminal careers. They conclude that offending is concentrated in a small deviant minority of high-rate offenders. The earlier they commence delinquent activity, the more offences they commit and the longer their criminal careers. Participation in offending peaks between the ages of 15 and 18 years. Males have a higher rate of offending than females regardless of age and ethnicity.

An example of an important longitudinal study is the work of Farrington & West (1990), in which 411 randomly selected juveniles in a south London area have been followed up from age 8 to 32 years. Four independent factors were identified as predicting offending at 21 years:
1 Socioeconomic deprivation.
2 Family history of criminality.
3 Poor parental child rearing.
4 School problems, for example low IQ.
The relative importance of these factors in influencing criminal behaviour is difficult to quantify. A term such as poor parental child rearing marks variation within it, ranging from passive neglect to active physical abuse or a combination of both. Clearly the influence of any one of the above factors will depend upon its severity and its interaction with psychological factors within the individual.

So far there has been no mention of mental disorder. The vast majority of criminals do not suffer from mental disorder, yet some of the factors identified in shaping a criminal career resur-

face when considering the development of some forms of mental disorder. These will now be examined.

### Social factors and antisocial personality disorder

Social disadvantage is important in the development of all forms of mental disorder, particularly where psychiatric diagnosis meets social problems, namely the areas of conduct disorder, antisocial personality disorder, alcoholism, and drug dependence. For the purposes of this chapter attention will be focused on antisocial personality disorder. The effects of social factors on classification of personality disorder are discussed in Chapter 8.

Section 1(2) of the Mental Health Act 1983 defines psychopathic disorder as 'a persistent disorder or disability of mind (whether or not including significant impairment of intelligence) which results in abnormally aggressive or seriously irresponsible conduct on the part of the person concerned'. The legal term psychopathic disorder may encompass all forms of personality disorder but is usually applied to those individuals who come within the psychiatric diagnosis of psychopathic or antisocial personality disorder.

The legal definition of psychopathic disorder suffers from the same limitation as the psychiatric definition, namely that '... mental abnormality is inferred from behaviour, while antisocial behaviour is explained by mental abnormality' (Wootton 1959). The same circularity is evident in the childhood diagnosis of conduct disorder, which is partly defined as a group of 'disorders mainly involving aggressive and destructive behaviour and disorders involving delinquency' (World Health Organization 1978). Thus delinquency becomes part of the definition of the disorder forming a link between criminal behaviour and mental disorder in childhood. Is there an association between childhood conduct disorder and adult antisocial personality disorder? The work of Robins (1966, 1978) is seminal in this respect.

Robins' original study was a follow-up of patients who attended the Municipal Child Guidance Clinic of St Louis, USA, in the 1920s (Robins 1966). The study arose fortuitously at a time when the clinic's records were about to be destroyed. Four hundred and thirty-six individuals who had been seen as children at the clinic were followed up over 30 years later.

The major finding of the study was that all types of antisocial behaviour in childhood predict a high level of antisocial behaviour in adults. Behaviours such as truancy, fighting, lying, vandalism and delinquency in childhood significantly predicted adult behaviour problems such as violence, alcoholism, drug abuse, job difficulties and delinquency. Further conclusions were drawn from the study:

1 Adult antisocial behaviour virtually requires childhood antisocial behaviour.

2 Most antisocial children do not become antisocial adults.

3 A variety of childhood antisocial behaviour is better than any particular behaviour at predicting adult antisocial behaviour.

4 Childhood behaviour is a better predictor than family background or social class of rearing.

5 Social class makes little contribution to the prediction of serious adult antisocial behaviour.

Although childhood antisocial behaviour was the most important predictor of adult antisocial behaviour, Robins also found various family variables had predictive value. These included an antisocial or alcoholic parent of either sex, divorce or separation of parents, living apart from both parents, poverty, number of siblings, and parental discipline. Robins' work carries greater weight as she has been able to replicate her findings in three other studies consisting of men of different racial backgrounds growing up and living in different parts of the USA.

Farrington (1990) has also recognized the importance of childhood conduct disorder in the development of adult criminality. He identified two further predictors of adult criminality:

1 Hyperactivity or attention deficit disorder in childhood.

2 Antisocial behaviour in childhood.

It is clear then that the work of Robins and West & Farrington overlaps to a considerable degree and can be summarized in Table 15.1. Social disadvantage in childhood is important in the development of criminal behaviour. In some in-

**Table 15.1** Childhood predictors of adult criminal and antisocial behaviour

*Childhood predictors of criminal behaviour*
Socioeconomic deprivation
Poor parental child rearing
Family history of criminality
School problems
Hyperactivity – impulsivity – attention deficit
Antisocial child behaviour

*Childhood predictors of adult antisocial behaviour*
Antisocial child behaviour
School problems
Socioeconomic deprivation
Divorce/separation of parents
Living apart from both parents
Poor parental discipline

*Note*: low social class is not predictive in either group

dividuals the interaction between social factors and psychological factors within the child result in the development of childhood conduct disorder which is crucial for the further development of antisocial personality disorder in adulthood.

### Theories and explanations

These studies have highlighted associations between social factors and the development of antisocial personality disorder and criminal behaviour. They have not sought to identify the possible mechanisms for this. Rutter & Giller (1983) have reviewed some of the theories from a biological, psychological and sociological perspective, which seek to explain the development of criminal behaviour. Any theory worth its salt has to try to account for some basic observations about delinquency. For example:

1 Most delinquents are male.

2 Half of all delinquents never return to court.

3 Delinquency decreases in early adult life.

4 The crime rate has risen dramatically in the last 50 years.

There is a need to move away from the notion of a single unifying cause of crime to multifactorial explanations. The question to be asked is not 'why is A delinquent and not B?', but 'why are A and B delinquent in some circumstances and not others?'.

This stresses the interaction between the individual and his social environment. It also must be recognized that factors which initiate criminal behaviour may differ from those which maintain it.

Sociological theories such as Merton's (1957) 'strain' theory, based on Durkheim's concept of 'anomie' postulate that delinquency results from the strain caused by the anomic disjuncture between cultural goals and the means available for their achievement. It is a class-based theory which fails to take into account the weak association between social class and criminal behaviour. An example of social learning theory is Sutherland's theory of 'differential association' (Sutherland & Cressey 1974) which postulates that criminal behaviour is learned through association with those who commit crimes. These two theories have been combined by Cloward & Ohlin (1960), who suggest that strain or anomie provides the potential for the development of delinquency whose expression is then dependent on the availability of illegitimate means and the opportunity for learning deviant roles.

Other social theories stress the importance of subcultural (Mays 1972), situational (Gibbons 1971) and labelling (West & Farrington 1973) effects on the development of offending. The influence of an individual's peer group, the specific situations which promote delinquency and the stigma of being labelled as deviant or delinquent are factors which initiate and maintain criminal behaviour.

Alternative social theories assume that everyone is born with the capacity to offend, and ask instead how individuals learn not to offend, which they postulate is through a process of internalized controls. Choice theories (Clarke 1982) postulate that individuals weigh up various factors before deciding whether to commit a particular offence. The focus is on the criminal event itself, emphasizing the individual's current circumstances and the immediate features of the setting. The 'new criminology' (Taylor *et al.* 1974) goes futher, focusing on the political economy of crime and the ways in which criminal laws maintain social divisions. The potential absurd end point of this approach is that 'there would be no crime without criminal laws'.

A complete contrast to these social theories is provided by biological theorists such as Eysenck (1977). He argues that antisocial criminal and psychopathic behaviour is related to genetically determined personality attributes which are modified by the social environment. Robins (1978) also recognizes the importance of personality characteristics and draws on life events research to postulate that the child's exposure to unusually severe stresses or an excess number of harmful life events in the family may promote childhood antisocial behaviour.

Psychoanalytical theories postulate that children are born with unconscious primitive urges which are modified by the development of internalized moral controls through the process of identification with parents. A failure in this process can lead to faulty personality development which in turn promotes antisocial behaviour. Psychoanalytical thinking stresses that unconscious mechanisms and intrapsychic conflict determine the nature and quality of delinquent behaviour which may have symbolic meaning for the individual. There is a lack of empirical substantiation of the role of the unconscious in delinquency and generally psychoanalytical theories have fallen out of favour in this area.

Finally the microsocial approach of Patterson (1982) deserves mention. He conducted a detailed analysis of natural family interactions within the home. He observed that parents of aggressive children tended to punish deviant behaviour more than parents of non-aggressive children, yet this seemed to encourage rather than suppress aggression. Family interaction generally consisted of frequent coercive interchanges with a lack of pleasurable or warm exchanges. He postulated that these families provided an inadequate and ineffective set of conditions for the learning of prosocial and the avoidance of antisocial behaviour.

In conclusion, theories and explanations abound in the study of antisocial behaviour and delinquency. No single theory is sufficient; the requirement is for a formulation which takes into account genetic, family and sociocultural factors and which is rooted in high quality empirical research.

## Criminal behaviour and mental disorder – an association?

In the eighteenth and early nineteenth centuries as forensic psychiatry began to develop, it was an accepted and undisputed belief that the mentally ill, having been robbed of reason by an unknown cerebral disease, were unpredictable, dangerous and violent to a great degree. An intimate relationship was assumed to exist between mental disorder and crime. Inferences were drawn from individual case studies, the more notorious the better, and famous cases which helped shape English legal concepts of criminal responsibility and insanity, such as Hadfield, Oxford and McNaughton, reinforced the link between mental illness and violence. Contemporary cases such as Peter Sutcliffe, the Yorkshire Ripper (Bavidge 1989), and Dennis Nilsen (Masters 1985) have done little to dispel this view, particularly in the public's mind.

Gradually the belief that mental disorder and crime, in particular violence, are inextricably linked has been challenged by the publication of a number of large-scale quantitative surveys. They can be broadly divided into those looking at populations of psychiatric patients to see how many have committed offences, for which they may or may not have been prosecuted, and estimates of mental disorder amongst prison populations charged or convicted of offences. These studies are highly relevant in the light of the current policy of treating the mentally ill in the community wherever possible. The public need to know whether their fears that hospitals will discharge a group of potentially violent people into their midst are justified. Some of these attitudinal issues are discussed later in the chapter.

### Studies of psychiatric populations

#### PRE-ADMISSION

There is evidence that mental illness is associated with a substantial risk of criminal behaviour prior to hospital admission. Admissions under the provisions of section 136 of the Mental Health Act 1983 usually result from some form of behaviour, whether violent or not, which has come to the attention of the police. Often the behaviour may be no more than a social nuisance, contravening the less serious sections of the Public Order Act 1986.

Szmukler *et al.* (1981) confirmed earlier findings (Rollin 1969, Kelleher & Copeland 1972) that patients brought to hospital by the police using their powers under section 136 are predominantly single, socially isolated, unsettled, and suffering from chronic mental illness, usually schizophrenia, with numerous previous hospital admissions and frequently with a criminal record.

Section 136 admissions form a minority of all admissions and cannot be seen as representative. However, Levine (1970) calculated that 70% of admissions to a state hospital exhibited behaviour considered a violation of the criminal law according to the local attorney. Lagos *et al.* (1977) in New Jersey studied 321 admissions, excluding those diagnosed as suffering from personality disorder and substance abuse, and found that 18% had been accompanied by actual violence and a further 18% had induced a fear of violence in others. A further American study by Post *et al.* (1980) looking at domestic violence estimated that 23% of patients had assaulted their partners at some stage. Tardiff & Sweillam (1980) analysed the records of 9000 patients admitted to public hospitals on Long Island and found that 12–14% had been assaultive in the two weeks before admission; schizophrenics were overrepresented in this group. In a study of first-episode schizophrenics admitted to hospital in the UK, 94 (37%) had been violent in the previous month (Johnstone *et al.* 1986) and 22% had been in contact with the police (MacMillan & Johnson 1987).

#### HOSPITAL VIOLENCE

Folkard's (1959) classic study of the sociology of violence at Netherne Hospital showed that violence occurred during the early stages of the hospital admission and was most likely to be perpetrated by schizophrenics acting on hallucinatory or delusional experiences. Numerous later studies have confirmed these findings, for example Tanke & Yesavage (1985) in the USA, and Fottrell (1980) and Noble & Rodger (1989) in the UK. The study of Noble & Rodger was carried out at the Bethlem Royal & Maudsley Hospitals and showed that most violent incidents were minor in nature, only 2% resulting in major physical injuries requiring subsequent medical treatment. However, serious violence including homicide, in hospital, although extremely rare, is not unknown. Ekblom (1970) identified 25 serious assaults in Swedish hospitals between 1955 and 1964, of which 8 resulted in fatalities, 7 on other patients.

Most studies of hospital violence are retrospective case note or violent incident register analyses and may suffer from inaccurate reporting. One prospective study by Edwards *et al.* (1988) however confirms the findings. Two studies disagree with the overrepresentation of schizophrenics in violent hospital incidents. One found an excess of manic patients (McNeil & Binder 1987), the other organic and personality disorder diagnoses (Evenson *et al.* 1974).

Finally, there is some evidence that imminent discharge from hospital may precipitate a violent incident amongst patients attached to the hospital and fearful of living in the community. Stein (1982) described one case of serious assault and Geller (1984) two cases of arson in psychotic patients who were predischarge or recently discharged. This problem may be exacerbated as the policy of deinstitutionalization is pursued.

COMMUNITY

The policy of closing the long-stay mental hospitals pursued vigorously in the USA and latterly in the UK has provided the impetus to assess the impact of transferring large numbers of previously hospitalized psychiatric patients to the community. This has been well reviewed by Rabkin (1979).

Early surveys of psychiatric patients discharged from hospitals in the USA showed arrest rates for offences lower than in the general population (Cohen & Freeman 1945, Brill & Malzberg 1962). This may have been due to their careful selection for discharge and subsequent effective supervision. Later surveys, however, have been less optimistic. Zitrin *et al.* (1976) in New York followed up 433

schizophrenics for 2 years and found 10% were arrested for violent and 11% for non-violent offences. The schizophrenics were mostly young men, often abusing drugs and alcohol. Their arrest rates were higher than the rates in the general population for the area, but lower for those suffering from alcoholism or drug dependence. In California, Sosowsky (1980) found that 25% of a predominantly schizophrenic population were convicted of a violent and 23% of a non-violent offence during an 8-year period. Allowing for age, sex and ethnic origin, patients had higher arrest rates than the general public.

Steadman *et al.* (1978) have shown that arrest rates are higher in ex-hospital patients than the general population of New York State and are increasing, but have challenged the interpretation that this points to an association between mental disorder and crime. They point out that the proportion of patients entering hospital who had a previous history of arrest rose from 15% in 1947 to 40% in 1975. One of the best predictors of future offending is past offending, therefore the apparent increase in arrest rates was simply a reflection of their recidivism. When the sample was divided according to the presence or absence of an arrest record the rates of subsequent arrest had remained stable. Although the arrest rates in the general population had been rising as well, it had not risen as much as the hospital population which suggests that hospitals might have been taking a different clientele, perhaps of patients who would otherwise have gone to prison (Melick *et al.* 1979). In other words, it may have been that hospitals in the USA were previously medicalizing criminal behaviour but the balance has now shifted. This will be discussed in more detail in the next section.

An important Swedish longitudinal study (Lindqvist & Allebeck 1990) has followed up 644 schizophrenics in Stockholm over 15 years and found a similar crime rate for males compared to the general population, but schizophrenic women had double the crime rate of normals. However, when violent offences only were considered there was a four-fold overrepresentation of schizophrenics, although most offences were of a minor nature.

Finally a dramatic opportunity to observe the consequences of the wholesale precipitous discharge of a group of convicted psychiatric patients from a state mental hospital was provided by the US Supreme Court in 1966. The detention of a convicted epileptic Johnnie K. Baxstrom in Dannemara State Mental Hospital following the expiry of his prison sentence was declared illegal; his release and that of another 920 men and 47 women was ordered, some to civil mental hospitals but many to the community. The vast majority suffered from schizophrenia or other psychoses (Steadman & Halfon 1971). Twenty-five per cent had committed homicide or other serious assault and they had spent an average of 18 years in prison or hospital at the time of release. Over the next 4 years they did better than other chronic adult mental patients in New York State and their level of dangerousness was surprisingly low.

Cocozza & Steadman (1974) identified variables associated with re-offending, namely previous criminal history and age. Those who had an early onset of offending with convictions for violence and were aged under 50 years at the time of release were more likely to re-offend; factors which also predict recidivism in criminals without mental disorder. Thornberry & Jacoby (1979) were able to replicate the Baxstrom study following a similar abrupt discharge of 586 patients from Fairview, a maximum security hospital in Pennsylvania, in 1971. Twenty-four per cent were arrested within the next 4 years, comparable to the arrest rate for released prisoners.

These last two studies have provided support for the view that 'there is no consistent evidence that the true prevalence rate of criminal behaviour among former mental patients exceeds the true prevalence rate of criminal behaviour among the general population, matched for demographic factors and prior criminal history' (Monahan & Steadman 1983).

## Studies of offender populations

In the USA only 1% of arrests end in a prison sentence (Stone 1984) and selection bias operates at every level of the criminal justice system. Similar bias is likely in this country and it may result in an overrepresentation of the mentally disordered in prison for reasons such as their greater ease of detection rather than any direct association between criminal behaviour and mental disorder. The most unbiased offender population to study would be a consecutive sample of attenders at court, although even this would lead to bias from those offenders who escape detection.

Psychiatric examinations have been carried out on two large samples of offenders appearing at the Court of General Sessions in New York. Bromberg & Thompson (1937) reported 9958 examinations between 1932 and 1935 and Messinger & Apfelburg (1961) an unspecified number between 1935 and 1957. The studies showed similar results, a level of psychosis of around $1-1.5\%$ and mental handicap at 2%. Serious psychiatric morbidity is of roughly the same prevalence as in the general population. The studies differed widely in their prevalence of psychopathic disorder, making interpretation of their figures difficult.

Bearing the caveats about bias in mind, most studies of offending and mental disorder have been conducted in prison populations which can be divided into remand and sentenced prisoners.

### REMAND PRISONERS

There has been no national survey in the UK of mental disorder within the remand population. However, there is good reason to believe that the prevalence of all types of mental abnormality is high, especially in London (Gibbens *et al.* 1977).

A study carried out in Brixton prison, a large remand prison in south London, systematically examined the records of 1241 men (Taylor & Gunn 1984) from whom a sample of 203 were interviewed (Taylor 1985). The prevalence of psychosis was 8.7%, of whom 70% were schizophrenic. Of those remanded for homicide the prevalence of schizophrenia was 11%, a substantial overrepresentation compared to the general population. A further 9% of the total sample were suffering from the effects of drug or alcohol withdrawal.

SENTENCED PRISONERS

Coid (1984) has compared the prevalence rates of mental disorder in 11 surveys of sentenced prisoners spanning 62 years in the UK and USA. Generally major psychosis was no more common than in the general population, but mental handicap, epilepsy and substance abuse were overrepresented. However, there was enormous variation between the surveys, for example a range from 5% to 78% for a diagnosis of personality disorder. This probably reflects different methodology and diagnostic criteria across the studies.

The most comprehensive study of sentenced prisoners in England and Wales has examined a 5% sample of the total sentenced population (Gunn *et al.* 1991). Of 1769 male prisoners, 37% had a psychiatric disorder, of whom 34 (2%) had psychoses and 15 (0.8%) had organic brain disorders, a total of 2.8% with serious mental illness. A further 407 (23%) had a primary diagnosis of alcohol or drug dependence, 177 (10%) personality disorder and 105 (6%) neurotic disorder. The authors judged that 52 (3%) required transfer to hospital for psychiatric treatment.

Finally mention must be made of Hafner & Boker's large-scale survey of crimes of violence by mentally abnormal offenders in West Germany (1982). They examined 533 mentally ill or defective individuals who had committed a crime of violence against the life of another person over a ten-year period commencing 1955. A crime of violence was defined as 'an attack on a human being which either led to the death of the victim or would have done so if circumstances outside the control of the person committing the attack had not intervened' (Hafner & Boker 1982a).

Only those suffering from a major mental disorder, namely psychosis, severe brain damage, epilepsy or mental handicap, were included. Those with a primary diagnosis of substance abuse and psychopathy were excluded. This group was then compared with convicted mentally normal offenders, non-violent mentally abnormal individuals both in hospital and in the community, and the general population over the age of criminal responsibility. The study produced a wealth of data and results but only a few conclusions can be presented here.

1 During the study period mentally abnormal violent offenders represented 3% of the total number of comparable violent offenders. According to the authors this is a comparable figure to the percentage of mentally abnormal individuals in the general population and they conclude that 'the mentally abnormal in general are not more likely and are in fact less likely to commit violent crime than are the mentally normal' (Hafner & Boker 1982b).

2 Fifty-three per cent of the mentally abnormal violent offenders had a diagnosis of schizophrenia, an overrepresentation compared to mentally abnormal non-offenders. The violent schizophrenics more often suffered delusions that were systematized with themes such as jealousy and persecution compared to the non-violent schizophrenics. In about 50% of violent offenders there was a delusional relationship between offender and victim. Taylor (1985) found a similar result in her survey of violent schizophrenics on remand: 46% were probably or definitely motivated by their psychotic symptoms.

3 The risk of violence in schizophrenia was calculated at 0.05%. This corresponds to five violent offenders per 10 000 suffering from schizophrenia. For affective psychoses the risk was 0.006%. The risk of suicide was vastly increased, by a factor of 100 in schizophrenia and 10 000 in affective psychoses, compared to homicidal violence.

4 When compared to the general population the age of onset of offending was significantly higher in the mentally abnormal violent group and tended to occur a number of years after the onset of the illness. This has been confirmed by Gibbens & Robertson (1983). Taylor & Parrott (1988) have shown that the proportion of offenders with mental disorder increases with age.

It is difficult to draw any specific conclusions from the disparate body of research reviewed here which seeks to establish a link between criminal behaviour and mental disorder. Part of the problem is that research may be conducted from a criminological or psychiatric perspective and results will tend to reflect a fundamental difference in approach (Wessely & Taylor 1991). In general most offenders do not suffer from mental disorder and most mentally disordered individuals do not commit offences. Generally mentally disordered offenders have more in common with other offenders than with mentally disordered non-offenders. The main area of overlap between offending and mental disorder is for those individuals suffering from psychopathic personality disorder, alcoholism and drug abuse (Guze 1976).

Nevertheless, there is a small but important group of violent, mentally ill, mainly schizophrenic, offenders whose violence is primarily a consequence of the psychotic symptoms they experience.

### Criminalization of the mentally ill

'Since 1954, 75 000 patients have been discharged from long stay beds in psychiatric hospitals. Where have they all gone? – those that are not dead that is' (Weller & Weller 1988). According to the Wellers there is only one answer – prison.

The purpose of this section is to examine the proposition that the closure of long-stay psychiatric hospitals through the policy of deinstitutionalization has led to the translocation of large numbers of mentally disordered offenders in prison. The notion of 'transcarceration' – the shift of this population from one institution to another – is not new. In 1939 Lionel Penrose, a devotee of social hygiene theory, who firmly believed mental disorder predisposed to crime, published a comparative study which included data on mental institution and prison populations in various European countries. He found an inverse relationship between the number of people in institutions for the insane and mentally defective and the number of sentenced prisoners. He concluded '. . . there is a definite incompatibility between the development of mental health services and the need for accommodation in prisons' (Penrose 1939).

Penrose himself stressed the need for caution in interpreting his findings and recommended more detailed research; however, he later stated: 'the prevalence of serious crimes, especially those which imply violence against the person, appears to be much more marked in countries which provide relatively few beds for mental patients' (Penrose 1943).

Penrose makes two assumptions that can be criticized. First that the amount of crime and mental disorder in a country can be measured by looking at the numbers in mental institutions and prisons, and secondly that an inference can be drawn from a seemingly inverse relationship between them.

Nevertheless, Penrose's assertion has achieved the status of a law enthusiastically adopted by those opposed to the policy of deinstitutionalization. Weller & Weller (1988) plotted residents in psychiatric hospitals from 1950 to 1984 against the number of prison inmates. They found a straight line best fit and a correlation coefficient of $-0.94$. They commented 'Of course an association does not establish a causal relationship but it is difficult to put forward convincing explanations for this exceedingly strong relationship, probably unprecedented in demographic data, except by postulating there is some decanting from the psychiatric hospitals to the prisons'.

Weller (1989) goes further, pointing out that as psychiatric hospitals close, the British Government is embarking on a large-scale prison building programme, using the site of recently closed Banstead Hospital for one of the new prisons.

It is unfortunate that the views of Penrose have been retrieved from obscurity to fuel this debate, because they are based on the outdated presumption that a strong association exists between mental disorder and crime which evidence shows is not the case.

Nevertheless there is mounting concern about the fate of patients discharged into the community from long-stay mental hospitals, both in the UK (Lowry 1989) and the USA (Jones 1983). The increasing number of homeless people on the streets of major cities is assumed to include recently discharged psychiatric patients amongst their swollen ranks serving as a vivid reminder of the failure of community care. It does not seem unreasonable to assume that some of them will subsequently become ensnared by the criminal justice system and end up in prison.

These two propositions will now be examined in some detail. First that there has been a shift of population from one institutional setting to another – the transcarceration hypothesis. Secondly, that the homeless contain large numbers of previously hospitalized psychiatric patients.

*Transcarceration hypothesis*

This section inevitably requires consideration of numbers to compare trends in the institutional population. Figures for the USA will be presented first since their policy of deinstitutionalization has taken place earlier and more rapidly than the programme in the UK.

There has been a dramatic shift in institutional populations in the USA over the last two decades. Steadman *et al.* (1984) write: 'at the end of 1968, there were 399 000 patients in state mental hospitals and 168 000 inmates in state prisons. Within a decade, the hospital population fell 64% to 147 000 and the prison population rose 65% to 277 000'. This dramatic increase in the prison population seems even more significant given that it had remained virtually constant in the decade prior to 1968.

Deinstitutionalization occurred rapidly across the USA fuelled by concern for the civil rights of the mentally ill, therapeutic optimism due to pharmacological advances, more stringent admission criteria with greater legal safeguards, and a shift of funding from hospitals to the community (Gudeman & Shore 1984). The closure programme comprised two distinct phases. First the discharge of long-stay patients into the community with hospital back-up for the new community facilities. Secondly, an overall decline in hospital admissions with emphasis on short-term crisis-led admissions and an avoidance of potentially lengthy admissions. These phases have been referred to as 'opening the back doors' and 'closing the front doors' respectively (Steadman & Morrissey 1984).

The transcarceration hypothesis requires evidence of two separate populations in prison, reflecting the phases described. The first consists of inmates who were previously psychiatric patients before the process of deinstitutionalization began. The second comprises a group of mentally disordered offenders with no previous psychiatric hospitalization who are being imprisoned. The implication with the second group is that previously they would have gone to hospital, a premise very difficult to prove hence the lack of research in this area. More attention has been paid to the group of previously hospitalized patients and some of the research has already been reviewed in the previous section. Generally it has shown that although arrest rates for previously hospitalized psychiatric patients may be higher than in the general population, it is still only a minority who are arrested for offences and they tend to have previous criminal histories. There is no evidence to support any large-scale transfer of psychiatric patients from hospital to prison, leading Teplin (1985) to conclude that the criminalization of the mentally ill is a dangerous misconception.

Turning to the position in England and Wales, a policy of community care has existed since 1959 reflecting the therapeutic optimism created by the introduction of phenothiazines in the mid 1950s. The 1962 Hospital Plan envisaged a massive reduction in hospital beds based on Tooth & Brooke's influential report (1961). The political conviction that the old mental hospitals no longer provided acceptable care was proclaimed by Enoch Powell in his famous 'Water Towers' speech delivered to the MIND Annual General Meeting in March 1961. This policy has recently been restated in the Government's response to the report 'Community care – agenda for action' (Griffiths 1988).

The move to the community, as well as being based on ideological grounds may have also reflected the desire to reduce investment in the country's large dilapidated Victorian mental hospitals and to fund the 'cheaper option' of treatment in the community with relatively low-cost medicines (Jones 1988). Furthermore, it must not be forgotten that the move from hospitals to the community was to some extent patient led. As Rollin (1969) pointed out: 'with a great sense of urgency ward doors were unlocked and blocks removed from windows . . . as freedom came in through the open doors security went out through the windows'. In other words patients voted with their feet and rejected hospital treatment which previously they had received compulsorily.

Anecdotal reports supporting the transcarceration hypothesis have been provided by doctors working in the Prison Medical Service who state they are seeing former mental patients appearing in prison with greater frequency, but what evidence in this country exists to support this view? Fig. 15.1 charts the decline in the mental hospital and mental handicap hospital population and the rise in the remand and sentenced prison population from 1962 to 1986. The combined psychiatric inpatient population fell from 196 234 to 100 863, a 49% reduction. The combined prison population rose from 31 063 to 46 974, an increase of 51%. Although the percentage changes are very similar the gross numbers differ widely – a 15 911 increase in prisoners and a 95 371 decrease in all patients. Thus this initial crude look at the figures shows clearly there has been no wholesale shift of psychiatric patients to prison (Fowles 1990).

Gross trends can be misleading. It is necessary to divide the prison population into its two distinct subgroups, those on remand awaiting trial or sentence and those who are serving a sentence. We shall see later that mentally ill offenders might well be remanded in custody for the preparation of psychiatric reports even when charged with relatively minor offences for which they would be unlikely to receive a custodial sentence, hence the mentally disordered may appear disproportionately in the remand population.

The number of prisoners under sentence increased from 28 258 in 1962 to 36 655 in 1986, while the remand population rose much faster from 2805 to 10 319 over the same period. Is this due to an influx of the mentally disordered? If one looks at the number of individuals remanded for the preparation of psychiatric reports, the answer appears to be no. In 1960 about 6000 reports were prepared, increasing to a peak of 14 000 in 1970, with a steady decline back to a figure of approximately 6000 in 1988/89. These figures have been taken from the annual reports of the Prison Department for the relevant years. Although the prevalence rates of mental disorder are higher in the remand population than the general population (Taylor 1985), this does not answer the question whether the figure has been recently increasing or whether rates of mental disorder have always been high.

The figures considered so far chart the decline in psychiatric hospital population which relates mainly to the phase of deinstitutionalization termed 'opening the back doors'. In the USA there has also been a decline in admissions to hospital. This has not occurred here. There has been a rise in

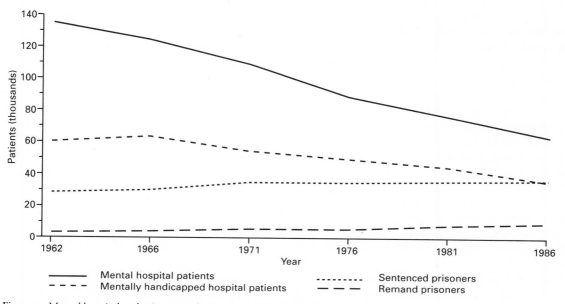

Fig. 15.1 Mental hospital and prison populations in England and Wales, 1962–86.

annual admissions to psychiatric hospitals, including mental handicap hospitals, to a total of nearly
250 000 per annum in 1986. It is not possible
to state how many of these admissions are readmissions of the same patient during the year,
but it is clear that psychiatric hospitals are still
admitting patients; the 'closing the front door'
phase has not developed as far as in the USA.
Nevertheless if the total population is declining
whilst the number of admissions is increasing, this
suggests there has been a shift to short-term admissions for the purpose of crisis intervention or
brief respite care.

Annual receptions into prison have also risen
both for sentenced and remand prisoners, with
figures of 86 153 and 75 657 respectively in 1986
(Fowles 1990). How many of the prison receptions in one year are also admitted to psychiatric
hospital in the same year? Unfortunately this
question is yet to be answered; a longitudinal
study of the institutional careers of patients is
required. In the meantime, an indirect answer can
be provided by looking at one basic demographic
characteristic about hospital and prison populations, namely their sex. During the decline in
hospital populations the sex ratio has remained
virtually constant, 58% female, 42% male. In
contrast women comprise a very small proportion
of both the sentenced and remand populations of
prisons, about 5%. Turning to annual admissions
to hospital, the increases in receptions of male
and female patients are largely in step with each
other, apart from an increase in male admissions
recently. Receptions of sentenced prisoners show
a greater increase for men over women, and for
remands a plateau for men and a decrease for
women. At no stage does the sex distribution
of the prison population compare with that of
hospitals.

In conclusion, an analysis of population trends
in mental hospitals and prison provides little evidence for the transcarceration hypothesis. The
increase in the remand and sentenced prison population cannot be accounted for by admission or
discharge policies of psychiatric hospitals. Other
factors such as the tendency to impose longer and
more frequent custodial sentences for serious offences, for example, for rape, and the increased

committal of offences to the crown court previously dealt with summarily, such as theft and
assault, superimposed on a dramatic increase in
the crime rate over the last 20 years has largely
accounted for the increase in both the sentenced
and remand populations.

Yet the nagging feeling remains that there are
mentally disordered offenders who previously
have or would have been admitted to hospital,
who now face rejection by psychiatric services.
Some evidence for this view is provided by Coid
(1988) who carried out a retrospective case note
study of all (362) mentally disordered men remanded to Winchester prison for psychiatric reports over the 5 years 1979–83. He found that
20% were rejected for treatment by their catchment area hospital, particularly those with chronic
psychoses or mental handicap. They posed the
least threat to the community yet were more likely
to receive a custodial sentence. He then compared
rejection rates across the two health regions which
received most of the referrals. The region without
a secure unit rejected significantly more referrals
than the region with such a unit, and referred
more prisoners to special hospitals. Coid felt the
attitudes of hospital staff was an important factor
as patients from the more rejecting region were
perceived as being potentially disruptive and aggressive and more likely to be labelled as having
psychopathic or personality disorder. He concluded: 'by finding their way into prison many are
obtaining the only care and treatment anyone is
prepared to offer them'.

Coid's study is retrospective in nature and is
therefore limited in drawing conclusions about
changes in the institutional careers of his sample
over time. By comparing practices across two
health regions however, he shows important differences between them. Clearly one region is less
willing to admit patients than the other, but
whether that implies the mentally ill of that region
have been criminalized is another matter. Coid
has little to say about the previous psychiatric
history of his sample, but does report that 82 of
the men had a history of absconding from hospital
or persistently failing to attend all outpatient
appointments. In addition, 57 had a history of
violence or seriously disruptive behaviour while

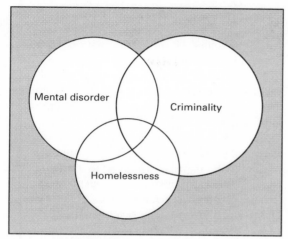

**Fig. 15.2** Relationship between mental disorder, criminality and homelessness.

in an NHS psychiatric hospital. In that respect they may resemble the patients referred to as 'incurable or incorrigible' (Rollin 1969), unsuitable for admission to any unlocked conventional mental hospital. Many of this group may end up on the streets or in the common lodging houses of large cities and will be considered below.

## Homelessness, mental disorder and crime

There is a complex relationship between homelessness, mental disorder and criminal behaviour. This can be represented rather simply as shown in Fig. 15.2. There are areas of overlap between each component and a central area denoting mentally disordered homeless criminals. These individuals are society's rejects increasingly visible on the streets of large cities in the UK and particularly in the USA.

Studies of the homeless are bedevilled by methodological problems, most notably lack of stringent diagnostic criteria applied to poorly representative samples of homeless people. There is no general agreement as to what constitutes homelessness, whether it refers to a complete lack of accommodation, a temporary roof over one's head, or whether it is a broader term embracing the concept of an unsettled rootless disaffiliated way of life. Not surprisingly estimates of the number of homeless people vary widely depending on the definition chosen (see also Chapter 21). A recent survey by the Salvation Army estimated that there were approximately 75 000 people who could be broadly categorized as homeless in London alone (Canter *et al.* 1989).

**Table 15.2** Prevalence of mental disorder in samples of homeless people in the UK and USA

| Author | Site | No. | Primary diagnosis | | |
| | | | Neurosis/ personality disorder | Schizophrenia | Substance abuse |
| --- | --- | --- | --- | --- | --- |
| Lodge-Patch 1970 | Salvation Army Hostel, London | 123 | 50 | 15 | 21 |
| Priest 1971 | Lodging Houses, Edinburgh | 77 | 18 | 32 | 18 |
| Tidmarsh & Wood 1972 | Camberwell Reception Centre | 130* 171† | 16 19 | 22 14 | 14 37 |
| Lipton *et al.* 1983 | Hospital Emergency Room, NYC | 100 | 12 | 72 | 9 |
| Arce *et al.* 1983 | Night Shelter, Philadelphia | 193 | 6 | 35 | 23 |
| Bassuk *et al.* 1984 | Night Shelter, Boston | 78 | 21 | 30 | 29 |
| Koegel *et al.* 1988 | Skid Row, Los Angeles | 328 | 31 | 12 | 31 |
| Joseph *et al.* 1990 | Medical Centre, London | 260 | 20 | 24 | 17 |

\* New cases.
† Casuals.

Notwithstanding the methodological difficulties, all samples of homeless people surveyed include a proportion who are mentally disordered and some of these have criminal convictions. Table 15.2 provides a summary of some surveys in the UK and USA.

The homeless mentally disordered are a heterogeneous group. Fischer & Breakey (1986) have subdivided them into four main groups: the chronic mentally ill, alcoholics, situationally distressed, and street people. Two further categories may be added, the new mentally ill and those who might be described as disaffected youth, namely young people often with a history of separation from parents, institutional upbringing, delinquency, who have been rejected by family and migrate to large cities with little clear idea about their future plans. They tend to be labelled as personality disordered when they come into contact with psychiatric services who are usually quick to reject them. Of course these categories are not mutually exclusive and it is a feature of the homeless mentally ill that they often have multiple handicaps, for example a schizophrenic illness complicated by a sociopathic personality and dependence on alcohol.

It is not possible to look in detail at the factors which lead to homelessness, bearing in mind the diversity of individuals who fall under this broad heading (some of these issues are discussed in Chapter 21). Generally there will be an interaction between social factors and individual psychological factors. Although any individual could conceivably become homeless, attention will be focused on those whose mental disorder appeared to be the most important precipitating factor. Tidmarsh & Wood (1972) in their large study of destitute men residing at the now closed Camberwell reception centre in south London showed that for those with a history of psychiatric hospitalization, 87% of the mentally ill, 59% of those with personality disorder, and 50% of alcoholics were living in settled accommodation either with family or alone, prior to hospital admission. Looked at another way, those with psychosis tended to become of no fixed abode on average 7.3 years after their first hospital admission, compared to 4.6 years for the personality

disordered, but for alcoholics the reverse was noted, admission occurring on average 2.4 years after their loss of settled accommodation. For psychotics and those with personality disorder their psychiatric problems predated their homelessness, whereas for alcoholics their alcoholism became a greater problem following their homelessness.

Lamb & Lamb (1990) have identified particular factors contributing to homelessness amongst the mentally ill, namely disorganized thinking and actions, poor problem solving, depression, and paranoia. Other associated factors were substance abuse and a lack of comprehensive health care.

The relationship between crime and homelessness is also complex. Homelessness itself has been criminalized to varying degrees since the Middle Ages. Two main offences under the Vagrancy Act 1824 are begging and sleeping out. Recorded convictions for these offences have varied greatly over the last century, with the main peak before World War I. During the 1920s and 1930s numbers were high and fairly constant, but never reaching pre-war levels. A graphic account of homelessness between the wars has been provided by Orwell (1933). After World War II prosecutions dropped markedly and the numbers of homeless sleeping out almost disappeared, partly due to the National Assistance Act 1948. This led the then London County Council to suspend its annual homeless census. In the 1980s there has been a reversal of this trend and although prosecutions for sleeping out have remained very low, probably due to a deliberate policy of not arresting those sleeping rough, the number of prosecutions for begging has begun to creep up.

Of perhaps more importance is the propensity of the homeless single person to commit crimes outside the vagrancy statutes. Such crimes may themselves lead to the breaking of ties with society and the descent into unsettledness, or they may be encouraged by this way of life and in either case may hinder escape from it. In earlier times the band of 'sturdy rogues' roaming the country, causing havoc and spreading panic, were a real menace to society, but today's single homeless person is likely to be a recidivist petty offender.

Studies of the criminal records of the homeless

show high rates of criminality. The large single homeless persons survey of 1966 showed that 60% of reception centre residents admitted to a prison record, with 9.4% having been released from prison in the preceding two months (National Assistance Board 1966). Edwards *et al.* (1968) found that a similar figure (59%) of their Camberwell reception centre sample had been imprisoned, but noted the longest sentence averaged 12.4 months with an average number of 7.4 sentences, suggesting multiple petty offences were being committed. It appears that figures for those sleeping out might be higher (Edwards *et al.* 1966). More recently Marshall (1989) found 48% of hostel dwellers in Oxford had previously been imprisoned.

Tidmarsh (1977) analysed the criminal careers of his Camberwell reception centre residents according to psychiatric diagnosis. Those with no psychiatric diagnosis had the lowest rate of previous convictions (38%). The mentally ill were next with a 55% rate, followed by those with personality disorder who had 69%, and the group with the highest rate were the alcoholics at 76%. Tidmarsh also found that the more handicaps suffered by an individual, for example, mental illness, alcoholism, personality disorder, the higher the rate of criminality. The most common offences were theft, criminal damage and vagrancy offences; violence was much less likely although higher than would be expected for the general population. Tidmarsh went further and looked at the hospital careers of his homeless men. He showed that for those with a diagnosis of mental illness or alcoholism, a history of imprisonment was associated with previous hospital admission. Support for Tidmarsh's findings comes from the USA where a survey of 529 homeless adults in Los Angeles showed a higher rate of criminality and longer period of homelessness in the previously hospitalized homeless than the rest of the sample (Gelberg *et al.* 1988).

In conclusion, although we have seen little evidence for the transcarceration hypothesis when looking at gross numbers, the situation is different in the disadvantaged world of the homeless mentally ill. The reasons for this are partly related to the multiple handicaps from which they suffer,

but also due to the administrative barriers which hinder their access to health care. Once homeless the mentally ill are seriously disadvantaged when they seek medical care. Their lack of accommodation makes it difficult for them to register with GPs, and even when that has been accomplished, the slavish adherence by psychiatric hospitals to catchment area boundaries may curtail further progress. This has been recognized by Government which has funded a primary care service for the homeless in central London (El-Kabir 1982) where a drop-in psychiatric clinic is attached (Joseph *et al.* 1990). Furthermore, funds have been made available to develop high care hostel facilities for the homeless with psychiatric multi-disciplinary support. Some have suggested that this will further marginalize the homeless (Lowry 1990), yet it seems the only way to provide health care for a group already shunned to some extent by psychiatric services which do not include the homeless in their financial budgeting.

In some cases hospitals may exacerbate homelessness by discharging patients to temporary hostel accommodation or even to the streets. Marshall's (1989) survey of Oxford hostel residents revealed that 48 of 146 residents showed persistent severe mental disability, yet 90% had previously been in psychiatric hospital, many as long-term patients. Marshall concluded: 'The two hostels, staffed by psychiatrically untrained workers and volunteers were effectively attempting to do the work equivalent to that in two long-stay psychiatric wards.... We are witnessing the inadvertent creation of mini-institutions in hostels'.

It has to be recognized that such individuals, having offended, will inevitably become ensnared in the criminal process due to administrative failure, negative attitudes and resource deficiencies. The next part of the chapter will consider how they can then be diverted from custody and the courts.

### Diversion from custody

The purpose of this section is to explore the interaction between psychiatry and the law when considering the disposal of the mentally disordered offender. The intention is to demonstrate that factors which criminalize mental disorder, are opposed by other factors which medicalize criminal behaviour. The system is a dynamic one and the pendulum may swing over time influenced by public policy, attitudes and legislative changes.

Melick *et al.* (1979) have argued that criminal behaviour has been medicalized in the past, thus those discharged psychiatric patients who subsequently offended had previous criminal histories and perhaps should not have been admitted to hospital in the first place. This view is held by some in the UK when considering patients with a diagnosis of psychopathic disorder. Mawson (1983) has argued that offenders classified as suffering from psychopathic disorder within the terms of the Mental Health Act 1983 should receive a custodial sentence, following which transfer to hospital under the provisions of section 47 of the Mental Health Act 1983 can be effected if hospital treatment is required. Although superficially attractive, in practical terms this leads to the rejection of such patients by psychiatric services. For example, the annual number of male admissions to Broadmoor special hospital detained under the legal category of psychopathic disorder has dropped steadily from 50 in 1973 to 4 in 1984, and yet the number of prison transfers

of such patients has remained fairly constant. In other words, offenders who are sentenced to prison when they might previously have received a hospital order are not subsequently transferred to hospital during their sentence.

Diversion from the criminal justice system takes two forms. First, diversion altogether, for example by discontinuing the case, or by the use of a hospital order under section 37 of the Mental Health Act (1983). Secondly, diversion from custody, for example using sections in Part 3 of the Mental Health Act 1983 or under provisions of the Bail Act 1976. Fig. 15.3 shows the potential points of diversion from the criminal justice system.

The first point of potential diversion arises with the police. Statutory provisions have been in existence for well over a hundred years to allow the police to convey mentally disordered persons from public places to a hospital or previously a workhouse. Section 136 of the Mental Health Act 1983 describes the latest version of this police power and studies show police referrals have high rates of chronic serious mental illness frequently requiring emergency psychiatric admission (Fahy 1989). Unfortunately the conclusion that is often drawn is that the police are skilled in recognizing mental illness, whereas perhaps a more cautious

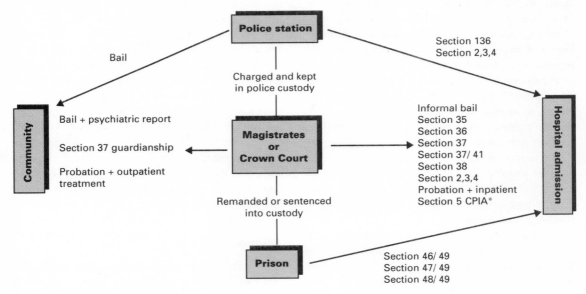

**Fig. 15.3** Diversion to psychiatric care from the criminal justice system. (Reproduced with permission from Joseph 1990.) Section numbers refer to the Mental Health Act (1983). * Criminal Procedure Insanity Act (1964).

interpretation would be that the police are missing many other cases of mental illness, hence the lack of false positives in their referrals. Certainly the use of section 136 is a first step to ensure diversion from the criminal justice system, but its use by the police is patchy and inconsistent and varies across the country (George 1972, Department of Health & Social Security 1986) and undoubtedly mentally disordered offenders will continue to be arrested and charged.

It is not uncommon for there to be an inordinate delay following remand in custody whilst awaiting psychiatric assessment, with no guarantee of subsequent hospital admission (Bowden 1978). The process can be speeded up considerably by arranging for psychiatrists to conduct assessments at court rather than in prison. This has been shown by a study currently being undertaken at two inner London magistrates courts (Joseph & Potter 1990). A psychiatric assessment service has been available at Bow Street and Marlborough Street magistrates' courts for 18 months, and during that time 180 mentally disordered petty offenders have been referred for psychiatric assessment by the magistrates, probation service and duty solicitors. Of the first 80 offenders assessed, 47% were suffering from schizophrenia. Thirty per cent of the total had been admitted directly to hospital from the court, mainly on a civil section of the Mental Health Act 1983, or on bail. A further 51% of defendants have been released and 19% have been returned to custody. A total of 35% of cases have been discontinued by the Crown Prosecution Service using their powers under section 23 of the Prosecution of Offences Act 1985. The advantage of this court-based psychiatric assessment service has been to allow a dialogue to take place between the psychiatrist and the Crown Prosecution Service regarding the suitability of discontinuing the case. Cases have been particularly likely to be discontinued if a hospital bed is available.

Legislation currently exists to allow the diversion of mentally ill offenders from the criminal justice system. Unfortunately the provisions which exist to divert the mentally ill are underused, primarily because there is a fundamental lack of communication between the mental health and criminal justice systems. Once the mentally disordered petty offender has been ensnared by the criminal process considerable delay may ensue, aggravated by the wait for psychiatric assessment before diversion can be achieved. Part of the problem is that psychiatrists assess mentally ill defendants who are remanded in custody in prison whilst the legal action takes place at the court. The way forward is for psychiatrists to shift their focus of assessment from the prison to the court particularly for the petty offenders, thereby reducing the time spent in custody.

### Social aspects of treatment

Having examined social factors implicated in the development of criminal behaviour and mental disorder, and having considered social and administrative policy and its impact on the mentally disordered offender particularly regarding access to health care, it remains finally to review social aspects of the various treatment settings available bearing in mind throughout the question, 'Is there any place for the treatment of the mentally disordered offender in prison?'

For serious offenders security considerations and protection of the public are paramount. The criminal justice and psychiatric systems reflect this and varying degrees of security are available for both.

#### *Special hospitals*

Section 4 of the National Health Act 1977 requires the Secretary of State to provide and maintain special hospitals for patients 'who in his opinion require treatment under conditions of special security on account of their dangerous, violent or criminal propensities'. It must be remembered 'special hospitals are not prison hospitals, there are no prison officers and all patients are detained under mental health legislation' (Hamilton 1985). Nevertheless, the nursing staff tend to be members of the Prison Officers Association and security considerations take precedence over the treatment ethic. In many respects the special hospitals retain features of a 'total institution' (Goffman 1961), and although part of the National Health Service, their management structure has distanced them from the rest of psychiatric services. However, there is change in the air with the creation of the new Special Hospitals Service Authority on 1 July 1989, which sees as one of its aims to make special hospitals an integral component of psychiatric services and to develop more effective links. A major research study funded by the Department of Health is currently being undertaken to assess the needs of the present inpatient population of 1700, particularly the level of security required for their safe containment. Preliminary findings suggest that half the inpatients are being treated in special hospitals when in fact their level of dangerousness does not warrant it (*The Guardian*, 20 September 1990).

Similar concerns have been expressed in Dell & Robertson's detailed study of the characteristics, attitudes and treatment of patients admitted to Broadmoor Hospital (1988). They interviewed patients and their responsible medical officers and divided them into those detained under the legal category of mental illness and those categorized as psychopathic disorder. Only 28% of the mentally ill needed the degree of security provided by Broadmoor and nearly 50% were rated as definitely or probably suitable for treatment in conditions of less security. A majority of the psychopaths felt that being in Broadmoor was a more comfortable and relaxed way of doing their time than being in prison but only a third were satisfied with the treatment they were receiving. The majority were not receiving any treatment other than the effect of being in Broadmoor and their length of stay was related to the seriousness of their index offence rather than psychiatric factors. The authors concluded that many of the psychopaths had in effect been sentenced to hospital and were not receiving any specific psychiatric help.

Nevertheless it can be argued that admission to special hospital, even if of doubtful value for some psychopathic patients, may offer protection from the more brutalizing effects of prison which might lead to a worsening of their condition.

### Regional secure units

Following the report of the committee on mentally abnormal offenders, known as the Butler Report (Home Office: Department of Health & Social Security 1975), resources were made available by the Regional Health Authorities for the building of regional secure units (RSU) to bridge the 'yawning' gap between the maximum security special hospitals and the low security general psychiatric hospitals of which many no longer have locked facilities. The building of these units has progressed very slowly and only half or so of the total of 1000 beds envisaged by the Butler committee have been opened. This has jeopardized the intention that the RSUs should take patients from court who might previously have been admitted to special hospital and also to help relocate those patients in high security who no longer require it. Part of the reason that the special hospitals have an excess of patients who no longer require high security is that they can wait years for transfer to the RSUs. A further problem is that the RSUs are reluctant to admit patients for more than two years and therefore some patients will be rejected unless there are clear indicators that their mental disorder is amenable to treatment.

The RSUs are in a difficult position. An attempt is made to create a therapeutic atmosphere with the emphasis on individual and group therapy for a mixed group of patients, both in terms of diagnosis and mode of admission, in whom security considerations are also important. The same staff carry out these diverse functions which can lead to role confusion and exploitation by some patients. Patient cliques may develop which can considerably disrupt the running of a small unit. Patients admitted from special hospital may have expected an early discharge and will resent a long stay. The pressures from within the RSU are matched by external pressures from special hospitals and general psychiatric wards to take patients. Although the characteristics of patients admitted to RSUs, their treatment and length of stay have been reviewed by Treasaden (1985), there is as yet little in the way of adequate follow-up of such patients to assess outcome. Finally, these units are expensive to run and some health authorities are more prepared to fund patients in the expanding private secure unit market than their own facilities. It is unlikely that the figure of 1000 beds will be reached.

## Prison

In a well-known and controversial study Zimbardo, the American social psychologist, and his colleagues, constructed a simulated prison and recruited Stanford University undergraduates who were randomly assigned the role of prisoner or guard (Haney *et al.* 1973). Those who were guards became brutal and punitive whilst the prisoners were subjugated and humiliated. The intensity of the behaviours displayed by the two groups took the researchers by surprise and at times it was felt that the experiment should be abandoned because of the ill-treatment of the prisoners.

This study highlights the importance of situational factors in shaping behaviour in institutions such as prisons. The atmosphere of 'us and them' permeates the prison environment, with rigid boundaries drawn on both sides and constant provocation between the two groups. All this can spill over easily into anarchy and chaos as shown by the riots at HM Prison Strangeways in Manchester which started on Sunday 1 April 1990 and lasted for 25 days before prison staff regained control. According to the then governor of the prison Brendan O'Friel, 'There has been a major act of violence that has been of a magnitude and size that is quite difficult to comprehend...an explosion of evil took place on Sunday' (*The Guardian*, 5 April 1990).

It is into this environment that the mentally disordered offender may well be consigned, often in the words of the Bail Act 1976 'for his own protection'. If his behaviour is particularly disturbed or bizarre he is likely to find himself placed in the so-called 'special medical room' commonly known as the 'strip-cell'. A visiting psychiatrist at Brixton Prison has written:

> These rooms are bare apart from a mattress, extremely dirty and faeces-smeared as a result of the patient's mental state, and stiflingly hot in summer and cold in winter. Patients often are naked because of their mental condition and have only a canvas blanket with which to keep warm. They may remain in this condition for some considerable time.
> (Herridge 1989)

Suicide in prison is a matter of increasing concern and a source of acute embarrassment to the prison authorities. Most studies have been conducted in the USA (Reiger 1971, Danto 1973), although Dooley (1990) has carried out a large retrospective case-note survey of 295 suicides in prisons in England and Wales between 1972 and 1987. This period has witnessed an increase in the suicide rate far in excess of the rise in the prison population. The most common method of suicide was by hanging, usually at night. There was an excess of suicide amongst prisoners on remand but others took place many years after reception into prison. Although many of those who killed themselves had a history of self-injury or psychiatric treatment, only 16% had been specifically noted as being at risk by prison staff. Dooley suggested that there should be greater trust and communication between inmates and staff to facilitate disclosure of problems, but there seems little chance of this in the current prison climate of tension and serious overcrowding. Since the vast majority of hangings were from the cell window bars, Dooley's more practical suggestion that cell windows should be redesigned to make it impossible to tie a knot seems a better alternative.

There are some rays of hope in the treatment of the mentally disordered in prison. HM Prison Grendon was opened in 1962 to provide treatment for those mentally disordered prisoners who did not require transfer to a psychiatric hospital. The ethos of the prison reflects the East & Hubert report (1939), which advocated psychological treatment based on analytical principles for offenders. Crucial to the regime at Grendon is the extensive use of group psychotherapy. Inmates are encouraged to become actively involved in each other's therapy and peer group pressure and influence is of great importance. Other therapeutic procedures include sex education, social skills training and psychodrama. A detailed description of both the regime and inmates has been provided by Gunn *et al.* (1978).

Despite many of the problems encountered by the special hospitals and regional secure units there is a vast difference between what they offer and the general conditions and treatment of the mentally disordered in prison. Since the riot at

Strangeways prison and subsequent copycat riots at other establishments, an inquiry has been set up, chaired by Lord Justice Woolf (Home Office 1991), to examine the prison system. There have been stinging criticisms of the overcrowded and squalid buildings with minimal provision for occupation and recreation (Report of HM Chief Inspector of Prisons 1989). Questions have also been asked about the calibre and experience of many of the applicants for jobs in the prison medical service, a branch of medicine where recruitment is difficult (Bluglass 1990). Finally the prison medical service has been subject to an internal scrutiny (Home Office 1990), which recommends the contracting out of prison medicine to the National Health Service, with greater emphasis on training for prison medical officers.

On the face of it there seems to be overwhelming support for the view that mentally disordered offenders should not receive psychiatric treatment in prison unless as a short-term emergency whilst hospital transfer is arranged. This view is reinforced by a recent High Court judgment that prison hospitals could not be expected to provide the same standard of care as National Health Service hospitals (Bynoe 1990). Yet in spite of all this the Chief Inspector of Prisons, Judge Tumim, advocates the setting up of prison hospitals where the Mental Health Act would apply. This view is not new. The importance of stimulating therapeutic endeavours within the prison system was felt strongly by Scott (1974), who wrote:

> It would perhaps help if approved parts of the prison system could be designated as hospitals . . . so hospital orders could be effected either in prison or in hospital . . . The prison medical service should merge with the National Health Service, and the forensic psychiatrists, instead of running esoteric little units in the Health Service, should treat patients in prison thus bringing a benevolent medical influence within the reach of any prisoner needing it . . .

The concern of this author for Scott's view is that courts will sentence the mentally disordered offender to prison to receive treatment which is unavailable elsewhere. The distinction between punishment and treatment will be blurred which

apart from being morally objectionable may encourage courts to pass exemplary sentences using treatment as an excuse for prolonged incarceration. The courts with their adversarial system of justice and their need to apportion blame and responsibility force a choice between badness or madness (Bowden 1983). Clearly this is a false dichotomy, individuals may be bad, mad, both or neither and may vary over time. However, this is the way the courts operate at trial and it is unlikely they can adopt a different framework during the sentencing stage. One has to accept the limitations of the criminal justice system in this respect and not expect a more subtle interplay between treatment and punishment. In essence, prison is for punishment and evidence of mental illness can excuse or mitigate liability to punishment. We have already seen how the presence of mental illness puts the petty offender at greater risk of a remand in custody. The psychiatric services, however underresourced, need to send a clear message to the courts that they are prepared to accept responsibility for the treatment of mentally disordered offenders when indicated and as quickly as possible. In the meantime the conditions in prison generally should be improved with the provision of facilities for the emergency treatment of mentally ill prisoners under common law without recourse to the Mental Health Act 1983.

## Conclusion

'Red monster lures young men to their deaths in homosexual house of horror' (Masters 1985). This is how Dennis Nilsen who confessed to a total of 15 homicides over a four-year period described himself in response to tabloid newspaper headlines.

Forensic psychiatry is a medical specialty whose patients are largely shunned and ignored by society, apart from the dramatic exception who is thrust, vilified, to the centre of attention. Unfortunately the sensational few cases of serious crimes committed by the mentally disordered influence the public's mind and can exert a disproportionate effect on public policy. Sometimes the effects can be beneficial, for example the case of the poisoner Graham Young, discharged from Broadmoor

Hospital only to re-offend, prompted an inquiry into overcrowding at the special hospitals which culminated in the creation of regional secure units on the recommendation of the Butler Report (Home Office: Department of Health & Social Security 1975). Regrettably the usual official response to allay anxiety about mentally disordered offenders is either to do nothing or to take retrogressive action emphasizing security and protection of the public over treatment needs.

This chapter has presented perspectives from criminology, social psychology and sociology to show that social factors are intimately associated with all aspects of forensic psychiatry and that social disadvantage shadows the mentally disordered offender throughout relationships with family, institutions and the wider public. The response to these 'outsiders' provides a litmus test measuring the degree to which society can call itself tolerant or humane. Changes in legislation and public policy can have a disastrous effect on the provision of services in an area already seriously underresourced. The public's appetite for lurid sensational stories of murder and mayhem eclipses the cautious, epidemiologically based research reviewed here which contradicts the popular myth that the mentally ill are unpredictable and dangerous.

The importance of further careful research is not only to influence the public, but also to challenge the attitudes of the funders and providers of health care, many of whom retain a simplistic view of crime and mental disorder which leads to the ostracism of both the mentally disordered offender and forensic psychiatry from mainstream services. This is particularly evident for the homeless who have no catchment area and for the petty offender whose only treatment is available in prison. It is in these areas that integration is required as a matter of urgency.

## Acknowledgments

Many thanks are due to Graham Robertson for his help in preparing this chapter.

## References

Arce A., Tadlock M., Vergare M. & Shapiro S. (1983) A psychiatric profile of street people admitted to an emergency shelter. *Hospital and Community Psychiatry* 34, 812–817.
Bassuk E., Rubin L. & Lauriat A. (1984) Is homelessness a mental health problem? *American Journal of Psychiatry* 141, 1546.
Bavidge M. (1989) *Mad or Bad?* Classical Press, Bristol.
Bluglass R. (1990) Recruitment and training of prison doctors. *British Medical Journal* 301, 249–250.
Bluglass R. & Bowden P. (1990) *Principles and Practice of Forensic Psychiatry*. Churchill Livingstone, Edinburgh.
Bowden P. (1978) Men remanded into custody for medical reports: the selection for treatment. *British Journal of Psychiatry* 132, 320–331.
Bowden P. (1983) Madness or badness? *British Journal of Hospital Medicine* 30, 388–394.
Brill H. & Malzberg B. (1962) *Statistical Report on the Arrest Record of 5354 Male Ex-patients Released from New York State Mental Hospital During the Period 1946–1948. Mental Hospital Service supplement 153.* American Psychiatric Association, Washington DC.
Bromberg W. & Thompson C. (1937) The relation of psychosis, mental defect and personality types to crime. *Journal of Criminal Law and Criminology* 28, 70–89.
Bynoe I. (1990) The prison medical wing: a 'place of safety?'. *Journal of Forensic Psychiatry* 1, 251–257.
Canter D., Drake M., Littler T., Moore J., Stockley D. & Ball J. (1989) *The Faces of Homelessness in London. Interim report to the Salvation Army.* University of Surrey, Department of Psychology.
Clarke R. (1982) Crime prevention through environmental management and design. In Gunn J. and Farrington D. (eds) *Abnormal Offenders: Delinquency and the Criminal Justice System*, pp. 213–230. Wiley, Chichester.
Cloward R. & Ohlin L. (1960) *Delinquency and Opportunity*. Free Press, Chicago.
Cocozza J. & Steadman H. (1974) Some refinements in the measurement and prediction of dangerous behaviour. *American Journal of Psychiatry* 131, 1012–1014.
Cohen L. & Freeman H. (1945) How dangerous to the community are state hospital patients? *Connecticut State Medical Journal* 9, 697–700.
Coid J. (1984) How many psychiatric patients in prison? *British Journal of Psychiatry* 145, 78–86.
Coid J. (1988) Mentally abnormal prisoners on remand: I – Rejected or accepted by the NHS. II – Comparison of services provided by Oxford and Wessex regions. *British Medical Journal* 296, 1779–1784.
Danto B. (1973) *Jail House Blues*. Epic Publications, Orchard Lake, Michigan.
Dell S. & Robertson G. (1988) *Sentenced to Hospital. Maudsley Monograph No. 32.* Oxford University Press, Oxford.
Department of Health & Social Security (1986) *Mental*

*Health Statistics for England: Booklet 11.* Government Statistical Service, London.

Dooley E. (1990) Prison suicide in England and Wales, 1972–87. *British Journal of Psychiatry* 156, 40–45.

East W. & Hubert N. (1939) *Psychological Treatment of Crime.* HMSO, London.

Edwards G., Hawker A., Hensman C. & Williamson V. (1966) London's skid row. *Lancet* i, 249–252.

Edwards G., Williamson V., Hawker A., Hensman C. & Postoyan S. (1968) Census of a reception centre. *British Journal of Psychiatry* 114, 1031–1039.

Edwards J., Jones D., Reid W. & Chu C. (1988) Physical assaults in a psychiatric unit of a general hospital. *American Journal of Psychiatry* 145, 1568–1571.

Ekblom B. (1970) *Acts of Violence by Patients in Mental Hospitals.* Scandinavian University Press, Stockholm.

El-Kabir D. (1982) Great Chapel Street medical centre. *British Medical Journal* 284, 480–481.

Evenson R., Altman H., Stetten I. & Brown M. (1974) Disturbing behaviour: a study of incident reports. *Psychiatry Quarterly* 48, 266–275.

Eysenck H. (1977) *Crime and Personality.* Paladin, London.

Fahy T. (1989) The police as a referral agency for psychiatric emergencies – a review. *Medicine Science and the Law* 29, 315–322.

Farrington D. (1981) The prevalence of convictions. *British Journal of Criminology* 21, 173–175.

Farrington D. (1990) Implications of criminal career research for the prevention of offending. *Journal of Adolescence* 13, 93–113.

Farrington D., Ohlin L. & Wilson J. (1986) *Understanding and Controlling Crime: Toward a New Research Strategy.* Springer-Verlag, New York.

Farrington D. & West D. (1990) The Cambridge study in delinquent development: a long term follow-up of 411 London males. In Kerner H. & Kaiser G. (eds) *Criminality: Personality Behaviour Life History.* Springer-Verlag, Heidelberg.

Fischer P. & Breakey W. (1986) Homelessness and mental health: an overview. *International Journal of Mental Health* 14, 6–41.

Folkard M. (1959) *A Sociological Contribution to the Understanding of Aggression and its Treatment.* Coulsdon, Surrey, Netherne Hospital.

Fottrell E. (1980) A study of violent behaviour among patients in psychiatric hospitals. *British Journal of Psychiatry* 136, 216–221.

Fowles A. (1990) The Mentally Abnormal Offender in the Era of Community Care. Paper Presented to the Cropwood Round Table Conference, Cambridge.

Gelberg L., Linn L. & Leake B. (1988) Mental health alcohol and drug use and criminal history among homeless adults. *American Journal of Psychiatry* 145, 191–196.

Geller J. (1984) Arson: an unforseen sequela of deinstitutionalisation. *American Journal of Psychiatry* 141, 504.

George H. (1972) A Study of Police Admissions to Psychiatric Hospitals. MD Thesis, University of London.

Gibbens T. & Robertson G. (1983) A survey of the criminal careers of hospital order patients. *British Journal of Psychiatry* 143, 362–369.

Gibbens T., Soothill K. & Pope P. (1977) *Medical Remands in the Criminal Court.* Maudsley Monograph No. 25. Oxford University Press, Oxford.

Gibbons D. (1971) Observations on the study of crime causation. *American Journal of Sociology* 77, 262–278.

Goffman E. (1961) *Asylums.* Penguin, London.

Griffiths R. (1988) *Community Care – Agenda for Action.* HMSO, London.

Gudeman J. & Shore M. (1984) Beyond deinstitutionalisation: a new class of facilities for the mentally ill. *New England Journal of Medicine* 311, 832–836.

Gunn J., Maden A. & Swinton M. (1991) Treatment needs of prisoners with psychiatric disorders. *British Medical Journal* 303, 338–341.

Gunn J., Robertson G., Dell S. & Way C. (1978) *Psychiatric Aspects of Imprisonment.* Academic, New York.

Guze S. (1976) *Criminality and Psychiatric Disorders.* Oxford University Press, Oxford.

Hafner H. & Boker W. (1982a) *Crimes of Violence by Mentally Abnormal Offenders. A Psychiatric and Epidemiological Study in the Federal German Republic,* p. 52. Cambridge University Press, Cambridge.

Hafner H. & Boker W. (1982b) *Crimes of Violence by Mentally Abnormal Offenders. A Psychiatric and Epidemiological Study in the Federal German Republic,* p. 280. Cambridge University Press, Cambridge.

Hamilton J. (1985) The special hospitals. In Gostin L. (ed.) *Secure Provision. A Review of Special Services for the Mentally Ill and Mentally Handicapped in England and Wales.* Tavistock, London.

Haney C., Banks W. & Zimbardo P. (1973) Interpersonal dynamics in a simulated prison. *International Journal of Criminology and Penology* 1, 69–79.

Herridge C. (1989) Treatment of psychotic patients in prison. *Psychiatric Bulletin* 13, 200–201.

Home Office (1990) *Report on an Efficiency Scrutiny of the Prison Medical Service.* Internal Home Office Document.

Home Office (1991) *Prison Disturbances April 1990. Report of an Inquiry.* Cmnd 1456. HMSO, London.

Home Office: Department of Health and Social Security (1975) Report of the Committee on mentally abnormal offenders. Cmnd 6244. HMSO, London.

Johnstone E., Crow T., Johnson A. & MacMillan F. (1986) The Northwick Park study of first episodes of schizophrenia. I: Presentation of the illness and problems relating to admission. *British Journal of Psychiatry* 149, 51–56.

Jones K. (1988) *Experience in Mental Health Community Care and Social Policy.* Sage, London.

Jones R. (1983) Street people and psychiatry: an introduction. *Hospital and Community Psychiatry* 35, 899–907.

Joseph P. (1990) Mentally disordered offenders: diversion

from the criminal justice system. *Journal of Forensic Psychiatry* 1, 133–138.

Joseph P., Bridgewater J., Ramsden S. & El-Kabir D. (1990) A psychiatric clinic for the single homeless in a primary care setting in Inner London. *Psychiatric Bulletin* 14, 270–271.

Joseph P. & Potter M. (1990) Mentally disordered homeless offenders – diversion from custody. *Health Trends* 2, 51–53.

Kelleher M. & Copeland J. (1972) Compulsory psychiatric admissions by the police: a study of the use of section 136. *Medicine, Science and the Law* 12, 220–224.

Koegel P., Burnam A. & Farr R. (1988) The prevalence of specific psychiatric disorders among homeless individuals in the inner city of Los Angeles. *Archives of General Psychiatry* 45, 1085–1092.

Lagos J., Perlmutter K. & Saexinger H. (1977) Fear of the mentally ill: empirical support for the common man's response. *American Journal of Psychiatry* 134, 1134–1137.

Lamb H. & Lamb D. (1990) Factors contributing to homelessness among the chronically and severely mentally ill. *Hospital and Community Psychiatry* 41, 301–305.

Levine D. (1970) Criminal behaviour and mental institutionalisation. *Journal of Clinical Psychology* 26, 279–284.

Lindqvist P. & Allebeck P. (1990) Schizophrenia and crime. A longitudinal follow-up of 644 schizophrenics in Stockholm. *British Journal of Psychiatry* 157, 345–350.

Lipton F., Sabatini A. & Katz S. (1983) Down and out in the city: the homeless mentally ill. *Hospital and Community Psychiatry* 34, 818–821.

Lodge-Patch I. (1970) Homeless men: a London survey. *Proceedings of the Royal Society of Medicine* 63, 437–441.

Lowry S. (1989) Concern for discharged mentally ill patients. *British Medical Journal* 298, 209–210.

Lowry S. (1990) Health and homelessness. *British Medical Journal* 300, 32–34.

MacMillan J. & Johnson A. (1987) Contact with the police in early schizophrenia: its nature frequency and relevance to the outcome of treatment. *Medicine, Science and the Law* 27, 191–200.

McNeil D. & Binder R. (1987) Predictive value of judgements of dangerousness in emergency civil committment. *American Journal of Psychiatry* 144, 197–200.

Marshall M. (1989) Collected and neglected: are Oxford hostels for the homeless filling up with disabled psychiatric patients? *British Medical Journal* 299, 706–709.

Masters B. (1985) *Killing for Company: The Case of Dennis Nilsen*, p. 20. Jonathan Cape, London.

Mawson D. (1983) 'Psychopaths' in special hospitals. *Bulletin of the Royal College of Psychiatrists* 7, 178–181.

Mays J. (ed.) (1972) *Juvenile Delinquency: The Family and the Social Group; A Reader*. Longmans, London.

Melick M., Steadman H. & Cocozza J. (1979) The medical-isation of criminal behaviour among mental patients. *Journal of Health and Social Behaviour* 20, 228–237.

Merton R. (1957) *Social Theory and Social Structure*. Free Press, New York.

Messinger E. & Apfelburg B. (1961) A quarter century of court psychiatry. *Crime and Delinquency* 7, 343–362.

Monahan J. & Steadman H. (1983) Crime and mental illness: an epidemiological approach. In Morris N. & Tonry M. (eds) *Crime and Justice*, vol. 4. University of Chicago Press, Chicago.

National Assistance Board (1966) *Homeless Single Persons*, p. 58. HMSO, London.

Noble P. & Rodger S. (1989) Violence by psychiatric in-patients. *British Journal of Psychiatry* 155, 384–390.

Orwell G. (1933) *Down and Out in Paris and London*. Penguin, Harmondsworth.

Patterson G. (1982) *Coercive Family Processes*. Castalia, Eugene, Oregon.

Penrose L. (1939) Mental disease and crime: an outline of a study of European statistics. *British Journal of Medical Psychology* 18, 1–15.

Penrose L. (1943) A note on the statistical relationship between mental deficiency and crime in the United States. *American Journal of Mental Deficiency* 47, 462–466.

Post R., Willet A., Franks R., House R., Back S. & Weissberg M. (1980) A preliminary report on the prevalence of domestic violence among psychiatric inpatients. *American Journal of Psychiatry* 137, 974–975.

Priest R. (1971) The Edinburgh homeless: a psychiatric survey. *American Journal of Psychotherapy* 25, 194–213.

Rabkin J. (1979) Criminal behaviour of discharged mental patients: a critical appraisal of the research. *Psychological Bulletin* 86, 1–27.

Reiger W. (1971) Suicide attempts in a federal prison. *Archives of General Psychiatry* 24, 532–535.

Report of HM Chief Inspector of Prisons (1989) HMSO, London.

Robins L. (1966) *Deviant Children Grown Up*. Williams and Wilkins, Baltimore.

Robins L. (1978) Sturdy childhood predictors of adult anti-social behaviour: replications from longitudinal studies. *Psychological Medicine* 8, 611–622.

Rollin H. (1969) *The Mentally Abnormal Offender and the Law*. Pergamon, Oxford.

Rutter M. & Giller H. (1983) *Juvenile Delinquency. Trends and Perspectives*. Penguin, Harmondsworth.

Scott P. (1974) Solution to the problem of the dangerous offender. *British Medical Journal* 4, 640–641.

Sosowsky L. (1980) Explaining the increased arrest rate among mental patients: a cautionary note. *American Journal of Psychiatry* 137, 1602–1605.

Steadman H., Cocozza J. & Melick M. (1978) Explaining the increased arrest rate among mental patients: the changing clientele of state hospitals. *American Journal of Psychiatry* 135, 816–820.

Steadman H. & Halfon A. (1971) The Baxstrom patients:

backgrounds and outcomes. *Seminars in Psychiatry* 3, 376–385.

Steadman H., Monahan J., Duffee B., Hartstone E. & Robbins P. (1984) The impact of state hospital deinstitutionalisation on United States prison populations 1968–1978. *Journal of Criminal Law and Criminology* 75, 474–490.

Steadman H. & Morrissey J. (1984) The impact of deinstitutionalisation on the criminal justice system: implications for understanding changing modes of social control. In Lowman J., Menzies R. & Palys T. (eds) *Transcarceration: Essays in the Sociology of Social Control*. Gower, Aldershot.

Stein G. (1982) Dangerous episodes occurring around the time of discharge of four chronic schizophrenics. *British Journal of Psychiatry* 141, 586–590.

Stone A. (1984) *Law, Psychiatry and Morality*. American Psychiatric Press, Washington DC.

Sutherland E. & Cressey D. (1974) *Criminology*, 9th edn. Lippincott, Philadelphia.

Szmukler G., Bird A. & Button E. (1981) Compulsory admissions in a London borough: I Social and clinical features and a follow-up. *Psychological Medicine* 11, 617–636.

Tanke E. & Yesavage D. (1985) Characteristics of assaultive patients. *American Journal of Psychiatry* 142, 1409–1413.

Tardiff K. & Sweillam A. (1980) Assault, suicide and mental illness. *Archives of General Psychiatry* 37, 164–169.

Taylor I., Walton P. & Young J. (1974) *The New Criminology*. Harper and Row, New York.

Taylor P. (1985) Motives for offending among violent and psychotic men. *British Journal of Psychiatry* 147, 491–498.

Taylor P. & Gunn J. (1984) Violence and psychosis. I – Risk of violence among psychotic men. *British Medical Journal* 288, 1945–1949.

Taylor P. & Parrott J. (1988) Elderly offenders: a study of age-related factors among custodially remanded prisoners. *British Journal of Psychiatry* 152, 340–346.

Teplin L. (1985) The criminality of the mentally ill: a dangerous misconception. *American Journal of Psychiatry* 142, 593–598.

Thornberry T. & Jacoby J. (1979) *The Criminally Insane. A Community Follow-up of Mentally Ill Offenders*. University of Chicago Press, Chicago.

Tidmarsh D. (1977) Psychiatric Disorder in a Population of Homeless Destitute Men. Unpublished MD Thesis, University of Cambridge.

Tidmarsh D. & Wood S. (1972) Psychiatric aspects of destitution: a study of the Camberwell reception centre. In Wing J. & Hailey A. (eds) *Evaluating a Community Psychiatric Service*. Oxford University Press, London.

Tooth G. & Brooke E. (1961) Trends in the mental hospital population and their effect on future planning. *Lancet* i, 710–713.

Treasaden I. (1985) Current practice in regional interim secure units. In Gostin L. (ed.) *Secure Provision. A Review of Special Services for the Mentally Ill and the Mentally Handicapped in England and Wales*. Tavistock, London.

Weller M. (1989) Mental illness – who cares? *Nature* 339, 249–252.

Weller M. & Weller B. (1988) Mental illness and social policy. *Medicine Science and the Law* 28, 47–53.

Wessely S. & Taylor P. (1991) Madness and crime: criminology versus psychiatry. *Criminal Behaviour and Mental Health* 1, 193–228.

West D. & Farrington D. (1973) *Who Becomes Delinquent?* Heinemann Educational, London.

Wootton B. (1959) *Social Science and Social Pathology*. George Allen & Unwin, London.

World Health Organization (1978) *Mental Disorders: Glossary and Guide to their Classification in Accordance with the Ninth Revision of the International Classification of Diseases (ICD-9)*. WHO, Geneva.

Zitrin A., Hardesty A., Burdock E. & Drossman A. (1976) Crime and violence among mental patients. *American Journal of Psychiatry* 133, 142–149.

# Chapter 16
# Social Psychiatry of Eating Disorders

G.F.M.RUSSELL

To examine eating disorders from the perspective of social psychiatry carries several advantages. The role of sociocultural influences in causing and moulding the expression of eating disorders is at least as powerful as in most other psychiatric illnesses. Hence, the approach of this book lends itself to a timely focus on the sociocultural aspects of anorexia nervosa and bulimia nervosa. However, the writer and the reader must guard themselves against the dangers that such a focused approach might obscure other causal factors. The most salient clinical feature of anorexia nervosa is severe emaciation and malnutrition. Even if the simplistic view is taken that this malnutrition is a wholly secondary consequence of the psychological disturbances, it assumes enormous importance in the pathogenesis of the illness, its perpetuation and its dangers. There are further reasons for accepting that biomedical factors play a crucial part in the genesis of eating disorders and this issue will be returned to later in this chapter. Suffice it to stress at this stage that a multidimensional approach to the understanding of eating disorders is imperative. Arguments for viewing anorexia nervosa as a multidetermined disorder have already been cogently presented by Garfinkel & Garner (1982). A related and overlapping concept is that of 'pathoplasticity' which helps us to evaluate those factors which act as predisposing or provoking agents, or exert a moulding influence on the illness (Russell 1985a). Pathoplasticity is a concept which helps us to grasp why an eating disorder such as bulimia nervosa should appear, with apparent suddenness, and yet retain a nosological connection with anorexia nervosa. Most important in our assessment of the problems presented by individual patients is the construction of a clinical formulation in depth, or in 'layers' to use Kretschmer's term of 'Schichtdiagnose' (quoted by

Bleuler 1937). This requires us to bear in mind the possible role of the patient's constitutional make-up (including the genetic constitution and personality traits), sociocultural nexus and personal experiences. Not only may these factors have an additive effect, but they may combine in a specific manner causing the patient to become ill:

> It is the interaction and timing of these phenomena in a given individual which are necessary for the person to become ill. In this sense, anorexia nervosa is a final common pathway, the product of a group of interacting forces. (Garfinkel & Garner 1982)

I shall now outline the contents of this chapter. The main eating disorders to be discussed are anorexia nervosa and bulimia nervosa. Obesity will not be considered even though sociocultural factors such as race, gender and economic status influence the prevalence of being overweight (Van Itallie & Woteki 1987). Genetic factors probably have an even greater importance in causing obesity (Bray 1987, Stunkard 1988). The overriding reason for omitting obesity from this chapter is the lack of firm evidence for any association with psychological disturbances or psychogenesis (Crisp & McGuiness 1976).

An appraisal of eating disorders in the context of social psychiatry is entirely apposite when the definition and scope of social psychiatry are carefully considered. Crisp's definition, on behalf of the British Association for Social Psychiatry, is suitably broad. It encompasses the study of the social determinants, influences and consequences of psychiatric disorders, and he adds furthermore the application of preventive measures and social interventions (1988). The contents of this book fit within this appropriately flexible framework. The subject matter of this chapter on eating disorders will concentrate on the epidemiology and socio-cultural determinants of anorexia and bulimia nervosa. The transcultural aspects of anorexia nervosa will also be discussed. The modern history of anorexia nervosa will be reviewed because of the evidence that the illness has changed during recent decades. A 'corrective' section on the multi-dimensional causation of anorexia nervosa will be added so as to remind readers that a sociocultural and biomedical synthesis is necessary for the proper understanding of eating disorders. The chapter will end with a short section on prevention which has proved elusive so far.

A consistent and striking observation is the very high predominance of female over male patients in both anorexia nervosa and bulimia nervosa, probably in all age groups. Garfinkel & Garner (1982) indicated that 90–95% of patients reported in most studies were female. The predominance of female patients in both anorexia and bulimia nervosa has led to a convention of referring to patients in the feminine gender, and this practice will be adopted in this chapter.

### Clinical features of eating disorders

Anorexia nervosa and bulimia nervosa are both relatively easy to diagnose. There are few psychiatric disorders whose clinical features and diagnostic criteria can be defined so precisely as these two eating disorders. In particular, their diagnostic criteria are *necessary* criteria in the sense that they must all be present if the diagnosis is to be sustained.

#### Anorexia nervosa

In the case of anorexia nervosa the basic diagnostic criteria which have stood the test of time were first put forward in 1970 (Russell 1970) and endorsed in a report from the Pathology of Eating Group at a Dahlem Conference (Garrow *et al.* 1976). The criteria were three-fold:
1 A self-imposed avoidance of 'fattening foods' leading to a marked loss of body weight and malnutrition.
2 An endocrine disorder which manifests itself in the female by a cessation of menstruation, or in

the male by a loss of sexual interest and a lack of potency.
3 A psychological disorder consisting of an over-valued idea expressed as a morbid fear of fatness associated with a fear of losing control over eating.

Since then, DSM-III-R (see Appendix to this chapter) has adopted similar criteria specifying, however, a weight loss of at least 15% as necessary for the diagnosis and adding a disturbance of the way the patient experiences her own body. ICD-10 (see Appendix) also lists the essential three criteria, but adds that the body mass index (BMI = weight in kg/(height in m)$^2$) should fall to 17.5 or less, and elaborates the different methods of weight loss (e.g. self-induced vomiting or purging, exercise, etc.). There are exceptions to the three necessary criteria listed above, and these exceptions are taken care of in ICD-10. For example, menstrual bleeding may persist when the patient is given hormonal replacement therapy or takes a contraceptive pill. Another important modification of the diagnostic criteria allows for an early onset of the illness before the completion of puberty. In children the pubertal sequence may be delayed (growth ceases; in girls the breasts do not develop and there is a primary amenorrhoea; in boys the genitals remain juvenile) (Russell 1985b, World Health Organization 1992).

#### Bulimia nervosa

The three necessary diagnostic criteria for bulimia nervosa remain much the same as when the disorder was first described (Russell 1979):
1 The patients suffer from powerful and intractable urges to overeat.
2 They seek to avoid the 'fattening' effects of food by inducing vomiting or abusing purgatives or both.
3 They have a morbid fear of becoming fat.
The last criterion is shared with uncomplicated anorexia nervosa.

The original version of DSM-III (American Psychiatric Association 1980) introduced a relatively wide set of 'criteria' for a disorder named 'bulimia', and this resulted in the overdiagnosis of behaviours which were less clear-cut than bulimia nervosa. This was corrected in DSM-III-R (American Psychiatric Association 1987) (see Appendix) and the original more satisfactory term, bulimia nervosa, accepted. This version contains the original three necessary criteria but refers to the episodes of overeating by the unattractive word 'binges' which is defined and quantified (at least two binge episodes a week for at least three months). ICD-10 (World Health Organization 1992; see Appendix) also includes the three essential criteria but adds an 'optional' feature, namely that the patient may recount a history of an earlier episode of anorexia nervosa.

In this chapter, the close relationship between anorexia nervosa and bulimia nervosa will be taken for granted. Both disorders share a common psychopathology – a morbid dread of fatness. Patients may develop bulimia nervosa having experienced a preliminary phase of anorexia nervosa. In rarer instances, the course may be in the reverse direction – a patient with bulimia nervosa may avoid food, lose weight and eventually meet the criteria of anorexia nervosa. It was because of this overlap of the two disorders that bulimia nervosa was originally described as a variant of anorexia nervosa (Russell 1979).

## Epidemiology of eating disorders

Epidemiology is an important tool to advance knowledge in social psychiatry. As with other psychiatric disorders, epidemiological methods have yielded valuable information on the distribution of eating disorders and the factors which influence this distribution (see also Chapters 3 and 4). So far the contributions of epidemiology have been greater in anorexia nervosa than bulimia nervosa. Almost certainly this is because bulimia nervosa has only recently been described, and the specific diagnostic criteria previously outlined were only incorporated in the revised form of DSM-III in 1987. The original definitions of DSM-III were too broad and led to diagnostic disagreements between different observers. Moreover, bulimia nervosa does not lend itself as readily to categorization as anorexia nervosa in which severe weight loss and amenorrhoea provide clear

cut-off points. In comparison, the clinical elements of bulimia nervosa are quantitatively distributed and may occur less severely in the normal population.

The principal aims of an epidemiological approach to eating disorders can be considered under a series of headings. The fulfilment of each aim will be summarized in anticipation of a more detailed description further on.

1 The first aim is to provide numerical data on the incidence and prevalence of anorexia nervosa and bulimia nervosa in the general population and within given populations. Several studies dating from 1970 have provided such data, mainly for anorexia nervosa. The most interesting and challenging finding is that the incidence of anorexia nervosa has increased markedly from the 1950s or early 1960s until the late 1970s or even later (Theander 1970, Kendell *et al.* 1973, Jones *et al.* 1980, Willi & Grossman 1983, Szmukler *et al.* 1986, Willi *et al.* 1990).

2 At a causal level, epidemiology aims at detecting associations between the eating disorders and other factors, thus suggesting hypotheses on aetiology and pathogenesis. So far the results have been meagre, merely confirming associations which were already known from clinical studies. Thus, anorexia nervosa occurs mainly in adolescent girls and young women, is commoner in higher or professional social classes and is rare among ethnic minorities. A recent new observation that bulimia nervosa is more prevalent in large cities than in rural areas (Hoek 1991) is thought-provoking and still requires to be explained.

3 Epidemiological research can help complete the clinical picture of disorders. Follow-up studies of 'cases' of anorexia nervosa detected by screening a general population may demonstrate a more favourable outcome than among patients diagnosed in hospital clinics, especially if they were inpatients (Szmukler 1985). So far most long-term follow-up studies have been hospital-based. Their findings suggest much variation in the clinical course of anorexia nervosa, best explained by the operation of selection biases which influence the severity of the illness in the patient population under study (Russell 1991).

**4** It is reasonable to attempt the prevention of eating disorders in populations shown by means of epidemiological studies to be particularly at risk (Slade 1988). A preventive approach would probably require a reduction in the prevalence of hazardous dieting (Patton 1988). This would demand profound cultural changes in defiance of current fashions and would pose serious difficulties (Szmukler 1985). 'Secondary prevention', by the early detection and treatment of established cases, may be a more profitable approach (Slade *et al.* 1990).

**5** Epidemiological research should serve as a guide to the medical and supportive services required to treat and manage eating disorders. Studies along these lines are extraordinarily sparse. One study in the UK under the aegis of the Royal College of Psychiatrists is currently in progress. In the USA much of the treatment is provided through the private sector. It is this author's impression that in most countries therapeutic facilities have arisen haphazardly and are often very scarce.

### Methodology

POPULATIONS STUDIED BY
EPIDEMIOLOGICAL METHODS

### General population surveys

Although a general population survey is said to be ideal from a methodological point of view, there are often problems which render this impracticable, especially when somewhat rare conditions are the subject of the survey (Henderson 1988). Large clinical studies mounted in the community encounter considerable difficulties. The large number of false positives causes time-consuming work, and provides low yields in terms of numbers of cases, thereby limiting useful conclusions (King 1989). How, therefore, does the prospective investigator respond to the criticism that the epidemiology of eating disorders has relied too heavily on clinical descriptions derived from hospital populations (Williams *et al.* 1982, King 1989)? A useful compromise may be that of surveying populations of patients who consult their GPs.

### Surveys of primary care populations

General practices have increasingly provided useful populations for epidemiological surveys, including surveys of eating disorders (Meadows *et al.* 1986, King 1989, Hoek 1991). The earlier studies have proved relatively ineffective in detecting 'cases' with the fully expressed disorder. For example, Meadows *et al.* found only one case of anorexia nervosa and one of bulimia nervosa through their survey, and King failed to detect any case of anorexia nervosa whereas he succeeded in identifying a reasonable number of cases of bulimia nervosa. Hoek's study has been the most successful of these three studies in as much as he obtained credibly high detection rates for both anorexia nervosa and bulimia nervosa.

It is useful to compare these three studies as regards their methodology before examining their findings in greater detail. The first two studies were undertaken in UK general practices. They relied on the use of screening questionnaires, mainly the Eating Attitudes Test (EAT, Garner & Garfinkel 1979). In the first study the questionnaires were mailed to 634 women aged 18–22 years, and the return rate was only 70% (Meadows *et al.* 1986). In the second study, the questionnaires were handed to 748 general practice attenders of both sexes aged 16–35 years and the much higher response rate of 96% was obtained (King 1989). In both studies subjects who scored above a threshold EAT score of 30 were invited to a psychiatric interview: the response rate was only 54% in the first study, but 91% in the second. The first study was therefore seriously marred by the overall poor response rate. The second study may also have missed cases of anorexia nervosa. The author attributed this to 'denial' on the part of anorectics who may have been missed.

These two English studies lacked the advantages built into the Dutch study (Hoek 1991) which was based on 58 general practices and required the GPs themselves to be responsible for diagnosing and registering patients with eating disorders over the course of two years (1985–86). The population under survey covered 151,781 people, the study was part of a continuous morbidity registration in The Netherlands, and the GPs had been instructed in the recognition of eating disorders. The Dutch population under study covered all ages including young adolescents among whom anorexia nervosa is most prevalent. The methodology of the Dutch study therefore commends itself for future surveys based on primary care populations.

## Surveys of populations thought to be particularly at risk

Informative surveys aimed at measuring the prevalence of eating disorders in vulnerable populations have been carried out for anorexia nervosa since the late 1970s and for bulimia nervosa since the early 1980s. Surveys of ballet and modelling students were conducted by Garner & Garfinkel (1980), Szmukler (1983), and Szmukler *et al.* (1985). These investigators predicted that there would be a high prevalence of anorexia nervosa among these students because of the powerful pressures exerted on them by their teachers to maintain a slim figure, in keeping with their professional image.

Populations of adolescent schoolgirls have also been surveyed so as to measure the prevalence of anorexia nervosa among them, as their susceptibility might be raised by virtue of their gender and age, and further increased if dieting was widely practised within the school population (Crisp *et al.* 1976, Mann *et al.* 1983, Szmukler 1983). As in the case of primary care surveys, schoolgirl surveys are likely to identify subjects with an incomplete clinical picture ('subclinical or partial syndromes'). Thus the distinction between those affected and those unaffected becomes less clear (Szmukler 1985). Nevertheless, in ideal circumstances, valuable and near-complete findings can be obtained as in the survey of 15-year-old schoolchildren in Göteborg, Sweden (Råstam *et al.* 1989). The investigators screened this population not only by means of questionnaires but also by using school growth charts for weight and height, and individual school nurse reports. The children screened out by this procedure underwent a full clinical examination and their mothers were interviewed. This thoroughness sets a model for community-based surveys.

## Surveys based on case registers and hospital records

Although these studies have been criticized for relying heavily on hospital records, they have proved their usefulness in providing the earliest estimate of the incidence of anorexia nervosa in different countries (Theander 1970, Kendell *et al.* 1973, Jones *et al.* 1980). Moreover, these estimates were informative in guiding the debate initiated by clinicians who believed that anorexia nervosa had presented more commonly from the 1960s onwards. The core of the data was usually derived from patients referred to inpatient and outpatient psychiatric services, at times supplemented by data on patients who had consulted paediatricians, general medical services or gynaecologists (Szmukler *et al.* 1986, Willi *et al.* 1990). Hospital-based records have not provided useful epidemiological data on bulimia nervosa.

## SCREENING AND ASCERTAINING EATING DISORDERS

Studies based on case registers and hospital records depend on the clinical evaluations made by experienced clinicians which can usually be accepted as reliable if they have adhered to recognized diagnostic criteria. Other surveys which seek to identify cases of anorexia nervosa and bulimia nervosa from sizeable populations usually adopt the strategy of screening out likely 'cases' of one or other disorder. This is followed by clinical interviews of the suspect cases who have scored above a given threshold on the screening test. Structured interviews can be used to advantage at this stage. The most commonly used screening test is the EAT (Garner & Garfinkel 1979). The EAT originally included 40 questions but has been modified and reduced to 26 questions which remain highly predictive of the total EAT-40 score. Thus, the EAT was utilized in the British primary care surveys (EAT-40 by Meadows *et al.* 1986, EAT-26 by King 1989). The following surveys of vulnerable populations also relied on the EAT for initial screening: ballet and modelling students (Garner & Garfinkel 1980, Szmukler *et al.* 1985) and schoolgirls (Mann *et al.* 1983, Szmukler 1983, Eisler & Szmukler 1985).

Although the EAT is the most frequently utilized screening test, doubt has been expressed about its predictive value in the very populations where its use has been popular. These are the populations in which the disorder under scrutiny appears uncommonly – at a rate of less than 10% (Williams *et al.* 1982). Williams and his colleagues have recommended that the Positive Predictive Value (PPV) be calculated for the EAT in the given population to which this test is being applied. The PPV is defined as the probability that a respondent with an above-threshold score on the screening questionnaire is actually a 'case' (in this instance a case of an eating disorder). It is calculated as follows:

$$\frac{\text{Number of identified cases of eating disorders}}{\text{Number of above-threshold scorers on the EAT}}.$$

It transpires that, in the population surveys of students and schoolgirls previously cited, the PPV ranges from 0.19 for the modelling students of Garner & Garfinkel to 0.04 for the girls attending state schools in England (Eisler & Szmukler 1985). These figures signify that only 19–4% of the EAT-screened positive scorers will actually have an eating disorder. These low percentages are a feature of surveys for disorders that have a low prevalence in the given populations. The relationship has been expressed mathematically by Shrout & Fleiss (1981):

$$PPV = \frac{P \times Se}{(1 - Sp) + P(Se + Sp - 1)},$$

where $P$ = prevalence, $Se$ = sensitivity and $Sp$ = specificity of the screening test (see also Chapter 3).

If the prevalence for an eating disorder is less than 10% the PPV of the EAT would inevitably be less than 50%, i.e. over half of the high scorers would not have an eating disorder.

The lessons from these observations are clear: the EAT has limited usefulness in surveys of populations which differ in the true prevalence of eating disorders. Comparisons should not be made on test scores alone. More detailed assessments, including clinical assessments, are essential

(Williams *et al.* 1982, Szmukler 1985, King 1989). Eisler & Szmukler (1985) also found that social class is a confounding variable in the EAT. They found that the mean EAT score was higher in state schools than in private schools, even though the number of cases of anorexia nervosa identified by means of individual interviews was much lower in the state schools. The discrepancy was due to systematic differences in the way the girls responded to different sets of questions of the EAT. Another caution about the EAT as a screening instrument has been expressed by King & Bhugra (1989) regarding its application to populations differing from those for which it was originally devised. Some of the questions in the EAT might be interpreted differently for linguistic, social or religious reasons, thereby weakening the comparability of the instrument for cross-cultural epidemiological research. It should be noted that, even with large populations, screening using more objective methods than questionnaires is possible and can yield impressive results. The study by Råstam *et al.* (1989) is a good example: 4291 schoolchildren were initially screened by means of school weight and growth charts and discussions with school nurses.

Surveys depending on initial screening by questionnaire also run the risk of failing to detect the very cases being sought. If the initial response rate to a questionnaire falls short of 100%, the non-respondents are precisely those subjects who conceal their disorder, even if they are currently receiving active treatment (Johnson-Sabine *et al.* 1988). It is also necessary to achieve a near-total success in interviewing high scorers on screening tests. King (1989) found that the 3 general practice patients who refused to be interviewed out of a possible 76 had previously consulted their GP because they were worried about their weight and had requested diets. These observations recognize Fairburn's view (1990) that eating disorders may be more common among those who choose not to cooperate with prevalence studies. Fairburn proposes that a satisfactory methodology must include a two-stage design – a structured interview to follow the self-report screening instrument. Such a structured face-to-face interview is necessary to elicit the key features of bulimia nervosa and thus

**Table 16.1** The incidence of anorexia nervosa

| Area | Authors | Period | Incidence per 100 000 population per annum |
|------|---------|--------|------------|
| Southern Sweden | Theander 1970* | 1931–40 | 0.08 |
| | | 1941–50 | 0.19 |
| | | 1951–60 | 0.45 |
| North-east Scotland | Kendell et al. 1973[†] | 1966–69 | 1.60 |
| | Szmukler et al. 1986[†] | 1978–82 | 4.06 |
| Zurich canton | Willi & Grossmann 1983* | 1963–65 | 0.55 |
| | | 1973–75 | 1.12 |
| | Willi et al. 1990* | 1983–85 | 1.43 |
| Monroe County, USA | Kendell et al. 1973[†] | 1960–69 | 0.37 |
| | Jones et al. 1980*[†] | 1970–76 | 0.64 |
| Denmark (nationwide) | Nielsen 1990[‡] | 1973–87 | 1.00 |
| Wellington, New Zealand | Hall & Hay 1991[§] | 1977–86 | 5.00 |
| Rochester, Minnesota, USA | Lucas et al. 1991[¶] | 1935–79 | 8.20 |
| Netherlands (general practice) | Hoek 1991[¶] | 1985–86 | 6.3 |

* Based on hospital records: admissions only, but including medical, paediatric, gynaecological as well as psychiatric admissions.
[†] Case-register studies.
[‡] Nationwide register of psychiatric admissions.
[§] Based on the referrals to the one available service in the treatment of eating disorders.
[¶] Community surveys, including non-hospitalized patients.

permit a correct diagnosis. Moreover, the screening instrument itself should be evaluated. For example, it must be ascertained whether a number of cases may not have been interviewed because they escaped detection by the screening instrument.

### Results of epidemiological surveys

#### INCIDENCE OF ANOREXIA NERVOSA

Table 16.1 lists estimates of the incidence of anorexia nervosa in different countries as reported by named researchers. The incidence rates found at specified periods of time are shown in the last two columns. The most informative data are provided from the studies which were repeated over different periods of time. The footnotes summarize the methodology and population for each study, as outlined earlier in this chapter. Table 16.1 includes only well-executed studies as defined by a careful methodology, the use of defined diagnostic criteria and a survey of a sufficiently large population (at least 50 000 people). An attempt will now be made to interpret the wide range of incidence rates that have been reported.

### Variations in incidence in different countries

It is likely that the different countries listed in Table 16.1 resemble each other in those sociocultural features that influence the appearance of eating disorders. The variations in the incidence of anorexia nervosa are more readily explained by factors other than national differences, especially those of methodology and differences in the patient population surveyed.

### Variations attributable to methodology and patient populations

The studies which counted only hospitalized patients with anorexia nervosa tended to yield low estimates of its incidence (Theander 1970, Willi & Grossman 1983, Nielsen 1990). Estimates based on case registers of psychiatric patients similarly yielded fairly low but variable incidence rates (Kendell *et al.* 1973, Jones *et al.* 1980). An exception was an incidence of 5.0 per year per 100 000 found in The Netherlands, but based on a relatively small population (Hoek & Brook 1985). In contrast, the incidence rates obtained from community-based studies were by far the highest (Lucas *et al.* 1988, Hoek 1991), presumably because they included less severe cases who were not admitted to hospital nor seen by specialists.

### Changes attributable to time

In view of the wide variations between studies, attributable to differences in methodology and populations surveyed, it is best simply to interpret the changes of incidence occurring in the same population surveyed at repeated intervals. This is possible with the surveys conducted in southern Sweden, north-east Scotland, Switzerland, Monroe County, USA, and Rochester, Minnesota, USA. In the first four of these serial surveys the researchers applied the same methodology to a similar population. Thus many of the other variables were controlled for, leaving the passage of years as the main factor influencing the incidence of anorexia nervosa. In the first four of these areas there was a clear trend of a progressive increase in incidence over successive years.

Theander (1970) was the first investigator to observe an increased incidence of anorexia ner-

vosa over three successive decades (1931–60). He was extremely cautious in interpreting his finding. The other investigators who found a similarly rising incidence tended to attribute this to changes in culturally determined attitudes or behaviour patterns over time (Kendell *et al.* 1973, Szmukler *et al.* 1986).

An initially discrepant finding was reported by Lucas and his colleagues in their first publication (Lucas *et al.* 1988). Contrary to their expectations, they did not find that the incidence of anorexia nervosa was any higher during recent years (1965–79) than in the earlier period of their study (1935–49). It should be noted that theirs was the highest estimate yet obtained (8.2 per 100 000 per annum). This high rate is probably explained by the wide scope of the study which concentrated on the population of Rochester, Minnesota (58 000 in 1980), and derived its data from the epidemiology archives at the Mayo Clinic. The diagnoses made at every centre of medical care in Rochester and the surrounding Olmsted County were entered into the archives: they were established during office consultations, house calls, emergency room visits as well as hospital admissions.

Lucas *et al.* (1991) recalculated their data, separating female patients who fell into the 15–24-year age band (61%) from the remaining (mainly older) patients. When the incidence rates for each five-year period from 1935–39 to 1980–84 were plotted, an increase was established after all in this younger group. Lucas concluded that this increase in incidence rates over successive half-decades reflected the greater vulnerability of the younger female subjects to adverse social factors. He further concluded that anorexia nervosa in older age groups might represent a different form of the disorder, possibly one more determined by biological factors.

The question of the rise in incidence of anorexia nervosa will again be discussed in a broader context later in this chapter.

**Table 16.2** The prevalence of anorexia nervosa in vulnerable female populations

| Subjects | Area | Age (years: mean or range) | Prevalence rate (%) |
|---|---|---|---|
| Ballet students | Toronto, Canada* | 18.6 ± 0.3 | 6.5 |
| | South-East England[†] | 15.6 ± 1.6 | 7.0[‡] |
| Modelling students | Toronto, Canada* | 21.4 ± 0.3 | 7.0 |
| Dietitians | UK[§] | 20–39 | 2.3 |
| Schoolgirls | London – private schools [‖][¶] | 16+ | 1.0 |
| | | 16–18 | 1.1 |
| | London – state schools [‖][¶] | 16+ | 0.2 |
| | | 16–18 | 0.14 |
| | London – state schools** | 15 | 0 |
| | Göteborg, Sweden[††] | 15 and under | 0.84 |
| | Rome, Italy[‡‡] | 13–20 | 0.8 |
| | South Australia[§§] | 12–18 | 0.1 |

* Garner & Garfinkel (1980).
[†] Szmukler *et al.* (1985).
[‡] Described as 'possible cases', see text.
[§] Morgan & Mayberry (1983).
[‖] Crisp *et al.* (1976).
[¶] Szmukler (1983).
** Mann *et al.* (1983).
[††] Råstam *et al.* (1989).
[‡‡] Cuzzolaro *et al.* (1990).
[§§] Ben-Tovim & Morton (1990).

## PREVALENCE OF ANOREXIA NERVOSA IN VULNERABLE POPULATIONS

Table 16.2 lists the findings of prevalence surveys in populations selected according to predicted degrees of risk for developing anorexia nervosa. All the populations consisted of female subjects.

The first survey of ballet and modelling students was carried out by Garner & Garfinkel (1980). The prevalence rates found in the ballet students (6.5%) and the modelling students (7%) were in keeping with their prediction that they were highly at risk because of professional and competitive pressures to acquire and maintain a slim figure. Moreover, most of these students were enrolled at a young age (10–12 years) and developed the disorder later on, while actively training in ballet. A similar study was undertaken in an English ballet school by Szmukler *et al.* (1985). They also found a high prevalence of 'possible' cases of anorexia nervosa but drew a distinction from patients presenting clinically, because at the end of one year's follow-up these 'possible' cases had all improved without any medical intervention.

These two studies were carefully executed. The students were screened by means of the EAT and they were all weighed and measured. Students who obtained a high score on the EAT were clinically interviewed and a number of 'cases' of anorexia nervosa identified, yielding the prevalence rates for the disorder shown in Table 16.2.

An equally exact methodology was not used in the study on British dietitians who were invited to return a questionnaire (Morgan & Mayberry 1983). The response rate was only 51%. No interviews were carried out and the subjects were simply asked if they had suffered from any of a number of illnesses listed in the questionnaire. The prevalence rate of anorexia nervosa shown in Table 16.2 is calculated for the younger respondents from the data provided by the authors. These is thus an apparent increased frequency of anorexia nervosa among British dietitians, but the study could not ascertain whether sufferers from the disorder were attracted into the profession or whether the recruits to dietetics developed the illness subsequently.

The other surveys listed in Table 16.2 were all concerned with ascertaining the prevalence of eating disorders in schoolgirls. Most of them utilized the screening procedure already described: high scorers on the EAT questionnaires were subsequently interviewed (Mann *et al.* 1983, Szmukler 1983, Ben-Tovim & Morton 1990). The weakness of this screening method has already been pointed out, and there is also the risk that some patients concealed their disorder ('denial' as suggested by King (1989)). The method of Crisp *et al.* (1976) differed in that there was no systematic screening. A 'case spotting' exercise was achieved through interviews with key staff in the schools – physical training teachers, matrons and school medical officers – and this led to frank cases of anorexia nervosa being identified.

There is a fairly wide variation among the prevalence rates reported (from 0 to 1.1%). More informative, however, is the consistent difference in prevalence rates in the English studies between private schools where a 1% rate was found and state schools where a low rate (0–0.2%) was obtained. This result is consistent with the view that social class influences the prevalence of anorexia nervosa, higher rates being manifest among the daughters of middle-class and professional English parents who tend to educate their children in private schools.

Such a social class distinction was not found to operate in the Swedish study (Råstam 1990). The overall prevalence of 0.84% for the total population of 2136 schoolgirls in Göteborg up to and including 15 years of age, represents a high frequency for anorexia nervosa (Råstam *et al.* 1989). This result indicates that the disorder is more common in this young population than had been thought by previous investigators. This relatively high prevalence rate can be taken as probably the most accurately determined result so far. It should be noted that a similarly high prevalence rate was obtained in a population of Rome schoolgirls, but their age range was much wider, thus increasing the chances of a relatively high rate being detected.

**Table 16.3** The prevalence of bulimia nervosa in women

| Subjects | Area | Age (years: range) | Prevalence rate (%) |
| --- | --- | --- | --- |
| Schoolgirls | London* | 16–18 | 0.37 |
| | London[†] | 14–16 | 0.99 |
| General practice | London[‡] | 16–35 | 1.00 |
| Urban population | Christchurch, New Zealand[§] | 18–44 | 0.70 |

\* Szmukler 1983.
[†] Johnson-Sabine *et al.* 1988.
[‡] King 1989.
[§] Bushnell *et al.* 1990.

Finally, it may be mentioned that most of these surveys identified subjects with less severe, subclinical forms of anorexia nervosa which have been named 'partial syndromes' (Szmukler 1985, Råstam *et al.* 1989).

## PREVALENCE AND INCIDENCE STUDIES IN BULIMIA NERVOSA

In spite of numerous studies during the past ten years, there have been few solid advances in our knowledge of the epidemiology of bulimia nervosa. Fairburn (1990) has reviewed the reasons for limited progress and attributed this to defects of methodology. The early studies relied exclusively on self-report questionnaires and unrepresentative populations – especially college students in the USA. Moreover, the diagnostic criteria then used in the USA were those of DSM-III for 'bulimia', which were insufficiently specific and permitted the inclusion of subjects who would not have met the criteria of bulimia nervosa as originally described (Russell 1979), or those of DSM-III-R or ICD-10. Thus, the results of these early studies yielded improbably high prevalence rates, e.g. 4.5% among 'freshman' college students (Pyle *et al.* 1983) and 5% among high-school girls (Johnson *et al.* 1984). An even higher figure (12%) was found for self-induced vomiting in female students (Halmi *et al.* 1981). Fairburn has reviewed the few studies that have used a more satisfactory two-stage methodology, and relied on the diagnostic criteria of Russell (1979) or DSM-III-R. The improved methodology has resulted in lower estimates of the prevalence of bulimia nervosa, which have been fairly consistent – about 1% among adolescents and young adult women (Fairburn 1990).

Some of the better prevalence studies were based on schoolgirl and general practice populations (Table 16.3). Szmukler (1983) investigated younger schoolgirls in England. Only 1 in 270 girls was diagnosed as suffering from bulimia nervosa, and he expressed the reservation that the severity of their disorder was generally less than in cases encountered clinically. In another, but larger, survey of London schoolgirls, a prevalence rate of 0.99% was detected for bulimia nervosa, and additionally 1.78% for 'partial syndrome' (Johnson-Sabine *et al.* 1988). Meadows *et al.* (1986) followed the recommended two-phased approach for their survey of general practices in Leicester. Unfortunately, it was marred by relatively low response rates, both for returning the EAT questionnaire and accepting the clinical interviews when high scorers indicated the need for an interview. A prevalence of only 0.25% was found for bulimia nervosa but there were several additional 'cases of partial syndrome'. The survey by King (1989) of eating disorders in a general practice population in south London yielded higher response rates and arguably more reliable results. One per cent of women aged between 16 and 35 years had bulimia nervosa and a further 3% had a partial-syndrome eating disorder.

Three further studies merit description because they sampled a wider cross-section of the population, and in the case of the first two relied on a methodology which differed from that recommended by Fairburn. The first, based on general practices in The Netherlands, depended on diagnoses made by the GPs themselves (Hoek 1991). The design permitted calculations of an incidence rate for the whole population at all ages, which resulted in a figure of 9.9 cases of bulimia nervosa per 100 000 population (Table 16.4). The point prevalence of bulimia nervosa was 20.4 per 100 000. The majority (71%) were aged over 25 years. The second study relied not on a community sample but on the clinical diagnoses made by the only available psychiatric specialist in eating disorders for the population in the Wellington region of New Zealand which numbered 340 000. The

authors described a sharply rising incidence of bulimia nervosa over the years 1976–86, culminating in a rate of 6.0 per 100 000 by the end of the survey (1985–86) (Table 16.4). The incidence rate for females aged 15–29 years at that time was 44 per 100 000. The third study, again from New Zealand, made use of a sampling strategy involving 'primary sampling units' from the census tracts of the entire Christchurch urban area (Bushnell *et al.* 1990). There were two interviews in subjects suspected of bulimic symptomatology: both used the Diagnostic Interview Schedule (DIS). The first was by a lay interviewer who was trained in the use of the DIS; the second was a clinician who applied appropriate sections of the DIS including the bulimia section. The finding varied according to which set of diagnostic criteria was used and whether recent or lifetime prevalence was sought. For women aged 18–44 years the prevalence of recent disorder was 0.2% for DSM-III bulimia, 0.5% for DSM-III-R bulimia nervosa and nil for Russell's criteria. The last finding arose because none of the cases admitted to vomiting or purging. The authors conclude that a true bulimia syndrome is far from common, although disturbed eating behaviour was widespread in their population.

### Conclusions drawn from epidemiological surveys

The causal associations discovered from epidemiological surveys can be briefly summarized. Fairburn (1990) believes that so far these surveys have contributed little in terms of aetiological explanations for bulimia nervosa. On the other hand, Johnson-Sabine *et al.* (1988) concluded that risk factors for eating disorders could be identified, in particular a history of being overweight or a general psychiatric morbidity. The remainder of this section will be concerned with conclusions drawn from surveys in anorexia nervosa.

#### AGE AND SEX

The epidemiological surveys yielded no surprises and confirmed established clinical opinion that anorexia nervosa commences most frequently in

Table 16.4 The incidence of bulimia nervosa

| Area | Authors | Incidence per 100 000 per annum |
|------|---------|----------------------------------|
| Netherlands | Hoek 1991 | 9.9 |
| New Zealand (Wellington) | Hall & Hay 1991 | 6.0 |

the young, especially within a few years of puberty. The two community-based surveys, having examined the most representative populations, are arguably the best source of evidence. In the Rochester (USA) study, half the cases in females occurred before the age of 20 years and at a rate 3.1 times greater than for females aged 20–59 years (Lucas *et al.* 1988). Among 'new patients' (with a recent onset) in The Netherlands, 63% were aged less than 20 years.

The marked predominance of female over male patients was also confirmed. The percentage of female patients was 88% in Rochester; 88% in Wellington, New Zealand; 92% in north-east Scotland (Szmukler *et al.* 1986); 92% in Denmark (Nielsen 1990); and 90% of the children in Göteborg (Råstam 1990). The predominance of females has been less in some of the clinical series of children with anorexia nervosa: 14 out of 20 prepubertal children reported by Jacobs & Isaacs (1986) and 35 out of 48 early-onset patients described by Fosson *et al.* (1987).

SOCIAL CLASS AND
SOCIOECONOMIC STATUS

Received wisdom from clinicians tells us that anorexia nervosa occurs predominantly in patients from middle-class backgrounds. For example, an observation made in 1880 was firm on the point that anorexia nervosa 'is much more common in wealthier classes of society than amongst those who have to procure their bread by daily labour' (Fenwick 1880). This view was apparently confirmed by clinicians working from specialist centres who reported on series of patients. Adopting the Registrar-General's five categories based on parental occupation, several investigators found an overrepresentation of patients in social classes I and II. The combined percentages of patients in these two social classes came to 66% in the series of Morgan & Russell (1975) and 74% in that of Crisp *et al.* (1980). In contrast, the combined social classes I and II comprised 27% of the general population in the UK in the 1981 Census. This conventional view of an upper social class predominance among anorexia nervosa patients has been challenged and attributed to a selection

bias operating for patients referred to specialist centres (Szmukler *et al.* 1986). This bias would be less powerful among patients listed on psychiatric case registers. Indeed, a high social class predominance was not found in the two studies utilizing the case register for north-east Scotland: social class I and II patients totalled only 34% in 1963–71 (Kendell *et al.* 1973) and 46% in 1978–82 (Szmukler *et al.* 1986). However, in another investigation utilizing a psychiatric case register in Zurich, Switzerland, a higher social class distribution was once again found by the researchers who utilized socioeconomic status of patients' fathers in categories of their own design (Willi *et al.* 1990). It must, therefore, be conceded that epidemiological surveys aimed at wider populations leave the question of the social class distribution in anorexia nervosa somewhat equivocal. On the other hand, prevalence surveys focused on school populations reinforce the clinical impression of a higher social class predominance, as demonstrated by high prevalence rates in private schools compared with state schools (Crisp *et al.* 1976, Szmukler 1983, Råstam 1990).

HAS THE INCIDENCE OF ANOREXIA
NERVOSA INCREASED SINCE THE 1950S?

As long ago as 1965, clinicians expressed the view that anorexia nervosa was no longer a rare disorder, but had increased in frequency, for example in Germany (Von Baeyer 1965) and in Japan more specifically since World War II (Ishikawa 1965). Hilde Bruch said the same in 1965, and by 1978 she wrote in more dramatic terms: 'One might speak of an epidemic illness, only there is no contagious agent; the spread must be attributed to psycho-social factors'.

As she believed in the reality of the spread of anorexia nervosa within populations she was right to speak of an epidemic and perceptive in attributing it to psychosocial factors. But it is questionable whether the spread is so great numerically as to merit the description of an epidemic. Not surprisingly, the term was seized upon as an Aunt Sally by Williams & King (1987) who incorporated it in the provocative title of their dismissive article: 'The "epidemic" of anorexia nervosa: another medical myth?' Williams & King examined the number of patients aged 10–64 years, admitted with the diagnosis of anorexia nervosa to psychiatric hospitals and units in England and Wales during the decade 1972–81. They applied an intricate method of statistical analysis (age-period-cohort modelling). They concluded that the undoubted increase in first admissions of patients with anorexia nervosa over the ten years was due entirely to an increase in the number of young women (aged 15–24) in the population, rather than a true increase in morbidity risk. Yet an examination of the raw data, rather than the presence or absence of significant changes, shows that the increase of women aged 15–24 years amounted to 11.6%, only about half the increase of first admissions over the decade (about 21%). Their conclusions should also be questioned because solid criticisms can be levied against the quality of their primary data. They ignored patients managed in non-psychiatric settings, in psychiatric outpatient clinics and in general practice, who would outnumber by far those admitted to psychiatric hospitals. Moreover, the routine returns of the diagnostic data they obtained from the Department of Health and Social Security are subject to error, a fact these authors concede. The value of the study by Williams & King lies in their warning that a change in morbidity must be analysed in the context of possible changes in the population in which it occurs. The more recent epidemiological surveys have indeed adjusted their prevalence rates to reflect the size of the young female population under study (Lucas *et al.* 1988, Willi *et al.* 1990). The strictures of Williams & King against an increase in the incidence of anorexia nervosa should, therefore, be put aside to enable conclusions to be drawn from the large body of research summarized in Table 16.1.

Almost all these epidemiological studies confirm an increased incidence of anorexia nervosa dating from around the 1950s and accelerating in the 1970s. In the Rochester study, however, this increase applied only to younger patients, aged 15–24 years. Another exception arises from the survey in Zurich where the investigators concluded that the rising incidence of anorexia nervosa had levelled off by 1983–85 (Willi *et al.* 1990). The

high but level incidence rates found in Wellington, New Zealand, can also be attributed to a plateau having been reached by the time the data had been gathered (Hall & Hay 1991). It can be concluded that the incidence of anorexia nervosa did indeed rise from the 1950s until the late 1970s, confirming the impressions of clinicians practising in the field.

## ADVERSE SOCIAL FACTORS IN CAUSING ANOREXIA NERVOSA

When Garner & Garfinkel (1980) demonstrated a relatively high prevalence of anorexia nervosa and excessive dieting concerns among dance and modelling students, they concluded that these young women were reacting adversely to their professional environment. Both kinds of careers involved increased attention to their body shape and the need to bring it under personal 'control'. The investigators also found that the prevalence of anorexia nervosa was higher among dancers in highly competitive schools than in less competitive settings. On the other hand, a keenly competitive environment without the focus on body shape (a school of music) did not lead to anorexia nervosa nor excessive concerns with food and weight among the students. Thus, they concluded that individuals who are obliged to focus their attention on acquiring a slim body shape are at risk for anorexia nervosa. This research provided the first objective evidence in support of the thesis that adverse social pressures of a specific kind can lead to anorexia nervosa, at least in vulnerable subjects. Garner & Garfinkel elaborated their findings further into a general theory that anorexia nervosa was a multidetermined disorder, with an important role for sociopathogenesis. They recognized the powerful impact of the media in establishing role models for women with a thin body shape.

The London study on ballet students yielded similar results to the Toronto study in finding a raised prevalence of anorexia nervosa, amounting to 7% (Szmukler *et al.* 1985). On the other hand, these investigators qualified their findings by stressing that their 'cases' only just reached the criteria for 'caseness', functioned well physically and socially, and responded promptly to sensible advice from their teachers to regain weight. Thus, the value of simple early intervention was clear. The implications were that the social pressures of attending a competitive ballet school only led to a mild form of anorexia nervosa, so long as there were no additional adverse factors, either in the patient's environment or in her own motivation for capitalizing on the effects of continued weight loss. In spite of this reservation both studies confirmed that social pressures can induce women to adopt an idealized thinner body shape. Garner & Garfinkel went further and suggested that society's current idealization of thinness in women could be a determinant of the purported increase in the incidence of anorexia nervosa.

## Transcultural aspects of eating disorders

It has long been known that anorexia nervosa is not universal in its geographical distribution. It is recognized to occur with increasing frequency in westernized and industrialized societies, but still to be rare in Asia (particularly in India), the Middle East (with the exception of Israel), and generally in poorly developed countries. Clinical reports indicate that anorexia nervosa has long been recognized in Russia and in the modern Soviet Union, though the patients tend to come from prosperous, well-educated families (Di Nicola 1990).

### *Rarity among black subjects within western populations*

In recent years clinical reports have been supplemented by more systematic observations. In particular, *comparisons of ethnic or racial groups in the same country* have led to the recognition of eating disorders across different cultures. Anorexia nervosa was previously considered to be very rare in members of the black races. Thus, experienced clinicians in the USA whose treatment centres included large black populations could assert as recently as 1977: '...all the patients referred meeting the criteria of anorexia nervosa were Caucasian. There is not a single well-documented case in the literature of this illness occurring in a black' (Halmi *et al.* 1977). However, a number of case reports appeared in the early 1980s (Garfinkel & Garner 1982, Robinson & Andersen 1985, Thomas & Szmukler 1985). Hsu (1987) reviewed 18 cases and described 4 black patients with anorexia nervosa and 3 with 'bulimia'. A further series of 13 black patients (2 anorexia nervosa; 11 bulimia nervosa) from the Maudsley Hospital, London was published in 1988 (Holden & Robinson 1988). The authors of these two reports concluded that eating disorders were becoming more common in blacks.

Hsu attempted to explain the relative protection of blacks from eating disorders that had prevailed hitherto. He suggested that they were less often obese, less preoccupied with weight and shape, and less likely to diet. On the other hand, this relative protection may be diminishing because of increasing affluence among some blacks leading to the acquisition of white middle class values, and through the influence of the media. In London, however, the black patients came from families where divorce was more prevalent and the fathers were from a lower social class, as compared with a control group of white eating-disordered patients (Holden & Robinson 1988).

### *Effects of major cultural change: eating disorders in immigrants*

In a number of studies it has been demonstrated that younger female immigrants who move to a new culture may suffer from an increased prevalence of eating disorders. These studies have usually been initiated on the assumption that exposure to western culture would be the cause of this increased prevalence. Thus, Nasser (1986) compared two matched samples of Arab female students attending London and Cairo Universities. Abnormal eating attitudes were estimated on the EAT-40, and clinical cases of eating disorders were determined by means of the Eating Interview. A higher proportion of abnormal EAT scores was obtained with the London sample (22%) than the Cairo sample (12%). Among the 50 London Arab students, six satisfied diagnostic criteria for bulimia nervosa and five were thought to constitute a partial syndrome of anorexia nervosa. Among the

60 Cairo students, there were no cases of anorexia nervosa nor bulimia nervosa. The large differences were attributed to the westernization of the London Arab students whose dress, for example, was similar to that of European students, whereas the Cairo students were generally traditional in their dress, some even wearing the veil. Some of the London students disclosed they had had a prior contact with sufferers from bulimia, suggesting 'socially contagious behaviour'. It is fair to conclude from this study that migrants acquire a greater vulnerability to eating disorders than prevails in their original culture. However, Nasser's very high 'case' rates of bulimia nervosa may have been due to a selective recruitment of her subjects.

A surprisingly high rate of eating disorders among Asian schoolgirls in Bradford was reported by Mumford & Whitehouse (1988). Six hundred 14 to 16 year olds were screened using the EAT-26, and they found a higher percentage of Asian girls (15%) than white girls (12%) scoring above threshold (20). Seventy-five per cent of the high-scoring subjects agreed to be interviewed.

Bulimia nervosa was diagnosed in seven of the Asian and two of the white schoolgirls – a statistically significant difference; only one case of anorexia nervosa was diagnosed, and that was among the Asian girls. These transcultural studies have been criticized in that they rely a great deal on the EAT whose questions may be misconstrued by subjects from the Third World, and even structured clinical interviews may give rise to cultural misunderstandings (King & Bhugra 1989). The latter transcultural study also yielded prevalence rates which were surprisingly higher than in comparable English populations.

A somewhat different interpretation was put forward for the finding that anorexia nervosa was more prevalent in a sample of Greek girls in Germany (1.1%) than among Greek girls who remained with their families in Greece (0.42%) (Fichter *et al.* 1983). This difference was attributed to the new social influences that affected the families of migrant Greek workers, rather than changes in the ideology of slimness and the practice of dieting which were, if anything, stronger in Greece.

## Prevalence study in a Third World population

It would seem highly desirable to measure the prevalence of eating disorders in populations judged to be free from westernized cultural influences. Such studies have not been undertaken, presumably because of difficulties in funding them. One exception is a prevalence survey in a state secondary school on São Miguel Island in the Azores (Portuguese) in which 1234 pupils of both sexes, aged 12–30 years, were given the Diagnostic Interview for Children and Adolescents which leads to DSM-III diagnoses. The interviews were conducted by senior nursing students after a period of instruction. The pupils were all white and came from social classes III and IV (Pinto de Azevedo & Ferreira 1992). During the preceding decade, no clinical cases of anorexia nervosa nor bulimia had been identified by the sole specialist in psychiatry residing and practising in the island. The results showed that the full syndromes of anorexia nervosa and bulimia were rarely encountered. Among the schoolgirls, the prevalence of DSM-III bulimia was only 0.3%, and there was no full case of anorexia nervosa (even though for partial syndromes the prevalence was 0.76%).

The authors concluded that the lower prevalence rates found in this school population were due to cultural differences. The pupils resided in an isolated island community free from sociocultural pressures to control eating and weight, such as prevail in western industrialized countries.

## Is anorexia nervosa a culture-bound syndrome?

This question is certainly relevant in view of the preceding account of the influence of cultural factors on the expression of anorexia nervosa. Moreover, the proposition that anorexia nervosa is a culture-bound syndrome has been put forward by at least four writers. Wig (1983) did so because he thought that it was as logical to consider 'intense fear of becoming obese' culture-bound as 'fear about shrinking of the genitals' (Koro). Prince (1985) believed that anorexia nervosa is the culture-bound syndrome which is most understandable to a western audience: 'As Westerners we all experience first-hand the powerful anorexic influences that are currently playing upon us, particularly the Western female.' When considering whether culture-bound syndromes ever originated in western cultures, Leff (1988) indicated that anorexia nervosa is an obvious candidate. Di Nicola (1990) also welcomes the inclusion of anorexia nervosa within the culture-bound syndromes, but prefers the term culture-reactive syndrome as he argues that it occurs mainly during conditions of rapid culture change.

The term culture-bound syndrome is not, however, self-explanatory. Indeed, there is no consensus about its meaning (Simons 1985). Hence, an attempt should be made to explain its origin and reach the clearest possible definition. The expression originally came from the term 'atypical culture-bound psychogenic psychoses' coined by Yap in 1962. In 1969 he substituted the term 'the culture-bound reactive syndromes' to cover a wide range of exotic behavioural disorders or syndromes, including Amok, Koro and Latah. He considered them to be culture-bound variants of reactive psychosis. Since then, the concept of the culture-bound syndrome has broadened and the plainest definition has been put forward by Prince (1985):

> A culture-bound syndrome may be defined as a collection of signs and symptoms which is not to be found universally in human populations, but is restricted to a particular culture or group of cultures. Implicit is the view that cultural factors play an important role in the genesis of the symptom cluster . . .

Prince adds the refinement that cultural effects should be limited to their psychosocial aspects. Leff (1988) has also proposed that the cultural forces may unmask a psychopathology which would otherwise remain hidden. When it is expressed it fulfils a function for the individual or his social group. For example, when a man goes amok and acts on his murderous rage, his social group may condone in part his aggression as the consequence of provocation.

Anorexia nervosa does meet these criteria of a culture-bound syndrome. First, it is limited in its occurrence to westernized or industrialized nations. Secondly, it is evident that psychosocial

pressures on women to achieve and maintain thinness constitute the most powerful component of the cultural factors leading to anorexia nervosa. The drive for thinness is not necessarily the only pathogenic cultural influence: we have already seen that the studies on Greek immigrant students in Munich led the authors to conclude that there was not always a direct link between the ideology of slimness and anorexia nervosa (Fichter *et al.* 1983). Other cultural influences which have been adduced are the juxtaposition of affluence and anorexia nervosa, changes in family configurations (Selvini-Palazzoli 1974) and unease with society's definition of femininity (Orbach 1979).

In order to accommodate exceptions to the rule, when anorexia nervosa occurs in non-westernized countries or within hitherto-protected cultural subgroups, Di Nicola (1990) has suggested that the illness can best be construed as arising in cultures undergoing rapid culture change. He views anorexia nervosa as a 'culture-change syndrome', thereby explaining the increased incidence of eating disorders in Japan and Israel (Kaffman & Sadeh 1989) and their raised prevalence in immigrant groups.

The concept of rapid culture change may also fit in with the views of feminist writers regarding women's vulnerability to eating disorders. Orbach sees anorexia nervosa as a 'hunger strike' in protest against society's definition of femininity. The anorectic adopts a slender shape to express her ambivalence about her femininity and her sexuality. On the one hand thinness is demanded of modern woman; on the other hand, it precludes her functioning as a real woman. The puzzle is why anorexia nervosa should have become common in the very societies and times when women's opportunities and social positions have at last improved. The answer might lie in the rapidity of the social changes and the conflicting pressures generated in vulnerable young women. They may be unable to reconcile the older expectations that women should be passive, dependent and all-giving, with the more modern goals of becoming independent, successful and high achievers (Butler 1988). It has also been proposed that women who are eager to achieve professional competence and appear intelligent, tend to adhere to a slim standard of body attractiveness (Silverstein *et al.* 1986a,b).

## The modern history of anorexia nervosa

The evidence reviewed so far clearly indicates the power of sociocultural forces to modify anorexia nervosa in two important ways:

1  By increasing its incidence, and
2  By changing its clinical form.

Data have already been presented in support of the increased frequency of anorexia nervosa in Western Europe and North America since the 1950s. Within these areas, anorexia nervosa has spread to subgroups who were previously protected (blacks in the USA and the UK). It has also spread to countries where it was previously uncommon. The strongest evidence of a change in the clinical form of the illness comes from the emergence of bulimia nervosa, first described as a variant of anorexia nervosa in 1979 (Russell 1979). Thus, it may be argued that anorexia nervosa has become transformed over recent decades (Russell 1985a, Russell & Treasure 1989).

It has long been recognized that mental illness, and the neuroses in particular, may undergo transformation. Karl Jaspers (1959) contrasted the more stable features of an illness with what he called their 'contemporary style'. He recognized that neurotic disorders could take on different forms with the passage of time:

> . . . we can learn how the picture of illness shifts though scientifically the illness may be identical; the neuroses in particular have a contemporary style – they flourish in certain situations and are almost invisible in others.
>
> The general impression nowadays regarding neuroses is as follows: hysterias have greatly decreased . . . the compulsive neuroses on the other hand have greatly increased.

How far should we widen the scope for the diagnosis of anorexia nervosa without running the risk of a loss of clinical cohesion? The arguments for retaining bulimia nervosa within the generic field of anorexia nervosa have been presented before (Russell 1979, Russell & Treasure, 1989). In essence, the two disorders share important clinical similarities, especially the patients' dread of weight gain. Moreover, the same patient may suffer from both illnesses at different times: the sequence is most often from anorexia to bulimia nervosa, but it can also occur in the reverse direction (Fahy *et al.* 1989). There is, however, a limit to the elasticity of the diagnostic concept of anorexia nervosa. It is somewhat risky to attach a retrospective diagnosis of anorexia nervosa to every historical character thought to have deprived herself of food, whatever the reason and whatever her clinical condition. For example, saints and pious women from the thirteenth century onwards have been labelled cases of 'holy anorexia' (Bell 1985). The 'fasting girls' of the sixteenth to nineteenth centuries, sometimes known as the 'miraculous maids' or 'Anorexia Mirabilis' because they claimed to be able to subsist for months without food, have also been considered to be the forerunners of anorexia nervosa (Brumberg 1988). Thus, it is necessary to draw limits around case descriptions that can still reasonably qualify for a diagnosis of anorexia nervosa.

This task, though necessary, is not an easy one. Some of the sources of difficulty should be outlined. First, a reliable clinical diagnostic frame of reference should be adopted, yet accurate medical descriptions are relatively recent. William Gull (1874) and Charles Lasègue (1873) were the originators of the clinical entity now called anorexia nervosa, and their descriptions have generally stood the test of time. It is also reasonable to include the earlier well-documented case histories of Richard Morton (1689) and Louis Victor Marcé (1860) as is cogently argued by Silverman (1983, 1989). When the recorded medical facts depart from these classical accounts, a clear line must be drawn. An example of excessive diagnostic latitude is the contention by Loudon (1980) that chlorosis, prevalent during the early years of the twentieth century, preceded the emergence of anorexia nervosa. Yet neither Morton nor Lasègue had any hesitation in excluding the 'green sickness' as the cause of wasting in their patients. Chlorosis was later found to be due to iron-deficiency anaemia. It occurred mainly among poor working girls who generally remained well nourished (Christian 1942).

A second source of difficulty is the extremely wide frame of reference adopted by historians such as Brumberg for the retrospective labelling of anorexia nervosa. She provides us with a fascinating and scholarly account of fasting girls through past centuries. Her thesis has the great merit of opening our minds to the likelihood that the socio-cultural causes of fasting in women are likely to have changed radically during different historical times: 'from a historical perspective... certain social and cultural systems, at different points in time, encourage or promote control of appetite in women, but for different reasons and purposes.' (Brumberg 1988). In a compelling way she tries to bridge the gap between the medieval saints and the modern anorectics: 'In the earlier era (13th to 16th centuries) control of appetite was linked to piety and belief; ... the modern anorectic strives for perfection in terms of society's ideal of physical, rather than spiritual beauty.'

Brumberg's arguments may be valid in the case of saintly women whose lives were well documented. The behaviour of Saint Catherine of Siena, for example, was described in detail by her confessor, Raymond of Capua. According to him, St Catherine felt she had to expiate her sins by vomiting. As she was unable to vomit spontaneously, she 'let a fine straw or some such thing be pushed far down her throat to make her vomit' (Rampling 1985). Similar behaviours are now well recognized as typical of self-induced vomiting, practised by anorectics and by patients with bulimia nervosa. Moreover, Rampling argues that asceticism is characteristic of anorexia nervosa and can find its equivalent foundation in spiritual and religious states of mind. To some degree, therefore, it is fair to examine carefully the socio-cultural nexus that encourages self-starvation. But Brumberg goes too far in her diagnostic latitude when she declares: 'We should expect to see anorexia nervosa "present" differently, in terms of both predisposing psychological factors and actual physical symptoms.'

This elastic concept of anorexia nervosa transgresses the clinical diagnostic entity known under this name.

It is appropriate to illustrate these arguments with reference to the tragic story of Sarah Jacob known as the Welsh fasting girl. Her parents claimed she could subsist for long periods without food or drink. Their motives included a wish to attract public attention and financial gain. She began fasting in October 1867 when she was only 12 years old and had not yet begun to menstruate. Medical authorities who were consulted were so reckless as to institute a 'watch' during which a team of nurses from Guy's Hospital ensured she ingested neither food nor drink. She died in consequence, and an autopsy revealed she was not emaciated but had perished from water deprivation and renal failure (Cule 1967). The antecedents and the medical features are sufficiently well documented to exclude a diagnosis of anorexia nervosa.

Another source of difficulty in establishing a retrospective diagnosis of anorexia nervosa is its apparently shifting psychopathology. Modern diagnostic criteria are relatively precise as regards the psychological characteristics of the patient and range only from a disturbed experience of one's own body (Bruch 1966; DSM-III-R) to a 'morbid dread of fatness' (Russell 1970; ICD-10). But this was not always so. In fact, the originators of the clinical entity we now know as anorexia nervosa were themselves hesitant about the nature of the psychological disorder. Gull wrote simply of 'a morbid mental state', Lasègue proposed 'la perversion mentale... qui justifie le nom que j'ai proposé faute de mieux, d'anorexie hystérique'. Marcé ascribed the food refusal of his patients to hypochondriacal ideas and beliefs ('une forme de délire hypochondriaque'). In fact, it has been argued that the psychopathology of anorexia nervosa has changed, both in its form and content, since the descriptions by Gull and Lasègue (Russell 1985a, Russell & Treasure 1989).

If it is true that the psychopathology of anorexia nervosa is susceptible to change, two important consequences flow from this observation. First, the diagnosis of this disorder should not be rejected just because patients in the past expressed their preoccupations in a language differing from that of the modern anorectic. Secondly, it is precisely the modern anorectic's stated dread of fatness that is most congruent with today's social cult of thinness. It may therefore be deduced that modern societal pressures have not only increased the frequency of anorexia nervosa but have also determined the nature of our patients' preoccupations. The patient's own explanatory model for her behaviour is in terms compatible with society's demands, except that her beliefs are held obstinately and amount to overvalued ideas. These sociocultural forces therefore exert a pathoplastic influence. They may not amount to fundamental or necessary causes but they act as triggering agents and shape the form of the illness. They will certainly influence the psychological content of the illness; in addition they contribute to its colouring and its form (Birnbaum 1923, Shepherd 1975). Consequently, the cult of thinness in westernized societies has probably resulted in neurotic disorders expressing themselves more often in the form of anorexia nervosa or bulimia nervosa, without neurotic illnesses as a whole necessarily becoming more frequent.

So far, the pathogenic sociocultural causes of eating disorders have been subsumed under the general formula of 'the cult of thinness' espoused in westernized societies. Vulnerable patients responding to such pressures may experiment with weight-reducing diets, a common practice among young women (Nylander 1971), carrying an established degree of risk (Patton 1988, Patton *et al.* 1990). Anorexia nervosa is arguably but an extension of determined dietary behaviours. Bulimia nervosa can also be viewed as an escape or rebound from dietary restraint to 'binge eating', (Agras 1990, Blundell 1990, Treasure 1990, Tuschl 1990). The social pressures which sustain dietary restraint should be examined in greater detail and Brumberg has produced an impressive list:

1 The publications of books and magazines containing keys to calorie counting.
2 Pressures from the fashion industry which caters only for the slimmer figure.
3 The film industy and television, promoting the view that the svelte figure is associated with both sexual allure and professional success.

4 An emphasis on physical fitness and athleticism. Brumberg extends this list beyond the specific pressures which lead to dietary restraint:
5 Anorexia nervosa is a form of feminist politics, i.e. the young woman's protest against the patriarchy.
6 Brumberg finally allows herself to be carried away by an enthusiastic witchhunt against a wide range of society's agents. She seems to believe that there occurs a 'promotion' of anorexia nervosa by health professionals and medical researchers: 'Americans are competitive even about disease . . . the idea of promoting a disease is not unheard of, since medical researchers must routinely compete for funding.'
Is she not being unfair to Americans? She berates the 'army' of health professionals who aspire to test patients, and are responsible for a 'deluge of publications and conferences'. She wonders at the creation of a new journal – *The International Journal of Eating Disorders* – and remarks on the high level of professional competition in which each specialty apparently pushes for intellectual ascendancy. Moderation in all matters is a commendable virtue.

## The multidimensional causation of anorexia nervosa

The introduction to this chapter contained the warning that focusing on the sociocultural causes of eating disorders might lead to the neglect of the biomedical causes of anorexia nervosa. As a corrective, it is necessary to attempt a synthesis of all these causes. The most specific evidence adduced so far in favour of biomedical causes has come from comparisons of concordance rates in monozygotic (MZ) and dizygotic (DZ) twins. The significantly higher concordance rates in MZ twins (56%) compared with DZ twins (5%) strongly favour a genetic predisposition to anorexia nervosa (Holland *et al.* 1984, 1988). Holland *et al.* (1988) have put forward a multidimensional model whereby the genetic vulnerability to anorexia nervosa will only find expression in societies subject to the cult of thinness, in which dieting is common and weight reduction is encouraged. They suppose, moreover, that genetically predisposed individuals carry a weakness of the homeostatic mechanisms that normally ensure weight restoration after a period of weight loss.

## Prevention

The preceding review has identified the societal pressures which are likely to lead to excessive concern with body shape in women, injudicious dietary behaviours and frank eating disorders. In theory, therefore, a suitable health educational programme advising young women to shun unsupervised dieting should succeed in reducing the incidence of eating disorders. A number of specific proposals have indeed been put forward: the media should abandon the promotion of the thin body image; pressures on adolescent girls should be reduced (Huon 1988); children should be helped to become more assertive and independent` (Noordenbos 1988). In practice it would be extremely difficult to implement these approaches. The necessary educational programme would have to be extremely powerful to succeed in influencing public opinion.

A more focused approach has been advocated by Slade (1988). He suggests:

1 The identification of individuals at risk, and
2 Interventions applied early when they are most likely to succeed, i.e. in subjects still experimenting with dieting who have not yet developed a frank eating disorder.

Slade has proposed a model for anorexia nervosa which predicts that dieting behaviour will spiral into the illness if the subject's personality includes two traits:

1 General dissatisfaction with life and self.
2 Perfectionist tendencies.

He has devised a questionnaire (SCANS = Sub-Clinical Anorexia Nervosa Scale) to detect these character traits in populations of female, middle-class adolescents and young adults. The questionnaire has been partly validated by identifying a small percentage of subjects with 'partial' eating disorders, using the EAT interview (Szmukler 1983).

In spite of the difficulties, it is highly desirable to mount an experimental focused educational programme aimed at influencing healthy attitudes to food and body size, with an appraisal of its impact on a chosen section of the population at risk.

## Conclusions

Several epidemiological surveys have been conducted to estimate the incidence and prevalence of anorexia nervosa. In the case of bulimia nervosa these studies are still at a very early stage. Epidemiological surveys of eating disorders are fraught with difficulties. On the one hand, community studies relying on screening tests elicit a large number of false positives; on the other hand, cases are often missed because the non-respondents tend to include subjects who conceal their disorder. Nevertheless, some surveys have yielded valuable data on incidence and prevalence. These are the surveys which have relied on more objective and complete records in schools (the Göteborg study), systematic clinical archives (the Mayo Clinic) and clinical contacts in primary care (The Netherlands study). The best available information from epidemiological studies in Western Europe and North America points to an incidence of 4–8 per 100 000 population per annum for anorexia nervosa; prevalence rates in schoolgirls may be as high as 1%. The prevalence of bulimia nervosa is around 1% in adolescents and young adult women; it is higher among city-dwellers than in rural communities.

On the whole, epidemiological surveys have confirmed that the incidence of anorexia nervosa has risen from around the 1950s to the 1980s. The best evidence comes from centres where an increase in incidence has been recorded during successive surveys conducted with the same methods on similar populations (e.g. north-east Scotland, Zurich, Switzerland, Monroe County, USA). There is only partial confirmation of a predominance of anorexia nervosa among higher social classes. Prevalence studies of populations deemed at special risk have supported the view that certain professional environments may be harmful if they focus attention on body size and shape.

It is entirely appropriate to consider anorexia nervosa as a culture-bound syndrome. The evidence is that its incidence is high in westernized societies and has risen during times when a cult of thinness has prevailed. One study of a school population in an island in the Azores has revealed a low prevalence of eating disorders, in keeping with an absence of pressures to control eating and body weight. On the whole, eating disorders have been rare among black subjects within western populations. Eating disorders may affect immigrants from previously protected cultures as they come under the influence of a western culture (e.g. Egyptian students or Asian immigrants in England).

Anorexia nervosa is an illness which has changed not only in its incidence but also in its clinical presentation in recent decades. This is demonstrated by the emergence of bulimia nervosa in recent years, a disorder allied to anorexia nervosa, and one which clinicians believe has become commoner than the 'parent' disorder. The psychological preoccupations of anorexic patients have also changed to reflect the sociocultural emphasis on the value of thinness.

Whereas sociocultural influences are profoundly important in causing anorexia nervosa and moulding its clinical form, it is essential to maintain a multidimensional perspective of this illness. The prevention of eating disorders should be attempted by means of health educational programmes advising young women to avoid unsupervised dieting.

## Appendix

### Diagnostic criteria for anorexia nervosa

DSM-III-R

**A** Refusal to maintain body weight over a minimal normal weight for age and height, e.g. weight loss leading to maintenance of body weight 15% below that expected; or failure to make expected weight gain during period of growth, leading to body weight 15% below that expected.
**B** Intense fear of gaining weight or becoming fat, even though underweight.
**C** Disturbance in the way in which one's body weight, size or shape is experienced, e.g. the person claims to 'feel fat' even when emaciated, believes that one area of the body is 'too fat' even when obviously underweight.
**D** In females, absence of at least three consecutive menstrual cycles when otherwise expected to occur (primary or secondary amenorrhoea). (A woman is considered to have amenorrhoea if her periods occur only following hormone, e.g. oestrogen, administration.)

ICD-10

**A** There is a significant weight loss (body weight maintained at least 15% below that expected (either lost or never achieved) or Quetelet's body mass index, BMI, of 17.5 or less). Prepubertal patients may show failure to make the expected weight gain during the period of growth.
**B** The weight loss is self-induced by avoidance of 'fattening foods'. One or more of the following may also be present:* self-induced vomiting; self-induced purging; excessive exercise; use of appetite suppressants and/or diuretics.
**C** Body-image distortion in the form of a specific psychopathology whereby a dread of fatness persists as an intrusive over-valued idea, and the patient imposes a low weight threshold on herself.
**D** A widespread endocrine disorder involving the hypothalamic–pituitary–gonadal axis, manifest in women as amenorrhoea, and in men as a loss of sexual interest and potency (an apparent exception is the persistence of vaginal bleeds in anorexic women who are on replacement hormonal therapy, most commonly taken as a contraceptive pill). There may also be elevated levels of growth hormone, raised levels of cortisol, changes in the peripheral metabolism of the thyroid hormone, and abnormalities of insulin secretion.
**E** If onset is prepubertal, the sequence of pubertal events is delayed or even arrested (growth ceases; in girls the breasts do not develop and there is a primary amenorrhoea; in boys the genitals remain juvenile). With recovery, puberty is often completed normally, but the menarche is late.

### Diagnostic criteria for bulimia nervosa

DSM-III-R

**A** Recurrent episodes of binge eating (rapid consumption of a large amount of food in a discrete period of time).

* WHO (1992) contains a clinical error which has been corrected here.

B A feeling of lack of control over eating behaviour during the eating binges.
C The person regularly engages in either self-induced vomiting, use of laxatives or diuretics, strict dieting or fasting, or vigorous exercise in order to prevent weight gain.
D A minimum average of two binge eating episodes a week for at least three months.
E Persistent overconcern with body shape and weight.

ICD-10

All of the following are required:
A There is a persistent preoccupation with eating and an irresistible craving for food; the patient succumbs to episodes of overeating in which large amounts of food are consumed in short periods of time.
B The patient attempts to counteract the 'fattening' effects of food by one or more of the following: self-induced vomiting; purgative abuse; alternating periods of starvation; use of drugs such as appetite suppressants, thyroid preparations or diuretics. When bulimia occurs in diabetic patients they may choose to neglect their insulin treatment.
C The psychopathology consists of a morbid dread of fatness and the patient sets herself a sharply defined weight threshold, well below her premorbid weight which constitutes the optimum or healthy weight in the opinion of the physician.
D There is often, but not always, a history of an earlier episode of anorexia nervosa, the interval ranging from a few months to several years. This episode may have been fully expressed, or may have assumed a minor cryptic form with a moderate loss of weight and/or a transient phase of amenorrhoea.

## References

Agras W.S. (1990) Is restraint the culprit? *Appetite* 14, 111–112.

American Psychiatric Association (1980) *Diagnostic and Statistical Manual of Mental Disorders*, 3rd edn. APA, Washington DC.

American Psychiatric Association (1987) *Diagnostic and Statistical Manual of Mental Disorders*, 3rd edn revised. APA, Washington DC.

Bell R.M. (1985) *Holy Anorexia*. The University of Chicago Press, Chicago.

Ben-Tovim D.I. & Morton J. (1990) The epidemiology of anorexia nervosa in South Australia. *Australian and New Zealand Journal of Psychiatry* 24, 182–186.

Birnbaum K. (1923) *Der Aufbau der Psychose*, pp. 6–7. Springer, Berlin.

Bleuler E. (1937) *Lehrbuch der Psychiatrie*, 6th edn, p. 121. Springer, Berlin.

Blundell J.E. (1990) How culture undermines the biopsychological system of appetite control. *Appetite* 14, 113–115.

Bray G.A. (1987) Factors leading to obesity: physical (including metabolic) factors and disease states. In Bender A.E. & Brookes L.J. (eds) *Body Weight Control: The Physiology, Clinical Treatment and Prevention of Obesity*, pp. 53–61. Churchill Livingstone, Edinburgh.

Bruch H. (1966) Anorexia nervosa and its differential diagnosis. *Journal of Nervous and Mental Disease* 141, 555–566.

Bruch H. (1978) *The Golden Cage: The Enigma of Anorexia Nervosa*, p. viii. Open Books, London.

Brumberg J.J. (1988) *Fasting Girls: The Emergence of Anorexia Nervosa as a Modern Disease*. Harvard University Press, Cambridge, Massachusetts.

Bushnell J.A., Wells J.E., Hornblow A.R., Oakley-Browne M.A. & Joyce P. (1990) Prevalence of three bulimia syndromes in the general population. *Psychological Medicine* 20, 671–680.

Butler N. (1988) An overview of anorexia nervosa. In Scott D. (ed.) *Anorexia and Bulimia Nervosa: Practical Approaches*, pp. 3–23. Croom Helm, London.

Christian, H.A. (1942) *Osler's Principles and Practice of Medicine*, 14th edn, pp. 945–947. Appleton-Century, New York.

Crisp A.H. (1988) The 1988 social psychiatry conference in London, England. *International Journal of Social Psychiatry* 34, 3–4.

Crisp A.H., Hsu L.K.G., Harding B. & Hartshorn J. (1980) Clinical features of anorexia nervosa: a study of a consecutive series of female patients. *Journal of Psychosomatic Research* 24, 179–191.

Crisp A.H. & McGuiness B. (1976) Jolly fat: relation between obesity and psychoneuroses in general population. *British Medical Journal* 1, 7–9.

Crisp A.H., Palmer R.L. & Kalucy R.S. (1976) How common is anorexia nervosa? A prevalence study. *British Journal of Psychiatry* 128, 549–554.

Cule J. (1967) *Wreath on the Crown: The Story of Sarah Jacob, the Welsh Fasting Girl*. Gomerian Press, Llandysul.

Cuzzolaro M., Frighi L. & Petrilli A. (1990) Eating disorders: an epidemiological survey in Italy. In Frighi L., Cuzzolaro M. & Caputo G. (eds) *International Symposium: Anorexia, Bulimia, Obesity*, pp. 25–31. Università 'La Sapienza' di Roma, Rome.

Di Nicola V.F. (1990) Anorexia multiforme: self-starvation in historical and cultural context. *Transcultural Psychiatric Research Review* 27, part I, 165–196; part II, 245–286.

Eisler I. & Szmukler G.I. (1985) Social class as a confounding variable in the eating attitudes test. *Journal of Psychiatric Research* 19, 171–176.

Fahy T.A., de Silva P., Silverstone P. & Russell G.F.M. (1989) The effects of loss of taste and smell in a case of anorexia nervosa and bulimia nervosa. *British Journal of Psychiatry* 155, 860–861.

Fairburn C. (1990) Studies of the epidemiology of bulimia nervosa. *American Journal of Psychiatry* 147, 401–408.

Fenwick S. (1880) *On Atrophy of the Stomach and on the Nervous Affections of the Digestive Organs*, p. 107. Churchill, London.

Fichter M.M., Weyerer S., Sourdi L. & Sourdi Z. (1983) In Darby P.L., Garfinkel P.E., Garner D.M. & Coscina D.V. (eds) *Anorexia Nervosa: Recent Developments in Research*, pp. 95–105. Alan R. Liss, New York.

Fosson A., Knibbs J., Bryant-Waugh R. & Lask B. (1987) Early onset anorexia nervosa. *Archives of Disease in Childhood* 62, 114–118.

Garfinkel P.E. & Garner D.M. (1982) *Anorexia Nervosa: A Multidimensional Perspective*, p. 189. Brunner/Mazel, New York.

Garner D.M. & Garfinkel P.E. (1979) The Eating Attitudes Test: an index of the symptoms of anorexia nervosa. *Psychological Medicine* 9, 273–279.

Garner D.M. & Garfinkel P.E. (1980) Socio-cultural factors in the development of anorexia nervosa. *Psychological Medicine* 10, 647–656.

Garrow J.S., Crisp A.H., Jordan H.A. *et al.* (1976) In Silverstone T. (ed.) *Report on the Dahlem Workshop on Appetite and Food Intake, Berlin 1975* (Life Sciences Research Report 2), pp. 405–416. Dahlem Konferenzen Abakon Verlagsgesellschaft, Berlin.

Gull W.W. (1874) Anorexia nervosa (apepsia hysterica, anorexia hysterica). *Transactions of the Clinical Society of London* 7, 22–28.

Hall A. & Hay P.J. (1991) Eating disorder patient referrals from a population region, 1977–1986. *Psychological Medicine* 21, 697–701.

Halmi K.A., Falk J.R. & Schwartz E. (1981) Binge-eating and vomiting: a survey of a college population. *Psychological Medicine* 11, 697–706.

Halmi K.A., Goldberg S.C., Eckert E., Casper R. & Davis J.M. (1977) Pretreatment evaluation in anorexia nervosa. In Vigersky R.A. (ed.) *Anorexia Nervosa*, pp. 43–54. Raven, New York.

Henderson A.S. (1988) *An Introduction to Social Psychiatry*, p. 19. Oxford University Press, Oxford.

Hoek H.W. (1991) The incidence and prevalence of anorexia nervosa and bulimia nervosa in primary care. *Psychological Medicine* 21, 455–460.

Hoek H.W. & Brook F.G. (1985) Patterns of care of anorexia nervosa. *Journal of Psychiatric Research* 19, 155–160.

Holden N.L. & Robinson P.H. (1988) Anorexia nervosa and bulimia nervosa in British blacks. *British Journal of Psychiatry* 152, 544–549.

Holland A.J., Hall A., Murray R., Russell G.F.M. & Crisp A.H. (1984) Anorexia nervosa: a study of 34 twin pairs and one set of triplets. *British Journal of Psychiatry* 145, 414–419.

Holland A.J., Sicotte N. & Treasure J. (1988) Anorexia nervosa: evidence for a genetic basis. *Journal of Psychosomatic Research* 32, 561–571.

Hsu L.K. (1987) Are the eating disorders becoming more common in blacks? *International Journal of Eating Disorders* 6, 113–124.

Huon G.F. (1988) Towards the prevention of eating disorders. In Hardoff D. & Chigier E. (eds) *Eating Disorders in Adolescents and Young Adults*, pp. 447–454. Freund Publishing House, London.

Ishikawa K. (1965) Über die Eltern von Anorexia-nervosa Kranken. In Meyer J.-E. & Feldmann H. (eds) *Anorexia Nervosa*, pp. 154–155. Georg Thieme Verlag, Stuttgart.

Jacobs B.W. & Isaacs S. (1986) Pre-pubertal anorexia nervosa: a retrospective controlled study. *Journal of Child Psychology and Psychiatry* 27, 237–250.

Jaspers K. (1959) *Allgemeine Psychopathologie*, 7th edn pp. 732, 742. Manchester University Press, Manchester. (Translated by Hoenig J. & Hamilton M.W.)

Johnson C., Lewis C., Love S., Lewis L. & Stuckey M. (1984) Incidence and correlates of bulimic behaviour in a female high school population. *Journal of Youth and Adolescence* 13, 15–26.

Johnson-Sabine E., Wood K., Patton G., Mann A. & Wakeling A. (1988) Abnormal eating attitudes in London schoolgirls – a prospective epidemiological study: factors associated with abnormal response on screening questionnaires. *Psychological Medicine* 18, 615–622.

Jones D.J., Fox M.M., Babigian H.M. & Hutton H.E. (1980) Epidemiology of anorexia nervosa in Monroe County, New York: 1960–1976. *Psychosomatic Medicine* 42, 551–558.

Kaffman M. & Sadeh T. (1989) Anorexia nervosa in the kibbutz: factors influencing the development of a monoideistic fixation. *International Journal of Eating Disorders* 8, 33–53.

Kendell R.E., Hall D.J., Hailey A. & Babigian H.M. (1973) The epidemiology of anorexia nervosa. *Psychological Medicine* 3, 200–203.

King M.B. (1989) Eating disorders in a general practice population: prevalence, characteristics and follow-up at 12 to 18 months. *Psychological Medicine Monograph Supplement* 14, 1–34.

King M.B. & Bhugra D. (1989) Eating disorders: lessons from a cross-cultural study. *Psychological Medicine* 19, 955–958.

Lasègue C. (1873) De l'anorexie hystérique. *Archives Générales de Médecine* 21, 385–403.

Leff J. (1988) *Psychiatry Around the Globe: 2, The Culture-bound Syndromes*, chap. 2, pp. 11–23. Gaskell, London.

Loudon I.S.L. (1980) Chlorosis, anaemia and anorexia nervosa. *British Medical Journal* 2, 1669–1675.

Lucas A.R., Beard C.M., O'Fallon W.M. & Kurland L.T. (1988) Anorexia nervosa in Rochester, Minnesota: a 45-year study. *Mayo Clinic Proceedings* 63, 433–442.

Lucas A.R., Beard C.M., O'Fallen W.M. & Kurland L.T. (1991) 50-year trends in the incidence of anorexia nervosa in Rochester, Minn: a population-based survey. *American Journal of Psychiatry* 148, 917–922.

Mann A.H., Wakeling A., Wood K., Monck E., Dobbs R. & Szmukler G.I. (1983) Screening for abnormal attitudes and psychiatric morbidity in an unselected population of 15-year-old schoolgirls. *Psychological Medicine* 13, 573–580.

Marcé L.-V. (1860) Note sur une forme de délire hypochondriaque consécutive aux dyspepsies et caractérisée principalement par le refus d'aliments. *Annales Médicopsychologiques* 6, 15–28.

Meadows G.N., Palmer R.L., Newball E.U.M. & Kenrick J.M.T. (1986) Eating attitudes and disorder in young women: a general practice based survey. *Psychological Medicine* 16, 351–357.

Morgan H.G. & Mayberry J.F. (1983) Common gastrointestinal diseases and anorexia nervosa in British dietitians. *Public Health London* 97, 166–170.

Morgan H.G. & Russell G.F.M. (1975) Value of family background and clinical features as predictors of long-term outcome in anorexia nervosa: four-year follow-up study of 41 patients. *Psychological Medicine* 5, 355–371.

Morton R. (1689) *Phthisiologia, seu Exercitiones de Phthisi.* Smith, London.

Mumford D.B. & Whitehouse A.M. (1988) Increased prevalence of bulimia nervosa among Asian schoolgirls. *British Medical Journal* 297, 718.

Nasser, M. (1986) Comparative study of the prevalence of abnormal eating attitudes among Arab female students of both London and Cairo Universities. *Psychological Medicine* 16, 621–625.

Nielsen S. (1990) The epidemiology of anorexia nervosa in Denmark from 1973 to 1987: a nation-wide register study of psychiatric admission. *Acta Psychiatrica Scandinavica* 81, 507–514.

Noordenbos G. (1988) Possible preventive measures for anorexia nervosa. In Hardoff D. & Chigier E. (eds) *Eating Disorders in Adolescents and Young Adults*, pp. 437–446. Freund Publishing House, London.

Nylander I. (1971) The feeling of being fat and dieting in a school population. Epidemiologic interview investigation. *Acta Sociomedica Scandinavica* 3, 17–26.

Orbach S. (1979) Self-starvation – anorexia nervosa. In *Fat is a Feminist Issue*, pp. 161–174. Hamlyn, Paperbacks, London.

Patton G.C. (1988) The spectrum of eating disorder in adolescence. *Journal of Psychosomatic Research* 32, 579–584.

Patton G.C., Johnson-Sabine E., Wood K., Mann A. & Wakeling A. (1990) Abnormal eating attitudes in London schoolgirls – a prospective epidemiological study: outcome at twelve-month follow-up. *Psychological Medicine* 20, 383–394.

Pinto de Azevedo M.H. & Ferreira C.P. (1992) Anorexia nervosa and bulimia: a prevalence study. *Acta Psychiatrica Scandinavica* (in press).

Prince R. (1985) The concept of culture-bound syndromes; anorexia nervosa and brain-fag. *Transcultural Psychiatric Research Review* 22, 117–121 (author's abstract).

Pyle R.L., Mitchell J.E., Eckert E.D., Halvorson P.A., Neuman P.A. & Goff G.M. (1983) The incidence of bulimia in freshman college students. *International Journal of Eating Disorders* 2, 75–85.

Rampling D. (1985) Ascetic ideals and anorexia nervosa. *Journal of Psychiatric Research* 19, 89–94.

Råstam M. (1990) *Anorexia Nervosa in Swedish Urban Teenagers.* Thesis of the University of Göteborg, Göteborg, Sweden.

Råstam M. Gillberg C. & Garton M. (1989) Anorexia nervosa in a Swedish urban region. A population based study. *British Journal of Psychiatry* 155, 642–646.

Robinson P.H. & Andersen A. (1985) Anorexia nervosa in American blacks. *Journal of Psychiatric Research* 19, 183–188.

Russell G.F.M. (1970) Anorexia nervosa: its identity as an illness and its treatment. In Price J.H. (ed.) *Modern Trends in Psychological Medicine*, pp. 131–164. Butterworths, London.

Russell G.F.M. (1979) Bulimia nervosa: an ominous variant of anorexia nervosa. *Psychological Medicine* 9, 429–448.

Russell G.F.M. (1984) The modern history of anorexia nervosa. *Aktuelle Ernährungsmedizin* 9, 3–7.

Russell G.F.M. (1985a) The changing nature of anorexia nervosa: an introduction to the conference. *Journal of Psychiatric Research* 19, 101–109.

Russell G.F.M. (1985b) Premenarchal anorexia nervosa and its sequelae. *Journal of Psychiatric Research* 19, 363–369.

Russell G.F.M. (1991) The prognosis of eating disorders: a clinician's approach. In Herzog W. & Vandereycken W. (eds) *The Course of Eating Disorders: Long-Term Follow-up Studies of Anorexia and Bulimia Nervosa.* Springer, Berlin.

Russell G.F.M. & Treasure J. (1989) The modern history of anorexia nervosa: an interpretation of why the illness has changed. In Schneider L.A., Cooper S.J. & Halmi K.A. (eds) *The Psychobiology of Human Eating Disorders. Annals of the New York Academy of Sciences* 575, 13–30.

Selvini-Palazzoli M. (1974) *Self-starvation from the Intrapsychic to the Transpersonal Approach.* Chaucer, London.

Shepherd M. (1975) Epidemiologische Psychiatrie. In Kisker K.P., Meyer J.-E., Müller C. & Strömgren E. (eds) *Psychiatrie der Gegenwart Forschung und Praxis*, vol. 3, 2nd edn, pp. 119–149. Springer, Berlin.

Shrout P.E. & Fleiss J.L. (1981) Reliability and case detection. In Wing J.K., Bebbington P.E. & Robins L.N. (eds) *What is a Case? The Problem of Definition in Psychiatric Community Surveys*, pp. 117–128. Grant McIntyre, London.

Silverman J.A. (1983) Richard Morton, 1637–1698. Limner of anorexia nervosa: his life and times. A tercentenary essay. *Journal of the American Medical Society* 250, 2830–2832.

Silverman J.A. (1989) Louis-Victor Marcé, 1824–1864: anorexia nervosa's forgotten man. *Psychological Medicine* 19, 833–835.

Silverstein B., Peterson B. & Perdue L. (1986a) Some correlates of the thin standard of bodily attractiveness for women. *International Journal of Eating Disorders* 5, 895–905.

Silverstein B., Perdue L., Peterson B., Vogel L. & Fantini D.A. (1986b) Possible causes of the thin standard of bodily attractiveness for women. *International Journal of Eating Disorders* 5, 907–916.

Simons R.C. (1985) Sorting the culture-bound syndromes. In Simons R.C. & Hughes C.C. (eds) *The Culture-Bound Syndromes – Folk Illnesses of Psychiatric and Anthropological Interest*, pp. 25–38. D. Reidel, Dordrecht.

Slade P. (1988) Early recognition and prevention: is it possible to screen people at risk of developing an eating disorder? In Hardoff D. & Chigier E. (eds) *Eating Disorders in Adolescents and Young Adults*, pp. 427–435. Freund Publishing House, London.

Slade P., Dewey M.E., Kiemle G. & Newton M. (1990) Update on SCANS – a screening instrument for identifying individuals at risk of developing an eating disorder. *International Journal of Eating Disorders* 9, (5), 583–584.

Stunkard A.J. (1988) Some perspectives on human obesity: its causes. The Salmon Lecture. *Bulletin of the New York Academy of Medicine* 64, (8), 902–923.

Szmukler G.I. (1983) Weight and food preoccupation in a population of English schoolgirls. In Bargman J.G. (ed.) *Understanding Anorexia Nervosa and Bulimia: Report of 4th Ross Conference on Medical Research*, pp. 21–27. Ross, Columbus, Ohio.

Szmukler G.I. (1985) The epidemiology of anorexia nervosa and bulimia. *Journal of Psychiatric Research* 19, 143–153.

Szmukler G.I., Eisler I., Gillies C. & Hayward M.E. (1985) The implications of anorexia nervosa in a ballet school. *Journal of Psychiatric Research* 19, 177–181.

Szmukler G.I., McCance C., McCrone L. & Hunter D. (1986) Anorexia nervosa: a psychiatric case register study from Aberdeen. *Psychological Medicine* 16, 49–58.

Theander S. (1970) Anorexia nervosa: a psychiatric investigation of 94 female patients. *Acta Psychiatrica Scandinavica Supplementum* 214.

Thomas J.P. & Szmukler G.I. (1985) Anorexia nervosa in patients of Afro-Caribbean extraction. *British Journal of Psychiatry* 146, 653–656.

Treasure J. (1990) Comments on some theoretical considerations: dietary restraint to binge eating. *Appetite* 14, 131–132.

Tuschl R.J. (1990) From dietary restraint to binge eating: some theoretical considerations. *Appetite* 14, 105–109.

Van Itallie T.B. & Woteki C.E. (1987) Who gets fat? In Bender A.E. & Brookes L.J. (eds) *Body Weight Control: The Physiology, Clinical Treatment and Prevention of Obesity*, pp. 39–52. Churchill Livingstone, Edinburgh.

Von Baeyer W. (1965) Zur bedeutung sozialpathologischer Faktoren im Krankheitsbild der Anorexia Nervosa. In Meyer J.-E. & Feldmann H. (eds) *Anorexia Nervosa*, pp. 150–153. Georg Thieme Verlag, Stuttgart.

Wig N.N. (1983) DSM III: a perspective from the third world. In Spitzer R.L., Williams J.B.W. & Skodol A.E. (eds) *International Perspectives on DSMIII: Diagnostic and Statistical Manual of Mental Disorders*, pp. 79–89. American Psychiatric Press, Washington DC.

Willi J., Giacometti G. & Limacher B. (1990) Update on the epidemiology of anorexia nervosa in a defined region of Switzerland. *American Journal of Psychiatry* 147, 1514–1517.

Willi J. & Grossman S. (1983) Epidemiology of anorexia nervosa in a defined region of Switzerland. *American Journal of Psychiatry* 140, 564–567.

Williams P., Hand D. & Tarnopolsky A. (1982) The problem of screening for uncommon disorders – a comment on the Eating Attitudes Test. *Psychological Medicine* 12, 431–434.

Williams P. & King M. (1987) The 'epidemic' of anorexia nervosa: another medical myth? *Lancet* i, 205–207.

World Health Organization (1992) *The ICD-10 Classification of Mental and Behavioural Disorders: Clinical Descriptions and Diagnostic Guidelines*. WHO, Geneva.

Yap, P.M. (1962) Words and things in comparative psychiatry with special reference to exotic psychoses. *Acta Psychiatrica Scandinavica* 38, 163–169.

Yap P.M. (1969) The culture-bound reactive syndromes. In Caudill W. & Lin T.-Y. *Mental Health Research in Asia and the Pacific*, pp. 33–53. East-West Center Press, Honolulu.

# Chapter 17
# Psychological and Social Aspects of AIDS

MICHAEL B. KING

AIDS is a severe, infectious disorder of immune functioning in which the causative agent is transmitted by exchange of bodily fluids. Transmission occurs iatrogenically through the exchange of blood products, as a result of sexual behaviour or during the injection of drugs. Thus, the spread of the infection is often linked to behaviours which are misunderstood and socially unaccepted. The syndrome evokes a complex interplay of social, psychological and organic factors which provide a unique challenge to social psychiatry.

### Staging of the syndrome

The human immunodeficiency virus (HIV) is a retrovirus which not only causes immunosuppression but directly affects the central nervous system. The infection is classified, according to the Centers for Disease Control (CDC 1986), into four principal stages. Acute infection occurs in stage 1 which may be symptomless or, more rarely, present as a severe illness with measurable immunosuppression. Stage 2 consists of a latent period, in which there are no symptoms or signs, but people are none the less infectious. In stage 3 there is development of persistent lymphadenopathy at two or more extra-inguinal sites, an evolution which often goes undetected by the patient. Stage 4 is a collection of subcategories in which more generalized symptoms are present, ranging from constitutional malaise with fever and weight loss to pneumonias, cancers and neurological disease. Current estimates suggest that 54% of people infected with the virus will progress to AIDS within 11 years (Lifson *et al.* 1990).

Two years before the discovery of HIV in 1983, the syndrome of AIDS was described in homosexual men in North America and this original focus laid the basis for much of the myth and prejudice which surrounds the disorder today.

### Homosexuality

In western countries, social factors in AIDS are inextricably linked with attitudes towards male homosexual behaviour. There is good evidence that many people are aware of a homosexual component to their sexuality. Although earlier studies had already reached similar conclusions, the controversial work of Kinsey *et al.* (1948, 1953) first established in the public and scientific mind the definite possibility of a continuum of sexual response. In a study of 3392 women and 3849 men in North America, 50% of male and 28% of female subjects reported awareness of erotic responses to members of the same sex. Kinsey *et al.* postulated a universal gradation between homosexuality and heterosexuality and despite the obvious limitations of self-report, much subsequent work has confirmed the concept (McConaghy 1987). This hypothesis, however, has not gone unchallenged. A recent reanalysis of the Kinsey data (Van Wyk & Geist 1984) has led to a reassertion of the more traditional model of a dichotomous distribution between a vast majority of the population who are heterosexual and approximately 5% who are exclusively homosexual.

A major difficulty of definition concerns the need for a clear distinction between same-sex desire, responsiveness and fantasy on the one hand and actual sexual behaviour on the other. The reality is that only people with a strong homosexual drive will act against their social interests; those people who on the continuum theory would be predicted to have equal attraction to either sex, are likely to take the socially acceptable path of heterosexuality.

Whether or not a continuum exists between an exclusively heterosexual and homosexual response, there is little doubt that the adoption of a homosexual lifestyle, in contrast to the occasional homosexual act, incurs social disapproval and consequent stress. Although no society has ever actively favoured homosexuality, homosexual acts as a prelude to, or in the setting of, a heterosexual life-style, particularly among men, have received limited tolerance (Davenport-Hines 1990), or even encouragement (Stoller & Herdt 1985). An increasingly polarized conception of sexuality, originating in British society more than two centuries ago, has shaped our contemporary view of sexual orientation (Davenport-Hines 1990). Throughout the eighteenth century the marginalization of men who sought sexual outlets with other men gradually escalated and resulted in increasingly severe penalties against them. Paradoxically, despite the social and political headway which homosexuals have made in the past twenty to thirty years, gay political movements have promoted the view of homosexuality as something inherent and unmalleable (Bancroft 1975). Although perhaps a necessary step in mounting a cohesive campaign against repression, a price has been paid in relative disregard for the essential individuality of sexual orientation.

The belief that homosexuals were mentally ill emerged only towards the end of the last century with the widespread adoption of the linguistic misnomer homosexual (Davenport-Hines 1990). Much of the interest in homosexuality as a disorder originated from a wish to understand it, often in psychoanalytical terms, but also to modify or alter the orientation towards the preferred heterosexuality. The link between mental illness and homosexuality was inevitably widened in the assumption that homosexual people had unstable personalities and were more vulnerable to a range of psychiatric disorder. Such claims occasionally still appear in the medical literature (Atkinson *et al.* 1988), despite obvious errors of ascertainment and difficulties in obtaining a representative sample of homosexual and bisexual people in the community. Even within the past decade, review

articles have been published in which implicit assumptions are made that homosexual men are unassertive, prone to neurotic distress and drug use, have failed in the pursuit of women, and that sexual reconditioning or training in social skills may ameliorate what is regarded as an essential weakness of character (Macculloch 1981). If psychiatric illness is any more common among homosexuals, this may be largely a result of the pressures that remain against them in modern society (Remafedi 1987). Unfortunately, negative attitudes of doctors towards homosexuality (Pauly & Goldstein 1970, Bhugra & King 1989) has generated a lack of trust in medicine on the part of homosexuals (Owen 1980).

A combination of forces in the 1960s and 1970s, including disillusionment with psychoanalytical theories, reactions against the negative effects of labelling, failure of the medical model to explain sexuality and the rise in gay political power resulted in the gradual dismantlement of illness theories (Israelstam & Lambert 1983). In 1973 the classification 'homosexuality' was replaced in the *Diagnostic and Statistical Manual II* (DSM-II) of the American Psychiatric Association (1973) with the category 'sexual orientation disturbance'. Despite considerable opposition from some quarters (Bayer & Spitzer 1982), this was later further modified in DSM-III (American Psychiatric Association 1980) to 'ego-dystonic homosexuality', a category retained to meet the requirements of homosexuals who are conflicted about their sexual identity. There is no a priori reason, however, why such a category should not also apply to heterosexuals in a similar predicament. This point has been accepted in the field trial version of the tenth edition of the *International Classification of Diseases* in which psychological and behavioural problems associated with sexual development and orientation are possible for heterosexual, homosexual and bisexual alike (World Health Organization 1992).

Hostile attitudes toward sufferers with HIV infection are rooted in the fertile ground of opposition to homosexuality. Unfortunately some of the animosity which has been rekindled by the AIDS pandemic emanated from the medical profession itself (Douglas *et al.* 1985, Matthews *et al.* 1986,

Seale 1987), although there is recent evidence that this has eased (Prichard *et al.* 1988, King 1989a). Negative public attitudes were focused in religiose condemnation of AIDS as a just penalty for perverse behaviour (Eisenberg 1986), with little recognition of the stigmatization such fallacious ideas brought in their wake (Murphy 1988). 'At risk groups' were convenient targets for reducing the sense of threat to the wider community, but did little to reduce the real threat (Ostrow & Gayle 1986). Ironically, HIV infection appeared in the homosexual community just as repression was easing. Since then, in Britain more than any other European country, there has been a retrenchment of conservative attitudes with government action to limit the support of activities or education that in any way encourage or 'promote' homosexuality and a wave of increasing physical violence against individuals identified as homosexual.

Patients with HIV infection have been stigmatized for their homosexuality as much as for the HIV infection itself (King 1989b). Although this has not always resulted in frank psychiatric disorder, it has created enormous difficulties for sufferers and carers. I have witnessed, on rare occasions, haemophiliac patients infected with the virus refusing to share hospital wards with homosexual patients whom they regard as having brought the epidemic on the world in the first place. The parallels with leprosy are more accurate than those who made them might realize. Leprosy was for many years confused with syphilis and was thought to be transmitted sexually (Kampmeier 1984).

Unfortunately, similar reactions have occurred against drug-users who have formed the so-called second pattern of the disorder in many countries and who are much less well organized politically to resist faulty and dangerous prejudice. Despite the increasingly positive approaches to the care of drug-users, they remain a singularly unpopular minority.

### Intravenous drug-users

Prevalence of HIV infection in people who inject themselves with illicit drugs varies widely, even between adjacent geographical areas, and depends on the extent of sharing of needles and syringes and the mobility of users (Brettle 1987). In New York, the incidence of new cases of AIDS is now greater in drug-users than homosexual men (Dole 1989). At least one-third of patients in Scotland are women whose infection arises from drug abuse or sexual contact with users (Brettle 1987). Women face particular difficulties of stigma and the dilemmas of pregnancy (Bradbeer 1989, Selwyn *et al.* 1989, Mellors & King 1992). It is estimated that 20 000 prisoners who have taken illicit drugs pass through the prison system in the UK every year (Trace 1990). It is also estimated that about two-thirds will inject drugs while in prison, over half of whom will share equipment (Carvell & Hart 1990). It is therefore obvious that the spread of HIV infection in people who inject illicit drugs is complicated by many individual and social factors.

There is a paradox at the heart of drug dependence. The drug-abuser is essentially an economic slave, supporting a huge market from which money is effectively laundered to provide employment and free spending for many (Dole 1989). Despite efforts against drug use by governments all over the world, abuse of drugs has escalated throughout the second half of this century. Although legislation had been enacted in the nineteenth century to control the use of opium, governmental control of a range of drugs of dependence was first introduced into the UK in 1920. Doctors continued, however, to have the power to prescribe controlled drugs even to drug-abusers if it was deemed necessary. Such wholesale medical freedom was soon questioned, however, and the Rolleston Committee published a report in 1926 (Ministry of Health 1926) which led to the introduction of stricter guidelines for doctors but did not prohibit prescribing. Public perception in the 1960s of increasing drug abuse and excessive prescribing by a small number of doctors, led to sharp legal restrictions on the prescribing of heroin and cocaine to special settings (Ministry of Health and Scottish Home and Health Department 1965). Drug treatment centres were established within the National Health Service and a system of notification of drug-users was developed (Ministry of

Health 1968). Legislation was finally brought into one Act, The Misuse of Drugs Act of 1971.

Throughout the 1970s and 1980s the Advisory Council on the Misuse of Drugs has monitored developments and recommended changes, particularly an emphasis on prevention (Home Office 1984). More recently it is clear that the philosophy of care of drug-users has altered profoundly. In a first report on the implications of HIV infection for services for drug misusers, published in 1988, the Department of Health and Social Security (1988) concluded: 'HIV is seen as a greater threat to public and individual health than drug misuse'. Although abstinence from drugs and prevention of drug use remains a priority, the emphasis had shifted towards harm reduction and the containment of infection.

During the last five years there has been an unprecedented attempt in western countries to reach drug-users in the community with education about safer injecting and safer sex, and the supply of needles and syringes. Community drug teams have become the model for this form of care in the UK. Although a policy of supplying syringes had been undertaken in Britain in the 1960s and 1970s to prevent hepatitis B and other infections, this practice had all but disappeared with the move to oral methadone. Reports from Edinburgh in 1986, however, suggested that high prevalence rates of HIV in drug-users were due to a lack of syringes and a large expansion in exchange schemes occurred. Unfortunately, the evidence that such programmes prevent spread of HIV is patchy and unconvincing. Sharing may persist with trusted friends or sexual partners, among people introduced to drugs for the first time, in prisons, or when 'scoring' from dealers (Stimson 1989). In other countries of Europe there have also been rare attempts, such as the recent one in Zurich, Switzerland, to ease the legislation on drug use in certain demarcated areas to counteract the underworld pattern of use with all its inherent dangers. These latter initiatives have had only limited success, perhaps as a result of their isolation.

Whether the care of drug-users should be the responsibility of medicine, and particularly psychiatry, remains unresolved. Sterile arguments over social versus medical models of drug dependence and whether certain personality types predispose to drug use have not been universally helpful. In the eyes of some, the medical profession has abdicated its role with drug-users by abandoning their care to other professions, mainly those in the social services (Dole 1989). There is considerable evidence that they are not welcomed by doctors and are considered unrewarding to treat (Glanz 1986, King 1989a). The public and the media unfortunately see only the failures of drug treatment programmes. The majority of users do not conform to the so-called junkie stereotype of the chaotic user with many psychological and social problems, but lead a stable existence usually on a contract of continuing treatment. Careful studies using matched populations have demonstrated that drug-users are no more likely than other groups to suffer psychiatric disorder (Neville *et al.* 1988), although there is often a history of dishonest or violent behaviour.

For most psychiatrists contact with drug-users will usually occur when major psychiatric problems such as psychotic and confusional states occur as a consequence of the drug use itself. When chaotic drug use, HIV infection and possible neuropsychiatric complications coincide, major difficulties for the liaison psychiatrist are likely to ensue. Interpretation of deficits on cognitive testing must take account of prior drug abuse which may have caused impairment on psychomotor tasks well before infection with HIV (Egan *et al.* 1990). Impairment on neuropsychological testing may not herald the onset of HIV encephalopathy but, nevertheless, it may damage an individual's ability to cope with the stress of the illness. Cognitive impairment in HIV infection is considered more fully below. Bizarre, or otherwise unexplained, psychological symptoms, particularly in inpatients, may also be due to continued drug use, with supplies provided by visitors.

Appropriate placement of drug-users ill with AIDS who may, hitherto, have lived in inadequate housing or on the streets, poses enormous problems for carers. Patients may either reject offers of public housing or masquerade as seropositive in order to qualify for special consideration in obtaining such accommodation. Perhaps the most successful social and psychological support can arise from specialized counsellors who have formerly used drugs themselves.

## Transmission by blood products

AIDS was recognized among recipients of blood or blood products by early 1983. Up to 12 000 people in the USA were infected via transfused blood before screening began (Friedland & Klein 1987). In the USA donated blood and plasma was first screened for antibodies to HIV in April 1985 and heat treatment of clotting factors, together with screening of donors and discouragement of donors who might be at risk, has subsequently reduced risk of transmission by this route to almost zero (Friedland & Klein 1987).

Haemophilia is a life-threatening, sex-linked, inherited condition for which there is supportive treatment by replacement of clotting factors VIII or IX, but no cure. Because many donors contribute to the plasma pool from which these products are obtained, the chances of virus transmission are increased. Until the early 1980s, the UK imported many blood products from the USA, a country in which blood donors are paid for their donation. Financial incentives increase the likelihood that unsuitable donors such as those who have abused drugs might be included. Seventy to eighty per cent of persons with haemophilia in the USA have been infected with the virus. In the UK, infection rates reported are between 6% and 59% depending on the severity of the haemophilia and the origin of the blood products used (AIDS Group of the UK Haemophilia Centre Directors 1988). This had enormous medicolegal implications and despite goverment attempts to compensate patients, led to attempts at litigation organized by patient groups, who claimed that the British Government should have acted earlier to screen blood and prevent imports of blood products, particularly from the USA (Dyer 1989).

Although haemophiliac patients do not carry the additional stigma of drug use or homosexuality and are sometimes regarded as 'innocent victims' (Curran et al. 1984), they and their families have been rejected for fear of the disease itself. Fear of contamination presents the commonest reason for the marginalization of adults and chil-

dren with HIV infection, despite clear evidence from western (Friedland et al. 1986) and African countries (Mann et al. 1986) that even close personal contact presents no risk to other people. Haemophiliac families must face the fact that their HIV infection occurred as a result of medical treatment and that this may have also occurred throughout their extended family due to the inheritable nature of haemophilia. They will also have the responsibility of telling children who may themselves be infected, and who may eventually be bereaved of their father (Miller & Harrington 1989).

## Fear of infection with HIV

Hypochondriacal fears focused on HIV infection are relatively common and present most often in general medical settings. Recent interviews with several hundred London GPs revealed that over half had patients under their care who were constantly fearful of having contracted AIDS (King 1989a). These concerns may become entrenched and lead to psychiatric referral. There is little to distinguish such patients from those expressing phobias of other disorders, and the model of abnormal illness behaviour is particularly applicable (Pilowsky 1978). Although hypochondriacal fears about AIDS are often difficult to treat, limited success has been claimed using a cognitive-behavioural approach, on the basis that such patients have many features in common with obsessive-compulsive disorder. Ruminative thoughts about infection lead to compulsive checks for possible bodily signs and the seeking of reassurance. Such ritual behaviour only temporarily relieves tension and may positively reinforce the occurrence and expression of both thought and ritual. Prevention of reassurance seeking in the face of cues to do so is a major part of the therapeutic contract (Miller et al. 1988). Patients are taught to reinterpret their symptoms as manifestations of anxiety rather than HIV and to cope more appropriately with circumstances which trigger the ruminations and compulsive behaviours.

When the fear of infection becomes delusional conviction there is an increased risk of self-harm. Patients suffering a major affective disorder may present with a conviction that they have AIDS, when they are at no apparent risk for HIV (Mahorney & Cavenar 1988). Alternatively, the delusional symptom may be one part of a more extensive psychosis. Treatment with antidepressant or antipsychotic medication is indicated, although the anxieties of the patient must be addressed by clear instruction about the nature of AIDS.

## Psychological distress in asymptomatic HIV infection

Psychological reactions to the diagnosis of HIV infection may be severe. People often react to the news with an acute anxiety response alternating with periods of denial. Often there is an impulse to confide in others which may have disastrous results. There may be withdrawal from friends and family and complete loss of sexual interest. Although HIV infection carries its own particular connotation in terms of prejudice and stigmatization, reactions to it are similar to responses to other serious illnesses in young people (Lloyd 1977, Maguire 1985). There is a mixture of anxiety and depression and, particularly in AIDS, guilt and self-blame relating to internalized public attitudes to sexual behaviour and drug misuse. People given the diagnosis may react against their homosexuality or drug use and blame themselves for past behaviour.

Reactions such as these are not universal, however, and may be short-lived. With adequate counselling, HIV testing can lead to an amelioration of psychological distress in many individuals, regardless of the test result, and does not appear to greatly aggravate distress in those who are found to be positive (Perry *et al.* 1990a). What may be crucial is the extent of past psychiatric history in individuals who present for testing. Several reports have indicated that people at risk for HIV have high rates of lifetime psychiatric disorder (Atkinson *et al.* 1988, Perry *et al.* 1990b), although methods of ascertainment of subjects in these studies are open to criticism. Whereas suicidal thoughts are frequent at the time of testing, there is now reassuring evidence that these are not intensified by testing and may actually decrease

within two months of the test result, even in those found to be HIV positive (Perry *et al.* 1990c). With the advent of increasingly effective preventative and supportive treatments it is imperative that HIV status is known and monitored.

Severe reactions to the diagnosis are more likely when there is a past history of decompensation under stress, counselling before and after the diagnosis is inadequate, the test is performed without the patient's knowledge or consent, and there is poor social support or frank rejection by others (King 1989b). It is particularly important that those who counsel patients newly diagnosed with HIV infection are fully cognisant of the disease itself. Much of this counselling involves medical education and is often more didactic than reflective (Miller & Bor 1988).

## Persisting psychiatric disorder in HIV infection and AIDS

Despite the nature of the disorder and its poor prognosis, a protracted psychiatric disorder is less common than has often been claimed (Atkinson *et al.* 1988). Early in the pandemic, reports of series of patients referred to psychiatrists led some to fear that psychological reactions were common and severe. More systematic work has revealed that psychiatric disorder, usually adjustment reactions and persisting depression, occur with approximately the same frequency as in other major and life-threatening illnesses (Devlen *et al.* 1987, King 1989b). The nature of the diagnosis given may be critical. For those assigned a diagnosis of AIDS, whether or not they knew of their HIV antibody status beforehand, the implication is graver and the consequent risk of suicide elevated. Although not always a clear finding from case series referred to psychiatrists (Sno *et al.* 1989), there is now clear epidemiological evidence that the rate of suicide in those with an AIDS diagnosis is 30–40 times higher than comparable groups of men in the general population. Although the profile of the typical individual with AIDS in North America who commits suicide is reported to be that of an unmarried, white, homosexual man who is 37 years old and who has known of the diagnosis for less than 6 months (Marzuk *et al.*

1988), this is hardly helpful in that it merely characterizes the most common patient with the disease in many parts of that country.

Reports of cross-sectional data have shown that perceived lack of social support is correlated with depression and hopelessness (Zich & Temoshok 1987). Extensive social support appears to be readily available to gay men, particularly among those who are open about their homosexuality (Hart *et al.* 1990). However, support outside the family may be less easily maintained in the face of chronic illness (Fitzpatrick *et al.* 1988). Drug-users who usually have less stable social support are especially vulnerable if they become ill. Important social factors which may precede onset of a psychiatric disorder, particularly an adjustment reaction, are loss of a love relationship and housing or financial crises (Baer 1989). Perhaps surprisingly, the occurrence of overt social stigmatization because of homosexuality, AIDS or both is not itself associated with psychological difficulties (King 1989c).

Cross-sectional data are limited to demonstrating association rather than causation. The social networks of ill people are often depleted and this is particularly so in AIDS where patients' peers may also be ill or dying. Although *perceived* adequacy of social support in terms of its availability, desirability, frequency of use and usefulness, avoids the difficulties of whether it is objectively adequate or not, dissatisfaction with social support may be the result of psychological difficulty rather than its cause. This dilemma is inherent to work on social relationships and life events in other fields (see also Chapter 10). Longitudinal data provide clues to risk factors for development of psychological problems and results have borne out many of the associations described in cross-sectional studies. Predictors for depression in a three-year cohort study of gay men in the San Francisco Mens' Health Study included loss of a lover or friend to AIDS, previous depression, loneliness and low satisfaction with social support (Castro *et al.* 1989).

Persisting psychological problems in HIV infection are related more to symptoms and perceived health status (Castro *et al.* 1989, Chuang *et al.* 1989, King 1989b, Ostrow *et al.* 1989), than

to actual stage of infection (King 1989b). *Self-reported* symptoms such as swollen glands, weight loss and fever are associated with greater distress, irrespective of verification of those symptoms (Ostrow *et al.* 1989). Perceived incapacity for work or social functioning, regardless of objective impairment, is also associated with psychological disorder (King 1989b). It may well be that men already predisposed to depression are more sensitive to bodily symptoms. Regardless of the explanation, ruminations about health and a lowering of perceived health status are important indicators of psychological distress, as they are in other serious illness (Derogatis *et al.* 1983, Devlen *et al.* 1987).

There is far less understanding of the psychological and social problems faced by people with haemophilia who are seropositive or have HIV disease than by homosexual men and drug-users. This is somewhat surprising in that the haemophiliac population is well defined and allows for representative sampling. Nevertheless, an important study of 75 haemophilic men, 31 of whom were HIV positive, recently demonstrated that seropositive men have increased levels of depression, anxiety and anger (Dew *et al.* 1990). Factors found to be associated with depression and anxiety included a personal history of psychiatric distress, a family history of psychiatric illness, lower levels of education, low support from wives, family or friends, a poor sense of mastery or recent life events involving loss. Although the study was cross-sectional in design, the authors claimed that overall levels of past psychiatric disorder did not differ between HIV-positive and -negative men, implying that current distress was a reflection of positive serostatus. These data are consistent with reports for homosexual men where perceived social support is a critical factor in psychological health. A prospective comparison of haemophiliac men and gay men in Oxford, England also reported that levels of psychological distress were higher in those haemophiliac or gay men who were seropositive at initial interview (Catalan *et al.* 1989). At 18-month follow-up, however, all psychological differences between seropositive and seronegative haemophiliac men had disappeared. Only concerns about sexual activity and the risk of infecting a partner remained as significantly different in the seropositive group (Catalan 1990). Although Catalan speculated that the improvement at 18 months may have been associated with less media coverage than at the outset of the study or improving medical care by health workers in the haemophilia field, the exact reasons for the change remained unclear.

The majority of patients with psychological problems are managed appropriately without recourse to psychiatric referral. Principal diagnoses in those referred for psychiatric help are adjustment disorders, major depression, psychotic states and organic brain syndromes (Perry & Tross 1984, Dilley *et al.* 1985, Buhrich & Cooper 1987, Baer 1989, Sno *et al.* 1989). Uncertainty over the course of the illness, perceived isolation, and illness as retribution for past behaviour are the commonest themes raised by patients (Dilley *et al.* 1985). Although psychotic states are more often of an affective type there is no evidence for a specific 'AIDS psychosis' (Halstead *et al.* 1988, Sno *et al.* 1989). Unfortunately we lack prospective epidemiological data on the incidence and prevalence of psychotic disorders in people with HIV disease as compared to the general population (Busch 1989).

The treatment of major psychiatric syndromes such as severe depression or psychosis follows traditional lines. Although antipsychotic and antidepressant drugs should be used judiciously in AIDS because of possible sensitivity to CNS effects and their anticholinergic effects on oral and bronchial secretions, it is clear that antidepressants are safe, efficacious and have no effect on immune function (Manning *et al.* 1990, Rabkin & Harrison 1990). Electroconvulsive therapy has been used successfully in HIV patients with severe depression who do not have major organic brain syndromes (Schaerf *et al.* 1989). Delusional states, particularly if complicated by AIDS encephalopathy, can be resistant to treatment with antipsychotic medication. This is particularly the case in people who have abused drugs. The resulting behavioural disturbance can be extremely difficult to manage in the side-rooms of medical wards, and transfer to psychiatric facilities, where the patient may be nursed less restrictively, yet nevertheless in a controlled environment, is often necessary.

## Involvement of the central nervous system in HIV disease

HIV enters the brain shortly after first infection, probably carried within macrophages which cross the blood—brain barrier. Virus released from these macrophages may cause a clinical or subclinical meningoencephalitis from which the patient recovers. With a later fall in immune competence, HIV begins to replicate in the brain (Perry 1990). In the mid 1980s the term AIDS dementia complex was first applied to the constellation of clinical and pathological findings that resulted from direct HIV involvement of the central nervous system (CNS) (Navia *et al.* 1986a,b). CNS pathology associated with HIV disease includes neoplasms, opportunistic infections, vascular lesions and a characteristic multinucleate giant cell encephalitis (Lantos *et al.* 1989). In the latter, there is relative sparing of the cortex with changes in the central white matter and deep grey structures, such as the basal ganglia. Research into this aspect of neurological AIDS has received an enormous investment of time and resources. Despite criticism of the term dementia applied in this setting, chronic loss of global cognitive functioning with apathy, withdrawal and deterioration of personality occurs in advanced HIV disease and is a source of great concern for patients and carers.

No consensus has been reached as to the most reliable and valid tests of cognitive function to apply. Neuropsychological testing may also have no direct relationship to actual organic impairment (Perry 1990). The tests may be insensitive to subtle impairment, or a highly intelligent individual may notice some deterioration in function and yet still remain within the normal range for that instrument. Results may be confounded by the influence of past drug or alcohol abuse (Egan *et al.* 1990), or patients fearing the onset of dementia may complain of cognitive deficit simply because they are depressed or otherwise emotionally distressed (Herns *et al.* 1989, Canick & Temoshok 1990). Even lack of sleep can impair performance on psychological testing (Idzikowski 1984).

Early reports of neuropsychological impairment in asymptomatic infection (Grant *et al.* 1987) have not been confirmed in larger studies in which standardized instruments and appropriate comparison groups have been used. Despite some persisting reports to the contrary (Naber *et al.* 1990), and despite the difficulty of interpreting the results of neuropsychological tests, current evidence indicates that people with asymptomatic HIV infection have no greater impairment on detailed neuropsychological assessment than HIV-negative controls (Carne *et al.* 1989, Goethe *et al.* 1989, Janssen *et al.* 1989, McArthur *et al.* 1989, Clifford *et al.* 1990, Egan *et al.* 1990, Riccio *et al.* 1990).

A neuropsychological assessment is an important part of the mental state examination of any patient with HIV disease, but is vital where there are vague signs such as fatigue, forgetfulness, distractibility, irritability or change in personality. The disinterest and withdrawal characteristic of HIV encephalopathy may be mistaken for depressive symptoms. Computerized scanning and electroencephalography are essential investigations, whenever organic impairment is suspected. A more difficult problem is the choice of cognitive assessment. Tests of verbal and visual memory, psychomotor coordination and word fluency are recommended as well as some assessment of premorbid intelligence. Clinicians should familiarize themselves with a brief battery of tests, remain aware of the limits of testing, and apply them regularly to monitor any change which may herald a deterioration in CNS function.

AIDS encephalopathy is the cause of major social problems for patients and their carers. Patients may neglect themselves, misunderstand or refuse medical and nursing care, or even create a danger to others through their chaotic behaviour. Application of the Mental Health Act of England and Wales may be unfamiliar in this setting, although technically there is no reason why patients cannot be removed compulsorily to medical wards of National Health Service Hospitals for physical treatment (Fenton 1987). Before taking this serious step, which is often distressing for friends and relatives, all other means of persuasion to help the patient must be employed. Occasionally, however, it may be urgently necessary to move a patient to a place of safety and resort to Common Law or the application of a Mental Health Section may be unavoidable (Department of Health and Welsh Office 1990, Jelley 1990.)

Treatment of organic brain syndromes in HIV disease will depend on careful delineation of the underlying problem. It is essential to establish the patient's level of functioning and arrange that he or she be cared for in a suitably structured environment with assistance for individual deficits. Relatives and friends should be taught about the nature of the disorder and the lack of control patients may have over certain aspects of their behaviour. This often involves a team of health workers with individual skills who cooperate with relatives and friends. It is a reasonable goal to maximize the patient's independence, albeit that eventually it may be impossible to maintain. The confusion which results from HIV encephalopathy should respond to small does of phenothiazines, although idiosyncratic reactions to these drugs are more common than usual and, for reasons which remain unclear, occasional patients need very high doses. In any case, the level of competence may fluctuate with the course of the illness. There is equivocal evidence that zidovudine, the principal drug which acts against the retrovirus, may arrest the progression of the dementing process (Portegies *et al.* 1989).

Psychiatrists may be called upon to assess testamentary capacity in the final stages of the illness. Questions of mental competence in the realm of personal and financial affairs should be handled in the same way as for other illnesses. Patients are competent to dispose of their possessions if there is no evidence for a major mental illness (including dementia) which *impairs their orientation or understanding of what is entailed.* They must know what a will is, have a rational idea of the assets at their disposal and know to whom they would reasonably be expected to leave possessions and the claims of each. Although patients must not suffer from delusions or obsessions which would pervert their judgement in disposing of property, the mere presence of paranoid ideas would not of themselves invalidate a will. Finally patients should not have been victims of undue influence (Rentoul & Smith 1973, Sanders 1984). These judgements must not be made narrowly. Every patient should be given the opportunity to decide for themselves. Eccentricity or a will made against the wishes of those closest to the patient are insufficient grounds on which to regard the patient as incompetent. It is worth keeping in mind that the doctors may be called upon to back their assessments in court if a will is challenged (Fraser 1987).

## Stress and immunity

There is a close and interdependent relationship between the CNS, hypothalamus–pituitary–adrenal axis and the immune system. Receptors for neurohormones exist on lymphocytes and many of these hormones are able to influence lymphocytic function (Perez & Farant 1988). Although stress may have a direct effect on behaviour, neurohormone release and immune response, the relationships are complicated and do not allow simple explanations of the direct influence of stress on immune function or vice versa (Dorian & Garfinkel 1987). Any investigation of stress and immune function must control for baseline levels of ambient stress, the nature, inherent meaning and duration of the stressor, and circadian or seasonal fluctuations in immunological functioning. Stress itself is a subjective phenomenon which is difficult to define or measure. The clearest evidence linking immunity with stress comes from studies of bereavement, in which it has been demonstrated that death of a spouse or close family member may impair both humoral and cell-mediated immunity in the bereaved (Linn *et al.* 1982, Schleifer *et al.* 1983).

Despite popular belief on the part of patients and some of their carers, the evidence in HIV infection that psychological or social factors have an important influence on immune competence, or progression of the disorder, remains to be demonstrated (Temoshok 1988). There is some evidence linking stressful life events with an elevated risk of illness onset in previously well seropositive men (Kessler *et al.* 1989), but careful prospective work correlating psychological and social variables with CD4 lymphocyte counts (the principal lymphocyte

infected by HIV) has not established any direct association (Perry *et al.* 1990d). Thus, it is not yet possible to attribute disease progression to the direct effects of emotional distress on the immune system. Studies are hampered by confounding influences on immune function such as alcohol and drug abuse, previous infections and current treatments. Furthermore, the time-lag between a stressor and its possible effects, and the role of homeostatic mechanisms in correcting imbalances caused by stress, are unknown.

## Consequences for partners, families and friends

The social stigma of HIV extends well beyond the person infected with the virus. There is evidence that people with close ties to patients suffer considerable distress for many of the same reasons as patients. The social and psychological impact of the disorder may spread beyond partners and families to include schools, the health-care system, employers and fellow employees, churches and other social institutions. Families may be collectively ostracized, or children left outcast in the wake of the epidemic (Carswell 1988, Quinn *et al.* 1989). In western countries these issues are most clearly seen in the families of haemophiliacs where both children and their parents may be infected. There may be secrets within families with dread of telling children their diagnosis, relative neglect of seronegative siblings and consequent jealousy, ostracism or teasing of children by peers and the complications of developing sexuality in affected adolescents (Miller *et al.* 1989). It has been reported from at least one prospective family study of haemophiliacs that marriages may be under stress because of poor communication between partners who may keep the facts from their children. There may also be increased use of alcohol and drugs.

Partners of people with HIV infection are subject to pressures both in relation to their need to care for and support the patient, but also as regards their own fears of contamination. In a study in which primary care physicians in London were interviewed about their care of people with HIV infection, doctors reported that the commonest reason why they were consulted by relatives and friends of patients with HIV, was concern about contracting the virus (King 1989a). Heterosexual partners may have to cope with revelations concerning the sexual or drug habits of their loved one, as well as the prospect of losing them. The wives of haemophiliac men who appear to be already under stress because of their husbands' haemophilia (Klimes *et al.* 1989) may face a further burden with HIV infection which has resulted directly from medical treatment. All sexual partners of infected individuals must face the possibility of viral transmission through sexual contact, and cope with the impact of this threat on the relationship. Homosexual partners are sometimes excluded by families who do not understand or accept the nature of their relationship with the patient and next-of-kin status may be denied them (Ostrow & Gayle 1986).

Bereavement issues are compounded when the cause of death is stigmatized. In a detailed North American study of mainly white homosexual men, it was reported that men bereaved of a lover or close friend with AIDS experienced symptoms of a post-traumatic stress response with intrusive thoughts and emotions about AIDS (Martin 1988). Bereaved men were vulnerable to demoralization and sleep problems. They were more likely to use sedatives and attend psychological services primarily for AIDS concerns. These findings remained significant after controlling for effects of their own compromised health status and appraised threat of AIDS. It should be reiterated here that seropositive men bereaved of their partner present a definite suicidal risk.

Although homosexual men often receive support from the gay community (Hart *et al.* 1990), they may be required to conceal the extent of their grief from others in their social network who are unaware of the true nature of their relationship with the deceased. The young heterosexual man who loses a wife will receive considerable understanding from acquaintances and work colleagues and will be allowed a period of reduced responsibility within which to resolve his grief. Not so for the homosexual man who may have to hide his loss, or who may in any case receive less sympathy because of an implicit assumption that homosexual relationships are less profound than heterosexual marriage.

In attempting to hide the true cause of death from relatives, family members may experience a secretive and protracted grief. Thus, parents suffer both the strain of loss and the consequences of only partial disclosure to those in their family who could help them most (Shearer & McKusick 1986). The death certificate, however, may betray even the most careful attempts to maintain privacy and in its present form in Britain offers no confidentiality after death (King 1989d). There are indications following the recent discussion document on Death Certification in England and Wales (Her Majesty's Government 1988) that a two-part certificate is about to be introduced. One part will not contain the cause of death and may be used by relatives for the required administrative procedures. This will go some way to increasing confidentiality for relatives, although the second part containing the cause of death will remain a public document to which journalists and others may gain access (King 1989d).

## Consequences for care-givers

In common with other serious diseases, caring for patients with HIV disease carries a psychological and social burden. The early hostility of medical, nursing and paramedical staff towards patients with active disease was partly based upon prejudice against homosexuals and drug-users, and partly on fear of contamination (Cecchi 1986, Gillon 1987, Kelly *et al.* 1987). Although this apprehension has abated somewhat, fear may remain in certain quarters even extending to the families and partners of those who treat patients.

It is obvious that caring for young people whose prognosis is poor is very stressful for carers. Severe stress can occur in individuals and teams of carers, particularly those dealing with advanced cases where death with its implicit sense of medical failure is a daily experience (Horstman & McKusick 1986, Ross & Seeger 1988, Volberding 1989). In the particular case of haemophilia, staff who may have cared for patients for years must confront HIV infection as something introduced, albeit inadvertently, by their own treatments. Although the burden of working with patients include fear of death, anxiety and overwork, there are also the positive aspects of an intellectual challenge and career satisfaction. The instinct in psychiatry, at least, is to assume that support groups will assist in dealing with these aspects of patient care, but there is evidence that health professionals are less convinced and may prefer to cope with the emotional aspects of their work by talking with friends, lovers and family members (Horstman & McKusick 1986). This may relate, however, to the type of care offered and support groups have been successful when focused and personal (Volberding 1989).

## Psychological sequelae of treatment

With increasingly effective prevention and treatment of complications, HIV disease is becoming a chronic disorder. Regular, supportive follow-up inevitably leads to a degree of dependency which may manifest itself as anxiety, hostility or depression appearing at times of interruption in the pattern of care such as holidays for members of the team, a change of personnel or as the time for discharge approaches. Patients may regress into a child-like state, inducing the doctor or team to take over all responsibility and refusing any therapeutic role for themselves. They may express emotions such as anger in inappropriate situations, thus damaging other areas of their lives. For example, they may walk out on a job, or become drunk or aggressive at home. A third possibility is one of splitting, in which care-givers are regarded by the patient as 'good' or 'bad', creating considerable strain within the team. Patients with HIV infection might be expected to be at greater risk for dependency than other people with chronic health problems because of possible social isolation, the gravity of the illness and its uncertain outcome. Although dependency does arise, the majority of patients appear to adapt to their condition in a mature way seeking more, rather than less, responsibility for their own health and future prospects (King 1989b).

Most patients with symptomatic HIV disease receive 3'-azido-3'-deoxythymidine (zidovudine) which prevents replication of HIV (Weller 1988).

The side-effects of zidovudine constitute a serious problem (Richman *et al.* 1987). Although the psychiatric side-effects of this drug have not been systematically documented, two cases of mania associated with zidovudine therapy have been reported (Maxwell *et al.* 1988). The more recently developed purine analogue 2'3'-dideoxyinosine (ddI) also has toxic side-effects, and psychological reactions to the drug include anxiety, irritability and headaches (Yarchoan *et al.* 1990). The role of exogenous interferons in HIV infection remains unresolved (De Wit *et al.* 1988). Their disadvantage is a tendency to produce neuropsychiatric side-effects. Patients usually report an influenza-like state shortly after injection, but more persistent complaints of poor concentration, fatigue and dysphoria may follow. Electroencephalographic changes can also occur. A marked increase in psychiatric symptoms occur during treatment but reverse on stopping interferon administration (McDonald *et al.* 1987). Physicians need to be aware of these complications which can be severe enough to require specific psychiatric help.

As a means of establishing the efficacy of new drugs in AIDS, the double-blind cross-over trial has come under increasing criticism. Patient advocacy groups have opposed clinical scientists in a battle which has enormous ethical and social implications (Swan 1989). Although effective treatments should not be withheld unnecessarily, it remains essential that clinical trials are properly conducted to establish that new medications are at least not positively harmful. It is just as essential, however, that the social implications of such a trial are fully explained. Patients entering a trial must balance potential benefit from treatment against unnecessary toxicity or even the development of potential resistance to the drug which might reduce its efficacy later in the course of the disease (Lee *et al.* 1989).

## Conclusions

HIV disease presents new challenges to society and medicine. Psychiatrists have had to address social factors which may induce both psychological disorder and a decline in physical health, ethical problems which accompany a stigmatized disease, neurotropism of a virus which can lead to organic brain syndromes, reactive stress in care-givers, and the toxic and debilitating effects of treatment. HIV infection has provided renewed impetus to research into the interface between social stress, psychological disorder and immunity. Despite a reawakening of prejudice against homosexuality, it has led to greater openness about sexual life-styles and a vastly increased vigour to gay political and patient advocacy groups. It has clarified our management of drug dependence, forced upon us a new tolerance of individual behaviour and made explicit the current moral and ethical assumptions underlying much of our health care.

# References

AIDS Group of the United Kingdom Haemophilia Centre Directors with the co-operation of the United Kingdom Haemophilia Directors (1988) Prevalence of antibody to HIV in haemophiliacs in the United Kingdom: a second survey. *Clinical and Laboratory Haematology* 10, 187–191.

American Psychiatric Association (1973) *Diagnostic and Statistical Manual*, 2nd edn. APA, Washington DC.

American Psychiatric Association (1980) *Diagnostic and Statistical Manual*, 3rd edn. APA, Washington DC.

Atkinson J.H., Grant I., Kennedy C.J., Richman D.D., Spector S.A. & McCutchan J.A. (1988) Prevalence of psychiatric disorders among men infected with human immunodeficiency virus. *Archives of General Psychiatry* 45, 859–864.

Baer J.W. (1989) Study of 60 patients with AIDS or AIDS-related complex requiring psychiatric hospitalisation. *American Journal of Psychiatry* 146, 1285–1288.

Bancroft J. (1975) Homosexuality and the medical profession: a behaviourist's view. *Journal of Medical Ethics* 1, 176–180.

Bayer R. & Spitzer R.L. (1982) Edited correspondence on the status of homosexuality in DSMIII. *Journal of the History of the Behavioural Sciences* 18, 32–52.

Bhugra D. & King M.B. (1989) Controlled comparison of attitudes of psychiatrists, general practitioners, homosexual doctors and homosexual men to male homosexuality. *Journal of the Royal Society of Medicine* 82, 603–605.

Bradbeer C. (1989) Mothers with HIV. *British Medical Journal* 299, 806–807.

Brettle R.P. (1987) Drug abuse and immunodeficiency virus infection in Scotland. *Journal of the Royal Society of Medicine* 80, 274–278.

Buhrich N. & Cooper D.A. (1987) Requests for psychiatric consultation concerning 22 patients with AIDS and ARC.

*Australian and New Zealand Journal of Psychiatry* 21, 346–353.

Busch K.A. (1989) Psychotic states in human immunodeficiency virus illness. *Current Opinion in Psychiatry* 2, 3–6.

Canick J.D. & Temoshok L. (1990) The Longitudinal Assessment of Perceived and Objective Cognitive Impairment in Symptomatic HIV Seropositive Men. Paper (F.B.366) presented at the 6th International Conference on AIDS, San Francisco, June 1990.

Carne C.A., Stibe C., Bronkhurst A. *et al.* (1989) Subclinical neurological and neuropsychological effect of infection with HIV. *Genitourinary Medicine* 65, 151–156.

Carswell J.W. (1988) Impact of AIDS in the developing world. *British Medical Bulletin* 44, 183–202.

Carvell A.L.M. & Hart G.J. (1990) Risk behaviours for HIV infection among drug users in prison. *British Medical Journal* 300, 1383–1384.

Castro F., Coates T.J. & Ekstrand M. (1989) Prevalence and Predictors of Depression in Gay and Bisexual Men During the AIDS Epidemic: The San Francisco Men's Health Study. Presented at the Vth International Conference on AIDS, Montreal, Canada. Book of abstracts WBO.40. International Development Research Centre, Canada.

Catalan J. (1990) Psychiatric Problems in HIV Infected Men with Haemophilia. Paper presented at Conference on Neurology and Psychiatry of AIDS, Monterey, California, 16–19 June.

Catalan J., Klimes I., Bond A., Garrod A., Day A. & Rizza C. (1989) Psychosocial and Neuropsychological Status of Haemophiliacs and Gay Men with HIV Infection: A Controlled Investigation. Presented at the Vth International Conference on AIDS, Montreal, Canada. Book of abstracts ThBP.31. International Development Research Centre, Canada.

Cecchi R.L. (1986) Heath care advocacy for AIDS patients. *Quarterly Review Bulletin* August 297–303.

Centers For Disease Control (1986) Classification system for human T-lymphocyte virus types III/lymphadenopathy-associated virus infection. *Morbidity and Mortality Weekly Report* 35, 334–339.

Chuang H.T., Devins G.M., Hunsley J. & Gill M.J. (1989) Psychosocial distress and well-being among gay and bisexual men with human immunodeficiency virus infection. *American Journal of Psychiatry* 146, 876–880.

Clifford D.B., Jacoby R.G., Miller J.P., Seyfried W.R. & Glicksman M. (1990) Neuropsychiatric performance of asymptomatic HIV-infected subjects. *AIDS* 4, 767–774.

Curran J.W., Lawrence D.N., Jaffe H. (1984) AIDS associated with transfusions. *New England Journal of Medicine* 310, 69–75.

Davenport-Hines R. (1990) *Sex, Death and Punishment*. Collins, London.

Department of Health and Social Security (1988) *AIDS and Drug Misuse Parts I and II*. HMSO, London.

Department of Health and Welsh Office (1990) *Code of Practice*. HMSO, London.

Derogatis L.R., Morrow G.R., Fetting J. *et al.* (1983) The prevalence of psychiatric disorders among cancer patients. *Journal of the American Medical Association* 249, 751–757.

Devlen J., Maguire P., Phillips P. & Crowther D. (1987) Psychological problems associated with diagnosis and treatment of lymphomas. II: a prospective study. *British Medical Journal* 295, 955–957.

Dew M.A., Ragni M.V. & Nimorwicz P. (1990) Infection with human immunodeficiency virus and vulnerability to psychiatric distress. *Archives of General Psychiatry* 47, 737–744.

De Wit R., Boucher C.A.B., Veenhof K.H.N., Schattenkerk J.K.M., Bakker P.J.M. & Danner S.A. (1988) Clinical and virological effects of high-dose recombinant interferon-X in disseminated AIDS-related Kaposi's sarcoma. *Lancet* ii, 1214–1217.

Dilley J.W., Ochitill H.N., Perl M. & Volberding P.A. (1985) Findings in psychiatric consultations with patients with acquired immune deficiency syndrome. *American Journal of Psychiatry* 142, 82–86.

Dole V.P. (1989) Methadone treatment and the acquired immunodeficiency syndrome epidemic. *Journal of the American Medical Association* 262, 1681–1682.

Dorian B. & Garfinkel P.E. (1987) Stress, immunity and illness – a review. *Psychological Medicine* 17, 393–407.

Douglas C., Kalman C. & Kalman T.P. (1985) Homophobia among physicians and nurses: an empirical study. *Hospital and Community Psychiatry* 36, 1309–1311.

Dyer C. (1989) Haemophiliacs sue British government. *British Medical Journal* 299, 700–701.

Egan V.G., Crawford J.R., Brettle R.P. & Goodwin G.M. (1990) The Edinburgh cohort of HIV-positive drug users: current intellectual function is impaired, but not due to early AIDS dementia complex. *AIDS* 4, 651–656.

Eisenberg L. (1986) The genesis of fear: AIDS and the public's response to science. *Law, Medicine and Health Care* 14, 243–249.

Fenton T.W. (1987) Practical problems in the management of AIDS-related psychiatric disorder. *Journal of The Royal Society of Medicine* 80, 271–274.

Fitzpatrick R., Newman S., Lamb R. & Shipley M. (1988) Social relationships and psychological well-being in rheumatoid arthritis. *Social Science and Medicine* 27, 399–403.

Fraser M. (1987) *Dementia. Its Nature and Management* John Wiley, Chichester.

Friedland G.H. & Klein R.S. (1987) Transmission of the human immunodeficiency virus. *New England Journal of Medicine* 317, 1125–1135.

Friedland G.H., Saltzmann B.R., Rogers M.F. *et al.* (1986) Lack of transmission of HTLV-III/LAV infection to household contacts of patients with AIDS or AIDS-related complex with oral candidiasis. *New England Journal of Medicine* 314, 344–349.

Gillon R. (1987) Refusal to treat AIDS and HIV positive patients. *British Medical Journal* 294, 1332–1333.

Glanz A. (1986) Findings of a national survey of the role of general practitioners in the treatment of opiate misusers: views on treatment. *British Medical Journal* 293, 543–545.

Goethe K.E., Mitchell J.E., Marshall D.W. *et al.* (1989) Neuropsychological and neurological function of human immunodeficiency virus seropositive asymptomatic individuals. *Archives of Neurology* 46, 129–133.

Grant I., Hampton Atkinson J., Hesselink J.R. *et al.* (1987) Evidence for early central nervous system involvement in the acquired immunodeficiency syndrome (AIDS) and other human immunodefiency virus (HIV) infections. *Annals of Internal Medicine* 107, 828–836.

Halstead S., Riccio M., Harlow P., Oretti R. & Thompson C. (1988) Psychosis associated with HIV infection. *British Journal of Psychiatry* 153, 618–623.

Hart G., Fitzpatrick R., McLean J., Dawson J. & Boulton M. (1990) Gay men, social support and HIV disease: a study of social integration in the gay community. *AIDS Care* 2, 163–170.

Her Majesty's Government (1988) *Registration: A Modern Service*. HMSO, London, CM531.

Herns M., Newman S., McAllister R., Weller I. & Harrison M. (1989) Mood State, Neuropsychology and Self Reported Cognitive Deficits in HIV Infection. Paper presented to the Vth International Conference on AIDS, Montreal, Canada, 4–9 June. *Montréal Abstract Volume* WBP 185. International Development Research Centre, Canada.

Home Office (1984) *Prevention: Report of the Advisory Council on the Misuse of Drugs*. HMSO, London.

Horstman W. & McKusick L. (1986) The impact of AIDS on the physician. In McKusick L. (ed.) *What To Do About AIDS*. University of California Press, California, pp. 63–74.

Idzikowski C. (1984) Sleep and memory. *British Journal of Psychology* 75, 439–449.

Israelstam S. & Lambert S. (1983) Homosexuality as a cause of alcoholism: a historical review. *International Journal of the Addictions* 18, 1085–1107.

Janssen R.S., Saykin A.J., Canon L. *et al.* (1989) Neurological and neuropsychological manifestations of HIV-1 infection: association with AIDS-related complex but not asymptomatic HIV-1 infection. *Annals of Neurology* 26, 592–600.

Jelley M. (1990) Common law and the 'Code of Practice' – a commentary. *Bulletin of the Royal College of Psychiatrists* 14, 449–451.

Kampmeier R.H. (1984) Early development of knowledge of sexually transmitted diseases. In: Holmes K.K., Mardh P., Sparling P.F. & Wiesner P.J. (eds) *Sexually Transmitted Diseases*, pp. 19–29. McGraw Hill, New York.

Kelly J.A., St Lawrence J.S., Smith S., Hood H.V. & Cook D.J. (1987) Stigmatization of AIDS patients by physicians. *American Journal of Public Health* 77, 789–791.

Kessler R., Joseph J., Ostrow D., Phair J., Chmiel J. & Rusk C. (1989) Psychosocial Co-factors in Illness Onset Among HIV Positive Men. Paper presented at the 5th International Conference on AIDS, Montréal, Canada, June

1989, *Montréal Abstract Volume* MAO48, pp. 53. International Development Research Centre, Canada.

King M.B. (1989a) Psychological and social problems in HIV infection: interviews with general practitioners in London. *British Medical Journal* 299, 713—717.

King M.B. (1989b) Psychosocial status of 192 out-patients with HIV infection and AIDS. *British Journal of Psychiatry* 154, 237—242.

King M.B. (1989c) Prejudice and AIDS: the views and experiences of people with HIV infection. *AIDS Care* 1, 137—143.

King M.B. (1989d) AIDS on the death certificate: the final stigma. *British Medical Journal* 298, 734—736.

Kinsey A.C., Pomeroy W.B. & Martin C.E. (1948) *Sexual Behaviour in the Human Male.* W.B. Saunders, Philadelphia.

Kinsey A.C., Pomeroy W.B., Martin C.E. & Gebhard P.H. (1953) *Sexual Behaviour in the Human Female.* W.B. Saunders, Philadelphia.

Klimes I., Catalan J., Bond A., Garrod A., Day A. & Rizza C. (1989) Psychosocial Status of Partners of Haemophiliacs with HIV Infection. Paper presented at the 5th International Conference on AIDS, Montréal, Canada, June 1989. *Montréal Abstract Volume*, E507, pp. 887. International Development Research Centre, Canada.

Lantos P.L., McLaughlin J.E., Scholtz C.L., Berry C.L. & Tighe J.R. (1989) Neuropathology of the brain in HIV infection. *Lancet* i, 309—311.

Lee C.A., Miller R. & Goldman E. (1989) Treatment dilemmas for HIV infected haemophiliacs. *AIDS Care* 1, 153—158.

Lifson A.R., Hessol N., Rutherford G. *et al.* (1990) Natural History of HIV Infection in a Cohort of Homosexual and Bisexual Men: Clinical and Immunologic Outcome. Paper (Th.C.33) presented at the 6th International Conference on AIDS, San Francisco, June 1990, Abstract vol. 1, p. 142.

Linn B.S., Linn M.W. & Jensen J. (1982) Degree of depression and immune responsiveness. *Psychosomatic Medicine* 44, 128—129.

Lloyd G.G. (1977) Psychological reactions to physical illness. *British Journal of Hospital Medicine* October, 352—356.

McArthur J.C., Cohen B.A., Selnes O.A. *et al.* (1989) Low prevalence of neurological and neuropsychological abnormalities in otherwise healthy HIV-1-infected individuals: results from the multicenter AIDS cohort study. *Annals of Neurology* 26, 601—611.

McConaghy N. (1987) Heterosexuality/homosexuality: dichotomy or continuum. *Archives of Sexual Behaviour* 16, 411—424.

Macculloch M.J. (1981) Male homosexual behaviour. *The Practitioner* 225, 1635—1641.

McDonald E.M., Mann A.H. & Thomas H.C. (1987) Interferons as mediators of psychiatric morbidity. An investigation in a trial of recombinant interferon in hepatitis-B carriers. *Lancet* ii, 1175—1178.

Maguire P. (1985) The psychological impact of cancer. *British Journal of Hospital Medicine* August, 100—103.

Mahorney S.L. & Cavenar J.O. (1988) A new and timely delusion: the complaint of having AIDS. *American Journal of Psychiatry* 145, 1130—1132.

Mann J.M., Quinn T.C., Francis H. *et al.* (1986) Prevalence of HTLV-III/LAV in household contacts of patients with confirmed AIDS and controls in Kinshasa, Zaire. *Journal of the American Medical Society* 256, 721—724.

Manning D., Jacobsberg L., Erhart S., Perry S. & Frances A. (1990) The Efficacy of Imipramine in the Treatment of HIV-related Depression. Paper (Th.B.32) presented at the 6th International Conference on AIDS, San Francisco, June 1990.

Martin J.L. (1988) Psychological consequences of AIDS-related bereavement among gay men. *Journal of Clinical and Consulting Psychology* 56, 856—862.

Marzuk P.M., Tierney H., Tardiff K. *et al.* (1988) Increased risk of suicide in persons with AIDS. *Journal of the American Medical Association* 259, 1333—1337.

Matthews W.C., Booth M.W., Turner J.D. *et al.* (1986) Physicians' attitudes toward homosexuality – survey of a California county medical society. *West Journal of Medicine* 144, 106—110.

Maxwell S., Scheftner W.A., Kessler H.A. & Busch K. (1988) Manic syndrome associated with Zidovudine treatment. *Journal of the American Medical Association* 259, 3406—3407.

Mellors J. & King M.B. (1990) A Controlled Study of the Psychiatric and Social Problems in Women with HIV Infection. Research Report, Academic Department of Psychiatry, Royal Free Hospital School of Medicine.

Miller D., Acton T.M.G. & Hedge B. (1988) The worried well: their identification and management. *Journal of the Royal College of Physicians of London* 22, 158—165.

Miller R. & Bor R. (1988) *AIDS: A Guide to Clinical Counselling.* Science Press, London.

Miller R., Goldman E., Bor R. & Kernoff P. (1989) AIDS and children: some of the issues in haemophilia care and how to address them. *AIDS Care* 1, 59—65.

Miller R. & Harrington C. (1989) HIV and haemophilia. *AIDS Care* 1, 212—215.

Ministry of Health (1926) *Report of the Departmental Committee on Morphine and Heroin Addiction.* HMSO, London.

Ministry of Health (1968) *The Rehabilitation of Drug Addicts: Report of the Advisory Committee on Drug Dependence.* HMSO, London.

Ministry of Health and Scottish Home and Health Department (1965) *Drug Addiction: The Second Report of the Interdepartmental Committee.* HMSO, London.

Murphy T.F. (1988) Is AIDS a just punishment? *Journal of Medical Ethics* 14, 154—160.

Naber D., Perro C., Schick U. *et al.* (1990) Psychiatric symptoms and neuropsychological deficits in HIV infection. In Bunney/Hippius/Laakman/Schmauss (eds) *Neuropsychopharmacology.* Springer-Verlag, Heidleberg, pp. 745–755.

Navia B.A., Jordan B.D. & Price R.W. (1986a) The AIDS dementia complex: I. Clinical features. *Annals of Neurology* 19, 517–524.

Navia B.A., Cho E.S., Petito C.K. & Price R.W. (1986b) The AIDS dementia complex: II. Neuropathology. *Annals of Neurology* 19, 525–535.

Neville R.G., McKellican J.F. & Foster J. (1988) Heroin users in general practice: ascertainment and features. *British Medical Journal* 296, 755–758.

Ostrow D.G. & Gayle T.C. (1986) Psychosocial and ethical issues of AIDS health care programs. *Quarterly Review Bulletin* August, 284–294.

Ostrow D.G., Monjan A., Joseph J. *et al.* (1989) HIV-related symptoms and psychological functioning in a cohort of homosexual men. *American Journal of Psychiatry* 146, 737–742.

Owen W.F. (1980) The clinical approach to the homosexual patient. *Annals of Internal Medicine* 93, 90–92.

Pauly I.B. & Goldstein S.G. (1970) Physicians' attitudes in treating male homosexuals. *Medical Aspects of Human Sexuality* 4, 27–45.

Perez M. & Farant J. (1988) Immune reactions and mental disorders. *Psychological Medicine* 18, 11–13.

Perry S.W. (1990) Organic mental disorders caused by HIV: update on early diagnosis and treatment. *American Journal of Psychiatry* 147, 696–710.

Perry S.W., Jacobsberg L.B., Fishman B. *et al.* (1990a) Psychological responses to serological testing for HIV. *AIDS* 4, 145–152.

Perry S.W., Jacobsberg L.B., Fishman B., Francis A., Bobo J. & Jacobsberg B.K. (1990b) Psychiatric diagnosis before serological testing for the Human Immunodeficiency Virus. *American Journal of Psychiatry* 147, 89–93.

Perry S., Jacobsberg L. & Fishman B. (1990c) Suicidal ideation and HIV testing. *Journal of the American Medical Association* 263, 679–682.

Perry S., Jacobsberg L. & Fishman B. (1990d) Relationship between CD4 Lymphocytes and Psychosocial Variables Among HIV Seropositive Adults. Paper (Th.B.27) presented at the 6th International Conference on AIDS, San Francisco, June 1990.

Perry S.W. & Tross S. (1984) Psychiatric problems of AIDS inpatients at the New York Hospital: preliminary report. *Public Health Reports* 99, 201–205.

Pilowsky I. (1978) A general classification of abnormal illness behaviours. *British Journal of Medical Psychology* 51, 131–137.

Portegies P., de Gans J., Lange J.M.A. *et al.* (1989) Declining incidence of AIDS dementia complex after introduction of zidovudine treatment. *British Medical Journal* 299, 819–821.

Prichard J.G., Lanyard L.K., Holloway R.L., Mosely M., Bale R.M. & Kaplowitz H.J. (1988) Attitude of family medicine residents toward homosexuality. *Journal of Family Practice* 27, 637–639.

Quinn T.C., Zacarias F.R.K. & St John R.K. (1989) AIDS in the Americas. *New England Journal of Medicine* 320, 1005–1007.

Rabkin J.G. & Harrison W.M. (1990) Effect of imipramine on depression and immune status in a sample of men with HIV infection. *American Journal of Psychiatry* 147, 495–497.

Remafedi G. (1987) Homosexual youth. A challenge to contemporary society. *Journal of the American Medical Association* 258, 222–225.

Rentoul E. & Smith H. (1973) *Glaisters Medical Jurisprudence and Toxicology.* Churchill Livingstone, Edinburgh.

Riccio M., Jadresic D., Hawkins D., Wilson B. & Thompson C. (1990) The Neuropsychology and Psychiatry of HIV Infection in Asymptomatic Gay Men – St Stephen's Cohort Study. Paper (F.B.363) presented at the 6th International Conference on AIDS, San Francisco, June 1990.

Richman D.D., Fischl M.A., Greigo M.A. *et al.* (1987) The toxicity of AZT in the treatment of patients with AIDS. *New England Journal of Medicine* 317, 192–197.

Ross M.W. & Seeger V. (1988) Determinants of reported burnout in health professionals associated with the care of patients with AIDS. *AIDS* 2, 395–397.

Sanders S.C. (1984) Testamentary capacity. In Grimley-Evans J.G. & Caird F.I. (eds) *Advanced Geriatric Medicine.* Pitman, London.

Schaerf F.W., Miller R.R., Lipsey J.R. & McPherson R.W. (1989) ECT for major depression in four patients infected with human immunodeficiency virus. *American Journal of Psychiatry* 146, 782–784.

Schleifer S.J., Keller S.E., Camerino M., Thornton J.C. & Stein M. (1983) Suppression of lymphocyte stimulation following bereavement. *Journal of the American Medical Association* 250, 374–377.

Seale J.R. (1987) Kuru, AIDS and aberrant behaviour. *Journal of the Royal Society of Medicine* 80, 200–202.

Selwyn P.A., Carter R.J., Schoenbaum E.E., Robertson V.J., Klein R.S. & Rogers M.F. (1989) Knowledge of HIV antibody status and decisions to continue or terminate pregnancy among intravenous drug users. *Journal of the American Society* 261, 3567–3571.

Shearer P. & McKusick L. (1986) Counseling survivors. In: McKusick L. (ed.) *What To Do About AIDS.* University of California Press, California, pp. 163–169.

Sno H.N., Jitschak G., Storosum G. & Swinkels J.A. (1989) HIV infection: psychiatric findings in the Netherlands. *British Journal of Psychiatry* 155, 814–817.

Stimson G.V. (1989) Syringe-exchange programmes for injecting drug users. *AIDS* 3, 253–260.

Stoller R.J. & Herdt G.H. (1985) Theories of origins of male homosexuality. *Archives of General Psychiatry* 42, 399–404.

Swan N. (1989) Patient power at AIDS conference. *British Medical Journal* 298, 1602–1603.

Temoshok L. (1988) Psychoimmunology and AIDS. In Bridge T.P., Mirsky A.F. & Goodwin F.K. (eds) *Psychological, Neuropsychiatric and Substance Abuse Aspects of AIDS.* Raven Press, New York, pp. 187–197.

Trace M. (1990) HIV and drugs in British prisons. *Druglink* 5, 12–15.

Van Wyk P.H. & Geist C.S. (1984) Psychosocial development of heterosexual, bisexual and homosexual behaviour. *Archives of Sexual Behaviour* 13, 505–544.

Volberding P. (1989) Supporting the health care team in caring for patients with AIDS. *Journal of the American Medical Society* 261, 747–748.

Weller I.V.D. (1988) Treatment of infections and antiviral agents. In: Adler M.W. (ed.) *ABC of AIDS*. British Medical Journal, London, pp. 33–36.

World Health Organization (1992) *The ICD-10 Classification of Mental and Behavioural Disorders: Clinical Descriptions and Diagnostic Guidelines*. WHO, Geneva.

Yarchoan R., Pluda J.M., Thomas R.V. *et al.* (1990) Long-term toxicity/activity profile of 2'3'-deoxyinosine in AIDS or AIDS-related complex. *Lancet* 336, 526–529.

Zich J. & Temoshok L. (1987) Perceptions of social support in men with AIDS and ARC: relationships with distress and hardiness. *Journal of Applied Social Psychology* 17, 193–215.

# Chapter 18
# Social Factors and Old Age

## BRICE PITT

The expansion in the world's elderly population is perhaps the most remarkable demographic event of the latter part of the twentieth century. The total world population will have increased by 26% between 1980 and 2000, while that of the population over the age of 65 will have risen by more than 53%. At present, while the population of developing countries is almost three times that of those regarded as developed, the respective populations over 65 years of age are equal. However, while the elderly population of the developed countries will have increased by 29.4% in the 20 years 1980–2000, that of the developing countries will have increased by 77% (United Nations 1979). So, although the developed countries are, and will for a long time remain, far more aged than the developing (in England and Wales, for example, 15% of the population are aged 65 or more, Fig. 18.1), the problems (as well as the benefits) of the ageing population are by no means confined to the more advantaged nations.

The 'aged dependency ratio' is defined as the population aged 65 and over as a percentage of the population aged 15–64 (deemed to be of working age). In the UK this is at present 23. By 2030 it is expected to be 31. Where there are now 5 people of working age for every 1 aged 65 years or more, there will then be only 3 (Department of Health 1991).

The population over the age of 65 has a span of about 35 years, so general statements about the elderly can be misleading. For example, there is far more disability among 'old old' people, 75 and over, than those who are younger. The OPCS disability surveys of 1984/85 found the prevalence of the most severe levels of disability to be 3 per 1000 for adults under 50, 16 per 1000 for those in their sixties and 133 per 1000 for those 80 and over (Martin et al. 1988). The risk of dementia increases exponentially with ageing over 65 (see below). Consequently it is as important to know the age structure of the over-65 population as well as the numbers and the proportion they form of the total population. Thus, while the total population of the British Isles over 65 is expected to increase by 2% between 1981 and 2001:

Those 65–74 will decrease by 9%,

Those 75–84 will increase by 11%, and

Those 85+ will increase by 67%.

(Government Actuary, Population Projection Series, No. 13)

As those over 85 are by far the most disabled, considerable concern has been expressed about this two-thirds increase in 20 years. (However, Jefferys (1988) points out that this is a numerical increase of only approximately 400 000.)

In a useful review of the social psychiatry of later life, Henderson (1990) notes that the number and proportion of old people in the world is now without precedent. This means, among other things, an increased responsibility for social psychiatry, which has accumulated a reasonable body of knowledge about the distribution of mental disorders in the elderly and about social factors influencing that distribution. He lists the following variables to be considered:

1 Sociodemographic factors.

2 Experiential variables: life events, social support, social stimulation, illness and disability.

3 Physical exposures: diet, medications, toxins.

4 Macrosocial changes, e.g. economic.

5 Social consequences of mental disorder on patients, family and the community.

6 Services – what proportion of elderly with mental illness reach their GPs, how appropriate are services given by GPs, hospitals, institutions?

7 Social treatments.

8 Prevention.

**UK 1891**

Population pyramid (millions). *Source: Census 1891*

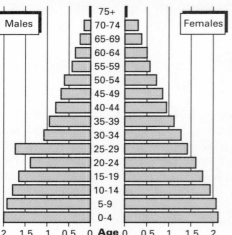

**UK 1988**

Population pyramid (millions). *Source: Eurostat*

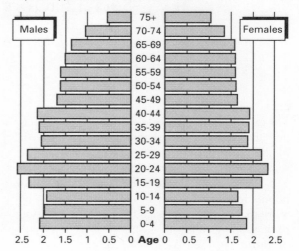

**Fig. 18.1** The ageing of the UK.

Much of this scheme will be used as the basis for this chapter, but first it is necessary to give an idea of the likely prevalence of psychiatric disorder among the elderly in the community.

Numerous studies since the classic survey of old age psychiatry in Newcastle upon Tyne (Kay *et al.* 1964) have achieved greater consistency as sampling, standardization for differences in age and sex distribution, and case definition have become more uniform (Brayne & Ames 1988). Among recent studies, that by Lindesay *et al.* (1989) in Southwark and North Lewisham is reasonably representative. This showed that among those aged 65 or more on GPs' lists, 5% were demented, 13% were depressed (4% major depression) and 12% had anxiety states (7% phobic).

Other important disorders in psychogeriatric practice (e.g. delirium, paraphrenia, personality and behaviour disorder) were much less prevalent, and are therefore given less attention in the consideration of social factors in this chapter.

## Dementia

It is not yet clear whether the severe cases of dementia seen, especially in hospitals and homes, represent a disease or one extreme of a continuum

of cognitive impairment associated with ageing (Brayne & Calloway 1988). Nor is it clear that mild cognitive impairment ('benign senescent forgetfulness' (Kral 1962), age-associated memory impairment (Crooke *et al.* 1986) or mild dementia) are early stages of more severe dementia or remain static. O'Connor *et al.* (1991b) followed up 31 cases of mild dementia over 75 years of age in the community for 2 years, and found that only 14 (45%) progressed to severe dementia.

Case definitions of dementia, however, emphasize disability. The *Diagnostic and Statistical Manual of Mental Disorders*, revised 3rd edition (DSM-III-R) of the American Psychiatric Association (1987) states as the first criterion for dementia: 'loss of intellectual abilities severe enough to interfere with social functioning'. The Royal College of Physicians (1981) defined dementia as 'the global impairment of higher mental function including memory, the capacity to solve the problems of day to day living, the performance of learned skills, the correct use of social skills and control of emotional reactions, without clouding of consciousness. It is often irreversible and progressive.' The Cambridge Examination for Mental Disorders of the Elderly (CAMDEX, Roth *et al.* 1986) gives operational diagnostic criteria for dementia which include, after 'global deterioration of the patient's intellectual and (usually) emotional and motivational behaviour in a state of unimpaired consciousness over a period of at least 6 months' as the first criterion, 'progressive failure in performance at work and in the common activities of everyday life not due to impairment in health or physical handicap'.

It may also be noted that dementia comprises more than the cognitive impairment which is the focus of the great majority of screening tests in surveys. Behavioural change and reduced ability to carry out the activities of daily life are very much part of the syndrome, and require information from an informant, not just testing the subject. The Blessed dementia scale (Blessed *et al.* 1968), which asks questions on change in performance of the activities of daily living, habits, personality interests and drive, is thus a useful complement to cognitive tests such as the Mini Mental State Examination (Folstein *et al.* 1975).

## Ageing

Of the risk factors identified for dementia, the most powerful is undoubtedly ageing. There is an exponential increase in first admissions to psychiatric units in England and Wales from the age of 55 onwards (Department of Health & Social Security 1985). While such admission statistics may only crudely reflect what is happening in the community (widowing in late life might increase the chance of admission, while the availability of the alternative of residential and nursing homes might reduce it), the correlation seems, in fact, to be very close. In their Newcastle study, Kay *et al.* (1964) found the prevalence of dementia in the population aged 65 and over to be 5.5%, but in those over 80 it was 22%, and this finding has been consistently confirmed subsequently. Jorm *et al.* (1987) reviewed 47 prevalence studies conducted between 1945 and 1985, and concluded that the prevalence rate for dementia among the elderly doubles with every 5.1 years of ageing up to the age of 95.

Social factors in the ageing of populations include, of course, improvements in public health and the quality of life which enhance survival at all ages, and contraception, abortion and sterilization which reduce the birth rate.

## Sex differences

Age-related first admissions to psychiatric units for dementia in England and Wales (Department of Health & Social Security 1985) show a very similar pattern between the sexes, with a very slight excess of men at all ages. Some community surveys have reported higher rates of dementia (or impaired cognition) in women than men (e.g. Morgan *et al.* 1987), a few report higher rates in men (Pfeffer *et al.* 1987) and others equal rates in the sexes (Griffiths *et al.* 1987). The meta-analysis by Jorm *et al.* (1987) identified three studies allowing the comparison of rates of Alzheimer's disease between the sexes, which showed a higher prevalence in women (e.g. Molsa *et al.* 1982). However, a subsequent analysis of incidence data (Jorm 1990) showed no sex difference, suggesting that the higher prevalence in women is because they live longer than men.

## Morbidity in homes and hospitals

As old people's homes (residential and nursing) are full of old, old people (the average age of those who live in them being usually over 80) who are in this accommodation at least partly because of difficulty in managing in their own homes, a high morbidity for the disabilities associated with ageing, including dementia, is to be expected. Mann *et al.* (1984) found that two-thirds of the residents of 'Part III' (i.e. statutory local authority) old people's homes in the London Borough of Camden were demented; half were moderately or severely so, half mildly. This suggests that such homes (even though not designated for the care of the demented or elderly mentally infirm (EMI)) are probably the major institutional resource for those demented old people who cannot manage or be managed at home. While this comprises only about a fifth of all demented people at any one time (Kay *et al.* 1964), only one twentieth of the total elderly population are in any kind of institutional care. Dementia is therefore a significant factor in entering an institution for continuing care. Clearly surveys which do not take account of old people in homes will underestimate the prevalence of dementia.

Geriatric and psychogeriatric continuing care wards purposely provide for some demented elderly patients with, respectively, significant physical or associated psychiatric disorder. General hospital wards also appear, perhaps less wittingly, to contribute to the care of the demented old people whose capacity for self-care is seriously reduced by their disorder. They are liable to accidents, hypothermia, malnutrition and neglect of conditions like diabetes and heart failure requiring medication. Feldman *et al.* (1987) surveyed consecutive patients admitted to medical wards in Oxford with the Present State Examination: 31% of those over 70 showed organic brain syndrome, of whom almost half were demented. Johnston *et al.* (1987) in a period prevalence study of all patients over the age of 65 in the Royal Free Hospital, screened with the Clifton Assessment Procedures for the Elderly (CAPE – Pattie & Gilleard, 1979) and the Mini Mental State Examination (MMSE – Folstein *et al.* 1975) found 22% to exhibit organic brain syndrome, of whom the majority were demented. In a similar study of two general hospitals serving an East London district, screening inpatients over the age of 65 with the Brief Assessment Schedule (BAS – Macdonald *et al.* 1982), the prevalence of organic brain syndrome was 33%, and two-thirds of these were demented (Pitt 1991). Only 54% of these patients, compared with 88% of the mentally normal, were at home 6 months after the original assessment. They stayed in hospital twice as long, and were six times as likely to die.

Demented old people are thus major users of inpatient general hospital services. Social factors which increase their doing so are those which reduce effective care in the community. This is particularly a hazard for those 'difficult' old people who deny their disability and refuse help, and those whose carers fall sick or die. Old people admitted as a consequence of such circumstances are sometimes stigmatized as 'social admissions', and indeed in the East London study cited above (Pitt 1991) a quarter of demented patients, compared with none of those who were mentally

normal, had been admitted for no very clear medical disorder. The other stigmatizing term 'bed-blocker' reflects the fact that demented old people do stay in general hospital beds longer than their medical or surgical disorder strictly warrants, while time is taken to make suitable arrangements for their safe discharge. In a general hospital in England at present with, say, 500 beds (excluding paediatric, geriatric, obstetric and psychiatric) there could well be 100 elderly patients with psychiatric disorder, the majority suffering from dementia. As populations continue to age, and despite the development of psychogeriatric services, this is and will remain a fact of hospital life. Attitudes, programmes, resources and the training of doctors, nurses, social and paramedical workers need to accommodate this reality.

### Regional differences in prevalence rates

Usually differences in the prevalence of dementia in different surveys are attributable to differences in identifying the study population, sampling, refusal rates, standardization for age and sex, screening instruments or case definition. Surveys which surmount all these obstacles to comparability yet still show differences may point to possible causal factors.

One interesting difference is between the western world and Japan (Hasegawa *et al.* 1984, Shibayama *et al.* 1986). It appears that whereas overall rates of dementia are similar, the ratio of Alzheimer's disease (or senile dementia of the Alzheimer type – SDAT) to multi-infarct dementia (MID) in the west, where the former predominates, is reversed in Japan. It has been suggested that there might be a cultural preference for the diagnosis of MID, which could be associated with rich living, in Japan, rather than Alzheimer's disease (AD), which may be perceived as a disease of degeneration. Homer *et al.* (1988) have demonstrated how difficult it can be to make a clinical distinction between AD, MID and mixed cases, and how often the diagnostician is confounded by the post-mortem findings. However, Henderson (1990) states: 'Having examined the diagnostic criteria used I am persuaded that the rates for AD and MID are likely to be largely free of diagnostic artefact and are almost certainly valid estimates.' Risk factors for MID include obesity and smoking (both of which may be culturally determined), as well as hypertension, cardiac disease and diabetes. MID is also more prevalent among younger old than old old people (e.g. Sulkava *et al.* 1985), but in a rapidly ageing society like Japan this is unlikely to explain the excess of MID.

One of the most intriguing and tantalizing differences in the prevalence of dementia was that demonstrated in the US/UK study (Gurland *et al.* 1983, Copeland *et al.* 1987b) between New York and London. The same team used the same instrument (the Geriatric Mental State (GMS) and its computerized algorithm AGECAT (Copeland *et al.* 1986)) in each capital, yet, while the prevalence of depression was virtually the same, there was twice as much dementia in New York. Of London men over 65, 2.2% were demented compared with 5.4% in New York, and 5.7% of London women compared with 10.1% in New York. Yet no persuasive causal factors have been identified to explain the differences. A speculation that some of the demented people in New York might have been exposed to 'bathtub gin' at the time of Prohibition remains only that. The numbers of cases in the two capitals were quite small. Also, with a lower response rate, more communication problems, more probable response set biases, more black people and far fewer who had been born in the capital in New York, 'it is difficult to conclude that the observed difference remains a true finding' (Brayne 1991).

### Education and social class

Folstein *et al.* (1975) found a correlation of 0.78 between verbal IQ and performance on the MMSE. Less well educated old people perform cognitive tests less well than those who are better educated (Anthony *et al.* 1982, Holzer *et al.* 1984, Escobar *et al.* 1986, Fillenbaum *et al.* 1988, O'Connor *et al.* 1989). If the diagnosis is based on such tests alone, then poorer education and lower social class are risk factors for dementia. Mortimer's hypothesis (Ferny 1988) is that such factors 'primarily reduce the margin of intellectual reserve to a level where a more modest level of brain patho-

logy results in a diagnosable dementia'. If true, this would be extremely important, but there is a strong suspicion that less educated or less intelligent people are simply less at ease with tests, or, having fewer resources with which to mitigate the effects of dementia, are more conspicuous among the users of public services. However, Jorm & Korten (1988) reported equal correlations in poor and well educated groups between scores on a brief cognitive screening test and on a rating-scale of need for help with everyday tasks.

O'Connor *et al.* (1991c) compared subjects in a community survey who scored 23 or less out of 30 on the MMSE with a sample of those who scored 24 or 25, using a structured diagnostic interview (CAMDEX) given by a psychiatrist. Neither educational attainment nor social class had any influence on the likelihood that subjects would be diagnosed as demented. The authors conclude that social and psychological factors (including anxiety) contribute substantially to cognitive test scores, and emphasize the importance of detailed assessment procedures in epidemiological surveys of dementia.

> We think it unlikely that standard cognitive tests can be modified to reduce demographic bias without removing the more demanding items which help to ensure high levels of sensitivity . . . Questions about orientation are an essential part of any assessment because of their high face validity, but computerised testing and subtle tests of recall like those incorporated in the Rivermead Behavioural Memory Test (Wilson *et al.* 1985) might be less reminiscent of the classroom and provide a better measure of subjects' abilities to function in ordinary life.

### Mental stimulation

In 'De Senectute' Cicero implied that old men preserve their intellects if they preserve their interests. This 'if you don't use it you lose it' hypothesis may be of relevance to the discussion of the effects of intelligence, education and class on dementia, in that brighter, better educated, more affluent old people are likely to have more mental stimulation in old age than those who are less fortunate. This hypothesis is very difficult to test in people. However, Diamond (1985) reports experimental work with rats at Berkeley University which suggests that those given a more stimulating life-style die with larger brains than those of the same strain whose existence is monotonous which die at a similar age. McWhorter & White (1987) studied the Framingham cohort and found physical inactivity (as well as diabetes, heart failure and having less than one bowel movement a day) to be associated with the subsequent development of primary progressive dementia. A spell of apathy may precede signs of cognitive impairment, but this is much more likely to be a feature of early dementia than to contribute to its development.

The relationship of depressive illness (prominent features of which are anhedonia, anergy and apathy) to dementia is interesting. It could be a risk factor (French *et al.* 1985), an early symptom (Burns *et al.* 1990), secondary to ('organic depression'), or masquerade as dementia (pseudodementia – Wells 1979). There are cerebral changes in late-onset depression intermediate between those of normal ageing and dementia (Jacoby *et al.* 1983). There is also the theoretical possibility that antidepressant treatment with anticholinergic drugs could exacerbate the well-established cerebral acetylcholine deficiency in Alzheimer's disease, and perhaps precipitate or exacerbate dementia.

However, there is little convincing evidence that previous psychiatric disorder (including depression) and indeed stressful life events are significant factors in the genesis of dementia (Heyman *et al.* 1984). Where depression and subjective or objective cognitive impairment are associated, the likelihood is that the one is symptomatic of the other.

Forgetfulness and poor concentration are frequent complaints of depressed and dysthymic people, especially the elderly (Pitt 1986), often without there being any objective evidence of what they complain of (Kahn *et al.* 1975). McHugh & Folstein (1979) however found cognitive impairment in depressed subjects, whose scores on the MMSE improved after treatment. Depression is a not uncommon and readily comprehensible reaction to dementia, perhaps particularly multi-infarct. Roth (1983) noted that the onset of a depressive syndrome for the first time in late life occurs in 25% of cases of MID, while guilt, pessimism and a labile affect are common in the remainder.

### Trauma and toxic factors

Dementia pugilistica is the consequence of repeated severe blows to the head, and neuropathologically is associated with an excess of neurofibrillary tangles, but not of amyloid plaques. Heyman *et al.* (1984) and Mortimer *et al.* (1985) both demonstrated that a previous history of head injury (usually because of a road traffic accident) severe enough to cause loss of consciousness was more common in patients developing AD many years later than in age-matched normal people. However, Sulkava *et al.* (1985) found no history of brain contusion in a series of 66 patients with AD and 152 with MID.

Alcohol abuse has not been found to excess in the past history of patients with AD (Heyman *et al.* 1984, French *et al.* 1985) but is a risk factor for MID (Pinessi *et al.* 1983).

The aluminium story shows no signs of being over yet, though it may seem far-fetched. Dialysis dementia is due to aluminium toxicity, but is distinct from Alzheimer's disease. Workers in Newcastle (Candy *et al.* 1986) demonstrated aluminosilicates at the heart of the senile plaque, but the association could be secondary (Yates & Mann 1986).

Martyn *et al.* (1989) undertook an epidemiological study of the prevalence of CAT scan-diagnosed AD patients under the age of 70 (who would be more likely than older patients to have had a scan) in England and Wales in areas where the water supply contained varying quantities of aluminium, sometimes added to make the water clear. Although aluminium in the water would account for only a small proportion of the daily intake of aluminium, its bioavailability might be increased by its being in an acidified solution (Perl 1985). The study showed that the risk of AD was 1.5 times higher in districts where the mean aluminium concentration exceeded 0.11 mg/litre than where the levels were less than 0.01 mg/litre. Where levels exceeded 0.01 mg/litre relative risks ranged from 1.3 to 1.5. If patients over 65 were excluded the relative risk in the highest aluminium group (above 0.11 mg/litre) was 1.7, there being a gradient of risk with increasing aluminium concentration. Although an active public health response to this research may be premature, this remains a 'space to watch'!

### Dementia and the economy

Commenting on the demographic shift to larger numbers of dependent elderly and rather smaller numbers of dependent young, Jorm (1987) remarks:

> Whereas children are to a large extent supported by their families, the elderly rely more heavily on the public purse . . . We can therefore expect public health expenditure to rise considerably, and senile dementia will make a large contribution to these costs, particularly as it often requires hospital or nursing home care.
>
> To give an example of the magnitude of the problem, one estimate puts the cost of caring for demented patients in the United States in the year 2030 as $30 000 million in 1978-value dollars (Plum 1979). This vast sum is eight times the amount now spent annually on all medical and mental health research in the United States; it makes current expenditure on research into dementia look miniscule.

All the growth in institutional care to match the ageing of the population in Britain in recent years has been in the private sector (Grundy & Arie 1982). This has been subsidized by at first quite generous social security subsidies for indigent residents. However, an audit report in 1987 pointed out that the escalating cost of such subsidies could not go unchecked. Griffiths' report (1988) suggested that this centrally funded subsidy might be a 'perverse incentive' to local government to encourage old people to go into private homes rather than provide community services for them locally out of its own funds. He proposed that the money now spent on subsidies for private homes should be given to local government, 'ring-fenced' to prevent its diversion to other purposes (e.g.

education) and made available for tailored 'packages of care' best suited to the individual old person's needs, which might comprise various patterns of care at home or residential care.

Eventually the Government endorsed most of these proposals in the White Paper 'Caring for People' (Secretaries of State for Health, Social Security, Wales, Scotland 1990). However, they were not prepared to 'ring-fence' the money transferred from residential home subsidies. There are good ideas in 'Caring for People', but the primary impetus behind the paper is less to improve community care than to contain the cost of residential care. In fact Britain already uses such care less than most other developed nations, and the evidence that there are viable, cost-effective alternatives in community care for those admitted to homes because of dementia is lacking. Much attention has been given to the 'Kent experiment' where expert social workers devised packages of community care for old people who would otherwise have gone into residential homes and successfully kept them at home with a better quality of life at two-thirds of the cost (Challis & Davies 1980, 1986). However, these old people were not demented, and when a similar project (Askham & Thompson 1990) was tried which included demented old people it was not nearly as successful.

The unpleasant reality is that where there is a high aged dependency ratio and an economic depression or recession, the needs of the elderly who cannot fend for themselves will not be adequately met by the State. This means that they will either suffer from neglect (including starvation, hypothermia or succumbing to serious accidents or untreated medical disorder) or the burden of their care will fall still more heavily upon the family.

### The burden on carers

The classic study by Grad & Sainsbury (1968) demonstrated the emotional strain on the carers of demented patients in a community-orientated psychogeriatric service compared with one in which the threshold for admission to a mental hospital was much lower. Since this publication there has developed a copious literature documenting the emotional cost of informal care. Greene *et al.* (1982) found that apathy in demented people depressed their families, while unstable mood made them embarrassed, angry and accusing. Argyle *et al.* (1985) found that sleep disturbance, restlessness, urinary and faecal incontinence, aggression, abuse and wandering were particularly common and intolerable in demented people admitted to a psychogeriatric unit because their carers could no longer cope. The study of Levin *et al.* (1983) on the supporters of demented old people found that their mean age was 61, only about a third rated their health in the previous year as good, half had disabilities which limited their activities, and about a third reported a number of symptoms of acute stress sufficient to suggest a need for psychiatric attention. Gilleard (Gilleard *et al.* 1984, Gilleard 1987) used the General Health Questionnaire (GHQ – Goldberg 1978) to measure carers' distress, and found caseness levels in about two-thirds of those with a demented dependent, compared with 25% in the general population.

Since 'granny battering' was first described by Baker in 1975, the topic of 'elder abuse' has received attention, and a social services survey (Tomlin 1988) found that 5% of elderly clients were being abused. Homer & Gilleard (1990) assessed the prevalence in all patients referred for respite care to the geriatric wards of two South London geriatric hospitals. There was a high morbidity for dementia, the mean Mental Test Score (Hodkinson 1972) being 6.7/10. Almost half of the carers admitted to some kind of abuse – verbal more commonly than physical. Physical abuse was associated with high alcohol consumption in the carer, and poor communication by the patient. Verbal abuse was associated with poor premorbid relations between carer and cared-for, and depression and anxiety in the carers. Few patients admitted that they had been abused. The authors conclude their summary: 'even with increased provision of services, care in the community may not be the best solution for these people'.

Gilleard (1987) found that where the demented dependents of female carers attended a psychogeriatric day hospital for three months or more, the carers' GHQ scores were substantially reduced.

However, Wells *et al.* (1990) found that the high level of psychological symptoms in care-givers was not significantly reduced by day care for their elderly relatives, whereas full-time admission of demented people to a special nursing home for dementia sufferers substantially reduced the carers' symptoms (Wells & Jorm 1987). The implications for the limitations of community care are plain.

The carers in the survey by Levin *et al.* (1983) wanted:

1 Early identification of the dementia.
2 Comprehensive medical and social assessment.
3 Timely referrals by the primary health care team to other agencies.
4 Continuing back-up and reviews.
5 Active medical treatment for disabling physical conditions.
6 Information, advice and counselling.
7 Regular help with household and personal care tasks.
8 Regular financial support.
9 Respite and continuing institutional care when needed.

O'Connor *et al.* (1991a) conducted a controlled trial of the effect on demented old people in Cambridgeshire of early intervention by a multidisciplinary team offering a wide range of help (including financial benefits, psychiatric assessment, physical aids, home helps and respite admissions). The outcome measure was permanent admission to long-term care within two years after the diagnosis. Early admission did not affect admission rates in those living with supporters, while it was associated with far more admissions (64% of the action group, compared with 8% of the controls) among those who were moderately or severely demented and living alone. Again, the limitations of community care for the demented in the 'Caring for People' blueprint are manifest.

## Depression

One of the most intriguing features of depression in old age is how much there is of it, and yet how little!

Depressive illness is the commonest psychiatric disorder in old age – more than twice as common as dementia, except in the very old – prevailing at a rate of between 11% and 16% in the population over 65 years of age according to recent studies in Britain (Gurland *et al.* 1983 – 12.9% in London; Copeland *et al.* 1987a – 11.3% in Liverpool; Lindesay *et al.* 1989 – 13.5% in South London; Livingston *et al.* 1990 – 15.9% in North London). It is the commonest single cause of referral to a psychogeriatric service (Pitt 1982). According to the Mental Health Enquiry for 1982 (Department of Health & Social Security 1985), there is a steady increase with age in first admissions to psychiatric units in England both for 'affective psychosis' and for 'depressive disorders not elsewhere classified'. Female admissions for affective psychosis reach a lifetime peak of 21 per 100 000 at risk at 80, but fall off thereafter; for the same disorder, male admissions climb to 14 per 100 000 at 70, and then plateau. Women show the same pattern for 'depressive disorders n.e.c.', peaking at 43 per 100 000 at 80, then falling off. Male admissions, however, continue to climb till the very end of life, overtaking women and attaining a peak of 55 per 100 000 at risk over the age of 85. It would be far too cynical to explain these sex differences by suggesting that while widowing is a grevious loss for men, it might sometimes be a relief for women! Men are at their most suicidal towards the end of their life-span (20 per 100 000 over 65 years of age – three times the rate in men aged 15–24), women towards the end of middle life (Office of Population Censuses & Surveys 1977, Pitt & Nowers 1986). There is a close relationship between suicide in old age and depressive illness at the time of the act (Barraclough 1971, Pierce 1987).

These figures accord with the common view that there is plenty to be depressed about in old age: loss of occupation, reduced income and company, bereavement, isolation, infirmity, loss of independence, serious painful illness, reduced life-expectancy, probable loss of status. Yet studies which use the same instrument to determine the prevalence of depression in younger and older adults consistently find much less in the elderly. In the Epidemiological Catchment Area study in the USA, using diagnostic criteria derived from DSM-III, Robins *et al.* (1984) reported much lower rates for lifetime depression in elderly people than in

younger subjects (perhaps this was a survivor phenomenon, more depressed people having died before reaching old age), while Myers *et al.* (1984) found the six-month prevalence of depression in three sites, and (Regier *et al.* 1988) the one-month prevalence in all five sites of the study, to be lower in the elderly than younger adults. In the latter study the highest rate (6.4%) was in those aged 24–44, while the lowest (2.5%) was in those over 65.

In their Present State Examination (PSE) study of consecutive medical inpatients in Oxford, Feldman *et al.* (1987) found the prevalence of depression to be 18% in those aged 17–54, 12.5% in those aged 55–69 and only 5% in those over 70. It could be argued that criteria for use across the ages might miss some cases of depression in the elderly in whom such somatic symptoms as weight loss, anorexia, anergy and insomnia could be ascribed to ageing or physical disorder. The rationale of the Geriatric Depression Scale (GDS – Yesavage *et al.* 1983) is that it avoids such items. However, the Oxford finding for the prevalence of depression in medical wards in old age is consistent with that of Bergmann & Eastham (1974) – 5% – and the East London general hospital wards study (Pitt 1991) – 6.5%: these were those meeting DSM-III criteria for major depression, but an equal number were suffering from dysthymic disorder or adjustment disorder with depressed mood. The bulk of the depressed old people in the British community studies are likely to have belonged to these latter categories.

Even so, the relatively low prevalence of depression in old compared with young people in community studies does not accord with the frequency, severity and chronicity of depression in psychogeriatric practice, and remains a puzzle which requires a satisfactory explanation.

### The social origins of depression in old age

This is the title of the classic paper by Murphy (1982), who studied 100 patients referred to old age psychiatry services in East London and 19 picked up from a community sample and compared them with 200 mentally healthy age- and sex-matched residents in the community. An association was found between the onset of depression and severe life events, such as physical illness, separation, bereavement and, less often, financial loss, enforced change of residence and unpleasant disclosures. These occurred in the previous year in 80% of patients, and only 26% of controls. More than twice as many patients as control subjects suffered major social difficulties in the previous two years – mainly ill health of a person close to the subject and housing problems. Not surprisingly, perhaps, working class subjects, who were more liable to severe life events and social difficulties, were more liable to depression. Having someone in whom to confide offered some protection against depression, but this seemed to be an attribute of personality rather than good fortune. In a follow-up study, however, Murphy (1985) found that depressed patients who had recovered by the end of the year were more likely to report an improvement in the quality of their close relationships than those whose clinical outcome was poor. These changes were not only due to the effect of not being depressed on the quality of relationships, but also to independent subsequent life events which improved quality and frequency of contact.

The relationship between physical illness and the onset of depression has been noted previously, for example by Post (1962) and Kay & Bergmann (1966). Kukull *et al.* (1986) note that chronic obstructive airways disease, Robinson *et al.* (1983) that stroke, and Koenig *et al.* (1988) that myocardial infarction may be particularly likely to induce depression.

## Anxiety states

The importance of states of anxiety in the psychiatric morbidity of the elderly was recognized by Bergmann (1979) in a follow-up study of the Newcastle cohort (Kay *et al.* 1964), of whom 26% were depressed or neurotic. About half of these conditions had developed before, and a half after the age of 65. Of the early-onset cases, approximately half were suffering from anxiety states, and of the late-onset cases, about a third. Symptoms included hypochondriacal worries, tension, irritability, phobias, panics and palpitations.

Phobias were very prominent among elderly women in Baltimore in the National Institute of Mental Health/Epidemiological Catchment Area (NIMH/ECA) survey (Myers *et al.* 1984): 14.2% of women aged 65 and over were sufferers. In this country a comparable prevalence was found in South London by Lindesay *et al.* 1989: 12% of those over 65 suffered anxiety states, of whom the majority were agoraphobic. The main precipitants of recent phobic disorder were physical illness and the threat of 'mugging'.

Housebound old people are quite unlikely to be diagnosed as phobic unless discovered by such community surveys. Ageist expectations of the elderly are low, and it is very easy to ascribe such a sheltered life to infirmity, such as a past mild stroke or fall, myocardial infarction, arthritis, dizziness or giddiness. Such collusion in the patient's view of herself as a fragile invalid may limit the quality of life in old age, but as yet the treatment of such disorders has been barely addressed.

## Other psychiatric disorders

### *Alcohol abuse*

Alcohol abuse dwindles with ageing, especially in men (Mishara & Kastenbaum 1980). Iliffe *et al.* (1991a) found in a general practice survey that only 3% of the population aged 75 and over appeared to drink above safe limits, though Wattis (1981) found that it was a significant causal factor for mental illness in up to 15% of elderly patients referred to psychiatrists. Depression is thought to contribute to some alcohol abuse in late life, but there was no association between drinking alcohol and depression in the GP study.

### *Paraphrenia*

Life events are of much less importance in the precipitation of paraphrenia than depression in old age, and precede no more than a quarter of episodes, i.e. no more often than were experienced by the normal controls in Murphy's (1982) study of depression. Flint *et al.* (1991) argue a distinction between paranoia and paraphrenia in old age; they both exhibit delusions but the former lack hallucinations. The study suggests that social factors such as prolonged social isolation and never marrying are relevant to paraphrenia, whereas cerebral infarction is a potent risk factor for paranoia. Hearing loss has been regarded as a risk factor for paraphrenia (Cooper *et al.* 1974, Eastwood *et al.* 1981), but Kalayam *et al.* (1991) found depression a far more frequent consequence in a hearing clinic; they concede, however, that paranoid patients might not readily attend such a clinic! Paraphrenic patients often complain of their neighbours and either seek rehousing or are moved by housing departments as a social solution to their delusional complaints. This is not always ineffective. Sometimes the hallucinations seem to move with the patients, but sometimes the move gives a respite of weeks or months, though usually they return in the end.

## Personality disorder

Introversion tends to increase with ageing. Withdrawal is a feature of dementia, depression, paraphrenia and some phobic states, but may be unrelated to mental illness. Some elderly recluses lead very limited, self-deprived, miserly lives on the edge of malnutrition. The 'senile squalor' (Macmillan & Shaw 1966) or 'Diogenes' syndrome is one in which reclusiveness is associated with living apparently blithely in advanced squalor, with the hoarding of rubbish. Alcohol may play a larger part in this condition than had been supposed (Snowdon 1987).

## What do general practitioners know and what do they do?

In the British health care system the GP is the prime mover; if he is ignorant of his patients' illnesses they may well not get the help and treatment they need. A celebrated study of the patients of three GPs with age-sex registers in Edinburgh (Williamson *et al.* 1964) suggested that the GPs only knew about the tip of the iceberg of psychiatric disorder among the elderly on their lists. In the past 25 years, however, GP awareness appears to have improved. Hooper (1988) was able to check the awareness of the primary health care team in

her general practice (doctors, nurses, receptionists) of various health and social particulars of a sample of patients aged over 75 against the data obtained by a screening Care Team for the Elderly employed by the Health Authority. The GP team's information was accurate for over 95% of a range of mental health functions – memory, disorientation, depression, loneliness, alcohol abuse, how much the patients were at risk, and who was receiving psychiatric care.

O'Connor *et al.* (1988) compared GPs' awareness of dementia among patients over 75 in their practices with the findings from the CAMDEX survey. Overall they correctly diagnosed dementia, at least as a possibility, in 121 out of 208 (58.2%) of the cases found. They missed only 22% of those with severe dementia, 39% of those with moderate, 50% of those with mild dementia, and considered 21.6% of those who were not demented as possibly or definitely demented. In a smaller sample, community nurses correctly diagnosed 86% of all cases, and 96% of those with moderate or severe dementia. On the other hand they misdiagnosed 46% of those who were not demented as possibly or, occasionally, definitely demented. Among the not demented subjects misclassified by doctors and nurses were a number of functional psychiatric disorders, mainly depression. The authors comment that as the doctors diagnosed dementia partly because of relatives' reports, but mainly because of noting deterioration in patients for whom they had cared for years, were they also to use brief cognitive tests and question families about changes in memory, intellect and behaviour, their already reasonable diagnostic accuracy would improve considerably. GPs rarely discussed the diagnosis with the family or mentioned it on the frequent occasions that demented patients were referred to clinics or for admissions. However, they referred appropriately to the psychogeriatric service: 3 of the 96 mildly demented, 15 of the 85 moderately demented and 9 of the 27 severely demented patients had been seen by the service on domiciliary visits, as outpatients or in hospitals.

Macdonald (1986) found that GPs in South London correctly diagnosed 56 out of 68 (82%) of those elderly patients attending their surgery who were high scorers on a depression rating scale. Their motivation may have been stimulated by the presence of the researcher in the surgery, rating the patients before the GP saw them: a certain overeagerness is suggested by their having diagnosed depression in a substantial minority of those who were not rated as depressed. However, this diagnostic success was not followed by any treatment for the depression – social, psychological or pharmacological.

New conditions of service for GPs in England and Wales (Department of Health & the Welsh Office 1989) require them or their primary care teams to assess annually patients over the age of 75. This includes a home visit, the mental condition, continence, general functioning and the use of medication. Iliffe *et al.* (1991b) surveyed 1160 patients aged 75 and over on the age-sex register of 9 practices in North and West London, and gave a fuller interview to a random 1 in 5 sample. GPs had seen two-thirds of these in the 3 months prior to the study, the consultations being initiated by the patients and taking place in the surgery. One in five had evidence of depression (according to the comprehensive assessment and referral examination (CARE; Gurland *et al.* 1977)) and 15% had scores on the MMSE suggestive of cognitive impairment. 'Depression' was recorded in the medical notes of only 3 of 52 patients with depression, though antidepressants were prescribed for 6. 'Dementia' was recorded in the notes of 3 of 36 with dementia. The authors conclude that annual assessment would yield much new evidence of depression and dementia. Up to 30% of those screened for these disorders would require further assessment, though the benefits in consequence are as yet undetermined.

Finally, a study of data from the National Ambulatory Care Survey (NAMCS) in the USA (Larson *et al.* 1991) found that primary care practitioners were significant providers of mental health services to older Americans, most commonly prescribing psychotropic drugs. Compared with psychiatrists, primary care practitioners infrequently diagnosed a mental disorder when prescribing, especially for older people. Schulberg & Burns (1988), in reviewing an extensive series of investigations on primary care, state that approximately 25% of primary care patients have mental dis-

orders, and that physicians underdiagnose them. The NAMCS study suggests that GPs do not undertreat to the extent that they underdiagnose; consequently some of the medication which is prescribed may be inappropriate.

## Summary

The ageing of the world, not only of developed nations, presents a challenge to the health and welfare services. The social psychiatry of old age has a contribution to make, including epidemiological studies, the identification of risk factors, assessing the burden on carers and the community, evaluation of services, social treatments and prevention.

In the developed countries, dementia prevails at 5% in the population aged 65 and over, and increases exponentially with ageing. It is not yet clear whether dementia in old age is a distinct disease, or at one extreme of a continuum of cognitive impairment with ageing. Men and women are probably equally susceptible. Dementia is a major factor in the use of residential care and acute as well as continuing care hospital beds. There may be more multi-infarct dementia than Alzheimer's disease in Japan, but elsewhere the latter predominates. Poor education and lower social class affect performance on cognitive tests, but are probably not risk factors for dementia. Dementia can be heralded or followed by depression, but most depressed old people who complain of forgetfulness are not demented. The contribution of aluminium, perhaps in drinking water, to Alzheimer's disease is postulated, but unproven. With a substantial expected increase in the population aged 80 or more, the economic burden of dementia weighs heavily. In Britain the substitution of community for residential care may prove satisfactory for some elderly people, but less so for the demented. The emotional strain of caring for a demented relative is now well known, and occasionally manifest in elder abuse. Though many relatives and friends cope willingly, the most effective relief is provided by admitting the demented dependent to institutional care. Hopes that early identification and intervention will reduce the need for institutional care are not so far vindicated. In fact they may increase the use of such care by identifying the need for it sooner.

Although depression is allegedly less common in old age than in younger people in community studies, it is the commonest psychiatric disorder in old age, and first admissions for depressive illness increase with ageing. Social factors such as physical illness and bereavement precede the onset of depressive illness referred to a psychiatrist in 80% of cases. Anxiety states are no less common and often overlooked.

General practitioner awareness of mental disorder in old people has improved over the past 25 years, and is likely to improve further in Britain as a consequence of a contractual requirement to assess those aged 75 and over annually. It is to be hoped, but it has not yet been demonstrated, that this will lead to improved treatment and management.

## References

American Psychiatric Association (1987) *Diagnostic and Statistical Manual* 3rd edn. (revised). APA, Washington DC.

Anthony J., Leresche L., Niaz U. *et al.* (1982) Limits of the 'Mini-Mental State' as a screening test for dementia and delirium among hospital patients. *Psychological Medicine* 12, 397–408.

Argyle N., Jestice S. & Brook C. (1985) Psychogeriatric patients: their supporters problems. *Age and Ageing* 14, 355–360.

Askham J. & Thompson C. (1990) *Dementia and Home Care.* Age Concern, London.

Baker A. (1975) Granny battering. *Modern Geriatrics* August, 20–24.

Barraclough B. (1971) Suicide in the elderly. In Kay D.W.K. & Walk A. (eds) *Recent Developments in Psychogeriatrics.* Headley, London.

Bergmann K. (1979) Neurosis and personality disorder in old age. In Isaacs A.D. & Post F. (eds) *Studies in Geriatric Psychiatry.* Wiley, Chichester.

Bergmann K. & Eastham E. (1974) Psychogeriatric ascertainment and assessment for treatment in an acute medical ward setting. *Age and Ageing* 3, 174–188.

Blessed G., Tomlinson B. & Roth M. (1968) The association between quantitative measures and degenerative changes in the cerebral grey matter of elderly patients. *British Journal of Psychiatry* 114, 797–811.

Brayne C. (1991) A Study of Dementia in a Rural Population. MD Thesis, University of London.

Brayne C. & Ames D. (1988) The epidemiology of mental disorders in old age. In Gearing B., Johnson M. & Heller T. (eds) *Mental Health Problems in Old Age.* Open University: Wiley, Chichester.

Brayne C. & Calloway P. (1988) Normal ageing, impaired cognitive function and senile dementia of the Alzheimer's type: a continuum? *Lancet* i, 1265–1266.

Burns A., Jacoby R. & Levy R. (1990) Psychiatric phemonena in Alzheimer's disease. *British Journal of Psychiatry* 157, 72–94.

Candy J., Oakley A., Klinowski J. *et al.* (1986) Aluminosilicates and senile plaque formation in Alzheimer's disease. *Lancet* i, 354–357.

Challis D. & Davies B. (1980) A new approach to community care for the elderly. British Journal of Social Work 10, 1–18.

Challis D. & Davies B. (1986) *Case Management in Community Care.* Gower, Aldershot.

Cooper A.F., Curry A., Kay D. *et al.* (1974) Hearing loss in paranoid and affective psychosis of the elderly. Lancet ii, 851–854.

Copeland J., Dewey M. & Griffith-Jones H. (1986) Computerised psychiatric diagnostic system and case nomenclature for elderly subjects: GMS and AGECAT. *Psychological Medicine* 16, 89–99.

Copeland J., Dewey M., Wood N. *et al.* (1987a) Range of mental illness among the elderly in the community: prevalence in Liverpool using the GMS–AGECAT package. *British Journal of Psychiatry* 150, 815–823.

Copeland J., Gurland B., Dewey M. *et al.* (1987b) Is there more depression, dementia and neurosis in New York? A comparative community study of the elderly in New York and London, using the computer diagnosis AGECAT. *British Journal of Psychiatry* 151, 466–473.

Crooke T., Bartus R., Ferris S. *et al.* (1986) Age-associated memory impairment: proposed diagnostic criteria and a measure of clinical change – report of a NIMH work group. *Developmental Neuropsychology* 2, 261–276.

Department of Health (1991) *Epidemiological Overview of the Health of Elderly People.* Central Health Monitoring Unit, London.

Department of Health & Social Security (1985) *Inpatient Statistics from the Mental Health Enquiry for England, 1982.* HMSO, London.

Department of Health & the Welsh Office (1989) *General Practice in the National Health Service. A New Contract.* DOH & WO, London.

Diamond M.C. (1985) The potential of the ageing brain for structural regeneration. In Arie T. (ed.) *Recent Advances in Psychogeriatrics* I. Churchill Livingstone, Edinburgh.

Eastwood M., Corbin S. & Reed M. (1981) Hearing impairment and paraphrenia. *Journal of Otolaryngology* 10, 306–308.

Escobar J., Burnam A., Karno M. *et al.* (1986) Use of the Mini-Mental State Examination (MMSE) in a community population of mixed ethnicity. *Journal of Nervous and Mental Disease* 174, 607–614.

Feldman E., Mayou R., Hawton K. *et al.* (1987) Psychiatric disorder in medical in-patients. *Quarterly Journal of Medicine* 240, 301–308.

Ferny G. (1988) Alzheimer's Disease: a new age. *New Scientist* 12, (11), 44–47.

Fillenbaum G., Hughes D., Heyman A. *et al.* (1988) Relationship of health and demographic characteristics to Mini-Mental State Examination among community residents. *Psychological Medicine* 18, 719–726.

Flint A., Rifat S. & Eastwood M. (1991) Late-onset paranoia; distinct from paraphrenia. *International Journal of Geriatric Psychiatry* 6, 103–110.

Folstein M., Folstein S. & McHugh P. (1975) Mini-Mental State: a practical method of grading the cognitive state of patients for the clinician. *Journal of Psychiatric Research* 12, 189–198.

French L., Schuman L., Mortimer J. *et al.* (1985) A case-control study of dementia of the Alzheimer type. *American Journal of Epidemiology* 121, 414–421.

Gilleard C. (1987) Influence of emotional distress among supporters on the outcome of psychogeriatric day care. *British Journal of Psychiatry* 150, 219–223.

Gilleard C., Gilleard E., Gledhill K. *et al.* (1984) Caring for the elderly mentally infirm at home: a survey of the supporters. *Journal of Epidemiology and Community Health* 38, 319–325.

Goldberg D. (1978) *Manual of the General Health Questionnaire.* NFEA, Windsor.

Grad J. & Sainsbury P. (1968) The effects that patients have on their families in a community care and a control psychiatric service – a two-year follow-up study. *British Journal of Psychiatry* 114, 265–278.

Greene G., Smith R., Gardiner M. & Timbury G. (1982) Measuring behavioural disturbance of elderly demented patients in the community and its effects on relatives: a factor analysis study. *Age and Ageing* 11, 121–126.

Griffiths R. (1988) *Community Care: Agenda for Action.* HMSO, London.

Griffiths R.A., Good W., Watson N. *et al.* (1987) Depression, dementia and disability in the elderly. *British Journal of Psychiatry* 150, 482–493.

Grundy E. & Arie T. (1982) Falling rate of provision of residential care for the elderly. *British Medical Journal* 284, 799.

Gurland B., Copeland J., Kuriansky J. *et al.* (1983) *The Mind and Mood of Ageing.* Croom Helm, New York.

Gurland B., Kuriansky J., Sharpe L. *et al.* (1977) The comprehensive assessment and referral evaluation (CARE): development and reliability. *International Journal of Aging and Human Development* 8, 9–42.

Hasegawa K., Honma A., Sato H. *et al.* (1984) The prevalence study of age-related dementia in the community (Japanese). *Geriatric Psychiatric* 1, 94–105.

Henderson A.S. (1990) The social psychiatry of later life. *British Journal of Psychiatry* 156, 645–653.

Heyman A., Wilkinson W. & Stafford J. (1984) Alzheimer's disease: a study of epidemiological aspects. *Annals of Neurology* 15, 335–341.

Hodkinson H.M. (1972) Evaluation of a mental test score assessment of mental impairment in the elderly. *Age and Ageing* 1, 233–238.

Holzer C., Tischler G., Leaf P. *et al.* (1984) An epidemiological assessment of cognitive impairment in a community population. In *Research in Community and Mental Health*, 4. JAJ Press, Greenwich, Connecticut.

Homer A. & Gilleard C. (1990) Abuse of elderly people by the carers. *British Medical Journal* 301, 1359–1362.

Homer A., Honavar M., Lanton P. *et al.* (1988) Diagnosing dementia: do we get it right? *British Medical Journal* 297, 894–896.

Hooper J. (1988) Case finding in the elderly: does the primary care team already know enough? *British Medical Journal* 297, 1450–1452.

Iliffe S., Haines A., Booroff A. *et al.* (1991a) Alcohol consumption by elderly people: a general practice survey. *Age and Ageing* 20, 120–123.

Iliffe S., Haines A., Gallivan S. *et al.* (1991b) Assessment of elderly people in general practice. 1. Social circumstances and mental state. *British Journal of General Practice* 41, 9–12.

Jacoby R., Dolan R., Levy R. & Baldy R. (1983) Quantitative computerised tomography in elderly depressed patients. *British Journal of Psychiatry* 143, 124–127.

Jefferys M. (1988) An ageing Britain: what is its future? In Gearing B., Johnson M. & Heller T. (eds) *Mental Health Problems in Old Age.* Open University: Wiley, Chichester.

Johnston M., Wakeling A., Graham N. & Stokes F. (1987) Cognitive impairment, emotional disorder and length of stay of elderly patients in a district general hospital. *British Journal of Medical Psychology* 60, 133–139.

Jorm A. (1987) *Understanding Senile Dementia.* Croom Helm, London.

Jorm A. (1990) *The Epidemiology of Alzheimer's Disease and Related Diseases.* Chapman & Hall. London.

Jorm A. & Korten A. (1988) Assessment of cognitive decline in the elderly by informant interview. *British Journal of Psychiatry* 152, 209–213.

Jorm A., Korten A. & Henderson A. (1987) The prevalence of dementia: a quantitative integration of the literature. *Acta Psychiatrica Scandinavica* 76, 465–479.

Kahn R., Zarit S., Hilbent N. & Niederehe G. (1975) Memory complaint and impairment in the aged: the effect of depression and altered brain function. *Archives of General Psychiatry* 32, 1569–1573.

Kalayam B., Alexopoulos G. & Merrell H. (1991) Patterns of hearing loss and psychiatric morbidity in elderly patients attending a hearing clinic. *International Journal of Geriatric Psychiatry* 6, 131–136.

Kay D., Beamish P. & Roth M. (1964) Old age mental disorders in Newcastle upon Tyne. Pt. 1. A study of prevalence. *British Journal of Psychiatry* 110, 146–158.

Kay D. & Bergmann U. (1966) Physical disability and mental health in old age. *Journal of Psychosomatic Research* 10, 3–12.

Koenig H., Meador K., Cohen H. & Blazer D. (1988) Self-rated depression scales and screening for major depression in the older hospitalized patient with medical illness. *Journal of the American Geriatrics Society* 36, 699–706.

Kral V.A. (1962) Senescent forgetfulness: benign and malignant. *Canadian Medical Association Journal* 86, 257–260.

Kukull W., Koepsell T., Inui T.S. *et al.* (1986) Depression and physical illness among elderly general medical clinic patients. *Journal of Affective Disorders* 10, 153–162.

Larson D., Lyons J., Hohmann A. *et al.* (1991) Psychotropics prescribed to the US elderly in the early and mid 1980s: prescribing patterns of primary care practitioners, psychiatrists and other physicians. *International Journal of Geriatric Psychiatry* 6, 63–70.

Levin E., Sinclair A. & Gorbach P. (1983) The Supporters of the Confused Elderly at Home – Extract from the Main Report: Families, Services and Confusion in Old Age. Allen & Unwin, London.

Lindesay J., Briggs K. & Murphy E. (1989) The Guy's Age Concern Survey. Prevalence rates of cognitive impairment, depression and anxiety in an urban elderly community. *British Journal of Psychiatry* 155, 317–329.

Livingston G., Hawkins A., Graham N. *et al.* (1990) The Gospel Oak study: prevalence rates of dementia, depression and activity limitation among elderly residents in Inner London. *Psychological Medicine* 20, 137–146.

Macdonald A. (1986) Do general practitioners 'miss' depression in elderly patients? *British Medical Journal* 292, 1365–1367.

Macdonald A., Mann A., Jenkins R. *et al.* (1982) An attempt to determine the impact of four types of care upon the elderly in London by the study of matched groups. *Psychological Medicine* 12, 193–200.

McHugh P. & Folstein B. (1979) Psychopathology of dementia: implications for neuropathology. In Katzman R. (ed.) *Congenital and Acquired Cognitive Disorders.* Raven Press, New York.

Macmillan D. & Shaw P. (1966) Senile breakdown in standards of personal and environmental cleanliness. *British Medical Journal* 2, 1032.

McWhorter W. & White L. (1987) Risk Factors for Dementia in a National Longitudinal Study: Preliminary Findings. Paper presented to a NIMH workshop, Bethesda, 8–9 June (unpublished).

Mann A., Graham N. & Ashby D. (1984) Psychiatric illness in residential homes for the elderly: a survey in one London borough. *Age and Ageing* 13, 257–265.

Martin M., Meltzer H. & Eliot D. (1988) *OPCS Surveys of Disability in Great Britain, Report 1.* HMSO, London.

Martyn C., Barker D., Osmond C. *et al.* (1989) Geographical relation between Alzheimer's disease and aluminium in drinking water. *Lancet* i, 59–65.

Mishara B. & Kastenbaum R. (1980) *Alcohol and Old Age.* Grune and Stratton, New York.

Molsa P., Marttila R. & Rinne U. (1982) Epidemiology of dementia in a Finnish population. *Acta Neurologica Scandinavica* 65, 541–552.

Morgan K., Dallosso H., Arie T. *et al.* (1987) Mental health and psychological well-being among the old and very old living at home. *British Journal of Psychiatry* 150, 801–807.

Mortimer J., French L., Hutton J. & Schuman L. (1985) Head injury as a risk factor for Alzheimer's disease. *Neurology* 35, 264–267.

Murphy E. (1982) Social origins of depression in old age. *British Journal of Psychiatry* 141, 135–142.

Murphy E. (1985) The impact of depression in old age on close social relationships. *American Journal of Psychiatry* 142, 323–327.

Myers J., Weissman M. & Tischler G. (1984) Six-month prevalence of psychiatric disorders in three communities. *Archives of General Psychiatry* 41, 959–967.

O'Connor D., Pollitt P., Brook C. *et al.* (1991a) Does early intervention reduce the number of elderly people with dementia admitted to institutions for long term care? *British Medical Journal* 302, 871–874.

O'Connor D., Pollitt P., Hyde J. *et al.* (1988) Do general practitioners miss dementia in elderly patients? *British Medical Journal* 297, 1107–1111.

O'Connor D., Pollitt P., Hyde J. *et al.* (1991b) The progression of mild idiopathic dementia in a community population. *Journal of the American Geriatrics Society* 39, 246–251.

O'Connor D., Pollitt P., Treasure F. *et al.* (1989) The influence of education, social class and sex on Mini-Mental State scores. *Psychological Medicine* 19, 771–776.

O'Connor D., Pollitt P. & Treasure F. (1991c) The influence of education and social class on the diagnosis of dementia in a community population. *Psychological Medicine* 21, 219–224.

Office of Population Censuses and Surveys (OPCS) (1977) *Mortality Statistics.* HMSO, London.

Pattie A. & Gilleard C. (1979) *Manual of the Clifton Assessment Procedure for the Elderly (CAPE).* Hodder and Stoughton, Sevenoaks.

Perl D. (1985) Relation of aluminium to Alzheimer's disease. *Environmental Health Perspective* 63, 149–153.

Pfeffer R., Afifi A. & Chance J. (1987) Prevalence of Alzheimer's disease in a retirement community. *American Journal of Epidemiology* 125, 420–436.

Pierce D. (1987) Deliberate self-harm in the elderly. *International Journal of Geriatric Psychiatry* 2, 105–110.

Pinessi L., Rainero I., Angelini G. *et al.* (1983) I fattori di reschio nelle sindrome demenziali primarie. *Minerva Psychiatrica* 24, 87–91.

Pitt B. (1982) *Psychogeriatrics*, 2nd edn. Churchill Livingstone, Edinburgh.

Pitt B. (1986) Characteristics of depression in the elderly. In Murphy E. (ed.) *Affective Disorders in Old Age.* Churchill Livingstone, Edinburgh.

Pitt B. (1991) The mentally disordered old person in the general hospital ward. In Judd F.K., Burrows G.D. & Lipsitt D.R. (eds) *Handbook of Studies on General Hospital Psychiatry.* Elsevier, Oxford.

Pitt B. & Nowers M. (1986) Elderly would be suicides are more determined, still treatable. *Geriatric Medicine* 16, (10), 7–8.

Plum F. (1979) Dementia: an approaching epidemic. Nature

279, 372–373.

Post F. (1962) *The Significance of Affective Disorders in Old Age. Maudsley Monograph no. 10.* Oxford University Press, Oxford.

Regier A., Boyd J., Burke J. *et al.* (1988) One-month prevalence of mental disorders in the United States. *Archives of General Psychiatry* 45, 977–986.

Robins L., Helzer J., Weissman M. *et al.* (1984) Lifetime prevalence of specific mental disorders in the three sites. *Archives of General Psychiatry* 41, 949–958.

Robinson R., Starr L., Kubos K. *et al.* (1983) A two year longitudinal study of post stroke mood disorders; findings during the initial evaluation. *Stroke* 14, 736–741.

Roth M. (1983) In Angst (ed.) *The Origins of Depression: Current Concepts and Approaches.* Springer, New York.

Roth M., Tym E., Mountjoy C. *et al.* (1986) CAMDEX: a standardised instrument for the diagnosis of mental disorder in the elderly with special reference to the early diagnosis of dementia. *British Journal of Psychiatry* 149, 698–709.

Royal College of Physicians of London (Committee on Geriatrics) (1981) Organic mental impairment in the elderly. Implications for research, education and the provision of services. *Journal of the Royal College of Physicians of London* 15, 141–167.

Schulberg H. & Burns B. (1988) Mental disorders in primary care: epidemiological, diagnostic and treatment research directions. *General Hospital Psychiatry* 10, 79–87.

Secretaries of State for Health, Social Security, Wales, Scotland (1989) *Caring for People.* HMSO, London.

Shibayama H., Kasahara Y., Kobayashi H. *et al.* (1986) An epidemiological survey on the age associated dementia resided in the community in Aichi prefecture. *Geriatric Psychiatry* 3, 223–235.

Snowdon J. (1987) Uncleanliness among pensioners seen by community health workers. *Hospital and Community Psychiatry* 38, 491–494.

Sulkava R., Wilstrom J., Aromaa A. *et al.* (1985) Prevalence of severe dementia in Finland. *Neurology* 35, 1025–1029.

Tomlin S. (1988) *Abuse of Elderly People: An Unnecessary and Preventable Problem.* British Geriatrics Society, London.

United Nations (1979) *Age and Sex Composition by Country 1960–2000.* UN, New York.

Wattis J. (1981) Alcohol problems in the elderly. *Journal of the Geriatric Society* 29, 131–134.

Wells C. (1979) Pseudodementia. *American Journal of Psychiatry* 136, 895–900.

Wells Y. & Jorm A. (1987) Evaluation of a special nursing home unit for dementia sufferers. A randomized, controlled comparison with community care. *Australia and New Zealand Journal of Psychiatry* 21, 524–531.

Wells Y., Jorm A., Jordan F. & Lefroy R. (1990) Effects on care-givers of special day care programmes for dementia suffers. *Australia and New Zealand Journal of Psychiatry* 24, 82–90.

Williamson J., Stokoe I., Gray M. *et al.* (1964) Old people at home: their unreported needs. *Lancet* i, 1117–1120.

Wilson B., Cockburn J. & Baddeley A. (1985) *The Rivermead Behavioural Memory Test.* Thames Valley Test Company, Reading.

Yates P. & Mann D. (1986) Aluminosilicates and Alzheimer's disease. *Lancet* i, 681–682.

Yesavage J., Brink T., Rose T. *et al.* (1983) Development and validation of a geriatric depression screening scale: a preliminary report. *Journal of Psychiatric Research* 17, 37–49.

# Chapter 19
## Social Aspects of Mental Handicap

A. HOLLAND

## Introduction

Understanding the relative influences of environmental, social and biological factors on the intellectual development of any given person, or groups of people, requires an appropriate conceptual framework. Confusion arises because of different terminology, and also, because of a failure to appreciate the importance of a developmental perspective and how, over time, the relative importance of environmental and biological factors may change (see Hodapp *et al.* (1990) and Clarke & Clarke (1984a) for detailed reviews).

The group of people classified as having a mental handicap is very heterogeneous. At one extreme, early development may be markedly delayed, life-expectancy reduced and the person may have a minimal level of skills and language development. In comparison, those who may be considered to be 'mildly mentally handicapped' may be minimally delayed in their early development and only noticed to have 'learning difficulties' when they start school. The terms 'mental handicap', 'mental retardation' and 'mental deficiency' are inadequate labels for describing people from such a diverse population, and such terms cannot encompass the complex interaction between a number of possible biological factors affecting brain development and the social and environmental factors, which together give rise to the resultant limitations in a person's survival skills and the impact on his or her quality of life. Similarly, terms such as 'learning difficulties' or 'learning disabilities' are an inadequate description of people who are severely or profoundly developmentally disabled with very limited language development, and who never develop essential living skills.

The classification system proposed by the World Health Organization (1980) is discussed in detail below. However, it is important at this stage to be clear, in general terms, about the characteristics of the population referred to in this chapter. The term 'mental handicap' refers to a person who has a generalized impairment of intellectual development, which may have occurred for one of many possible reasons, or be due to a combination of factors. It may be suspected in childhood because the child's early developmental milestones are delayed or abnormal; for example, language development may be limited to a few single words and motor milestones delayed. This may be accompanied by a delay in, or failure to acquire, adequate social and living skills. They may be recognized as being in need of special educational help in childhood and may continue to have deficits in their social and intellectual abilities as adults. Assessment of the individual's intellectual abilities using standardized tests (e.g. the Wechsler Intelligence Scales for Children or Adults, WISC, WAIS-R), indicate that the child's or adult's abilities, on a variety of verbal and performance tasks, are at a low level in comparison to the established mean for a person of that age in the general population (see Berger & Yule 1985 for review).

The significance of many of these factors will depend critically upon the age of the person at the time. There is considerable variability in the age at which children reach specific milestones. The failure to say single words by three years may be indicative of a number of possible problems including deafness but also, if accompanied by a lack of normal childhood play and ritualistic behaviour, may be a component of autism. Limited language development, in the absence of a hearing impairment, together with the limited development of other aptitudes at age five or ten years, would be of still greater significance.

The terminology used will also depend upon who uses it, upon the question which is being asked at the time and may also be determined by any legal framework within which the terms are being employed (Gunn 1990). The parents of a child who is clearly delayed in his/her development are likely to want to know the cause of the delay. The recognition that the cause is a specific genetic disorder has considerable importance for counselling, may allow some statement to be made about the future prognosis and helps the family come to terms with having a child who has a particular disorder affecting their development (Bicknell 1988). Later the recognition of the presence of a 'learning difficulty' or of specific sensory impairments (Ellis 1986) are important as special educational help may maximize the child's abilities at different stages of development. In this context 'labels' and the various terminology, if appropriately used, are important as they may lead to specific positive interventions.

An understanding of how social factors are important, either as a major cause of developmental intellectual impairment and therefore of mental handicap, or in exacerbating the problem, has been confused, not only because of the difficulty of defining and recognizing 'mental handicap' but also because of an appropriate move away from a perspective dominated by the medical approach to diagnosis. Psychological assessment techniques have been developed and refined, a more systematic approach to skills training has minimized disabilities and, in England and Wales, the Education Acts have brought about major changes in the educational provision available to people with a mental handicap (Education (Handicapped Children) Act 1970, Education Act 1981). The importance of social factors can only be examined in the light of these historical changes as well as by the use of a better diagnostic framework.

This chapter examines the influence of social factors in two broad areas. The first is in the role that such factors might have in the aetiology of mental handicap and, in particular, the influence of social factors on the extent of any given impairment, disability and handicap in an individual. The second is how social factors and accompanying changes in perception of people who are mentally handicapped have influenced the 'care' of this group of people.

## Historical perspective

It has been acknowledged for several hundred years that there is a difference between those born with a disorder affecting mental development, which remains throughout life, and those who have a disorder which varies over time and is only temporary. The terms 'idiot' and 'lunatic' were used respectively to describe these two different groups. The care of the former group was often equated with the care of the 'poor', and in France, for example, this was carried out by the church: the term 'cretin' is a corruption of the French word 'chretien', meaning 'christian'. The care of people who were apparently incapable of looking after themselves became enshrined in legislation which required that more sophisticated methods of identifying the relevant population of people were developed. In England a series of Acts of Parliament were passed in an attempt to provide for the needs of those seen as being 'defective', including Education Acts (1870, 1899), the Idiots Act (1866) and later, following a Royal Commission, the Mental Deficiency Act (1913).

The subsequent development and changes in attitudes towards this population have been reviewed by others (Clarke & Clarke 1985, Craft 1985) and have been extensively discussed by Sarason & Doris (1969). A number of parallel developments occurred at the end of the nineteenth and beginning of the twentieth century, including the development of intelligence tests by Binet and the eugenics movement. The latter group were particularly concerned about what they saw as a relationship between pauperism and feeblemindedness. People who had previously been seen as in need of care and education were now also seen as a threat to society and in need of segregation.

Classification systems such as that used in the Mental Deficiency Act (1913) were developed for administrative purposes and the definitions were made sufficiently broad to enable compulsory admission to hospital for people who were considered socially deviant or undesirable, rather than in need of care by reason of developmental disability. The terminology used was 'arrested or incomplete development of mind' which was considered to be wider than the concept of intellectual development alone. Unlike the 1959 and 1983 English and Welsh Mental Health Acts (MHA), 'subnormality of intelligence' was not part of the definition. The existing Board of Control considered that antisocial characteristics in youth were sufficient to enable medical practitioners to certify a person as 'mentally defective'. O'Connor & Tizard (1954) found in a survey of inpatients in mental handicap institutions that the average IQ of younger adult 'feeble minded defectives' was just over 70, confirming the view that prior to the 1959 Mental Health Act many people compulsorily admitted to 'mental deficiency institutions' were not significantly intellectually impaired.

A further development during this period was the recognition of different syndromes associated with mental handicap, including, for example, Down's syndrome (.866) and inborn errors of metabolism (Garrod 1909), and thus an attempt was made to classify according to the likely cause of the disability. Refinements of the IQ tests made them less influenced by education and as a result strict classification systems were developed by groups such as the expert committee of the World Health Organization in 1969. Other methods of classification based on probable aetiology were also elaborated. Tredgold (1952) referred to primary and secondary amentia, the former being generally chromosomal or due to other genetic or constitutional disorders, the latter as a result of damage to the foetus, or infection in infancy. One of the most influential papers was that by Lewis (1933) who was at the time Commissioner for the Board of Control. He sought a solution to the social problems presented by people who were mentally defective and, whilst recognizing the importance of the classification system of Tredgold which was concerned with aetiology, felt that this had little value in terms of possible social solutions. However, Lewis himself emphasized the

variety of conditions and the range and types of disabilities encompassed by the term 'mental deficiency' and believed that 'mental deficiencies' was a more accurate description. In his paper he drew an analogy with the observed variations in height in any population. Variation in height is normally distributed: those who fall outside this distribution do so for pathological reasons (e.g. achondroplasia, or acromegaly causing excessive shortness and tallness, respectively). The majority of people however would cluster around the mean, variations about this probably being due largely to genetic factors. In the case of the mental deficiencies Lewis proposed a similar model in which there were the pathological types and the subcultural types. The former generally fell, in terms of intellectual ability, outside and at the lower end of the normal distribution of intellectual abilities. He recognized that, as with his example of height, there would be some degree of overlap between the two types. Lewis argued that genetic factors were in fact of particular importance in the less intellectually disabled subcultural group. He discussed the various social and economic influences which might interact with an inherited propensity to 'feeble-mindedness', and considered that this group presented with the greatest social problems. He did not see a solution in segregation and thought that education should be improved for all of society, thereby raising the abilities of those at the bottom. He did not offer specific solutions but it is likely that he was arguing strongly for good, universal education, improved housing, and a proper structure of social support. These earlier observations by Lewis were later shown to be substantially correct, yet the role of 'nature versus nurture' in the causation of mild developmental intellectual impairment became the source of considerable debate, eventually leading to major efforts at 'environmental' improvement through 'head start' programmes.

### The nature–nurture debate

The separation between 'pathological' and 'subcultural mental deficiency' suggested that different factors were important in the causation of the intellectual impairments in the two groups. One of the most extensive studies to examine the question was a large study of children in Aberdeen (Birch *et al.* 1970). Children with mild degrees of 'mental subnormality' came largely from families in the lower social classes. Furthermore, those affected who were not in this social group more often had evidence of neurological abnormality. In contrast, people born with disorders associated with severe degrees of 'mental subnormality' were found in all groups of society regardless of background. This excess of children with mild degrees of mental handicap in families in the lower social classes has been reported by others (Stein & Susser 1960, Rutter *et al.* 1970). These findings together with the observation that mean IQ scores in the population have increased over time (Scottish Council for Research in Education, 1953) led to debate about the relative importance of public health, educational and social policies as well as the role of genetic factors. The difficulty of interpreting the findings partly reflects the inadequacy of classification systems used at that time, but also illustrates the complex interrelationships present within any given family. Tizard (1974) in his analysis of longitudinal studies quotes the work of Birch who identifies a number of characteristics which may cluster together within any family with a mildly mentally handicapped child, including inadequate housing, poor nourishment, minimal education, family disorganization together with poor perinatal health. Such families may also be too disorganized to seek help which, if it was available, might have ameliorated the level of disability.

The 'nature-nurture' discussion as regards the cause of mild developmental intellectual impairment continues to this day. Environmental factors have been emphasized in the manual of the American Association on Mental Deficiency (Grossman 1983), but studies of the correlations of IQ scores between relatives have demonstrated convincingly that genetic factors are of considerable importance. The IQ scores of monozygotic (MZ) twins reared apart have correlations of greater than 0.70, and when reared together of over 0.80. Both these scores are considerably higher than the correlations for dizygotic (DZ) twins, or siblings (Vernon 1979). However the

difference between the correlations for MZ twins reared apart versus those reared together, indicate that environment is still important. When considering genetic/environmental influences it is also important to state that findings within a population cannot be directly applied to any given person. The relative influence of genetic effects may be very small in a poverty-stricken and deprived environment but large in an enriching environment.

As different disorders associated with developmental intellectual impairment become known and as people with specific syndromes have been assessed in more detail (see for example the study of IQ scores in people with Down's syndrome (Breg 1977), it is clear that, in terms of IQ scores, there is a considerable overlap between the two groups. As the study of Birch *et al.* (1970) elegantly showed, the role of abnormal brain development is of considerable importance at the more impaired end of the spectrum and becomes less so at the other end, where other studies have indicated that polygenic factors become more relevant. However, a distinction has to be drawn between the level of impairment and the level of disability: the latter may be considerably influenced by environmental and, by implication, social factors (see below).

## Social factors and the causes of mental handicap

Understanding the causes of mental handicap and the development of social policies and legislation to provide for the group of people affected has been complicated by changing attitudes and concepts. The refinement of definitions is needed so that a clearer understanding across disciplines can be achieved as to what social, psychological, medical and political interventions are appropriate to minimize the negative effects of being mentally handicapped and maximize the options for those concerned and their families.

### *Impairments, disabilities and handicaps*

The World Health Organization (1980) has proposed a more complex classification system which is particularly applicable to chronic disorders. In applying this system of classification to mental handicap it is necessary to ask what is the impairment, the disability and the handicap, and at each level to ask what is known about the likely causative factors. This is applicable in terms of population-based research or with a given individual and has the advantage that it provides a framework for all those working in this field regardless of discipline. It also can help to direct the form of any intervention. When asking the question 'What social factors are important in the causation of mental handicap'?, such a framework of classification allows a more sophisticated analysis. The definitions are given below, together with some of the evidence relating to social factors and their importance in understanding the aetiology of the problem.

## IMPAIRMENT

*Definition.* In the context of health experience, an impairment is any loss or abnormality of psychological, physiological, or anatomical structure or function.

*Characteristics.* Impairment is characterized by losses or abnormalities that may be temporary or permanent, and that include the existence or occurrence of an anomaly, defect, or loss in a limb, organ, tissue or other structure of the body, *including the systems of mental functioning.* Impairment represents exteriorization of a pathological state, and in principle it reflects disturbances at the level of the organ.

As has already been stated when referring to mental handicap, the disorder is developmental in nature and has its origins in childhood. At this level of classification there is an assumption that in any given individual there is a developmental and biologically determined limitation to the maximum level of intellectual ability which can be achieved. The extent of the biological restrictions placed upon any individual's intellectual abilities cannot be assessed other than by using standardized tests of intelligence. In this context they are not ideal as levels of performance and may be contaminated by educational effects, the state of the person on the day of the test and other factors (see Berger & Yule 1985). However, they are still the best measure available. It is clearly established that well-recognized disorders are associated with developmental intellectual impairment (e.g. Down's syndrome). In this group of people brain development is abnormal and observed low scores on intellectual assessment are likely to be largely a reflection of this.

In those disorders in which brain development is clearly abnormal the question remains as to what social factors might influence the occurrence of such disorders. The differentiation of neural tissue begins early in the first trimester and is followed by a period of rapid growth of the brain, which continues until 18 months of age (Dobbing 1984). Chromosomal and genetic disorders may have their effect at a very early stage, alternatively the effects of teratogens may influence differentiation of the brain structure or impair the growth of the brain. There may also be social influences which have their effect at this level. Down's syndrome is an important cause of mental handicap due to the inheritance of an extra chromosome 21 (trisomy 21), usually from the mother. The greater the maternal age at conception the higher the likelihood of chromosomal non-dysjunction, and social effects which influence family size could conceivably influence the prevalence of Down's syndrome births (Gath & Gumley 1986). The opportunity of antenatal screening for all mothers over the age of 35 or 37 years has decreased the number of Down's syndrome births, but the acceptance of such a service may be influenced by social variables. Owens *et al.* (1983) reported a decrease in the mean maternal age of mothers in Liverpool with a low rate of acceptance of amniocentesis and argued that the maternal age change was more likely to be the explanation of the reduced number of Down's syndrome births. In the USA the use of such services varies widely, amniocentesis being accepted by over ·30% of older women in New York state but only 5–6% in rural areas.

In contrast to clearly identified disorders of known chromosomal and genetic aetiology, disorders with environmental origins also have to be considered. A number of congenital infections are known to have effects on the foetus, including rubella (Miller *et al.* 1982), cytomegalovirus

(Reynolds *et al.* 1974) and toxoplasmosis (Wilson *et al.* 1980). Campaigns to encourage schoolgirls to be immunized against rubella have taken different forms in the USA and the UK, but their aim is to increase the general level of immunity against this disorder in females by the time they reach child-bearing age so that rubella infection is rare in expectant mothers, and maternal rubella as a cause of developmental intellectual impairment as well as hearing and visual impairment can be eliminated. Social factors may well be influential in the likelihood of maternal infections as well as in the acceptance of an immunization campaign.

The detrimental effects of excessive maternal alcohol consumption during pregnancy on the developing foetus are an important and preventable cause of developmental intellectual impairment (see also Chapter 11). Since the introduction of the term 'foetal alcohol syndrome' in 1973 by Jones & Smith, there has been considerable evidence of brain abnormalities and physical abnormalities in the affected child (Porter *et al.* 1984). The mechanism(s) whereby alcohol may result in damage to the developing foetus may be a combination of direct effects of alcohol as well as other psychosocial and nutritional factors which may well accompany alcohol abuse (Pratt 1984). Specific interventions warning mothers about the effects of alcohol on the developing foetus have been shown to have some effect (Little *et al.* 1984).

The occurrence of disorders, genetic or environmental, which result in abnormal foetal brain development or brain damage prenatally or in childhood may well be under social influences. A general recognition of the importance of good health during pregnancy, better obstetric and paediatric care, the offer of prenatal counselling to older mothers or to families with specific genetic disorders, and immunization campaigns are all ways in which society can reduce the general burden of developmental problems which affect intellectual development.

### DISABILITY

*Definition.* In the context of health experience, a disability is any restriction or lack (resulting from an impairment) of ability to perform an activity in the manner or within the range considered normal for a human being.

*Characteristics.* Disability is characterized by excesses or deficiencies of customarily expected activity, performance and behaviour, and these may be temporary or permanent, reversible or irreversible, and progressive or regressive. Disabilities may arise as a direct consequence of impairment or as a response by the individual, particularly psychologically, to a physical, sensory or other impairment. Disability represents objectification of an impairment and as such reflects disturbances at the level of the person.

For people with a developmental intellectual impairment, it is the resultant disability which has potentially the greatest impact on the individual's life. Disabilities may be varied and include the results of additional physical, psychological and sensory impairments. Among this group of people as a whole, a developmental learning disability will be universal as recognized by the need for special education. For some children, for example, it will take longer to acquire the skills to dress, or to acquire numeracy and literacy skills than a child without an intellectual impairment. It is the extent of disability or what has been referred to as 'secondary handicaps' which may be considerably influenced by social factors. One of the major debates has centred on whether disability can be reduced by early and long-term psychological and educational input. The question of early intervention is well reviewed in the paper by Zigler & Berman (1983). As is often the case in the field of mental handicap there is an assumption that somehow this population is different from the general population and that general commonsense rules do not apply. In an analysis of the effectiveness of intervention, the starting point must be that, for example, emotional deprivation, physical and/or sexual abuse, poor educational opportunities, lack of a supportive family structure will be at least as disadvantageous to a child with an intellectual impairment as to a child who is intellectually average (Clarke & Clarke 1984b). Those children with mild levels of intellectual impairment are particularly likely to come from families who are financially impoverished (Richardson 1981), and in which there is a poor quality of parental care (Stein & Susser 1960, Nihira *et al.* 1980). 'Head start' programmes may be of some value to children born not only with a developmental disorder, but also within disadvantaged families. Some support for early interventions comes from longitudinal studies of children with an established chromosomal cause for their developmental disorder, Down's syndrome (Ludlow & Allen 1979) and cri-du-chat syndrome (Wilkins *et al.* 1980). These studies have demonstrated some short-term benefits of early intervention but only limited lasting advantage following intensive educational and psychological input in early life. Study of children with Down's syndrome has also demonstrated that their is clearly a limit to the observed improvement, and the effect of being born with trisomy 21 is likely to be the most powerful influence on their development.

Early intervention strategies have increasingly focused on involving the parents so that they can learn the major principles and apply them throughout the child's life. For children living within socially disadvantaged homes, benefits from early intervention have been show to disappear if parents are not involved (Harris *et al.* 1981). Institutional settings are in themselves not necessarily disadvantageous but the extent of one-to-one contact, which is more likely to be greater in a home situation, is the significant factor (Tizard & Tizard 1974). Given the will and appropriate resources the disability of children with developmental disorders can be reduced (Hunt *et al.* 1976).

HANDICAP

*Definition.* In the context of health experience, a handicap is a disadvantage for a given individual, resulting from an impairment or disability, that limits or prevents the fulfilment of a role that is normal (depending on age, sex, and social and cultural factors) for that individual.

*Characteristics.* Handicap is concerned with the value attached to an individual's situation or experience when it departs from the norm. It is characterized by a discordance between the individual's performance or status and the expectations of the individual himself or of the particular group of which he is a member. Handicap thus represents socialization of an impairment or disability, and as such it reflects the consequences for the individual – cultural, social, economic, and environmental – that stem from the presence of impairment and disability.

The level of handicap occurring as a result of a developmental intellectual impairment and learning disability will not only be dependent on the extent of the impairment and the disability but also on the demands of the environment. Such demands may increase as society becomes more technological and there are greater expectations in terms of occupational ability. Interventions to minimize either the impairment and/or disability should result in a reduction of the handicap. For example, a child with a learning disability because of a visual impairment may be helped by glasses, thus reducing his/her handicap. If the visual impairment could not be helped by glasses, then braille books and special education could reduce the disadvantage or handicap that the child experiences. The provision of ramps for people in wheelchairs is also an example of how environmental change might reduce the impact of having an unchanging disability.

This classification system allows a more systematic examination of the complex interaction between social and biological factors associated with mental handicap. The advantage of such an approach is that it also helps to direct intervention. The presence of a particular genetic disorder affecting brain development may indicate the need for a particular approach at the level of brain structure and functioning. The resultant learning disability requires a different form of intervention. It clearly does not diminish the importance of special education or of modifying the environment to minimize disadvantage. All these are different levels of intervention which may diminish the level of actual handicap.

PREVALENCE OF DEVELOPMENTAL
INTELLECTUAL IMPAIRMENT, AND
RESULTANT DISABILITY
AND MENTAL HANDICAP

The accurate estimation of prevalence rates depends upon having an agreed definition of what is being measured and on that definition having adequate reliability. This has been a major problem in mental handicap.

The prevalence of developmental intellectual impairment is statistically defined. Using standard IQ tests (e.g. Wechsler Intelligence Scales), IQ scores within an unselected population are almost normally distributed and 2% of the population fall more than two standard deviations below the mean. For those tests with a mean of 100 and a standard deviation of 15, this is an IQ score of below 70 points. As is illustrated by Fig. 19.1, IQ

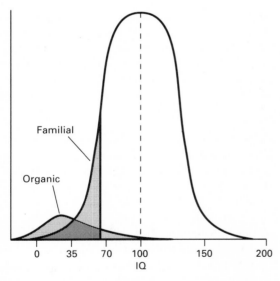

**Fig. 19.1** The near normal distribution of IQ scores from an unselected population. Approximately 2% of the population have an IQ score two standard deviations below the mean (<70). The distribution to the left is skewed, and represents a combination of those people whose developmental disorder is due to a specific disorder, for example Down's syndrome, and those who have a developmental intellectual impairment for familial reasons, either polygenic and/or environmental in origin.

scores have been shown to be normally distributed with a skew to the left caused by the 'pathological group'. Identified syndromes, inborn errors of metabolism and particular environmental factors account for much of the skew.

This population of people with a developmental intellectual impairment resulting in IQ scores below 70 will all have a learning disability, which is likely to require special help at school. In England and Wales this is recognized by the fact that those children who are 'statemented' as having 'special needs' because of their 'learning difficulty' have the right to special help and in some cases may stay at school until 19 years of age. Within the population as a whole there will be others who do not have a generalized intellectual impairment but have, for example, specific reading retardation, and as such have a learning disability. The percentage of the population who may therefore require special educational help due to specific or generalized learning disabilities is higher than the 2% with IQs below 70.

There has been considerable research which has attempted to quantify both the practical and psychological burden placed on a family with a mentally handicapped child. The level of disability associated with the presence of developmental intellectual impairment is primarily dependent on the presence or not of other impairments, including behavioural and psychiatric disorders, sensory impairments and social and language impairments characteristic of autism (Table 19.1). All these are more common among the developmentally intellectually impaired.

The resultant level of disadvantage or handicap due to the presence of a developmental intellectual impairment and learning disability is therefore a result of a complex interaction between an individual's various impairments, abilities and disabilities and society's response to them, and therefore cannot easily be quantified. However, the numbers of people with levels of disability requiring special service provision is known. These studies generally agree that 3–4 per 1000 of the population fall within the 'severely mentally handicapped' group (Birch *et al.* 1970) and under the World Health Organization's classification system would have an IQ below 50, would have a significant

**Table 19.1** The extent of different disabilities found within a mentally handicapped population in residential setting and those living at home by age group

|  | n | Disability* | | | | | |
|---|---|---|---|---|---|---|---|
|  |  | Non-ambulant | Problem behaviour | Incontinent | Needs assistance | No problems | Not assessed |
| *Home* | | | | | | | |
| 0–14 years | 49.24 | 10.4 (21) | 4.83 (10) | 5 (10) | 15.9 (32) | 12.29 (26) | 0.73 (1.5) |
| 15+ years | 71.65 | 3.2 (4) | 3.17 (4) | 1.69 (2) | 9.29 (9) | 53.90 (75) | 0.94 (1.3) |
| *Residential* | | | | | | | |
| 0–14 years | 19.96 | 6.1 (31) | 4.86 (24) | 3.65 (18) | 3.63 (18) | 1.69 (8) | 0.10 (0.5) |
| 15+ years | 96.19 | 7.23 (8) | 15.58 (16) | 0.15 (0.2) | 16.58 (17) | 49.36 (52) | 0.21 (0.2) |

The figures have been taken from the White Paper 'Better Services for the Mentally Handicapped' (1971) which combined the results of three epidemiological studies.
* The figures give the average numbers, with percentages in brackets, found to have one of a number of other impairments resulting in additional disabilities.

disability in living skills and communication and thus very likely be disadvantaged.

### Behavioural and psychiatric disorder

A further cause of disability is the occurrence of additional behavioural and psychiatric disorder. The presence of such additional problems can have a profound effect on the family (Carr 1990) and on the quality of life for both the individual and the family (Brown 1990). It is problems such as these which may require the intervention of psychologists and psychiatrists, but what additional factors, biological, developmental or environmental, contribute to such problems occurring is still far from clear.

The Aberdeen study (Birch *et al.* 1970) found high rates of psychiatric disorder among the children with 'mental subnormality'. When the group was divided on the basis of IQ, additional psychiatric disorder was present in 45% of those with IQ levels of less than 50, 48% of those with IQ levels of between 50 and 59, 21% with IQ levels between 60 and 69, and 7% in those with levels of IQ greater than 70. The authors noted that psychiatric disorder was most common in those with clear evidence of neurological abnormality, rather than in those with lesser degrees of handicap but who came from disadvantaged social situations. Other studies have also reported high rates of

additional psychiatric disorder, including behavioural problems, conduct and emotional disorders and psychiatric illness. Rutter *et al.* (1970a) in the Isle of Wight Study found that nearly 50% of 'brain damaged' children had additional psychiatric disorders compared to under 7% of the control group, and Corbett (1979) found similar rates of psychiatric disorder in children and adults with mental handicap. There are often differences in definition between studies but the findings among the more severely handicapped are likely to be reliable. However, establishing a definite base rate for 'mild mental handicap' within any given area is almost impossible, and as people with mild mental handicap and additional psychiatric disorder are more likely to be in contact with services than those without psychiatric disorder, reported rates of psychiatric disorder are likely to be higher than is actually the case.

The presence of additional behavioural problems for whatever reasons has been found to be one of the major factors in determining whether families can cope at home and whether an individual can live successfully in a community setting. Eyman & Call (1977) in a study of 7000 people living in the community or in institutions found much higher levels of maladaptive behaviour in the latter group. In a later study they concluded that it was the problem behaviour which resulted in admission to an institution, and not 'institutionalization' which resulted in problem behaviour (Eyman *et al.* 1981).

As with the causes of mental handicap itself, the factors which contribute to problem behaviour and psychiatric disorder are likely to be multiple. The application of both psychological and psychiatric models can contribute to the identification of these factors and to the use of particular treatments or appropriate management strategies to reduce their extent and severity (Holland & Murphy 1990).

## Social factors and their influence on the 'care' of people with mental handicap

To understand the causes of mental handicap it is necessary to categorize these according to specific physical and/or mental characteristics. Such categorization is fundamental to medical research both to aid in the identification of the aetiology of a particular illness or genetic disorder, and also in the testing of any specific treatment. As discussed earlier, methods of categorization were also used as a means of segregating a group of people thought to have 'arrested or incomplete development of mind' and who were perceived as being a threat to society. Large 'colonies' far from centres of population were seen to be the British answer and families were advised that it would be better if they forgot about their handicapped child and leave it to others to look after him or her. Although the majority of mentally handicapped people still continued to live at home, families had very little in the way of support and were often stigmatized by having, and caring for, their handicapped child. Mental handicap, mental deficiency and deviancy became intertwined so that one was invariably equated with the other.

Sociological research challenged the notion that 'deviance' in an individual was something which could be identified easily by a 'medically qualified practitioner' and was a result of some innate abnormality. It became important to examine the circumstances surrounding the use of such labels as 'mental deficiency' and to ask what in society determined that someone be so labelled (Alaszewski & Bie Nio Ong 1991). The result of being seen as 'stupid' in a society which valued intellectual ability was that people so labelled would be discriminated against in employment, for example, and would be further devalued by society (Dexter 1964). Much of the present-day arguments of what to call people with a developmental intellectual impairment has its origins in the subsequent radical and very necessary reappraisal of how society provides for its disadvantaged groups. A change in perception was necessary in order that new models of care could develop for people who clearly had 'special needs'.

Central to this change in philosophy was the concept of 'normalization', which arose in Scandinavia (Bank-Mikkelsen 1969, Nirje 1973), but which was developed by Wolfensberger (1972). The original concept was concerned with providing as normal an environment as possible for a person with mental handicap, and later was more focused on using as 'culturally normal means as possible' to bring about the necessary help. Later still the use of 'culturally valued' means to bring about a 'valued role in society' was emphasized. The changing emphasis has resulted in a change in terminology to that of 'social role valorization' (Wolfensberger 1983).

This whole debate started at a time when the means used to care for people with a mental handicap were far from 'normal' (i.e. institutional), and as such it has significantly changed the way services are provided. In the UK following a report on Ely Hospital, the 1971 White Paper 'Better Services for the Mentally Handicapped' ushered in major social changes which are only now coming to fruition. Increasing awareness that large institutions did not and could not provide an acceptable quality of life for those living there combined with a recognition that the apparent disability of people with a mental handicap could improve providing the means were there to help them, resulted in a recognition that quality services were required so that people with a mental handicap could live 'an ordinary life' (King's Fund Centre 1980). This publication stated three principles which should guide service development:
1 Mentally handicapped people have the same human value as anyone else.
2 Mentally handicapped people have a right and a need to live like others in the community.

3 Services must recognize the individuality of mentally handicapped people.

Government policy has continued to emphasize the importance of care in the community. The Jay Committee (1979) strongly supported a shift from hospital to community care and the need for a change of emphasis in training from primarily a nursing one to a social care model. A clear committment was made to the principles of locally based services in the Government papers 'Mental Handicap: Progress, Problems, and Priorities' (Department of Health & Social Security 1980) and in 'Care in the Community' (Department of Health & Social Security 1981).

## Services

The starting point for the consideration of the types of services people with a developmental intellectual impairment are likely to need must be the recognition that their needs are as similar and varied as the rest of the population, with the likelihood that, in addition, they may also have special needs. People with such developmental disabilities are very different from each other, and the recognition that service developments have to be determined by 'need' is in striking contrast to the days of large institutions where there was little recognition of individual need or of individual rights.

The recognition that people with a 'mental handicap' could learn and develop was crucial to the later development of appropriate models of 'care' (Tizard & O'Connor 1952, Clarke & Clarke 1954). This radically changed the perspective from that of a service which might provide for a person's basic needs over a lifetime, from childhood to old age, to the need for 'services' which would help maximize the individual's potential, and as with the non-disabled population would provide for the changing needs with the different stages in a person's life. A number of strategies and systems were devised to help staff identify individual need (Blunden 1981, O'Brien & Tyne 1981, Ward 1982, 1984, Shearer 1985).

The increasing acceptance of the importance of 'an ordinary life' (King's Fund Centre 1980) and the results of the evaluation of specific projects such as the Eastern Nebraska Community Office of Retardation (ENCOR) schemes (Thomas *et al.* 1978) provide a framework onto which specific services can be built. The provision of these needs involves a number of Government Departments and many different disciplines ranging from special health, through education to social welfare. These differing areas of need clearly interact and overlap. An individual's mental health needs cannot be divorced from the environment they live in, the social relationships they have and from, for example, the fact that they have a profound social impairment due to autism. In the field of mental health one of the major challenges is to know how to bring together the increasing recognition that people with specific intellectual and psychological disabilities may require very different service approaches. The needs of a child or adult who is autistic may be very different from a child or adult of equal intellectual level but who is not socially impaired.

The Independent Living Council for People with Mental Handicap (1986) and O'Brien (1987) put forward the idea that any service should have as its goal 'five accomplishments' for those using the service. These included: the right to mix in the community and not to be segregated, the opportunity to form valued relationships, the right of choice in matters of everyday life, help to develop competence through meaningful activity and the right to respect.

## Family needs

The social needs of the child or adult with a developmental intellectual impairment and resultant disability cannot be separated from the needs of their family. The process by which parents accept that their child is 'mentally handicapped' is likely to be a very individual one and will be influenced by their own perception of the problem, past experiences and the level of support available to them. The response to the news that a child has a disorder associated with mental handicap has been described as similar to a 'bereavement response', in this case the loss is that of the expected 'perfect child' (Solnit & Stark 1977), but the family may be so overwhelmed that there is a pathological adjustment (Bicknell 1983). The family needs will include information about their child imparted in an honest, supportive and appropriate manner (Carr 1984, Nursey *et al.* 1991). Knowledge about the cause of the child's developmental disorder can be crucial to help allay guilt, to allow the family to receive sound genetic counselling and also to help plan for the child's future needs.

Byrne & Cunningham (1985) have reviewed what is known about the effects of having a handicapped child on the family. They critically discuss the assumption that stress is inevitable, or that every family member will necessarily be similarly affected. Others have argued that the presence of 'unmet service needs' rather than having a child with a disability is the main stressor (Wilkin 1979). Increased levels of stress, as measured using the Rutter 'Malaise Inventory' (Rutter *et al.* 1970), have been found particularly in mothers of mentally handicapped children. Higher levels have also been associated with lower social class, one-parent families, low income and other variables such as the nature of the handicap and the presence, in older children, of additional problem behaviour, but Byrne & Cunningham (1985) have pointed out that different studies have found conflicting results. Studies which have examined the 'burden' of community care have shown that mothers take the major responsibility, with some support from fathers and sisters (Carey 1982). In other studies, the changing nature of the stress experienced by families is illustrated by, for example, the different concerns families have when their child is old enough to leave school as he or she is frequently unemployed, and also their concern about who will be responsible for their child's future care (Card 1983). Studies have attempted to identify the factors which predict successful coping by examining the characteristics of family members and the functioning of the family as a whole. The presence of both parents, a good marital relationship and support from other family members were found in the various studies to have been important (see review by Byrne & Cunningham 1985).

More recently it has been recognized that the presence or absence of additional problem be-

haviour or psychiatric disorder is a key factor in whether families can continue to support their child at home. Quine & Pahl (1985) found that mothers' scores on the 'Malaise Scale' were highly correlated with the presence of disordered behaviour, in contrast to other problems such as poor communication, limited mobility and incontinence. In a number of studies behaviour problems emerged as the most important stressful factor, together with night-time disturbance and social isolation of the mother (see Carr 1990 for review).

Families are faced with having to cope with their child's developing needs and with the different services responsible for meeting these needs, including local education departments, social services and various branches of the health service. In infancy practical help may be required at home, later special educational provision will be the major concern, and later still specialist residential services may be required.

## Conclusions

Study of the factors contributing to the level of any given person's intellectual ability, their disabilities and the resultant mental handicap illustrates the complexity of the interaction between biologically and environmentally determined factors. The development of any child is influenced by the development of their central nervous system and the environment they find themselves in at any given time. Social deprivation and neglect is damaging regardless of innate ability, or, for example, the presence or absence of a chromosomal disorder. More sophisticated classification systems enable the influence of different factors to be teased out and allow the development of appropriate intervention strategies which may minimize the level of disability and resultant handicap.

Social factors may influence the prevalence of specific causes of developmental intellectual impairment within a population. The extent to which expectant mothers drink alcohol, or are immunized against rubella are examples of this. The influence of social factors on the extent of disability is likely to be of greater importance, although 'head start' programmes have generally been disappointing. Perhaps the major change within a social perspective has been in terms of attitudes and service developments. Appropriate systems of classification have allowed the concept of 'deviance' to be separated from 'mental deficiency', and through lobbying and as a result of inquiries, governments in the UK, USA and elsewhere have recognized that this group of people have special educational, social and health needs as well as needs common to everybody.

Families continue to be responsible for the main burden of care and identification of those factors which might increase or decrease the stress in any given family or individual is becoming increasingly important. Additional problem behaviour and psychiatric disorder is a further burden and methods of assessment, effective intervention and support are required.

## References

Alaszewski A. & Ong B.N. (1991) From consensus to conflict: the impact of sociological ideas on policy for people with a mental handicap. In Baldwin S. & Hattersley J. (eds) *Mental Handicap Social Science Perspective.* Tavistock/Routledge, London.

Bank-Mikkelsen N.E. (1969) A metropolitan area in Denmark: Copenhagen. In Kreugel R. & Wolfensberger W. (eds) *Changing Patterns in Residential Services for the Mentally Retarded.* President's Committee on Mental Retardation, Washington DC.

Berger M. & Yule W. (1985) IQ tests and assessments. In Clarke A.M., Clarke A.D.B. & Berg J. (eds) *Mental Deficiency: The Changing Outlook.* J. Methuen, London.

Bicknell J. (1983) The psychopathology of handicap. *British Journal of Medical Psychology* 56, 167–178.

Bicknell J. (1988) The family and the mentally handicapped member. *Current Opinions in Psychiatry* 1, 553–557.

Birch H.G., Richardson S.A., Baird D., Horobin G. & Illsley R. (1970) *Mental Subnormality in the Community: A Clinical and Epidemiological Study.* Williams and Wilkins, Baltimore, Maryland.

Blunden R. (1981) *Individual Plans for Mentally Handicapped people. A Procedural Guide.* Mental Handicap in Wales, Applied Research Unit, Cardiff.

Breg W.R. (1977) A review of recent progress in research. *Pathobiology Annals* 7, 257–303.

Brown R.I. (1990) Quality of life for people with learning difficulties: the challenge for behavioural and emotional disturbance. *International Review of Psychiatry* 2, 23–32.

Byrne E.A. & Cunningham C.C. (1985) The effects of mentally handicapped children on families – a review. *Journal of Child Psychology and Psychiatry* 26, 847–864.

Card H. (1983) What will happen when we are gone? *Community Care* 471, 20–21.

Carey G.E. (1982) Community care – care by whom? Mentally handicapped children living at home. *Public Health* 96, 269–278.

Carr J. (1984) Family processes and parent involvement. In Dobbing J., Clarke A.D.B., Corbett J.A., Hogg J. & Robinson R.O. (eds) *Scientific Studies in Mental Retardation.* Royal Society of Medicine, London.

Carr J. (1990) Supporting the families of people with behavioural/psychiatric disorder. *International Review of Psychiatry* 2, 33–41.

Clarke A.D.B. & Clarke A.M. (1954) Cognitive changes in the feeble-minded. *British Journal of Psychology* 45, 173–179.

Clarke A.M. & Clarke A.D.B. (1984a) Constancy and change in the growth of human characteristics: the First Jack Tizard Memorial Lecture. *Journal of Child Psychology and Psychiatry* 25, 191–210.

Clarke A.M. & Clarke A.D.B. (1984b) Social influences in the aetiology and prevention of mild retardation. In Dobbing J., Clarke A.D.B., Corbett J.A., Hogg J. & Robinson R.O. (eds) *Scientific Studies in Mental Retardation.* Royal Society of Medicine, London.

Clarke A.M. & Clarke A.D.B. (1985) Criteria and classification. In Clarke A.M., Clarke A.D.B. & Berg J. (eds) *Mental Deficiency: The Changing Outlook.* Methuen, London.

Corbett J.A. (1979) Psychiatric morbidity and mental retardation. In Snaith P. & James F.E. (eds) *Psychiatric Illness and Mental Handicap.* Headley Brothers, Ashford.

Craft M. (1985) Classification, criteria, epidemiology and causation. In Craft M., Bicknell J. & Hollins S. (eds) *Mental Handicap.* Baillière, Tindall, London.

Department of Health & Social Security (1971) *Better Services for the Mentally Handicapped.* DHSS, London.

Department of Health & Social Security (1980) *Mental Handicap: Progress, Problems and Priorities.* DHSS, London.

Department of Health & Social Security (1981) *Care in the Community.* DHSS, London.

Dexter L.A. (1964) On the politics and sociology of stupidity in our society. In Becker, H.S. (ed.) *The Other Side: Perspectives on Deviance.* The Free Press, New York.

Dobbing J. (1984) Pathology and vulnerability of the developing brain. In Dobbing J., Clarke A.D.B., Corbett J.A., Hogg J. & Robinson R.O. (eds) *Scientific Studies in Mental Retardation.* Royal Society of Medicine, London.

Down J.L. (1866) Observations on an ethnic classification of idiots. *London Hospital, Clinical Lecture and Report,* 3, 259–262.

Education Act (1981) HMSO, London.

Education (Handicapped Children) Act (1970) HMSO, London.

Ellis D. (1986) *Sensory Impairments in Mentally Handicapped People.* Croom Helm, London.

344 *Chapter 19*

Eyman R.K., Borthwick S.A. & Miller C. (1981) Trends in maladaptive behaviour of mentally retarded persons in community and institutional settings. *Journal of Mental Deficiency* 85, 473–477.

Eyman R.K. & Call T. (1977) Maladaptive behaviour and community placement of mentally retarded persons. *American Journal of Mental Deficiency*, 82, 137–144.

Garrod A.E. (1909) *Inborn Errors of Metabolism*. Oxford University Press, London.

Gath A. & Gumley D. (1986) Family background of children with Down's syndrome and of children with a similar degree of mental retardation. *British Journal of Psychiatry* 149, 161–171.

Grossman H.J. (1983) *Classification in Mental Retardation*. American Association on Mental Deficiency, Washington DC.

Gunn M.J. (1990) The law and learning disability. *International Review of Psychiatry* 2, 13–21.

Harris S.L., Wolchik S.A. & Weitz S. (1981) The acquisition of language skills by autistic children. Can parents do the job. *Journal of Autism and Developmental Disorder* 11, 373–384.

Hodapp R.M., Burack J.A. & Zigler E. (1990) *Issues in the Developmental Approach to Mental Retardation*. Cambridge University Press, New York.

Holland A.J. & Murphy G. (1990) Behavioural and psychiatric disorders in adults with mild learning difficulties. *International Review of Psychiatry*, 2, 117–136.

Hunt J. McV., Mohandessi I.K., Ghodssi M. & Akiyama M. (1976) The psychological development of orphanage reared infants: interventions with outcomes (Tehran). *Genetic Psychology (Monographs)* 94, 177–226.

Idiots Act (1866) HMSO, London.

Independent Living Council for People with Mental Handicap (1986) *Pursuing Quality: How Good Are Your Local Services for People with Mental Handicap?* IDC, London.

Jay Committee (1979) *Report of the Committee of Enquiry into Mental Handicap Nursing and Care*. Cmnd. 7468. HMSO, London.

Jones K.L. & Smith D.W. (1973) Recognition of the foetal alcohol syndrome in early infancy. *Lancet* ii, 999–1001.

King's Fund Centre (1980) *An Ordinary Life: Comprehensive Locally Based Residential Services for Mentally Handicapped People*. King's Fund Centre, London.

Lewis E.O. (1933) Types of mental deficiency and their social significance. *Journal of Mental Science* 79, 298–304.

Little R.E., Young A., Streissguth A.P. & Uhl C.N. (1984) Preventing fetal alcohol effects: effectiveness of a demonstration project. In Porter R., O'Connor M. & Whelan J. (eds) *Mechanisms of Alcohol Damage in Utero. Ciba Foundation Symposium, 105*. Pitman, London pp. 254–257.

Ludlow J.R. & Allen L.M. (1979) The effect of early intervention and pre-school stimulus on the development of the Down's syndrome child. *Journal of Mental Deficiency Research* 23, 29–45.

Mental Deficiency Act (1913) HMSO, London.

Mental Health Acts (1959, 1983) HMSO, London.

Miller K., Craddock-Watson J.E. & Pollock T.M. (1982) Consequences of confirmed maternal rubella at successive stages of pregnancy. *Lancet* ii, 781–784.

Nihira K., Meyers C.E. & Mink I.T. (1980) Home environment, family adjustment and the development of mentally retarded children. *Applied Research in Mental Retardation* 1, 5–24.

Nirje B. (1973) The Normalization principle: implications and comments. In Gunzberg A.C. (ed.) *Advances in the Care of the Mentally Handicapped*. Bailliére, Tindall, London.

Nursey A.D., Rohde J.R. & Farmer R.D.T. (1991) Ways of telling new parents about their child and his or her mental handicap: a comparison of doctors' and parents' views. *Journal of Mental Deficiency Research* 35, 48–57.

O'Brien J. (1987) A guide to personal futures planning. In Bellamy G.T. & Wilcox (eds) *A Comprehensive Guide to the Activities Catalog: An Alternative Curriculum for Youth and Adults with Severe Disabilities*. Paul H. Brookes, Baltimore, Maryland.

O'Brien J. & Tyne A. (1981) *The Principles of Normalization. A Foundation for Effective Services*. Campaign for Mentally Handicapped People, London.

O'Connor N. & Tizard J. (1954) A survey of patients in twelve mental deficiency institutes. *British Medical Journal* 1, 16–18.

Owens J.R., Harris F., Walsker S., McAllister E. & West L. (1983) The incidence of Down's syndrome over a 19 year period with special reference to maternal age. *Journal of Medical Genetics* 20, 90–93.

Porter R., O'Connor M. & Whelan J. (eds) (1984) *Mechanisms of Alcohol Damage in Utero. Ciba Foundation Symposium, 105*. Pitman, London.

Pratt O.E. (1984) What do we know of the mechanisms of alcohol damage in utero. In Porter R., O'Connor M. & Whelan J. (eds) *Mechanisms of Alcohol Damage in Utero. Ciba Foundation Symposium, 105*. Pitman, London, pp. 1–7.

Quine L. & Pahl L. (1985) Examining the causes of stress in families with severely handicapped children *British Journal of Social Work* 15, 501–517.

Reynolds D.W., Stagno S., Stubbs K.G. et al. (1974) Inapparent congenital cytomegalovirus infection and elevated cord IgM levels: causal relation with auditory and mental deficiency. *New England Journal of Medicine* 290, 291–296.

Richardson S.A. (1981) Family characteristics associated with mild mental retardation. In Begas M.J., Haywood H.C. & Garber H.L. (eds) *Psychological Influences in Retarded Performance*. University Park Press, Baltimore.

Rutter M., Graham P. & Yule W. (1970a) *A Neuropsychiatric Study in Childhood*. Spastics International Medical Publications, London.

Rutter M., Tizard J. & Whitmore K. (1970b) *Education, Health and Behaviour*. Longman, London.

Sarason S.B. & Doris J. (1969) *Psychological Problems in Mental Deficiency*, 4th edn. Harper, New York.

Scottish Council for Research in Education (1953) *Social Implications of the Scottish Mental Health Survey*. University of London Press, London.

Shearer A. (1985) *The Leading Edge: Community-based Services for People with Mental Handicap*. Campaign for the Mentally Handicapped and King's Fund Centre, London.

Solnit A.J. & Stark M.H. (1977) Mourning and the birth of a defective child. In Eissler R.S. (ed.) *Physical Illness and Handicap in Childhood*. Yale University Press, New Haven, Connecticut.

Stein Z. & Susser M. (1960) The families of dull children. A classification for predicting careers. *British Journal of Preventative and Social Medicine* 14, 85–88.

Thomas D., Firth H. & Kendall A. (1978) *ENCOR – A Way Ahead*. Campaign for the Mentally Handicapped, London.

Tizard J. (1984) Longitudinal Studies: Problems and findings. In Clarke A.M. & Clarke A.D.B. (eds) *Mental Deficiency: The Changing Outlook*. Methuen, London.

Tizard J. & O'Connor N. (1952) The occupational adaption of high-grade defectives. *Lancet* ii, 620.

Tizard J. & Tizard B. (1974) The institution as an environment for development. In Richards M.P. (eds) *The Integration of the Child into a Social World*. Cambridge University Press, Cambridge.

Tredgold A.F. (1952) *Mental Deficiency*, 8th edn. Baillière, Tindall, London.

Vernon P.E. (1979) *Intelligence, Heredity and Environment*. Freeman, San Francisco.

Ward L. (1982) *People First: Developing Services in the Community for People with Mental Handicap*. King's Fund Centre, London.

Ward L. (1984) *Planning for People: Developing a Local Service for People with Mental Handicap 1: Recruiting and Training Staff*. King's Fund Centre, London.

Wilkin D. (1979) *Caring for the Mentally Handicapped Child*. Croom Helm, London.

Wilkins E., Brown J.A. & Wolf B. (1980) Psychomotor development in 65 home-reared children with *cri-du-chat* syndrome. Journal of Paediatrics 97, 401–405.

Wilson C.B., Remington J.S., Stagno S. & Reynolds D.W. (1980) Development of adverse sequelae in children born with sub-clinical congenital toxoplasma infection. *Pediatrics* 66, 764–774.

Wolfensberger W. (1972) *The Principle of Normalisation in Human Services*. National Institute on Mental Retardation, Toronto.

Wolfensberger W. (1983) 'Social Role Valorization': A proposed new term for the principle of normalization. *Mental Retardation* 21, 234–239.

World Health Organization (1969) *Manual of the International Statistical Classification of Diseases, Injuries and Causes of Death*, 8th edn. World Health Organization, Geneva.

World Health Organization (1980) *International Classifications of Impairments, Disabilities and Handicaps*. World Health Organization, Geneva.

Zigler E. & Berman W. (1983) Discerning the future of early childhood intervention. *American Psychologist* 38, 894–906.

# Chapter 20
# Urbanization and Mental Disorder

TRUDY HARPHAM

## Introduction

Urbanization (the relative increase in the urban population as a proportion of the total) and its consequences has been one of the most widely discussed social issues of the last three decades. At the beginning of the last century the world's urban population totalled less than 50 million; today it exceeds 1.6 billion and the United Nations predicts a figure of 2.92 billion by the year 2000 (World Health Organization 1990). In 1980 it was predicted that 'in the next two decades, the world will undergo, as a result of the urbanization process, the most radical changes ever in social, economic and political life' (UNFPA 1980). This chapter considers the association between urbanization and mental disorders. As the author's experience is mainly in developing countries this is the focus of the discussion. The chapter covers urbanization in developing countries; the increasing attention to physical health in urban areas of these countries; the lack of attention paid to mental health; the debates within the literature; studies of mental health in urban areas, and provides a case study of a research project on maternal mental health in Rio de Janeiro, Brazil.

## Urbanization in developing countries and increasing interest in the health of the urban poor

In developing countries it is estimated that 44% of the population will be living in urban areas by the year 2000. Some Third World cities are expected to reach extremely large sizes by the end of the century: Mexico City 31 million; Sao Paulo 25.8 million; Rio de Janeiro, Bombay, Calcutta and Jakarta each exceeding 16 million; Seoul, Cairo, Manila exceeding 12 million (World Bank 1984). By the year 2000 the developing world is projected

to triple its cities of 5 million or more to 45 out of a world total of 60. However, only 23% of the urban population in the Third World will be living in cities with 4 million or more inhabitants by 2000 – most of the urban population will be living in smaller towns and cities (Hardoy & Satterthwaite 1986).

Although the above figures are useful in indicating trends, certain caveats must be borne in mind when using them. The definition of urban varies from country to country. For example in Peru urban centres are those with 100 or more occupied dwellings; in India they are settlements with 5000 or more inhabitants. Mostly definitions of this lower range fall between 1500 and 5000 people, but there are undoubtedly problems when comparing urban populations.

During any discussion of urbanization it is important to keep in mind that, contrary to what is often supposed, natural increase and not migration is the major factor for population increases. Natural increase is responsible for an average of 61% of urban population growth in developing countries compared to only 39% from rural migration (United Nations 1980).

While the developing world is in general undergoing urbanization at a rapid rate, there are major differences between countries and regions. Generally speaking those regions with lower absolute levels of urbanization, such as sub-Saharan Africa and parts of Asia, are in fact experiencing some of the highest levels of migration from rural to urban areas and the most rapid relative rates of urbanization.

The rapid growth in cities has been accompanied by a rapid growth in urban inhabitants who live in grossly substandard, overcrowded conditions without the funds for decent housing.

The figures available from cities in developing countries indicate that in the 1970s and 1980s slum and shanty town dwellers represented on average 30–60% of the urban population. Estimates are that, at present, an average of 50% of the urban population live at the level of extreme poverty, with this figure rising as high as 79% in some cities like Addis Ababa (Donohue 1982). Assuming that in the year 2000 one-half of the urban population will still be of low income, over 1 billion people will be counted among the urban poor. Good, comprehensive accounts of urbanization in developing countries can be found in Gugler (1988) and Drakakis-Smith (1987).

This rapid urbanization in developing countries has received a growing amount of attention by health workers. Although in the 1970s and early 1980s primary health care in developing countries had a distinctly rural focus, there are now a number of research studies and health programmes focusing upon poor urban populations. Many of these studies and programmes are described in the two books that have been written about urban health in developing countries, by Harpham *et al.* (1988) and Tabibzadeh *et al.* (1989). Most of the studies reviewed in these books emphasize that the urban poor are at the interface between underdevelopment and industrialization and their disease patterns reflect the problems of both. From the first they carry a heavy burden of infectious diseases and malnutrition, while from the second they suffer the typical spectrum of chronic and social diseases (Rossi-Espagnet 1984). Ekblad (1990) similarly suggests that three major pathologies are emerging in low-income urban settlements:

1 Infectious and gastrointestinal diseases (often termed 'diseases of poverty').
2 Chronic degenerative diseases.
3 Conditions associated with the stress precipitated by social isolation, insecurity, dissolution of primary family relations and cultural conflicts.

Although studies and programmes recognize the wide range of health problems that the urban poor experience, action still focuses upon physical health while very little attention is paid to mental health. Mental health has not been brought into the domain of primary health care within these settings. Possible reasons for this include perceptions that it is difficult to measure the problem of mental ill-health and even if the extent of the problem was measured, there are few guidelines for action at the community level.

## Urbanization and mental health – the debates within the literature

### Urban–rural differences

When reviewing the literature on urbanization and mental health one finds several contradictory studies. Cheng (1989) points out that the notion that urbanization has adverse effects on mental health has been held by many medical and social scientists. The rapid urbanization described above is commonly associated with noise, people earning a low wage, high population density, social isolation and poor physical environment – factors which might well be related to an excess of psychiatric morbidity. In contrast, the supportive traditional rural life pattern is believed to be beneficial to mental health (Klerman 1969, Greenblatt 1970, Fromm 1973, Murphy & Taumoepeau 1980). Dohrenwend & Dohrenwend (1974) reviewing and summarizing data concluded that eight out of ten studies reported a higher frequency of mental disorder in urban populations than in rural ones, the increase being mainly in neuroses and personality disorders. However, Cheng (1989) found no rural–urban difference in overall minor psychiatric morbidity in Taiwan and pointed out that this was in agreement with surveys in developed countries including the USA (Comstock & Helsing 1976), Australia (Krupinski 1979) and Great Britain (Brown & Prudo 1981). Ekblad (1990) notes that culture might exert a strong influence on the relationship between urbanization and health and highlights the study by Shen *et al.* (1985) in China which also found lowest rates of psychiatric morbidity in urban areas. Cheng (1989) suggests that the notion of an adverse effect of urbanization on psychological wellbeing is probably misleading and stresses that social risk factors may be specific to a particular community. Burvill (1982) suggests that every society may produce its own specific stresses, and that these stresses are no more frequent in industrialized, urbanized society but merely different in type.

### Intra-urban differences

An increasing amount of studies are being undertaken to highlight differences *within* cities in terms of physical health (see Harpham *et al.* (1988) for a full review of these). For example, the urban poor can experience infant mortality rates which are nearly three times as high as the average figure given for a city as a whole (Manila); malnutrition and parasitic infections are severe health problems for the urban poor in contrast to their urban neighbours (Singapore, Delhi, Bogota, Manila); postneonatal mortality predominates over neonatal mortality among the urban poor while the reverse is true for the higher socioeconomic classes (Porto Alegre). Very little research is available on intra-urban differences in *mental* health. Ekblad (1990) provides a good summary of the issues of 'social drift' and 'social residue' which are key concepts in any discussion of intra-urban differences in mental health. Social drift is a tendency for people with particular characteristics to move to particular areas and social residue is the tendency for people with particular characteristics to be left behind when the better-adjusted members of the population move out. Ekblad explains that which of the two processes is more powerful may depend on whether migrants are primarily pushed (perhaps due to impoverished rural areas forcing them to move to shanty towns without much opportunity of improving their conditions) or pulled (as in many western societies, where people move with realistic aspirations, acquiring better jobs in urban areas). 'It . . . seems that explanations of area differences (in mental health) are likely to come from studies of the process whereby populations with particular characteristics come to inhabit particular areas rather than by focusing on the physical environment' (Ekblad 1990, p. 119). In other words, this moves us away from an 'environmental determinism' approach to one in which social, economic and political factors are viewed as key variables in the relationship between urbanization and mental health. There is a need for more research which addresses these

variables in an analysis of intra-urban differences in mental health. Such research will require community-based studies rather than clinic-based studies which are unrepresentative of the wider community.

### A review of selected studies of mental health in urban areas

Most of the studies which provide an indication of the prevalence of psychiatric morbidity in urban areas of developing countries use structured interviews, such as the Present State Examination (PSE) or an interview form of the Self Response Questionnaire – 20 items (SRQ20). A series of international collaborative studies conducted by the World Health Organization used these types of methods. Leff (1990) has pointed out that these methods have been criticized by advocates of the 'new cross-cultural psychiatry' for imposing western concepts of psychopathology on non-western populations – 'psychiatric imperialism'. Most of the studies reviewed here are open to this criticism and although Leff's (1990) suggestions of involving anthropologists and undertaking genuinely collaborative studies are welcomed, this approach to research is not yet widely developed. The studies reviewed below include a mixture of health service-based studies (e.g. clinic attenders) and population- or community-based studies (e.g. random household surveys).

Some of the more useful published studies of psychiatric morbidity in developing country urban settings include:
- Alam (1978) found a 39% prevalence of psychiatric morbidity in his general practice survey in Dhaka, Bangladesh.
- Busnello *et al.* (1983) reported a prevalence of 55.4% in their study of 242 consecutive attenders in a primary health care centre in Porto Alegre, Brazil.
- Sen *et al.* (1987) used a two-stage design (SRQ20) and the Clinical Interview Schedule (CIS) and found a prevalence of minor psychiatric morbidity of 46% in a study of primary medical care settings in Calcutta.
- Mari (1987) used the PSE and CIS with primary care attenders in Sao Paulo, Brazil and found a

prevalence of minor psychiatric morbidity of 45–63% in three clinics.

• Rahim & Cederblad's (1989) survey of 204 adults in Khartoum, Sudan in which a wide range of methods were used including the SRQ, found that 40% had at least one psychiatric symptom, in 23.7% this was mild but in the remaining 16.6% it was moderate to severe.

• Cheng (1989) used modified Chinese versions of the SRQ and CIS with 1050 randomly selected subjects from rural, suburban and urban Taiwan. There was no significant difference in minor psychiatric morbidity between the three communities, with an average of 24.1%.

• Chakraborty (1990) used a 'Household Survey Questionnaire and Interview' method in Calcutta with 13 335 persons and found 13.8% with a 'broad category of mental disorder'.

At this stage it is necessary to introduce a note of caution about the methods described above. Goldberg (1972) has referred to the kinds of methods used in most of the above studies as 'complaints inventories' and suggests that they 'merely represent a "tabulation of misery"' . . . especially true for individuals of low social class, since miseries and dissatisfaction are universally found in people of low status in industrial societies'. This point is likely to be even more pertinent for residents of slums in developing countries. Screening questionnaires can be regarded as useful survey instruments, but it remains unclear whether they measure psychiatric illness or part of the normal range of emotional responses to life events. Many of these illnesses are transient affective disorders (Goldberg 1972) and these assessments should not therefore be regarded as an index of permanent psychiatric disability. However, use of instruments like this is bound to increase, particularly when health professionals working in fields like 'urban health' are realizing the need to address issues of mental health and therefore the need to measure mental health in a community-based manner. It is vital that psychiatrists actively educate and update primary health care workers about the most useful assessment methods available. This requires psychiatrists to publish in non-specialized journals and to bring their knowledge to community health forums.

## The need to study risk factors – a case study in Rio de Janeiro

There is a need to move beyond studies which merely measure the prevalence of psychiatric morbidity in urban areas. The social risk factors which are associated with mental ill-health in urban areas need to be identified and communicated to primary health care workers. As Cheng (1989) has pointed out, these social risk factors may be specific to a particular community but this does not reduce their importance. Any attempt to generalize the results of studies again produces a confusion of literature. For example, in a review of the epidemiology of mental disorders in Latin America, Almeida-Filho (1987) dismisses migration as a factor associated with mental disorders but identifies the socioeconomic situation in which migration takes place as the main factor associated with mental disorder. However, the results of an earlier study of his (Almeida-Filho & Bastos 1982) showed a higher risk of depressive disorders among migrant women, even after controlling for occupation, educational status and marital status.

As an example of a study which analyses risk factors, a case study of maternal mental health in a large squatter settlement in Rio de Janeiro, Brazil is presented below. This research was conducted under the PhD programme at the London School of Hygiene and Tropical Medicine and full details of methods can be found in Reichenheim (1988).

Rocinha is the largest squatter settlement in Rio de Janeiro and occupies an area of about half a square kilometre in the core of the city's well-off district. The squatter settlement's population is a disputed issue. Census figures quote 32 966 inhabitants whereas locals estimate 300 000. According to this study the population is around 60 000. This in itself reflects the problems faced by the researchers in taking adequately representative samples.

Within Rocinha the population is quite heterogeneous. To put this differential into perspective, the average monthly earnings in a household of five individuals belonging to the lower-income quartile was £63, whereas the earning for a family of four in the upper-income quartile was £279.

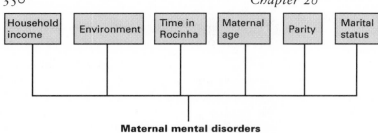

**Maternal mental disorders**                    Fig. 20.1  The variables in the study.

The variables considered within the study are presented in Fig. 20.1. The survey was carried out in two stages. First, a sampling frame of households with mothers rearing children under the age of five years was established by undertaking censuses in randomly selected areas of Rocinha. The first stage sampling frame consisted of the 30 enumeration districts of Rocinha used in the 1980 Brazilian Census. One thousand and forty-eight mothers with under-fives were found in the ten screened areas. Secondly, a structured questionnaire was administered at the household level to a subsample of 480 randomly selected mothers. The response rate was 95.8%. No information was available about the non-respondents.

Originally, the SRQ20 was conceived as a self-completion questionnaire. It has been recommended that in countries where the level of literacy is low, the indirect application of the SRQ20 by health workers is more suitable (Mari 1987). The SRQ20 was designed by Harding *et al.* (1980) and has been validated against in-depth psychiatric questionnaires in Colombia, Sudan, India and the Philippines, with sensitivities ranging from 73% to 83% and specificities ranging from 72% to 85%. The SRQ20 has been further validated in other studies in Kenya and Brazil with similar sensitivities and specificities. The confidence in the choice of using the SRQ20 comes from the fact that it has been tested and validated twice in Brazilian urban settings (Busnello *et al.* 1983, Mari 1987). Thus, it offered the advantage of being available in its Portuguese version without the need for field testing the translation.

The SRQ20 is composed of 20 yes/no questions – 4 on physical symptoms and 16 on psycho-emotional disturbances. For analytical purposes, low and high scorers were defined as mothers with scores less than or equal to seven, and equal to or above eight, respectively. This was accepted after Mari's (1987) findings that the 7/8 cut-off point was the best trade-off between high sensitivity and low false positives for the adult female population in urban Sao Paulo. One point must be borne in mind throughout the interpretation of the results. The finding is a *proportion of probable cases* and not an estimate of true prevalence of psychiatric disorders. The latter cannot be obtained from the present study because its calculation involves comparing the SRQ20 with a clinical examination. This again is a problem that social psychiatrists need to address. The other variables in the model were collected by a household questionnaire.

Table 20.1 shows the profile of the mothers according to each component of the SRQ20. The items that most frequently contributed to high scores were, in decreasing order, tenseness, sadness, frequent headaches, frequent frights, and thinking and decision-making difficulties. All these were present in more than 40% of mothers. Anxiety symptoms (questions 3, 4, 5, 6 and 8) were the most prevalent. Seventy-eight per cent of mothers answered they were nervous, tense or worried. This may be a manifestation following a state of hypervigilance coupled with the feelings of helplessness and dependency. The lack of control over the setting in which the stressor occurs is believed to be as important as the stressor itself (Stokols 1978).

Depression symptoms (questions 9–18 and 20), though not so frequent, are relevant for their salience. Crying more than usual, a feeling of worthlessness, inability to play a useful role in life culminating with thoughts of suicide is a gloomy picture affecting at least one-sixth of the mothers interviewed. This suggests a grave social and do-

**Table 20.1** Self Response Questionnaire (SRQ20) profile

| | | Yes | |
|---|---|---|---|
| | | No. | % |
| 1 | Do you often have headaches? | 212 | 46 |
| 2 | Is your appetite poor? | 139 | 30 |
| 3 | Do you sleep badly? | 125 | 27 |
| 4 | Are you easily frightened? | 209 | 45 |
| 5 | Do your hands shake? | 130 | 28 |
| 6 | Do you feel nervous, tense, worried? | 358 | 78 |
| 7 | Is your digestion poor? | 115 | 25 |
| 8 | Do you have trouble thinking clearly? | 186 | 40 |
| 9 | Do you feel unhappy? | 218 | 47 |
| 10 | Have you been crying more than usual? | 95 | 21 |
| 11 | Do you find it difficult to enjoy your daily activities? | 153 | 33 |
| 12 | Do you find it difficult to make decisions? | 196 | 43 |
| 13 | Is your daily work suffering? | 88 | 19 |
| 14 | Are you unable to play a useful role in life? | 89 | 20 |
| 15 | Have you lost interest in things? | 127 | 28 |
| 16 | Do you feel you are a worthless person? | 72 | 16 |
| 17 | Has the thought of ending your life been in your mind? | 68 | 15 |
| 18 | Do you feel tired all the time? | 150 | 33 |
| 19 | Do you have uncomfortable feelings in your stomach? | 119 | 26 |
| 20 | Are you easily tired? | 143 | 31 |

mestic state of crisis which deserves more attention than has been hitherto given.

The proportion of probable cases of mental disorders was 36%. Although in a strict clinical sense the states described above are different ones, the term mental disorders will be used below as a summary term meaning interchangeably the psychosomatic, depression and anxiety symptoms. This is acceptable for two reasons. First, because the distinction between depressive and anxiety states in the community setting is unclear (Goldberg & Huxley 1980). Second, as Webb (1984) argues, the combined use of psychological and psychosomatic symptoms has more validity when measuring the overall psychiatric health of a population than in institution-based data where there is a need to discriminate between the symptoms for therapeutic purposes.

This finding is striking if one considers that almost all other prevalence figures were collected in clinical settings which have a selection bias towards overestimation. Consistent with this study, are the clinically based findings of Busnello *et al.* (55.4%) and Mari (50%).

The factors tested for association with maternal mental disorders are presented in Table 20.2. The lower the household income, the worse the physical housing conditions and the less educated the mother, the higher the chance of being mentally disturbed. Marital status showed a borderline association with mental disorders due to the relatively small number of partnerless mothers. The direction of the association, though, agrees with theory showing an excess of mothers with mental disorders in the partnerless group. Parity and teenage (adolescent) motherhood were not associated with mental disorders. Length of residence in Rocinha – migration status – did not show a statistically significant association with mental disorder. The number of suicidal thoughts among mothers suggests an acute social and domestic state of crisis. The maternal mental health status in the lowest socioeconomic group is particularly critical, with probable mental disorders among nearly 50% of mothers.

This study indicates the extent of mental disorder in a poor urban community but also indicates the differences within a community (intra-urban

**Table 20.2** Bivariate associations with maternal mental disorders

| Variable | Cases per stratum | % with mental disorders | Relative risk | P-value of association |
|---|---|---|---|---|
| *Income per capita* | | | | |
| Low (lower quartile) | 112 | 47.3 | 1.6 | |
| Middle (mid quartiles) | 225 | 33.8 | 1.1 | 0.016 |
| High (upper quartile) | 123 | 30.3 | 1.0 | |
| *Environmental conditions** | | | | |
| Bad (score 0–8) | 87 | 48.3 | 1.4 | |
| Moderate (score 9–13) | 233 | 33.1 | 0.95 | 0.037 |
| Good (score 14–17) | 138 | 15.0 | 1.0 | |
| *Maternal education*[†] | | | | |
| Unschooled | 263 | 40.7 | 1.3 | |
| Schooled | 195 | 30.7 | 1.0 | 0.029 |
| *Maternal age* | | | | |
| Teenager (<20 years) | 31 | 35.5 | 0.97 | |
| Non-teenager (20+ years) | 428 | 36.4 | 1.0 | 0.785 |
| *Marital status* | | | | |
| Partnerless | 72 | 45.8 | 1.4 | |
| Living with partner | 376 | 34.0 | 1.0 | 0.056 |
| *Parity* | | | | |
| >3 offspring | 172 | 41.3 | 1.4 | |
| 2–3 offspring | 136 | 36.0 | 1.2 | 0.130 |
| 1 offspring | 145 | 30.3 | 1.1 | |
| *Maternal length of residence in Rocinha* | | | | |
| ≤3 years (recent migr.) | 109 | 37.6 | 1.2 | |
| 4 ≤ 9 years (intermed. migr.) | 137 | 40.1 | 1.3 | 0.292 |
| ≥10 years (long-term migr.) | 117 | 35.0 | 1.1 | |
| Naturals | 96 | 31.2 | 1.0 | |

* The overall environmental condition of a household was derived through a scoring system from the following conditions: crowding, housing material, floor material, availability of electricity, type of waste disposal facility inside the household, type of waste disposal facility outside the household, water source and garbage disposal facilities.
[†] Mothers were defined as unschooled if they were illiterate or if they had not finished primary school (first four years).
Source: Reichenheim & Harpham (1991).

differentials) and highlights the importance of certain social risk factors for mental disorder. The social risk factors that emerge in this study highlight the importance of maternal education which has, interestingly, also been identified as one of the main determinants of child survival (i.e. of infant and child mortality) in developing countries. (Cleland & van Ginneken 1989). The risk factors also include poverty and poor environmental conditions. These are factors which are repeatedly

identified as having an independent association with ill-health among the urban poor in general. Whether these risk factors for mental disorder are similar in different communities within countries, or even between countries, is not yet known and more research is needed in this area. Primary health care is increasingly important in rapidly growing poor urban communities in developing countries. If the wide range of health problems of the urban poor are to be addressed, health workers need to be presented with the results of the kind of research suggested above. In this way, in addition to developing our knowledge base about urbanization and mental disorder, research can play the vital role of stimulating action.

# References

Alam M.N. (1978) Psychiatric morbidity in general practice. *Bangladesh Medical Research Council Bulletin* 4, 38–42.

Almeida-Filho N. (1987) Social epidemiology of mental disorders: a review of Latin American studies. *Acta Psychiatrica Scandinavica* 75, 1–10.

Almeida-Filho N. & Bastos S.B. (1982) Estudo caso-controle da associacao entre migracao e desordens depressivas em mulheres. *Journal Brasileiro de Psiquiatria* 31, 25–29.

Brown G.W. & Prudo R. (1981) Psychiatric disorder in a rural and an urban population. 1. Aetiology of depression. *Psychological Medicine* II, 581–599.

Burvill P.W. (1982) The epidemiology of psychiatric illness in industrialized society. *Australia and New Zealand Journal of Psychiatry* 16, 144–151.

Busnello E.L., Lima B. & Bertolote J.M. (1983) Aspectos interculturais de classificacao e diagnostico. *Journal of Brazilian Psychiatry* 32, 207–210.

Chakraborty A. (1990) *Social Stress and Mental Health: A Social–psychiatric Field Study of Calcutta.* Sage, London.

Cheng T.A. (1989) Urbanization and minor psychiatric morbidity. *Social Psychiatry and Psychiatric Epidemiology* 24, 309–316.

Cleland J. & van Ginneken J. (1989) Maternal schooling and child mortality. In Hill A.G. & Roberts D.S. (eds) Health intervention and mortality change in developing countries. *Journal of Biosocial Research* (suppl 10), 13–14.

Comstock G.W. & Helsing K.J. (1976) Symptoms of depression in two communities. *Psychological Medicine* 6, 551–563.

Dohrenwend B.P. & Dohrenwend B.S. (1974) Psychiatric disorders in urban settings. In Arieti S. & Caplan G. (eds) *American Handbook of Psychiatry*, 2nd edn, vol. 29. Basic Books, New York.

Donohue J.J. (1982) Facts and figures on urbanization in the developing world. *Assignment Children* 57/58, 21–41.

Drakakis-Smith D. (1987) *The Third World City.* Methuen, London.

Ekblad S. (1990) Family stress and mental health during rapid urbanization. In Nordberg E. & Finer D. (eds) *Society, Environment and Health in Low-income Countries.* Karolinska Institute, Stockholm.

Fromm E. (1973) *The Anatomy of Human Destructiveness.*

Holt, Rinehart and Winston, New York.

Goldberg D.P. (1972) *The Detection of Psychiatric Illness by Questionnaire. Maudsley Monograph* 21. Oxford University Press, Oxford.

Goldberg D.P. & Huxley P. (1980) *Mental Illness in the Community: The Pathway to Psychiatric Care.* Tavistock, London.

Greenblatt M. (1970) The troubled mind in the troubled city. *Comprehensive Psychiatry* 11, 8–17.

Gugler J. (1988) *The Urbanization of the Third World.* Oxford University Press, Oxford.

Harding T.W., Arango M.V., Baltazar J. (1980) Mental disorders in primary health care: a study of the frequency and diagnosis in four developing countries. *Psychological Medicine* 10, 231–241.

Hardoy J.E. & Satterthwaite D.E. (1986) *Small and Intermediate Urban Centres in the Third World: Their Role in National and Regional Development.* Hodder and Stoughton, London.

Harpham T., Lusty T. & Vaughan P.J.V. (1988) *In the Shadow of the City: Community Health and the Urban Poor.* Oxford University Press, Oxford.

Klerman G.L. (1969) Mental health and the urban crisis. *American Journal Of Orthopsychiatry* 39, 818–826.

Krupinski J. (1979) Urbanization and mental health. *Australia and New Zealand Journal of Psychiatry* 13, 139–145.

Leff J. (1990) The new cross-cultural psychiatry: editorial. *British Journal of Psychiatry* 156, 305–307.

Mari J.J. (1987) Psychiatric morbidity in three primary medical care clinics in the city of Sao Paulo: issues on the mental health of the urban poor. *Social Psychiatry* 22, 129–138.

Murphy H.B.M. & Taumoepeau B.M. (1980) Traditionalism and mental health in the South Pacific: a re-examination of an old hypothesis. *Psychological Medicine* 10, 471–482.

Rahim S.I.A. & Cederblad M. (1989) Epidemiology of mental disorders in young adults of a newly urbanized area in Khartoum, Sudan. *British Journal of Psychiatry* 155, 44–47.

Reichenheim M. (1988) *Child Health in an Urban Context: Risk Factors in a Squatter Settlement of Rio de Janeiro.* PhD, London University.

Reichenheim M. & Harpham T. (1991) Maternal mental health in a squatter settlement in Rio de Janeiro. *British Journal of Psychiatry* 159, 683–690.

Rossi-Espagnet A. (1984) *Primary Health Care in Urban Areas: Reaching the Urban Poor in Developing Countries.* A state of the art report by UNICEF and WHO. Report number 2499M. World Health Organization, Geneva.

Sen B., Wilkinson G. & Mari J.J. (1987) Psychiatric morbidity in primary health care: a two stage screening procedure in developing countries – cost effectiveness and choice of instruments. *British Journal of Psychiatry* 151, 33–39.

Shen Y.C., Wang Y.F. & Yang X.L. (1985) An epidemiological investigation of minimal brain disfunction in six elementary schools in Beijing. *Journal of Child Psychology and Psychiatry* 1, 11–20.

Stokols D. (1978) Environmental psychology. *Annual Review of Psychology* 29, 253–295.

Tabibzadeh I., Rossi-Espagnet A. & Maxwell R. (1989) *Spotlight on the Cities: Improving Urban Health in Developing Countries*. World Health Organization, Geneva.

United Nations (1980) Patterns of urban and rural population growth. *United Nations Population Studies No. 68.* Department of International Economic and Social Affairs, United Nations, New York.

UNFPA (1980) *Rome Declaration on Population and the Urban Future*. International Conference on Population and the Urban Future, UNFPA, Rome, 1–4 September 1980.

Webb S.D. (1984) Rural–urban differences in mental health. In Freeman H.L. (ed.) *Mental Health and the Environment*. Churchill Livingstone, Edinburgh.

World Bank (1984) *World Development Report 1984*. Oxford University Press, New York.

World Health Organization (1990) *Global Estimates for Health Situation Assessment and Projections 1990*. Division of Epidemiological Surveillance and Health Situation and Trend Assessment, WHO, Geneva.

# Chapter 21

# Unemployment, Poverty and Homelessness

## DINESH BHUGRA

### Introduction

Unemployment, poverty and homelessness are three social factors that may occur separately, and singly or together produce enough psychological stress in the vulnerable to bring them to the psychiatrist. This chapter focuses on the psychological and psychiatric implications of these three states. We shall not review social policy responsible for these states here. It must be stated at the outset that the definitions of all these states vary according to authors and their professional background. Hence each section will start with an attempt at definition followed by the impact of each state. As Warr (1987) points out, the five components of mental health are: affective well-being, competence, autonomy, aspirations and integrated functioning. He goes on to draw a distinction between job-related mental health and context-free mental health.

Figure 21.1 illustrates various factors that may affect physical and mental health of the individual. Unemployment often leads to poverty which leads to poor health and higher mortality. In addition occasionally poverty may lead to homelessness. Living conditions, poor health and limited access to statutory health services can contribute to precipitation as well as perpetuation of ill-health. It must be emphasized that this chapter does not purport to offer a comprehensive review of these states (for these see Townsend 1979, Hayes & Nutman 1981, Kelvin & Jarrett 1983, Lamb 1984, Fryer & Ullah 1987, Warr 1987, Smith 1987, Dumont 1989).

### Unemployment

Unemployment has been distinguished from lack of work. Employment has been defined as 'the work we do for money whereas work is a much broader category' (Smith 1987). Unemployment is seen as a state of worklessness experienced by people who see themselves or are seen by others as potential members of the work-force (Hayes & Nutman 1981). This latter definition obviously includes perception of others, which as we shall see later is very much linked to the Protestant Work Ethic – thereby adding stigma to the consequences of unemployment. The notions of work have shifted from the productive effort itself to a predominantly social relationship. Job loss is defined as a premature involuntary termination of employment (Hayes & Nutman 1981). Thus a distinction needs to be made between those who retire voluntarily or retire involuntarily at the normal retirement age for their occupational group and those who have been made redundant or have never entered the job market. The individual's reactions to states vary, as will become clearer later in this section.

Employment is not itself an activity but an institutionalized social relationship (Fryer & Ullah 1987). It is argued that employment is a voluntary but institutionally regulated contractual exchange relationship between two parties, one of whom wishes to sell work and the other to buy it. This relationship entails rights and responsibilities, the province of powerful social norms and legislation on both sides (Fryer & Payne 1986). There are, however, several questions that need to be addressed in the relationship of unemployment with physical and mental ill-health.

### Historical studies

One of the earliest studies in the field of psychological consequences of unemployment was that of Jahoda and her colleagues (see Jahoda *et al.*

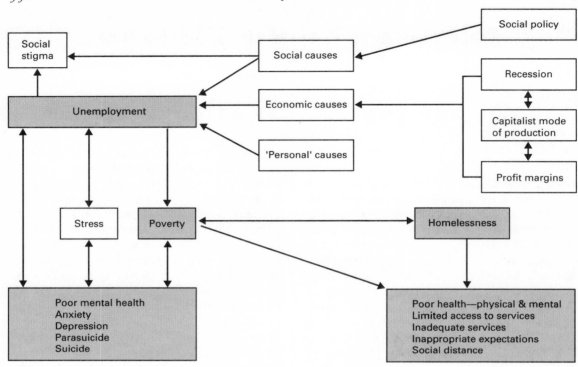

**Fig. 21.1** Interaction of unemployment, poverty, homelessness and poor health.

1933/1972, Fryer 1987, 1989, 1990 for further discussion). Marienthal (population 1986), a few miles south-east of Vienna, was clustered around a textiles factory which until 1922 provided employment for virtually the whole village. By 1930 the factory had completely shut down, by which time 77% of the families had not a single employed member. Most of the field-work for the Marienthal study was carried out in a period of six weeks, although 120 working days were spent there (Jahoda *et al.* 1933/1972). A thorough-going triangulation model was employed because 'psychological self-observations cannot be expected of working-class people' (Lazarsfeld 1932), and in addition it was necessary to avoid injuring the susceptibilities of the distressed population. The researchers became a part of the community, a method used again by Jahoda in Monmouth-shire a few years later (Jahoda 1987). The dominant finding was that of resignation – 70% of the families were placed into this category –

defined as 'no relation to the future, no hopes, extreme restriction of all needs beyond the bare necessities'. Despair and apathy were noted in smaller numbers though nearly a quarter of the families maintained household, care of the children, subjective well-being and hopes for the future (Jahoda *et al.* 1933/1972). The authors acknowledge that despair and apathy are probably two different stages of a process of psychological deterioration that is parallel to the narrowing of economic resources. Employment according to Jahoda (1979) offers six latent functions: imposing time structure on the working day; regular shared experiences and contact (often) outside the family; a link with transcending goals and purposes; definition of aspects of personal status and identity; enforced activity, and a control function (Jahoda 1986). Soon after her arrival in the UK, Jahoda was involved in a similar study in Monmouthshire (Jahoda 1987). Here, the Subsistence Production Society (SPS) was set up in 1935, with its central feature being cooperation of a number of unemployed men in producing goods to be used for their own subsistence and not for sale in the open market. Based on the ideas of the Order of Friends – the men got no wages – they purchased the products of their work and paid prices calculated on the basics of the cost of the raw materials plus 20% for overhead costs. They continued to receive their unemployment benefits. Buhler (1933) described the analysis of activity in various aspects of life and divided it into five stages: first stage of childhood and adolescence (dependency); period of transition (trial and error), leading on to third stage of full vitality (definite, settled characters); fourth stage was a decline in vitality (employment became the dominating feature) and last stage of restriction in vitality and work. Under normal circumstances most individuals go through these; however, when external economic conditions are stringent a straight passage though these stages is not possible. Interactions with external factors may lead to more stress (for further discussion see Jahoda 1987). Two additional spheres of action – 'abstract' thought processes dealing with ideology, be it political or religious, and 'real' thought processes which have to do with daily life, thereby directing actual behaviour – contribute to psychological functioning of the individual. Over a period of four years the work of SPS blossomed into a diversified production, distribution and consumption centre. Among the members once again resignation was noted. However, Jahoda (1987) reported that in Monmouthshire nothing worse than resignation was noted, and this was assumed to be due to the 'size and permanence of the unemployment allowance in Wales'. The difference in consumption power in the two communities was significant for psychological well-being (Fryer 1987).

In the 1930s, there were some impressive investigations into the psychological effects of unemployment (Bakke 1933, 1940a,b, Israeli 1935, Pilgrim Trust Report 1938). Bakke's field-work, initially in Greenwich, London and then in New Haven, used a combination of strategies – participant observation, interviews, time budget analysis and document analysis – and revealed widespread psychological debilitation, economic insecurity, exhaustion, poor self-esteem and reduced social contact and despondency. Hopelessness was a common theme running through these studies. Macky & Haines (1982) remark that today's psychology of unemployment is remarkably similar to that of earlier portrayals. A general conclusion was that the unemployed suffered emotional instability (Brandt 1932), general depression (Lewis 1935), reactive depression, loss of morale (Elderston 1931), poor occupational morale (Hall 1934), loss of self-confidence and status (Eisenberg & Lazarsfeld 1938), prestige (Pratt 1933) and self-esteem (Bakke 1933, Kardiner 1936). Individuals became fearful (Beckman 1933), discouraged, distrustful (Rundquist & Sletto 1936), bitter and antagonistic towards employing classes (Hall 1934), hopeless (Jahoda *et al.* 1933/1972) and aimless (Zawadski & Lazarsfeld 1935). A loss of sense of time (Fischer & Heimann 1933), and feelings of apathy (Zawadski & Lazarsfeld 1935) were reported.

## Psychological impact

In the mid 1980s with a massive increase in the numbers of unemployed, researchers started looking at various psychological sequelae of unemployment. In 1971, Murray Parkes had proposed the notion of psychosocial transitions defined as 'those major changes in life space which are lasting in their effects, take place over a relatively short period of time and which affect large areas of the assumptive world'. This concept is fairly similar to those of life events (also see Chapters 7 and 10). In life events terms loss of job rates fairly high and chronic unemployment would be construed as a chronic difficulty. We shall initially focus on unemployment as an acute job loss and its impact. Here parallels can be drawn with Bowlby's (1978) concept of loss. After initial shock in the newly unemployed, optimism yields to pessimism fairly soon and fatalism follows (Harrison 1976). Similarly Hill (1977, 1978) proposed three phases: initial response (possibly traumatic accompanied with denial); intermediate phase of a kind of inertia;

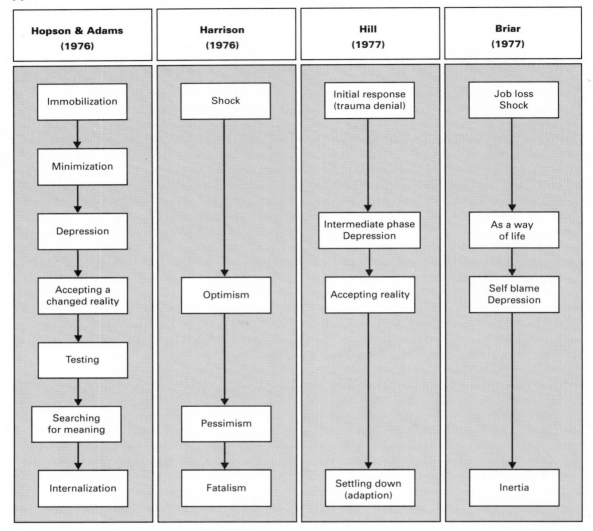

| Hopson & Adams (1976) | Harrison (1976) | Hill (1977) | Briar (1977) |
|---|---|---|---|
| Immobilization | Shock | Initial response (trauma denial) | Job loss Shock |
| Minimization | | | |
| Depression | | Intermediate phase Depression | As a way of life |
| Accepting a changed reality | Optimism | Accepting reality | Self blame Depression |
| Testing | | | |
| Searching for meaning | Pessimism | | |
| Internalization | Fatalism | Settling down (adaption) | Inertia |

**Fig. 21.2** Models of loss and phases post unemployment.

followed by a third phase of settling down to unemployment. Other authors (Eisenberg & Lazarsfeld 1938, Hopson & Adams 1976, Briar 1977) have reported similar phases (Fig. 21.2).

In the more recent studies the findings of psychological research on unemployment mirror those of the 1930s. Unemployment has been reported to be associated with unhappiness (Campbell *et al.* 1976), high rates of stress (Cobb *et al.* 1966, Cobb & Kasl 1977), psychiatric disorder (Fried 1969, Gove & Geerken 1977, Rueth & Heller 1981), psychiatric morbidity (Banks *et al.* 1980, Brenner & Bartell 1983, Kemp & Mercer 1983), depression (Fisher 1965, Hill 1977, Jackson & Warr 1983), externality (Tiffany *et al.* 1970, Kasl & Cobb 1971) and worry (Warr 1978). In addition poor subjective well-being (Miles 1983), emotional instability (Shanthamani 1973) hypochondria and anxiety (Fisher 1965) have been observed. On a more personal level low self-esteem (Sheppard 1965, Tiffany *et al.* 1969, 1970, Schlozman & Verba 1978), self-worth

(Harrison 1976), self-concept (Kingsley 1976, McGann & Kenny 1977), self-confidence (Jackson & Warr 1983), self-respect (Goffman 1969, Daniel 1972) and status (Hepworth 1980) have been reported. Dissatisfaction with accomplishment (Schlozman & Verba 1978), distrust (Cobb & Kasl 1977), insecurity and helplessness (Leavy & Freedman 1961, Payne *et al.* 1983) and narrow outlook (Gould 1971) have been reported with unemployment.

At a more epidemiological level Brenner's work (1971, 1973, 1976) has attracted quite a lot of attention. Using New York State's fluctuation in the employment index, Brenner (1973) found a strong inverse relationship between unemployment and physical and psychological morbidity. (For a critique of Brenner's methodology, see Kasl 1979, Marshall & Funch 1979.) Using historical data, Brenner (1971, 1976) reported an increase in murder, manslaughter, rape, robbery, embezzlement, fraud, arson, burglary and larceny as result of adverse change in employment and income in the USA, Canada, England and Wales and Scotland. Gravelle *et al.* (1981) argued that Brenner overestimated the mortality costs of high unemployment and reanalysed his data to show that there was no direct connection between the two during the period 1922–76.

Socioeconomic status prior to unemployment plays an important role in dealing with the effects of unemployment. The higher the socioeconomic status, the more support and financial resources there may be available, and therefore such individuals may be less exposed to deleterious life changes. Studies have shown that managers are less affected by unemployment than workers (Schlozman & Verba 1978, Buss & Redburn 1983). In one sample, 48% of the individuals expressed a positive attitude towards job loss (Little 1976), whereas 35% were noted to have a positive attitude in another sample (Fineman 1983). In the latter study anxiety levels were reported to be normal.

Low stress is thus related to control in terms of electing for redundancy and where personal involvement in the previous job was low. Also in such individuals, unemployment was seen in low-threat terms and belief in personal worth and confidence. More managers were less affected by steel plant closure than mill workers.

Prior high involvement in the job and belief in one's personal competence, associated domestic difficulties, repeated job application failure and inactive approaches are linked with stress accompanying unemployment (Fineman 1979, 1983). Schlozman & Verba (1979) noted that the more prestigious the job, the less psychologically devastating the response. This was said to be directly related to persistence of a sense of professional identity. On the other hand, Goodchilds & Smith (1963) observed that the longer the unemployment lasted, the more defensive and self-critical higher socioeconomic status subjects became. Atkinson *et al.* (1986) using longitudinal data to assess the social costs of unemployment found that with an increase in number of weeks following unemployment, a decrease in the quality of marital relationships was observed in white collar workers. Blue collar workers on the other hand showed a decrease in frequency of contact with network members. They reported that unemployment had a negative effect on marital and family support, in part through its effect on the husband's psychological well-being. Work is often seen as an important part of self-identity (Kelvin 1981).

Unemployed people are noted to show inactivity (see Fagin & Little 1984, Kelvin *et al.* 1985, Kilpatrick & Trew 1985) and social isolation (Trew & Kilpatrick 1984, Henwood & Miles 1987). Unemployed people are noted to be more anxious when compared to a matched group of employed folk (Banks & Jackson 1982, Jackson & Warr 1984, Payne 1988). Depression has been measured in this group using well-established, well-validated measures and has been shown to be higher in comparison with employed people (Cobb & Kasl 1977, Feather 1982, Finlay-Jones & Eckhardt 1981, Payne & Hartley 1984, Winefield *et al.* 1988). Kessler *et al.* (1987) from their community sample reported that the psychological impact of unemployment was to do with unemployment itself and not a selection bias. Melville *et al.* (1985) used a questionnaire with men attending a job centre in Southampton. A second interview looked at marital status; work history, income change and at this stage the subjects were given the Beck Depression Inventory (BDI) (Beck *et al.* 1961) and the General Health Questionnaire – 30 item version (GHQ-30) (Goldberg 1978). Ninety-eight men were then matched with employed men who were contacted by mail. The GHQ and BDI scores were higher in the redundant group, whereas no relationship was found between test scores and age, duration of employment, social class, marital status or decrease in income. Since self-rating scales were used and only 69% of respondents participated in the study, the finding from this study offers a limited insight. Jenkins *et al.* (1982) conducted a longitudinal study with a group of journalists when their newspaper was threatened with closure. A two-stage screening method was used. Initial GHQ screening was following by a clinical assessment interview. The period was divided into three phases: the first phase was the period of anticipated closure, two months prior to the set closure date and one month after all employees had received notice of redundancy; the second phase represented the period when redundancy notices were revoked, and the third phase represented the period three months after the threat of redundancy had been lifted when internal changes in the paper had been made. All 321 journalists were approached and a proportion of cases and non-cases were then interviewed. The most common symptoms displayed by the sample were complaints of poor sleep, depression and fatigue. Anxiety, poor concentration and irritability were also fairly common. A diagnosis of depressive neurosis was given to 26.5% individuals and another 12.2% were given the diagnosis of anxiety neurosis. Twenty-one per cent of the sample reported that the threat of redundancy had affected their marriage and another 17% noted its effects on their social lives. One-third of the respondents (37%) saw anticipated redundancy in terms of loss of status and job satisfaction.

Frese & Mohr (1987) relying on structured interviews, standardized testing procedures and a longitudinal analysis of 51 subjects over a period of 2 years, demonstrated that prolonged unemployment or re-unemployment led to depression,

reduced hope and increased financial problems. Being employed or retired produced a reduction in depression. They argued that problems associated with the daily hassles of unemployment, such as financial problems and disappointed hopes, play a role in the development of depression. Unlike some other studies, they observed that internal/external control, passivity, sickness and age do not influence the effects of unemployment on depression. As they conclude, 'Unemployment also means major identity loss. Whether we are able to handle these losses in an acceptable way is determined by the compensatory possibilities society offers us.' In another longitudinal study, this time from Sweden, it was observed that anxiety unfolded into more disabling states of depression, social isolation and alcoholism as time went on (Joelson & Wahlquist 1987). The workers adopted a sick role and shifted their self-descriptions from a group setting to an individual one. The anticipatory phase was found to be a very burdensome period of unemployment due to the prolonged uncertainty. Despite good compensation in economic terms depressive reactions were observed. In contrast in a group of 35 unemployed technical professionals, Jacobson (1987) found two models at work. The first was termed 'transactional' where the meaning of the event (in this case unemployment) was experienced in terms of its impact on resources and demands. The other one was called 'transitional' which involved a change in the framework of ideas, beliefs and values within which the individuals evaluated themselves.

As becomes obvious from this limited review, most of the work has been done among male unemployed. Women, youth and those of ethnic minorities also suffer from unemployment and the impact on them and their reactions are different. We shall now very briefly look at these groups.

## Women

Even though female employment has grown more rapidly them male employment over the postwar period, the proportion of women of working age in employment is still notably lower than that of men. As Henwood & Miles (1987) point out, despite these facts unemployment figures record men's unemployment as being much higher than women's (Allin & Hunt 1982, Joseph 1983). They argue that unemployment statistics only include the 'economically active' (those employed, or looking for employment, in the formal economy), which means that retired people and housewives who are not regarded as such do not appear in the figures. In addition, unemployment figures are compiled from those people actually registering themselves as available for employment.

Henwood & Miles (1987) also emphasize that the acceptance of a sexual division of labour which sees men as the breadwinner and the women as the carers is embodied in social policies. Henwood (1983) using postal questionnaires and home visits collected data from 107 women and 117 men. Seven groups of people formed the great majority of the sample. These were: full-time employed men and women; part-time employed women; unemployed women and men; self-defined housewives, and retired people. Nearly all women in part-time employment were married (or cohabiting) and three-quarters had children. Women in full employment were also more likely not to be married, to be younger and without children. The results showed a positive relationship between being in employment and access to certain categories of experience. Both employed men and women scored significantly higher on all categories of experience. When Henwood compared employed women with housewives she found that social contacts were seen as a major non-financial reason for women wanting paid work. Henwood & Miles (1987) concluded that many people lacking employment, whether formally unemployed or engaged in informal economic activities such as housework and child care, are failing to gain access to important categories of experience which contribute towards a sense of well-being. Miles & Howard (1984) also reported that registered unemployed differed from their employed peers in their well-being.

It is difficult to know whether women are being affected more now simply because of changing roles and expectations. Another complicating factor is the role of women as spouses and mothers of unemployed men. It is almost impossible to disentangle these factors. Quite apart from the economic nonsense of the wife's self-inflicted unemployment, it is tragic at a personal level (Kelvin & Jarrett 1985). There is evidence to suggest that single women are anxious to retain their independence that their employment allows them (Pilgrim Trust 1938) and, interestingly, failure as an unemployed woman does not rely on the social reality of a women being a breadwinner. This may be beginning to change. Feather & Barber (1983) and Feather & Bond (1983) reported that in their sample, women tended to score higher on Protestant Work Ethic and importance of employment than did the unemployed male. Others have shown that female school leavers are more affected (Banks & Jackson 1982). Another interesting aside is that most of the evidence (Rose 1955, Feld 1963, Radloff 1975) but not all (Sharp & Nye 1963, Pearlin 1975) indicates that married women who work are in better mental health than those who do not. Ensminger & Celentano (1990) interviewed a proportion of unemployed subjects they contacted through unemployment agencies. After selecting 100 unemployed respondents they completed interviews with 92 matched controls. Unmarried continuously employed men had lower GHQ scores than their female counterparts, giving some support for the added burden for solo parenting in these data. The authors were able to confirm that part of the psychological distress of unemployed women compared to employed men was due to their lower social support.

Brenner & Levi (1987) studied the effects of job loss and long-term unemployment among Swedish women (also see Levi *et al.* 1984). The study included four groups with 100 subjects each. The first group was that of unemployed people, predominantly women, who were studied from 1 month before to 2 years after job loss. The second group was employed women who were followed from 4 months after job loss to 18 months of unemployment. Two control groups — one in insecure jobs and the other one in jobs in expanding fields — were used. Various psychological measures including GHQ, BDI, self-esteem measures, biomedical measures, including

serum cortisol, human growth hormone, prolactin, and physical measures like blood pressure
and other indicators of physical health were
assessed. A sizeable proportion of the unemployed
persons (over 40%) reported pronounced depressive reactions (compared to 12% among the
employed). The authors concluded that effects of
long-term unemployment were largely those of
psychological nature and the Swedish welfare
system might account for some buffering effects of
long-term unemployment. Starrin & Larsson
(1987) interviewed 36 unemployed women, using
Wacker's (1977) and Olsen's (1982) models of
reactions to unemployment which include:

1 A confirmation of the sociocultural normative
orientation towards work
2 A refocusing of life interests
3 An incapacity to deal with (1) and action
possibilities
4 An innovative restructuring of the relation
between work and identity.

Starrin & Larsson (1987) reported that the
reactions to unemployment, their meaning and
their context were seen in relation to two core
variables demonstrated in their sample of 36 unemployed women: relation to wage labour and
relation to alternative activities leading to four
groups. These four groups were called the 'give
uppers', 'the clenchers', 'the refocusers' and 'the
ambivalent'. For the first two, the unemployment
brought a serious effect on their identity and
mental health, producing feelings of hopelessness
and depression. The 'refocusers' enjoyed their lives
and replaced work with meaningful activities.
Brinkmann (1981) reported from West Germany
that financial problems were often found to be
less severe for married unemployed women. Far
fewer women than men tended to blame themselves for being unemployed, and fewer women
than men blamed family conflicts on their unemployment. Women were also able to talk
easily to others. As noticed above, missing the
social contacts was a bigger psychological burden
of unemployment for women. These findings
need to be evaluated further in view of Brown
& Harris's (1978) findings about lack of a
confidant and unemployment as vulnerability
factors in working-class women. Heinemann *et al.*

(1980) reported that only 17% of the women
who were registered as unemployed at the time
of the first interview identified themselves as
housewives at their subsequent interview. Thus
changing self-ascription may contribute to preservation of self-respect and self-esteem. The
long-term unemployed women were less rational
and more often resigned and less emotionally
stable. Like the Brinkmann (1981) observation,
half of the interviewed housewives claimed to
want a job because they felt isolated and longed
to be among other people. They did not see a
retreat into the traditional female role as a viable
alternative.

Women's positions in the labour market are
different from those of men's and in addition
women are still expected to fulfil two roles
(Starrin & Larsson 1987). Women's unemployment can be perceived as a double bind. In
addition mental and physical health of women is
affected through their own unemployment as well
as through the unemployment of their partner or
children. The tensions between the couple and
family relationships are discussed later.

### Children and youth

The mental health of children and young adults
can also be influenced by parental unemployment.
After leaving school, lack of employment is bound
to affect their emotional and psychological
growth. Another complicating factor in youth
employment is the notion of 'permanent im-
permanence' (Carle 1987). In this group, periods
of joblessness are in general short and alternate
with job programmes and training or educational
programmes. The impact of unemployment on a
youth's growth cannot be underestimated. The
social effects, Carle (1987) argues, are primarily
of three kinds: those limited to the individual's
welfare, those concerning the individual's connection to his group and those concerning the
individual's relationship with society – expressed
sociomedically, sociopsychologically and socio-
culturally respectively. The young often have the
highest relative unemployment of all age groups
and within this group young women and immigrants often fare the worst. A lack of job oppor-

tunities and getting unemployed status soon after leaving school add to the complications. The consequences of unemployment on the youth are similar to those observed among the adults (Kannas & Hietaharju cited in Carle 1987). Decreased general hygiene, altered daily schedules, physical as well as psychological passivity and increase in sleep disorder occur in this group. Unemployment leads to a lack of self-confidence, apathy, isolation, and breaking up of social networks in the young in the same way that it does for the adult (for a full review see Carle & Schale 1982).

Cullen *et al.* (1987) reported on a sample of young people aged 16–23. The study involved young white-collar and blue-collar workers, trainees and young people who were unemployed. A total of 135 young adults of both sexes participated in the study. In addition to occupational and sociodemographic details the sample were interviewed on life stressors and satisfactions; job-seeking behaviour, locus of control, health-related behaviours and factors, social support and details of health status and general well-being. Unemployed females manifested relatively more caseness on depression and unemployed males were more likely to be cases on GHQ-12. Interestingly a significant association was observed between socioeconomic status of the father and employment status of the offspring. Another observation was that those unemployed who had lower levels of educational attainment tended to show higher levels of both suicidal ideation and depression. As the total number of episodes of unemployment increased, psychological health tended to decrease. Similar findings have been reported by Banks *et al.* (1980) and Banks & Jackson (1982).

Unemployment among the youth, as noted above, tends to affect relationships with others and the way the unemployed youth is perceived. It displaces the individual from a variety of settings and a variety of potential settings which would have been taken for granted. Thus a feeling of dislocation interacting with perception among others contributes to low self-esteem, self-worth and self-confidence. Feather (1982) found low self-esteem, high depression scores and more

apathy in 69 unemployed males and females in comparison to the employed controls. Gurney (1981) observed that the general effect of unemployment in youth is that of inhibiting development rather than inflicting trauma. In an earlier study Gurney (1980) had found that unemployed males showed mistrust. Young single unemployed who are still developing their interests and career aspirations and are financially cushioned by family can tolerate prolonged unemployment (Stevenson 1974). External factors may be blamed for one's unemployment (Feather & Davenport 1981). Layton (1984) in a study of school leavers demonstrated that the jobless suffered a loss of confidence, personal neglect and a degree of social dysfunction and were more inclined to attribute their plight to external causes. Among skilled and semi-skilled workers facing redundancy, Layton (1984) observed more anhedonia, loss of confidence and social dysfunction. For those who found employment mental health improved as did levels of state-anxiety. Extraversion, neuroticism, lie-scale, trait anxiety, impulsivity and intelligence were all found to be poor predispositional predictors of future status. Winefield & Tiggemann (1990) report that a curvilinear relationship existed between unemployment and psychological distress in their sample of school leavers. They followed the group longitudinally and each year's unemployed cohort was divided into those unemployed for less than three months, those unemployed from four to eight months and those unemployed for nine months or more. The subjects were given locus of control, depressive affect and self-esteem scales, along with GHQ-12 and other measures. On most of the dependent measures the nine-month group was significantly worse off than the other two groups. They reported that older persons had less social pressure to get jobs which enables them to adjust better to longer periods of unemployment like the teenagers, but the group in between suffers more.

### Ethnic minorities

Unemployment among ethnic minorities is noted to be high. The stigma of being unemployed, being dependent on social security and being black contribute to a tremendous feeling of rejection and despair. Ullah (1987) in an ethnographic study reported that for some of his subjects being unemployed was simply another feature of being black, in much the same way that bad housing and limited educational opportunities were. In some subjects unemployment may take a back seat to other forms of discrimination that may be piling up against them. Ullah *et al.* (1985) also reported that having someone to turn to for help with money and having someone to suggest things to do were significantly negatively associated with measures of stress.

### Unemployment and the family

Systematic research on the relationship between unemployment and the family is not a new phenomenon. However, the impact is individualistic and it would be foolish to make generalizations. Unemployed people are not a homogeneous group and neither are the families. There are different kinds of structures, dynamics and social networks. The personal meaning of unemployment depends upon changes in financial status and demands made upon such a source. However, the 'loss' affects tacitly the family and subsequently the society (see Fig. 25.3).

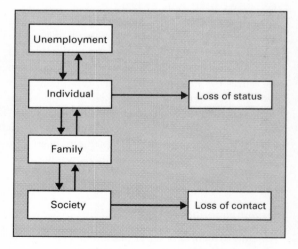

**Fig. 21.3** Interlinking of impact of unemployment.

Children coming from families where parents are unemployed have been shown to have poor scholastic performance and disturbed behaviour (Fagin 1981). In another study, children were noted to be more distrustful and avoided social interaction (Buss & Redburn 1983). Increased nervous disorder (Schneider 1932), emotional instability and antisocial behaviour (Brandt 1932), disobedience (Schumacher 1934), poor school work (Schneider 1932) and robbing of a sense of security among the children (Elderston 1931) have been reported. Brenner (1973) observed that infant mortality rates were related to economic recessions, with a lag of one to two years of the peak average mortality behind the peak of unemployment. Loss of ambition (Obermann 1931), apathy (Wunderlich 1934), maladjustment (Rundquist & Sletto 1936) and developmental problems in adolescence (Erikson 1956) have been observed.

In families where the home was good, unemployment brought the family together, whereas if the home was ready to break up, unemployment proved the last straw (Rogers 1933–34, Groves 1934–35, Rundquist & Sletto 1936). If father and son were both unemployed, parents lost their authority and the son lost a reference point on which to build his future. If the son was working, it increased his self-worth but reduced the father's self-esteem in the eyes of the family (Zawadski & Lazarsfeld 1935).

With trusted persons behind them unemployed males are able to cope with their unemployment (Brown *et al.* 1975) — support increases coping ability (Myers *et al.* 1975, Cobb 1976). In close marriages, tensions created by a husband's unemployment were ameliorated by a supportive wife who shared all the problems (Jenkins *et al.* 1982). If couples are not close, the pressures on both tend to be far worse. On the other hand, if the wife takes on a job role reversal the pressure of financial power can affect the dynamics even more strongly (Marsden & Duff 1975). It makes sense to observe that well organized families fare better than poorly organized families, largely because the former adjust realistically and provide practical support. Penkower *et al.* (1988) identified three major risk factors in the wives whose husbands had been laid off: family psychiatric history, financial difficulties and low social support from relatives. Another observation that has often been made is that blue-collar workers were more likely to keep in contact with each other and friends to get jobs (Harrison 1976, Banks *et al.* 1980). Fagin (1981) interviewed 22 families 6 months after registering as unemployed and 19 were revisited after another half year. While some families reported fewer health problems, most reported changes for the worse in the unemployed worker, his/her spouse and in the family's children. Headaches and backaches increased in both the partners. Clinical depression, lethargy and increased alcohol and tobacco consumption were reported in many of the men. Murphy *et al.* (1984) reported that non-employed women were more likely than employed women to be married to unemployed men. Smith (1987) emphasizes that one of the main ways in which unemployment harms families is through poverty. Economic factors do affect marriage and birth rates. Beale & Nethercott (1986) noted a significant rise in rates of pregnancy compared with controls when a factory closed. Such an increase itself may have implications for a possible increase in ambivalence or rejection towards such children and child abuse. Gayford (1975) reported in a study of 100 cases of wife battering that nearly half (48%) of partners had been unemployed at some time and more than a quarter (29%) were frequently or mostly unemployed. This is an area where links with other behaviour such as increased alcoholism, gambling and child abuse need to be explored further.

## Physical health and unemployment

Clinical evidence suggests that unemployment affects physical health. Smith (1987) draws our attention to the parallels between the sick role and the unemployed role. He reviews the evidence for a link between physical ill-health and unemployment, and concludes that as a group the unemployed are more unhealthy than the employed and clearly the unhealthy have a higher chance of becoming and staying unemployed. Brenner & Levi (1987) reported from their long-

term unemployed sample that unemployment lasting more than 9 months is accompanied by a significant decrease in lymphocyte reactivity, but after 24 months of unemployment this reactivity is restored (also see Arnetz *et al.* 1987). Cullen *et al.* (1987) reported that accidents requiring medical treatment within the previous 12 months were particularly evident among the unemployed sample. Other studies have shown a higher mortality for the unemployed over a long-term follow-up (Moser *et al.* 1984, 1986). The Select Committee of the House of Lords on Unemployment (1982) believed unemployment to be among the causes of ill-health, mortality, crime or civil disorder. Even though they caution that irrefutable proof in this area is virtually impossible, they found the evidence to be highly indicative for their conclusions.

Bartley (1988) argues that unemployment appears to be an 'indicator' of more general patterns of labour force participation in men which puts them at risk of cumulative disadvantages over time. The impact of unemployment on specific psychiatric disorders like suicide and parasuicide has been noted (see Platt 1984, Platt & Kreitman 1985).

In order to make any sense of the impact of unemployment, poverty and homelessness on an individual's mental and physical health, we need to employ our energies not only on cross-sectional and longitudinal studies but also, more importantly, on individual perceptions and individual contexts. In addition, unemployment needs to be reviewed less as abnormal and deviant, particularly during periods of economic recession in which a high proportion of the work-force is affected.

## Poverty

Unemployment and poverty may be linked in some cases. Unemployment may contribute to financial insecurity and inability to purchase goods. This link has to be studied further in order to understand the impact on self-esteem and support which occurs due to unemployment and/or poverty. Not all unemployed individuals are poor and neither are all poor individuals unemployed. The two states can be separate or linked and this is what makes understanding them so difficult.

Poverty can be defined objectively and applied consistently only in terms of the concept of relative deprivation. Individuals, families and groups in the population can be said to be in poverty when they lack the resources to obtain the types of diet, participate in the activities and have the living conditions and amenities which are customary or at least widely encouraged or approved of in the societies to which they belong (Townsend 1979).

Rowntree (1901) defined families whose 'total earnings are insufficient to obtain the minimum necessaries for the maintenance of merely physical efficiency' as being in primary poverty. Subsequent studies on poverty were greatly influenced by this definition which applied the concept of subsistence. Townsend (1979) recommends that absolutist definitions be abandoned and called for a new approach to both the definition and measurement of poverty. It is important to remember that one man's poverty may (still) be another man's riches. There has to be a fundamental distinction between actual and socially perceived needs as well as between objective and conventionally acknowledged poverty. Stouffer *et al.* (1949) introduced the concept of relative deprivation which was further elaborated by Merton (1957) and Runciman (1966). Relativity is an important facet in any definition of poverty simply because the frame of reference in adapting this approach can be regional, national or international since people are bound by the same economic trading, institutional and cultural systems.

If needs are perceived as relative to a given society, then these are also relative to the set of social subsystems to which the individual may belong. The resources of those conceived as poor are so seriously below those commanded by the average individual or family that they are, in effect, excluded from ordinary living patterns, customs and activities.

The impact of poverty can lead to deprivation in environment, deprivation in housing and deprivation at work (Fig. 21.4). A culture of poverty is not simply a matter of economic deprivation or low position on socioeconomic indicators. A culture is a set of acquired patterns of conduct, a way of life, that provides its participants with adaptive techniques to deal with a set of recurring problems according to Sarbin (1970). He then goes on to argue that viewed in this way the focus is less exclusively on the individual victims of poverty but rather on the social organization that creates specific social types that reproduce and maintain themselves with predictable regularity.

One of the major identifiable problems in studies on unemployment, poverty and homelessness is that quite often individual differences are ignored and interest is focused on social class as an independent variable largely because it is readily quantifiable. In addition, once an individual is classified as working class, his/her classification carries not only an expressed criterion of earnings but also tacit stereotypes of how such an individual behaves and how he/she ought to behave. A further complication identified by Sarbin (1970) is that the classification of such persons at the lower end of the dimension tends to homogenize the respectable poor and the degraded poor, whereas the latter are participants in the culture of poverty.

## Psychological impact of poverty

In addition to financial pressures contributing to the poor functioning of the individual or family unit under environmental stress, for example, poor inner city housing, increased pollution, lack of play facilities for children, limited personal and interpersonal space, specific psychological impacts have been monitored:

1 Conceptualization of time is different.

2 Linguistic code is restricted, relatively undifferentiated, simplex, lacking in modifiers and aimed at reinforcing and implementing the social structure rather than conveying information (Bernstein & Henderson 1969). This can lead to a circle of poverty of language, emotional and psychological expression thereby narrowing the repertoire hence making interventions difficult. It can be hypothesized that such a code will then

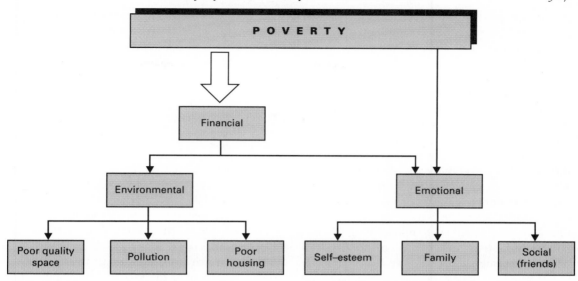

**Fig. 21.4** Impact of poverty.

lead on to externalization of locus of control.

3 This externalization is manifested by beliefs in fate and luck evidenced further through a lack of concern for upward mobility. This can be compared to Seligman's model (1975) of learned helplessness.

However, as we know from our experience, quite often individual differences play a very important role in development of self-esteem and breaking away from this circle of poverty.

Langner *et al.* (1970) randomly selected one child from each household containing one or more children between 6 and 18 years of age from a clustered random sample of 1034 households on the east and west sides of Manhattan, New York. They picked 400 subjects and even though they argue that their sample was representative, in reality nearly one-third of the sample was made up from the immigrant population. Half the mothers were employed. A 2-hour interview with mothers and 300 children demonstrated that absent fathers had a definite relationship to the child's impairment. Children with absent fathers were worse off in almost every impairment area, whether they were boys or girls, than those with fathers. However, the presence of a surrogate

father had a bimodal association with the degree of impairment. Boys without fathers were better off than those with a surrogate, while girls without fathers were better off with surrogates. The authors explain this discrepancy in terms of role modelling for the boys. However, low socio-economic status and ethnic background were associated with greater impairment in urban children. Even in those families with higher incomes, prejudice played an important role in ethnic minorities. Poverty and discrimination were important factors rather than immigration alone. Parents' education, interruption of maternal care, and number of different addresses at which the child had lived in the city bore a relationship to impairment. Low-income females showed almost twice the impairment of males.

Allen (1970b) argues that the types of evaluative decisions the psychiatrist makes (i.e. diagnosis) are a function of the conceptual and value systems he holds, which may be biased against behaviour of the poor even though this behaviour may be very adaptive in the lower class environment (see also Chapter 5). Lewis's (1961) work on personality profile of the poor defines it thus: 'a strong present-time orientation with little ability to defer gratification and plan for the future, a sense of resignation and fatalism ... a high tolerance for psychological pathology of all sorts ...'.

Greater premarital sexual experience among the poor (Kinsey *et al.* 1948), lower educational attainment (Strauss 1962), lack of financial savings and patterns of consumption (Schneider & Lysgarrd 1953) have been taken as evidence of their inability to postpone gratification (see also Mischel 1961). However, there are also cultural variables as shown in the differences between two black groups from the islands of Trinidad and Grenada – the latter were more willing to postpone gratification and had a greater trust in promise keeping. It has been argued that lower socioeconomic classes lay more emphasis on submissiveness and passive self-conception (Bieri & Loback 1961). Poverty is not necessarily related to negative self-concept.

Allen (1970a) has argued that the culture of poverty concept has the following running themes: strong feeling of fatalism and belief in chance; strong present-time orientation and short-term perspectives; impulsiveness or inability to delay present gratification or to plan for the future; concrete rather than abstract thinking processes, concrete verbal behaviour, feelings of inferiority; acceptance of aggression and illegitimacy and authoritarianism.

Poverty can best be appreciated in terms of the impact that it has on individuals and families rather than through statistical norms. A lack of resources as well as a denial of access to these resources compounds the problems of poverty. Individuals are affected by various types of poverty (as outlined by Townsend 1979), i.e. minority group poverty, subsistence poverty, starvation poverty, relative poverty – compared with others – and relative historical and mismanagement poverty. We have not looked at the impact of poverty on individual groups like the elderly, ethnic minorities, disabled, etc. The structure of poverty needs to be studied as well as individual characteristics and the interaction between the two. Often individuals and families are tied in an 'interlocking network of inequali-

ties' (Coffield 1983 in Madge 1983). As Andrews (1990) argues, the poor do not exist in a vacuum and any study of poverty has to look at the whole spectrum within communities, societies and nations.

## Homelessness

### Definition

Homelessness has been defined by various authors in various ways. There does not appear to be a consensus about its meaning. The definitions include: 'homeless', i.e. without a home; 'roofless'; 'rootless'; 'no fixed abode', etc. In reality as Lipton *et al.* (1983) suggest the term homeless is actually a catchword, a misnomer that focuses on only one aspect of the individual's plight; other aspects like job, financial aspects, social support, etc. are discounted. It is sometimes easy to define a syndrome or delineate a spectrum rather than be absolutely precise about the definition of homelessness. Clearly, to be homeless is to lack regular and customary access to a conventional dwelling unit (Wright 1989), and as Wright goes on to emphasize, the ambiguities arise in trying to define 'regular and customary access' and a 'conventional dwelling unit'. There is often an element of choice in some definitions of homelessness. Not all people who 'choose' to live in what may be termed as inadequate housing by any other standards will be seen as homeless. Wright (1989) draws attention to the distinction between the 'literally homeless' and the 'marginally housed', first proposed by Rossi *et al.* (1987). The literally homeless are the ones who have nowhere to go – no rented rooms, no squats, no friend's accommodation and thus either sleep on the streets or avail themselves of other space like shelters, hostels, etc. Marginally housed on the other hand according to Wright (1989) are those 'who have a more or less reasonable claim to a more or less stable housing situation of more or less minimal adequacy, being closer to the "less" than the "more" on one or all criteria'. However, Wright then goes on to call the literal homeless afflicted with the 'disease of homelessness'. Thus the problem of definition and 'medicalization' of the homeless lets the social policy off the hook – the policy that contributed to the numbers of the homeless. In the USA the policy of deinstitutionalization has been blamed for the increase in the numbers of the homeless. In Britain too the closure of the mental hospitals has been blamed for the purported increase in the numbers of homeless. However, a lack of cheap rented accommodation, fall in numbers of dwelling units available, an increase in unemployment, government policies and changes in social security benefits are some of the factors that would need to be considered to complete the picture. It is also important to remember that any data related to homelessness are subject to basic problems in defining the population of interest and sampling difficulties concerning selection and size. The figures in the following review should be taken as relative and not absolute, that is, they will not be applicable to all homeless populations (also see Yach *et al.* 1990).

Rossi *et al.* (1987) reported that being homeless was predominantly a male condition, and black and native Americans constituted considerably more than their proportionate share of the homeless, with whites and Hispanics proportionally underrepresented. The sample was chosen in Chicago. The 'literal' homelessness resulted from extreme poverty in housing markets with an inadequate supply of low-cost housing, especially for single persons. This burden according to Rossi *et al.* (1987) falls on the disaffiliated and upon those who have been extremely poor for a very long time.

The homeless traditionally have been seen as dropouts, skid-row alcoholics. This stereotype has changed dramatically in the last 20 years or so. Scott & Boustead (1990) reported four groups from their small sample of homeless people. This author is following the classification suggested by the Royal College of Psychiatrists' Working Party (Bhugra 1991). The three groups are:

1 Single homeless people.
2 Young homeless.
3 Homeless families.

Wright (1989) had further subdivided single homeless into the elderly, the veterans and the disabled. Within our categories further divisions

according to sex or disability are of course possible.

### Single homeless people

As noted earlier, this is the group most likely to be stereotyped. However, this is also the subgroup studied most energetically over the last three decades. Traditionally in this country this group has included white middle-aged males usually hailing from Ireland or Scotland. However, American as well as British studies have started noting the presence of homeless people from ethnic minorities.

Weller & Weller (1985) assessed the homeless at Crisis at Christmas and tapped such a group. In a subsequent study Weller *et al.* (1989) reported the cumulative results from 1985 to 1988 and were able to show that 22% of their sample were psychotic at the time of the interview and 41% gave a history of psychosis. It is important to note that other studies have found that the homeless schizophrenic has often not been in contact with the services in the first place (Dayson 1992). The TAPS (Team for the Assessment of Psychiatric Services) project (see also Chapter 32) found that only one patient in their sample of 278 patients discharged from the hospital had become vagrant. Varying rates of psychosis have been reported amongst this group (Tidmarsh & Wood 1972, Timms & Fry 1989). Rates of psychiatric morbidity have been reported from various locations, for example, hostels (Marshall 1989, Timms & Fry 1989), lodging houses (Priest 1971, Shanks 1984), reception centres (Tidmarsh & Wood 1972), no fixed abode admissions in psychiatric hospitals (Herzberg 1987), etc.

Studies from the USA have been numerous and often well designed. The most notable study was that of Breakey *et al.* (1989) which randomly selected 298 men and 230 women from various locations. A random subsample of 203 received extended PSE, full physical examination, Eysenck Personality Inventory (EPI), Short Michigan Alcohol Screening Test and other tests including breath alcohol. A minority of the sample was white. Nearly one-third of women and one-fifth of men were anaemic. To further complicate the issue, one-third of women had been raped and a vast majority (91% of men and 80% of women) had an axis 1 DSM-III disorder of anxiety and depression. Thus it becomes apparent that unlike the domiciled mentally ill, this group suffers from a multitude of problems including social, psychological and physical varieties.

Until recently homeless women have not been studied adequately, but recent evidence (Marshall & Reed 1992) suggests that they suffer from the same range of psychiatric problems as men. However, these authors go on to suggest that homeless women are younger and socially more stable but have a higher level of psychiatric morbidity. In addition, this group lacks confidence in male therapists which makes any therapeutic relationship more difficult to establish. Austerberry & Watson (1983) reported that the younger, employed women (though technically homeless) were more likely to stay with friends or to remain in unsuitable relationships when they lost accommodation, whereas the older, married and unqualified women who had little knowledge of the housing system were more likely to be living in a direct access hospital. Marshall & Reed (1992) found that 45 out of 63 women in their sample where a diagnosis could be made had a DSM-III-R diagnosis of schizophrenia. Two-thirds of this sample had seen a psychiatrist and a quarter had physical illness. In other studies these rates have varied tremendously (Table 21.1). La Gory et al. (1990) reported that 59% of their sample showed signs of 'probable clinical caseness' on depression. They found limited impact of social factors on depression among the homeless. The variable rates of major mental illness have suggested the vulnerability of the homeless, but it is depression which may be silent or subclinical and yet potentially serious. As Gory et al. (1990) state, 'The problem for the homeless is not one of unresponsive networks, rather social supports cannot reduce distress as effectively in this very needy population as in other groups'. Such high levels of depression along with high levels of reported suicide from Stockholm studies (Alstrom et al. 1975) should alert the clinicians and researchers alike to look into this area.

### Young single homeless people

The second broad group is that of young single homeless people (young here taken to mean below 25 years old). This group is becoming an increasingly visible problem and very little is known of the prevalence of psychiatric illness among them. However, in view of the fact that a high proportion may have come from broken homes or out of social services care, it would seem reasonable to assume that this group too would have a higher rate of mental distress. In addition, the hazards of eking out a living on the streets of cities will expose them to life events and stress and also introduce the clients to the drug and prostitution subculture. Workers in the field suggest that substance misuse is high in this group and sooner or later HIV status will become a major issue.

Studies from the USA have reported overrepresentation of young black men (Susser et al. 1989, Susser & Struening 1990). In a sample of 177 males (aged 17+) who were first-time users of homeless shelters, Susser et al. (1989) found that 71% had one or more of the following: definite or possible psychosis, multiple suicide attempts, a predilection for substance-abuse dependence and severe emotional distress. Those men who had been homeless for much of the previous five years showed more signs of psychopathology on every measure than those who were homeless 'for just a few times'. From Melbourne, Herrman et al. (1989) reported a near 50% rate of current psychopathology. Mundy et al. (1990) studied psychotic symptoms in 96 homeless adolescents aged between 12 and 17 years who were located in street sites or using shelter services. More than a quarter (29%) reported experiencing four or more psychotic symptoms. Cormier & Rochon (1988) were unable to correlate drug addiction and low self-esteem with vagrancy among young people (aged 15–25 years). In contrast, Ritter (1989) found that typical clients for crisis shelters were 17 and 18 year olds who used a combination of drugs and alcohol and engaged in commercial sex. Sexually transmitted diseases were common in this group. Raychaba (1989) drew attention to the similarities between the young in care and

**Table 21.1** Psychiatric morbidity among the homeless

| Authors | Number | Source | Group | Diagnosis | | | | | | Other factors |
|---|---|---|---|---|---|---|---|---|---|---|
| | | | | A Schizophrenia | B Affective disorder | C Personality disorder | D Substance abuse | E Other diagnosis | F No diagnosis | |
| Whiteley 1955 | 100 out of 130 (8.4% of all admissions) | Admissions from Reception Centre and Lodging House | Male | 32% | 14% | 19% | 14% | 21% | | Nearly half first referrals ethnic minority |
| Meyerson 1956 | 101 | Skid Row Rehab. | Male | 29% | | 61% | | | 10% | |
| Berry & Orwin 1966 | 135 (145 admissions) | NFA admissions | Male and female | 49% | 13% | 28% | | 10% | | Subnormality/alcohol/epilepsy associated with three main categories |
| Edwards *et al.* 1966 | 51 | Soup kitchen | Male | | | | 94% | 20% | 4% | Looking for alcoholics |
| Scott *et al.* 1968 | 310 | GP attenders | Male and female | 0.2% (psychiatric) | 0.2% (psychiatric) | | 9% | | | 50% had physical problems |
| Edwards *et al.* 1968 | 279 | Reception centre | Male | | | | 10% (alcohol) | | | 76% not been in hospital. 59% had been in prison |
| Crossley & Denmark 1969 | 51 | Hostel | Male | 19% | | 64% | | 6% | | 10% physical problem |
| Goldfarb 1970 | 200 | Admissions to alcoholic rehab. | | 33% | 18% | 38% | | 10% | | |
| Priest 1970 | 123 | Salvation Army hostels | Male | 15% | 8% | 50% | 1% | 15% | | 11% no mental problem |
| Priest 1976 | 79 | Lodging houses | Male and female | 32% | 5% | 18% | 18% | 9% | | 18% no problem |

*continued on p. 372*

**Table 21.1** (*continued*)

| Authors | Number | Source | Group | A Schizophrenia | B Affective disorder | C Personality disorder | D Substance abuse | E Other diagnosis | F No diagnosis | Other factors |
|---|---|---|---|---|---|---|---|---|---|---|
| Lodge Patch 1970, 1971 | 130 (new cases) | Reception centre | Male | Mental illness 22% | | 16% | 14% | | | 29% job problem |
| Tidmarsh & Wood 1972 | 50 | Lodging houses | Male | 25% | | | 47% | | | Nearly half legal problems |
| Lewis 1978 | 76 | Travellers Aid | | ——— 60% history psychiatric care* ——— | | | | | | |
| Chrmiel et al. 1979 | 35 | Emergency clinic | | 26% | 17% | | | | | |
| Streltzer 1979 | 114 | Emergency clinic | Male/female | 31% | 11% | | | 26% | 25% | 8% dissociative disorientation |
| Tabler 1982 | 269 | City shelter | | ——— 31% had psychiatric histories* ——— | | | | | | |
| Arce et al. 1983 (also see Vergare & Arce 1984) | 193 | Emergency shelter | Male/female | ——— '84% mental illness*† ——— | | | | | | 179 interviewed |
| Brown et al. 1983 | 150 + 195 | Food line users | Male/female | ——— 30% had history of institutionalization‡ ——— | | | | | | |
| Lipton et al. 1983 | 90 | Hospital | Male/female | 72% | | 11% | 9% | | 8% | |
| Bassuk et al. 1984 | 78 | Homeless shelter | Male/female (and children) | 40% | | 21% | 29% | | 9% | 44% had medical disorders |
| Fernandez 1984 | 256 | Admissions | Male/female | ——— 34% psychotic illness* ——— | | | | | | |
| Vergare & Arce 1984 | 193 | | | 48% | 5% | 11% | 12% | 12% | | 8% |
| Whitley et al. 1985 | 191 | Shelter/Hotel | | ——— 16% psychodynamic impairment* ——— | | | 15% | | | |
| Fischer et al. 1986 | 51 | Missions | Male/female | 2.0% | 14% | 16% | 70% | 39% | 21% | |
| Snow et al. 1986 | 164 + 767 | Range | Male/female | ——— 15% had mental illness* ——— | | | | | | |
| Herzberg 1987 | 140 | Hospital admission | 50 females 90 males | 42% 25% | 15% 5% | 33% 26% | 8% 35% | 2% 5% | | |

| Study | Sample | Location | Sex | A | B | C | D | Notes |
|---|---|---|---|---|---|---|---|---|
| Rossi et al. 1987 | 722 | Shelters Streets | Male/female | 23% | 47% | 33% | | 17% prisons 28% physical illness |
| Breakey et al. 1989 | 289 M 230 F | Various locations | | | 91% M 80% F | | | Quarter of women had been raped |
| Hamid & MacCarthy 1989 | 174 F 149 M | Various locations Service contact | Male/female | Behaviour 3–16% | Mood related 19–29% | | 8% | |
| Marshall 1989 | 43 | Hostels | Male/female | — 67% (floridly psychotic)† | 37% 'neurotic' | 48% | 12% | 71% had previous admission |
| Susser et al. 1989 | 223 | Shelters | Male | 8% (25% psychosis) | | 58% | | |
| Timms & Fry 1989 | 124 | Hostel | Male | 31% | 6% | 9.5% | 45% | |
| La Gory et al. 1990 | 150 | Shelter | Male/female | | 59% | | | |
| Mundy et al. 1990 | 96 | Shelter | Adolescents | ——— Mental Problem: not classified 29% had 4 or more psychotic symptoms‡ ——— | | | | |
| Susser & Struening 1990 | 223 (177 new) | Shelter | Male | Psychotics 8% definite, another 9% probable or possible | | | | |
| Scott & Boustead 1991 | 35 | Shelter | Male/female | 50% | | 14% | 7% | |
| Marshall & Reed 1992 | 70 | Hostel | Female | 71% | 3% | 10% | 9% | 23% physical illness |

* Refers to Diagnosis columns A–C.
† Refers to Diagnosis columns A and B.
‡ Refers to Diagnosis columns A–D.

homeless people. These included drug/alcohol use and abuse, transiency, emotional problems, lack of employment and social skills, and lack of social support systems. The study concluded that it was not entirely surprising (bearing the above in mind) that the scenario for young people leaving care sets the stage for them to become homeless individuals. Kufeldt & Nimmo (1987) urge a distinction between sporadic runaways and 'true' homeless. The former were more likely to be female and two major reasons for running away were poor communication in the home and some form of abuse (see also Powers *et al.* 1990). Hier *et al.* (1990) reported that among those who were thrown out ('throwaways') and those who left ('runaways'), females were more likely to be antisocial and males more hostile. Even though the sample size was small the average age was only 15. (On the same issue see also Council on Scientific Affairs 1989.)

More careful epidemiological work needs to be carried out to assess the full extent of the problems in this group.

### Homeless families

This group is becoming more visible and a major issue in management. Homeless families, though technically placed in bed and breakfast hotels and sometimes hostels, have the advantage of being able to register with a GP. However, in view of cramped conditions, limited facilities and whole families living in one room, a different set of problems emerges. Even though not enough epidemiological data are available, one would expect, given Brown & Harris's (1978) work, that there would be an increase in depression among single mothers. In addition, given the extremes of deprivation concerned, one would expect high rates of emotional and conduct disorders among children. Bassuk *et al.* (1986) and Bassuk & Gallagher (1990) reported from Massachusetts that in their sample of 80 homeless women and 151 children drawn from 14 family shelters, over two-thirds came from broken homes. The women were young (medium age 27 years), had a poor work record, few supports and long histories of residential instability. Nearly three-quarters (71%) were given a diagnosis of personality disorder. Among the children almost half of the 81 preschoolers tested suffered from developmental delays and one-third showed evidence of two major delays. The school-aged children were noted to be severely anxious and depressed. These authors also observed from anecdotal evidence that children often regressed and showed behaviours that were seen as attempts to cope with the stresses of homelessness generally and of shelter and living in hotels specifically. This was further confirmed by Boxill & Beaty (1990) who studied 40 homeless women and their children. They observed that these mothers and children were forced to build their relationships in an open and public 'personal space'. Six themes emerged from their study: an intense desire to demonstrate internalized values as a way of asserting self; questioning the certainty of anything and the ambiguity of everything; conflict over the need for attention and the experienced demand for independence; public mothering; unravelling of the mother role, and its experience of being externally controlled. Thus it is not surprising that an internalized confusion may arise both in the mothers and their children.

The reasons for homelessness in this group have been noted to be eviction, domestic conflict and unsafe living conditions (Mills & Ota 1989). Each unit therefore would have a different set of problems that need to be identified and worked with. Domestic conflicts also have implications for self-esteem and relationship difficulties. The children's physical and emotional growth is bound to be affected. Whitman *et al.* (1990) have reported language development delay in children of homeless families. Horowitz *et al.* (1988) compared three groups of children: 'hotel children' (i.e. those living in welfare hotels with their families); non-hotel children in an attendance improvement/dropout prevention programme, and non-hotel children in the community. School environment was observed as a 'facilitator' in hotel children's adaption to their environment. Problems in individuation and lack of effective models for young people will contribute to the psychological stress in the younger age group. Bassuk (1987) described the extent and origins of the problems of homeless families in Boston. Findings from her sample of 51 mothers and 78 children indicated chaotic developmental histories, long-term patterns of residential instability, minimal or absent supportive relationships, family violence, poor work histories and inadequate involvement with service agencies. Most of the work with this group in the UK has been carried out by GPs (see Stone 1989). Maternal depression was noted to be significantly increased amongst homeless mothers in London. When assessed by scoring specific questions it emerged that 16% were clinically depressed and another 19% could be classified as borderline depressives (Tempia M. 1991, personal communication). In addition to psychological problems, physical problems of living in a cramped space, and lack of adequate personal, medical and social facilities are bound to contribute to ill-health. The issues related to homelessness in ethnic groups are discussed by Tantam (1991). Susser *et al.* (1989) reported that blacks in their sample were overrepresented and they saw this as a reflection of culture where family networks may be weak.

### Psychiatric morbidity

As noted above, the estimates of psychiatric morbidity in the homeless vary a lot. This is a reflection of the source of the data collection as well as diagnostic criteria being employed (Table 21.1). Not all homeless people are mentally ill or have substance-abuse problems. The evidence of a correlation between homelessness and alcoholism or mental illness and homelessness does not mean that either factor is a cause or consequence of homelessness (Wright 1989).

A major problem in addition to the multiplicity of chronic or acute-on-chronic illnesses in this group is the inflexibility of psychiatric services delivery which prevents mental health workers from meeting the wide range of needs in this group. Not only do homeless people have multiple needs, they may also lack a 'social substrate' for

health. Furthermore, they display a limited trust in statutory services. On the other hand the inflexibility of services and strictness about catchment area provision make it more difficult for the homeless to be hooked into services. It has been noted that most subjects in one study obtained health services from their GPs (George *et al.* 1991). The changes in the NHS, with 'money following patient' may create additional difficulties since any definition of the 'last home' may prove difficult and unacceptable. Yet another complicating factor is the inability to register with primary care professionals which makes communication with the GP and continuity of care an impossible task. Williams & Allen (1989) reported from their study that in the Camden pilot scheme of health care for single homeless just over one-third were registered with a GP. On being interviewed a majority acknowledged that they had not tried to get themselves registered during the previous year because this was not a priority and others thought that registration was a waste of time given their mobility. Thus even if the services are available and willing, the potential consumers may not wish to take these on. The use of the Mental Health Act is often limited due to lack of contact with GPs and social services as well as the next of kin.

The psychiatric morbidity is often that of a chronic variety (for further discussion see Bachrach 1984). Figures from the Lewisham and North Southwark Homeless Team (Timms P. 1991, personal communication) suggest that the most commonly encountered form of schizophrenia is that of disorganized type characterized by thought disorder and hallucinations (using DSM-III-R criteria). Though this group is often identified with treatment resistance, clinical experience suggests that a majority will actually respond well to treatment if they can get it. The problems of minor psychiatric morbidity are complicated because of difficulties associated with negotiating with housing departments and other social agencies. Alcohol and drug abuse, sharing of needles and unsafe sex are bound to increase the neurological and psychiatric complications in this group.

*Management*

The first step in planning any intervention is to estimate the extent of the problem in any given catchment area. Numerous sources like the number registered with the local housing department, direct access hostel places, voluntary organizations and no fixed abode admissions can give an idea of the extent of homelessness. Multidisciplinary teams in general psychiatry settings are the most suitable agencies to provide help and manage mentally ill homeless people. A close liaison with the voluntary agencies and identification of a key worker are important aspects of the management. The key worker should be involved in assessment and discharge plans. Department of Health circulars HC(90)23 and HC(89)5 recommend guidelines to prevent patients from 'dropping through the net of care' and becoming or remaining homeless when they require adequate treatment and follow-up. As Bachrach (1984) recommends, the planning principles must have precise goals and objectives, comprehensive services with interagency co-operation, individualized programming, flexible format (of services) and cultural relevance. The Select Committee of the House of Lords (1982) recommended that the restoration of economic competitiveness is only one plank in the fight against unemployment. This chapter does not deal with social policy but it is important to remember that changes at both macro and micro levels in society are needed if the stigma and associated problems with unemployment are to be dealt with in a coherent manner.

# References

Allen V.L. (1970a) Psychology of poverty: problems and prospects. In Allen V.L. (ed.) *Psychological Factors in Poverty*. Markham, Chicago, pp. 367–383.

Allen V.L. (1970b) Personality correlates of poverty. In Allen V.L. (ed.) *Psychological Factors in Poverty*. Markham, Chicago, pp. 242–266.

Allin P. & Hunt A. (1982) Women in official statistics. In Whitelegg E. (eds) *The Changing Experience of Women*. Martin Robertson, Oxford.

Alstrom C.H., Lividelius R. & Salum I. (1975) Mortality among homeless men. *British Journal of Addictions* 70, 245–252.

Andrews M. (1990) Poverty – a multidimensional concept. *British Journal of Clinical and Social Psychiatry* 7, 176–181.

Arce A.A., Tadlock M., Vergare M.J. *et al.* (1983) A psychiatric profile of street people admitted to an emergency shelter. *Hospital and Community Psychiatry* 34, 812–817.

Arnetz B., Wasserman J., Petrini B. *et al.* (1987) Immune function in unemployed women. *Psychosomatic Medicine* 49, 1.

Atkinson T., Liem R. & Liem J.H. (1986) The social costs of unemployment: implications for social support. *Journal of Health and Social Behaviour* 27, 317–333.

Austerberry H. & Watson S. (1983) *Women on the Margins*. City University Housing Group, London.

Bachrach L. (1984) The homeless mentally ill and Mental Health Services: an analytical review of the literature. In Lamb H.R. (ed.) *The Homeless Mentally Ill*, pp. 11–54. APA Press, Washington DC.

Bakke W.W. (1933) *The Unemployed Man*. Nisbet, London.

Bakke W.W. (1940a) *The Unemployed Worker, A Study of the Task of Making a Living Without a Job*. Yale University Press, New Haven.

Bakke W.W. (1940b) *Citizens without Work*. Yale University Press, New Haven.

Banks M.H., Clegg C.W., Jackson P.R., Kemp N.J. & Stafford E.M. (1980) The use of the General Health Questionnaire as an indicator of mental health in occupational studies. *Journal of Occupational Psychology* 53, 187–194.

Banks M. & Jackson P.R. (1982) Unemployment and risk of minor psychiatric disorder in young people: cross-sectional and longitudinal evidence. *Psychological Medicine* 12, 789–798.

Bartley M. (1988) Unemployment and health: selection or causation – a false antithesis. *Sociology of Health and Illness* 10, 41–67.

Bassuk E.L. (1987) The feminization of homelessness. *American Journal of Social Psychiatry* 7, (1), 19–23.

Bassuk E.L. & Gallagher E.M. (1990) The impact of homelessness on children. *Child and Youth Services* 14, 19–33.

Bassuk E., Rubin L. & Laurait A. (1984) Is homelessness a mental health problem? *American Journal of Psychiatry* 141, 1546–1550.

Bassuk E., Rubin L. & Laurait A. (1986) Characteristics of sheltered homeless families. *American Journal of Public Health* 76, 1097–1101.

Beale N. & Nethercott S. (1986) Job loss and first pregnancy in young women. *British Medical Journal* 292, 799.

Beck A.T., Ward C.H., Mendelson M., Mock J. & Erbaugh, J. (1961) An inventory for measuring depression. *Archives of General Psychiatry* 4, 561–571.

Beckman R.D. (1933) Mental perils of employment.

Occupations 12, 28–35.

Bernstein B. & Henderson S. (1969) Social class differences in the relevance of language to socialisation. *Sociology* 3, 1–20.

Berry C. & Orwin A. (1966) No fixed abode: a survey of hospital admissions. *British Journal of Psychiatry* 112, 1019–1025.

Bhugra D. (1991) Psychiatric Care of the Homeless Mentally Ill. Report of a working party of the Royal College of Psychiatrists, London.

Bieri J. & Loback R. (1961) Self-concept differences in relation to identification, religion and social class. *Journal of Abnormal Social Psychology* 62, 94–98.

Bowlby J. (1978) *Loss: Sadness and Depression*. Penguin, Harmondsworth.

Boxill N.A. & Beaty A.L. (1990) Mother/child interactions among homeless women and their children in a public night shelter in Atlanta, Georgia. *Child and Youth Services* 14, 49–64.

Brandt L. (1932) *An Impressionistic View of the Winter of 1930–31 in New York City*. Welfare Council of New York, New York.

Breakey W.R., Fischer P.J., Kramer M. *et al.* (1989) Health and mental health problems of homeless men and women in Baltimore. *Journal of the American Medical Association* 262, 1352–1327.

Brenner M.H. (1971) *Time series analysis of the relationships between selected economic and social indicators*, vols I & II. National Technical Information Services, Springfields, VA.

Brenner M.H. (1973) Foetal, infant and maternal mortality during periods of economic instability. *International Journal of Health Services* 3, 145–157.

Brenner M.H. (1976) Effects of the economy on criminal behaviour and the administration of criminal justice in the US, Canada, England and Wales, Scotland. In *Economic Crisis and Crime*. United Nations Social Defense Research Institute, Rome.

Brenner S.O. & Bartell R. (1983) The psychological impact of unemployment: a structural analysis of cross-sectional data. *Journal of Occupational Psychology* 56, 129–136.

Brenner S.O. & Levi L. (1987) Long-term unemployment among women in Sweden. *Social Science and Medicine* 25, 153–161.

Briar K.H. (1977) The effect of longterm unemployment on workers and their families. *Dissertation Abstracts International* March 37, (9-A), 6062.

Brinkmann C. (1981) Finanzielle und psycho-soziale Belastungen wahrend der Arbeirslosigkert. In Wacker A. (ed.) *Vom Schock Zum Fatalismus?* Campus Verlag, Frankfurt.

Brown C., MacFarlene S., Paredes R. *et al.* (1983) *The Homeless of Phoenix: Who are They? And What Should be Done?* Phoenix South Community MHC.

Brown G.W. & Harris T. (1978) *Social Origins of Depression*. Tavistock, London.

Brown G.W., Ni Bhrolchain M. & Harris T. (1975) Social class and psychiatric disturbance among women in an urban population *Sociology* 9, 225–254.

Buhler C. (1933) *Der Menscliche Lebenslanf als psychologisches Problem*. Hirzel, Leipzig.

Buss T.F. & Redburn S. (1983) *Mass Unemployment: Plant Closing and Community Mental Health*. Sage, London.

Campbell A., Converse P.E. & Rodgers W.L. (1976) *The Quality of American Life*. Russell Sage, New York.

Carle J. (1987) Youth unemployment – individual and societal consequences and new research approaches. *Social Science and Medicine* 25, 147–152.

Carle J. & Schale C. (1982) *Unemployment – Problems, Actions and Effects*. National Swedish Social Welfare Board, Malino.

Chrniel A.J., Akhter S. & Morris J. (1979) The longdistance psychiatric patient in the emergency room. *International Journal of Social Psychiatry* 25, 38–46.

Cobb S. (1976) Social support as a moderator of life stress. *Psychosomatic Medicine* 38, 300–314.

Cobb S., Brooke G.W., Karl S.V. & Connelly W.E. (1966) The health of people changing jobs. *American Journal of Public Health* 56, 1476–1481.

Cobb S. & Kasl V. (1977) *Termination: The Consequence of Job Loss*. NIOSH Publication # 77–724, Cincinnati.

Cormier D. & Rochon J.P. (1988) L'errance, la toxicomanie et l'estime de soi chez les jeunes. *Revue Québecoise de Psychologie* 9, 111–122.

Council on Scientific Affairs (1989) Health care needs of homeless and runaway youths. *Journal of the American Medical Association* 262, 1358–1361.

Crossley B. & Denmark J.C. (1969) Community care: a study of the psychiatric morbidity of a Salvation Army Hostel. *British Journal of Sociology* 20, 443–449.

Cullen J.H., Ryan G.M., Cullen K.M., Ronayne T. & Wynne R.F. (1987) Unemployed youth and health: findings from the pilot phase of a longitudinal study. *Social Science and Medicine* 25, 133–146.

Daniel W.W. (1972) *Whatever Happened to the Workers in Woolwich?* Political and Economic Planning, London.

Dayson D. (1992) Crime, vagrancy, death and readmission of the long-term mentally ill during their first year of local reprovision. *British Journal of Psychiatry* Suppl. (in press).

Dumont M.P. (1989) Effects of unemployment on mental health. *Current Opinion in Psychiatry* 2, 287–290.

Edwards G., Hawder A., Williamson V. & Hensman C. (1966) London's skid row. *Lancet* i, 249–252.

Edwards G., Williamson V., Hawker A., Hensman C. & Postoyan S. (1968) Census of a reception centre. *British Journal of Psychiatry* 116, 1031–1059.

Eisenberg P. & Lazarsfeld P. (1938) The psychological affects of unemployment. *Psychological Bulletin* 35, 358–390.

Elderston M. (1931) *Case Studies of Unemployment*.

University of Pennsylvania Press, Philadelphia.

Ensminger M.E. & Celentano D.D. (1990) Gender differences in the effect of unemployment on psychological distress. *Social Science and Medicine* 30, 469–477.

Erikson E.H. (1956) Problem of ego-identity. *Journal of the American Psychoanalytic Association* 4, 56–121.

Fagin L. (1981) *Unemployment and Health in Families.* DHSS, London.

Fagin L. & Little M. (1984) *The Forsaken Families.* Penguin, Harmondsworth.

Feather N.T. (1982) Unemployment and its psychological correlates: a study of depressive symptoms, self-esteem, protestant ethic values, attributional style and apathy. *Australian Journal of Psychology* 34, 309–323.

Feather N.T. & Barber J. (1983) Depressive reactions and unemployment. *Journal of Abnormal Psychology* 92, 185–195.

Feather N.T. & Bond M.J. (1983) Time structure and purposeful activity among employed and unemployed university graduates. *Journal of Occupational Psychology* 56, 241–254.

Feather N.T. & Davenport P.R. (1981) Unemployment and depressive affect: a motivational analysis. *Journal of Personality and Social Psychology* 41, 422–436.

Feld S. (1963) Feelings and adjustment. In Nye F.I. & Hoffman L.W. (eds) *The Employed Mother in America.* Rand McNally, Chicago.

Fernandez J. (1984) In Dublin's Fair City: the mentally ill of no fixed abode. *Bulletin of the Royal College of Psychiatrists* 8, 187–190.

Fineman S. (1979) A psychosocial model of stress and its application to managerial unemployment. *Human Relations* 32, 323–345.

Fineman S. (1983) *White Collar Unemployment: Impact and Stress.* Wiley, New York.

Finlay-Jones R. & Eckhardt B. (1981) Psychiatric disorder among the young unemployed. *Australian and New Zealand Journal of Psychiatry* 15, 265–270.

Fischer P.J., Shapiro S., Breakey W.R., Anthony J.C. & Kramer M. (1986) Mental health and social characteristics of the homeless: a survey of mission used. *American Journal of Public Health* 76, 519–524.

Fischer R. & Heimann F. (1933) *Deutsche Kinderfibel.* Revohlt, Berlin.

Fisher A.L. (1965) Psychiatric follow-up of long-term industrial employees subsequent to plant closure. *International Journal of Neuropsychiatry* 1, 267–274.

Frese M. & Mohr G. (1987) Prolonged unemployment and depression in older workers: a longitudinal study of intervening variables. *Social Science and Medicine* 25, 173–178.

Fried M. (1969) Social differences in mental health. In Kova J. Antonensky A. & Zola I. (eds) *Poverty and Health: A Sociological Analysis.* Harvard University Press, Cambridge, Massachusetts.

Fryer D. (1987) Monmouthshire and Marienthal sociographic of two unemployed communities. In Fryer D. &

Ullah P. (eds) *Unemployed People*, pp. 74–93. Open University Press, Milton Keynes.

Fryer D. (1989) The Marienthal studies of unemployment. In Greif S., Holling H. & Nicholson N. (eds) *Work and Organisational Psychology: An International Handbook of Key Issues.* Psychologie Verlage Union, Munich.

Fryer D. (1990) The mental health costs of unemployment: towards a socio psychological concept of poverty. *British Journal of Clinical and Social Psychiatry* 7, 164–175.

Fryer D. & Payne R.L. (1986) Being unemployed: a review of the literature on the psychological experience of unemployment. In Cooper C.L. & Robertson I. (eds) *International Review of Industrial and Organisational Psychology*, pp. 235–278. Wiley, Chichester.

Fryer D. & Ullah P. (1987) *Unemployed People.* Open University Press, Milton Keynes.

Gayford J.J. (1975) Wife battering: a preliminary survey of 100 cases. *British Medical Journal* iii, 388–391.

George S.L., Shanks N.J. & Westlake L. (1991) Census of single homeless people in Sheffield. *British Medical Journal* 302, 1387–1389.

Goffman E. (1969) *Stigma.* Penguin, Harmondsworth.

Goldberg D.P. (1978) *Manual of the General Health Questionnaire.* NFER, Windsor.

Goldfarb C. (1970) Patients nobody wants: skid row alcoholics. *Diseases of the Nervous System* 31, 274–281.

Goodchilds J.D. & Smith E.E. (1963) The effects of unemployment as mediated by social status. *Sociometry* 26, 287–293.

Gould T. (1971) Out of work: the experience. *New Society* 20 May, 859–861.

Gove W.B. & Geerken M.R. (1977) The effect of children and employment on the mental health married men and women. *European Journal of Sociology* 56, 66–76.

Gravelle H.S.E., Hutchinson G. & Stern J. (1981) Mortality and unemployment: a critique of Brenner's time series analysis. *Lancet* ii, 675–679.

Groves E.R. (1934–35) Adaptations of family life. *American Journal of Sociology.* 40, 772–779.

Gurney R.M. (1980) Does unemployment affect the self-esteem of school leavers? *Australian Journal of Psychology* 32, 175–182.

Gurney R.M. (1981) Leaving school, facing unemployment and making attributions about the causes of unemployment. *Journal of Vocational Behaviour* 18, 79–91.

Hall O.M. (1934) Attitudes and unemployment: a comparison of the opinions and attitudes of employed and unemployed men. *Archives of Psychology* 165, 5–65.

Hamid W. & MacCarthy M. (1989) Community psychiatric care for homeless people in inner London. *Health Trends* 21, 67–69.

Harrison R. (1976) The demoralising experience of prolonged unemployment. *Employment Gazette* 84, 339–348.

Hayes J. & Nutman P. (1981) *Understanding the Unemployed.* Tavistock, London.

Heinemann K., Rohrig P. & Stadie R. (1980) *Arbeitslose*

*Frauen in Spanningsfeld von Erwebstattigkeit and Hausfrauenrolle.* Ernst Knoll, Melle.

Henwood F. (1983) Unemployment and Housework. Unpublished MSc Thesis, University of Sussex.

Henwood F. & Miles I. (1987) The experience of unemployment and the sexual division of labour. In Fryer D. & Ullah P. (eds) *Unemployed People*, pp. 94–110. Open University Press, Milton Keynes.

Hepworth S.J. (1980) Moderating factors of the psychological impact of unemployment. *Journal of Occupational Psychology* 53, 147–155.

Herrman H., McGory P., Bennett P., Van Riel R. & Singh B. (1989) Prevalence of severe mental disorders in disaffiliated and homeless people in inner Melbourne. *American Journal of Psychiatry* 146, 1179–1184.

Herzberg J. (1987) No fixed abode: a comparison of men and women admitted to an east London psychiatric hospital. *British Journal of Psychiatry* 150, 621–627.

Hier S.J., Korboot P.J. & Schweitzer R.D. (1990) Social adjustment and symptomatology in two types of homeless adolescents: runaways and throwaways. *Adolescence* 25, 761–771.

Hill J.M.M. (1977) *The Social and Psychological Impact of Unemployment.* Tavistock Institute of Human Relations, London. Doc #2T 74

Hill J. (1978) The psychological impact of unemployment. *New Society* 43, 118–120.

Hopson B. & Adams J. (1976) Towards an understanding of transition: defining some boundaries of transition dynamics. In Adams J., Hayes J. & Hopson B. (eds) *Transition*. Martin Roberston, London.

Horowitz S.V., Springer C.M. & Kose G. (1988) Stress in hotel children: the effects of homelessness on attitudes towards school. *Children's Environment Quarterly* 5, 34–36.

Israeli N. (1935) Distress in the outlook of Lancashire and Scottish unemployed. *Journal of Applied Psychology* 19, 67–68.

Jackson P.R. & Warr P.B. (1983) Age Length of Unemployment and Other Variables Associated with the Men's Ill Health During Unemployment. MRC/SSRC SYPY Memo 585.

Jackson P.R. & Warr P.B. (1984) Unemployment and psychological ill health: the moderating role of duration and age. *Psychological Medicine* 14, 605–614.

Jacobson D. (1987) Models of stress and meanings of unemployment: reactions to job loss among technical professionals. *Social Science and Medicine* 24, 13–21.

Jahoda M. (1979) The impact of unemployment in the 1930's and the 1970's. *Bulletin of the British Psychological Society* 32, 309–314.

Jahoda M. (1986) The social psychology of the invisible: an interview with Marie Jahoda by David Fryer. *New Ideas in Psychology* 4, 107–118.

Jahoda M. (1987) Unemployed men at work. In Fryer D. & Ullah P. (eds) *Unemployed People*, pp. 1–73. Open University Press, Milton Keynes.

Jahoda M., Lazarsfeld P.F. & Zeisel H. (1933/1972) *Marienthal: the Sociography of an Unemployed Community.* Aldine-Athenton, New York.

Jenkins R., MacDonald A., Murray J. & Strathdee G. (1982) Minor psychiatric morbidity and the threat of redundancy in a professional group. *Psychological Medicine* 12, 799–807.

Joelson L. & Wahlquist L. (1987) The psychological meaning of job insecurity and job loss: results of a longitudinal study. *Social Science and Medicine* 25, 179–182.

Joseph G. (1983) *Women at Work.* Philip Allan, Oxford.

Kardiner A. (1936) The role of economics security in the adaptation of the individual. *Family* 17, 187–197.

Kasl S.V. (1979) Changes in mental health status associated with job loss and retirement. In Jarrett J.E., Rose R.M. & Klerman G. (eds) *Stress and Mental Disorder*, pp. 179–200. Raven Press, New York.

Kasl S. & Cobb S. (1971) Physical and mental health correlates of status incongruence. *Social Psychiatry* 6, 1–10.

Kelvin P. (1981) Work as a source of identity: the implications of unemployment. *British Journal of Guidance and Counselling* 9, 2–11.

Kelvin P.M., Dewberry C. & Bunker N. (1985) Unemployment and the Use of Time. Paper presented at the BPS Annual Conference, Swansea.

Kelvin P. & Jarrett J. (1985) *Unemployment: Its Social Psychological Effects.* Cambridge University Press, Cambridge.

Kemp N.J. & Mercer A. (1983) Unemployment, disability and rehabilitation centres and their effects on mental health. *Journal of Occupational Psychology* 56, 37–48.

Kessler R.C., House J.S. & Turner J.B. (1987) Unemployment and health in a community sample. *Journal of Health and Social Behaviour* 28, 51–59.

Kilpatrick R.M. & Trew K. (1985) Life styles and psychological well being among unemployed men in Northern Ireland. *Journal of Occupational Psychology* 58, 207–216.

Kingsley S. (1976) An Investigation of Personal Instincts Concerning Unemployed Older Managers. Unpublished MSc Thesis, cited in Layton (1984).

Kinsey A.C., Pomeroy W.B. & Martin C.E. (1948) *Sexual Behaviour in the Human Male.* Saunders, Philadelphia.

Kufeldt K. & Nimmo M. (1987) Kids on the street: they have something to say. Survey of runaway and homeless youth. *Journal of Child Care* 3, 52–61.

La Gory M.L., Ritchey F.J. & Mullis J. (1990) Depression among the homeless. *Journal of Health and Social Behaviour* 31, 87–101.

Lamb H.R. (1984) *The Homeless Mentally Ill.* APA Press, Washington DC.

Langner T.S., Herson J.H., Greene E.L., Jameson J.D. & Goff J.A. (1970) Children of the City: affluence, poverty and mental health. In Allen V.L. (ed.) *Psychological*

*Factors in Poverty.* Markham, Chicago, pp. 185–209.

Layton C. (1984) Some Psychological Effects of Unemployment. Unpublished PhD Thesis, University of London.

Lazarsfeld P.F. (1932) An unemployed village. *Character and Personality* 1, 147–151.

Leavy S.A. & Freedman L.Z. (1961) Psychopathology and occupation. I Economic security. *Occupational Psychology* 35, 23–35.

Levi L., Brenner S., Hall E.M. *et al.* (1984) The psychological, social and biochemical impacts of unemployment in Sweden. *International Journal of Mental Health* 13, 18–34.

Lewis A. (1935) Neurosis and unemployment. *Lancet* ii, 293–297.

Lewis N. (1978) *Community Intake Services for the Transient Mentally Disabled.* San Francisco, Travellers Aid Society.

Lewis O. (1961) *The Children of Sanchez.* Random House, New York.

Lipton F.R.M., Sabatini A. & Katz S.E. (1983) Down and out in the city: the homeless mentally ill. *Hospital and Community Psychiatry* 34, 817–821.

Little C.B. (1976) Technical professional unemployment: middle class adaptability to personal crisis. *Sociology Quarterly* 17, 262–274.

Lodge Patch IC (1970) Homeless men. *Proceedings of the Royal Society of Medicine* 63, 437–441.

Lodge Patch IC (1971) Homeless men in London. *British Journal of Psychiatry* 118, 313–317.

McGann B. & Kenny U. (1977) *Significant Factors in the Thinking of Unemployed Executives.* Anco, Dublin.

Macky K. & Haines H. (1982) The psychological effects of unemployment: a review of the literature. *New Zealand Journal of Industrial Relations* 7, 123–125.

Madge N. (1983) *Families at Risk.* Heinemann, London.

Marsden D. & Duff E. (1975) *Workless: Some Unemployed Men and their Families.* Penguin, Harmondsworth.

Marshall J.R. & Funch D.P. (1979) Mental illness and the economy: a critique and partial replication. *Journal of Health and Social Behaviour* 20, 282–289.

Marshall J.E. & Reed J.L. (1992) Psychiatric morbidity in homeless women. *British Journal of Psychiatry* 160, 761–768.

Marshall M. (1989) Collected and neglected. Are Oxford hostels for the homeless filling up with disabled psychiatric patients? *British Medical Journal* 299, 706–709.

Melville D.I., Hope D., Bennison D. & Barraclough B. (1985) Depression among men made involuntarily redundant. *Psychological Medicine* 15, 789–793.

Merton R.K. (1957) *Social Theory and Social Structure.* Illinois, Glencoe.

Meyerson D.J. (1956) The 'skid row' problem. *New England Journal of Medicine* 254, 1168–1173.

Miles I. (1983) *Adaptation to Unemployment.* University of Sussex SPRU Technical Report, Brighton.

Miles I. & Howard J. (1984) A study of youth employment and unemployment (originally cited In Henwood F. & Miles I. *Unemployment and the Sexual Division of Labour*). In Fryer D. & Ullah P. (eds) *Unemployed People*, pp. 94–110. Open University Press, Milton Keynes.

Mills C. & Ota H. (1989) Homeless women with minor children in the Detroit metropolitan area. *Social Work* 34, 485–489.

Mischel W. (1961) Father absence and delay of gratification: cross-cultural comparisons. *Journal of Abnormal Social Psychology* 63, 116–124.

Moser K.A., Fox A.J. & Jones D.R. (1984) Unemployment and mortality in the OPCS longitudinal study. *Lancet* ii, 1324–1328.

Moser K.A., Fox A.J., Jones D.R. & Goldblatt P.O. (1986) Unemployment and mortality: further evidence from the OPCS longitudinal study 1971–1981. *Lancet* i, 365–367.

Mundy P., Robertson M., Robertson J. & Greenblatt M. (1990) The prevalence of psychotic symptoms in homeless adolescents. *Journal of the American Academy of Child and Adolescent Psychiatry* 29, 724–731.

Murphy J.F., Dauncey M., Newcombe R., Garcia J. & Elbourne D. (1984) Employment in pregnancy: prevalence, maternal characteristics, perinatal outcome. *Lancet* i, 1163–1166.

Myers J., Lindenthal J.J. & Pepper M.P. (1975) Life events, social integration and psychiatric symptomatology. *Journal of Health and Social Behaviour* 16, 121–127.

Obermann K. (1931) Jugend und Berof. *Monthly Magazine for the Advance of Vocational Counsel and the Vocational Improvement of Youth* 6, 93–95.

Olsen P. (1982) *Arbejdsloshedens social psykologi.* Dansk Psyokologisk Forlag, Kopenhaum.

Parkes C.M. (1971) Psycho-social transitions: a field for study. *Social Science and Medicine* 5, 101–115.

Payne R.L. (1988) A longitudinal study of the psychological well being of unemployed men and the mediating effect of neuroticism. *Human Relations* 41, 119–138.

Payne R.L. & Hartley J. (1984) Financial situation, health, personal attributes as predictors of psychological experience amongst unemployed men. *Journal of Occupational Psychology* 60, 31–47.

Payne R.L., Warr P.B. & Hartley J. (1983) Social Class and the Experience of Unemployment. MRC/SSRC SAPH Memo 549.

Pearlin L. (1975) Sex roles and depression. In: *Proceedings of the 4th Life Span Developmental Psychology Conference*, pp. 191–207.

Penkower L., Bromet E.J. & Dew M.A. (1988) Husbands' layoff and wives' mental health. *Archives of General Psychiatry* 45, 994–1000.

Pilgrim Trust (1938) *Men without Work.* Cambridge University Press, Cambridge.

Platt S. (1984) Unemployment and the suicidal behaviour: a review of the literature. *Social Science and Medicine* 19, 93–115.

Platt S. & Kreitman N. (1985) Parasuicide and unemployment among men in Edinburgh 1968–1982. *Psychological Medicine* 15, 113–123.

Powers J.L., Eckenrode J. & Jaklitsch B (1990) Maltreatment among runaway and homeless youth. *Child Abuse and Neglect* 14, 87–98.

Pratt, G.K. (1933) *Morale. The Mental Hygiene of Unemployment.* National Committee for Mental Hygiene, New York.

Priest R.G. (1970) Homeless in Chicago and Edinburgh. *Proceedings of the Royal Society of Medicine* 63, 441–445.

Priest R.G. (1971) The Edinburgh homeless. *American Journal of Psychotherapy* 25, 194–213.

Priest R.G. (1976) The homeless person and psychiatric services. *British Journal of Psychiatry* 128, 128–136.

Radloff, L. (1975) Sex differences in depression: the effects of occupation and mental status. *Sex Roles* 1, 249–265.

Raychaba, B. (1989) Canadian youth in care. *Children and Youth Services Review* 11, 61–73.

Ritter B. (1989) Abuse of the adolescent. *New York State Journal of Medicine* 89, 156–158.

Rogers D.B. (1933–34) Adjustments in the competent family. *Family* 14, 322–324.

Rose A.M. (1955) Factors associated with the life satisfaction of middle aged persons. *Marriage and Family Living* 17, 15–19.

Rossi P., Wright J., Fischer G. & Willis G. (1987) The urban homeless: estimating composition and size. *Science* 235, 1336–1341.

Rowntree B.S. (1901) *Poverty: A Study of Town Life.* Macmillan, London.

Rueth T. & Heller A. (1981) Unemployment: a factor in mental health crisis. *American Journal of Social Psychiatry* 3, 49–51.

Runciman W.G. (1966) *Relative Deprivation and Social Justice.* Routledge & Kegan Paul, London.

Rundquist E.A. & Sletto R.F. (1936) *Personality in the Depression: A Study in the Measurement of Attitudes.* University of Minnesota Press, Minneapolis.

Sarbin T.R. (1970) The culture of poverty, social identity and cognitive outcomes. In Allen V.L. (ed.) *Psychological Factors in Poverty.* Markham, Chicago, pp. 29–46.

Schlozman K.L. & Verba S. (1978) The new unemployment: does it hurt. *Public Policy* 26, 333–358.

Schlozman K.L. & Verba S. (1979) *Injury to Insult.* Harvard University Press, Cambridge, Mass.

Schneider L.S. & Lysgarrd S. (1953) The deferred gratification pattern: a preliminary study. *American Sociological Review* 18, 142–149.

Schneider O. (1932) Unemployment and the school child. *Zeitschrift für Gesundheit S uirwalt-ung* 3, 409–418.

Schumacher H.C. (1934) The depression and its effects on mental health of the child. *Mental Hygiene* 18, 287–293.

Scott J. & Boustead M. (1990) Characteristics of homeless adults in temporary accommodation. *British Journal of Clinical and Social Psychiatry* 7, 182–187.

Scott R., Gaskell P.G. & Morrell D.C. (1968) Patients who reside in common lodging houses. *British Medical Journal* 2, 1561–1564.

Select Committee of the House of Lords on Unemployment (1982) Report. HMSO, London.

Seligman M.E.P. (1975) *Helplessness,* pp. 253, 262. Freeman, San Francisco.

Shanks N.J. (1984) Mortality amongst inmates of a common lodging house. *Journal of the Royal College of General Practitioners* 34, 38–40.

Shanthamani V.S. (1973) Unemployment and neuroticism. *Indian Journal of Social Work* 34, 43–45.

Sharp L. & Nye F.I. (1963) Maternal mental health. In Nye F.I. & Hoffman L.W. (eds) *The Employed Mother in America,* pp. 309–319. Rand McNally, Chicago.

Sheppard H.L. (1965) Worker reaction to job displacement. *Monthly Labour Review* 88, 170–172.

Smith R. (1987) *Unemployment and Health.* Oxford University Press, Oxford.

Snow D.A., Baker S.G., Anderson L. & Martin M. (1986) The myth of pervasive mental illness among the homeless. *Social Problems* 33, 407–423.

Starrin B. & Larsson G. (1987) Coping with unemployment – a contribution to the understanding of the women's unemployment. *Social Science and Medicine* 25, 163–171.

Stevenson O. (1974) From the general to the specific. Cited in Harrison C.F. (1976) The demoralizing experience of prolonged unemployment. *Employment Gazette* 84, 339–348.

Stone R. (1989) The homeless: bed and breakfast families. In *Mental Health and Homelessness,* OP9. Royal College of Psychiatrists, London.

Stouffer, S.A., Suchman E.A., Devinney L.C., Stor S.A. & Williams R.M. (1949) *The American Soldier,* vol. 1. Princeton University Press, New Jersey.

Strauss M.A. (1962) Deferred gratification, social class and the achievement syndromes. *American Sociological Review* 27, 326–335.

Streltzer J. (1979) Psychiatric emergencies in travellers to Hawaii. *Comprehensive Psychiatry* 20, 463–468.

Susser E. & Struening E.L. (1990) Diagnosis and screening for psychotic disorders in a study of the homeless. *Schizophrenia Bulletin* 16, 133–145.

Susser E., Struening E.L. & Conover S. (1989) Psychiatric problems in homeless men: lifetime psychosis, substance use, and current desires in new arrivals at New York City shelters. *Archives of General Psychiatry,* 46, 845–850.

Tabler D.L. (1982) *Preliminary Report: Emergency Adult at Risk Shelter: A BCDSS Demonstration Project.* Department of Social Services, Baltimore.

Tantam D. (1991) High risk groups: the homeless and ethnic minorities. *Current Opinion in Psychiatry* 4, 295–303.

Tidmarsh D. & Wood S. (1972) Psychiatric aspects of destitution. In Wing J.K. & Hailey A.M. (eds) *Evaluating a Community Psychiatric Service.* Oxford University Press, Oxford, pp. 327–340.

Tiffany D.W., Cowan J.R. & Shontz F.C. (1969) Parts II and III in Final Report of a Vocational Rehabilitation Administration Research Project No. RD 2380, p. 672. Institute for Community Studies, Kansas City.

Tiffany D.W., Cowan J.R. & Tiffany P.M. (1970) *The Unemployed: A Social-psychological Portrait.* N.J. Prentice-Hall, Englewood Cliffs, New Jersey.

Timms P.W. & Fry A. (1989) Homelessness and mental illness. *Health Trends* 21, 70–71.

Townsend P. (1979) *Poverty in the United Kingdom.* Allen Lane, London.

Trew, K. & Kilpatrick R. (1984) *Daily Life of the Unemployed: Social and Psychological Dimensions.* Queen's University Department of Psychology, Belfast.

Ullah, P. (1987) Unemployed black youth in a Northern City. In Fryer D. & Ullah P. (eds) *Unemployed People*, pp. 111–147. Open University Press, Milton Keynes.

Ullah P., Banks M. & Warr P. (1985) Social support, social pressures and psychological distress during unemployment. *Psychological Medicine* 15, 282–295.

Vergare M.J. & Arce A.A. (1984) Unpublished data cited in Arce A.A. & Vergare, M.J. (1984) Identifying and characterizing the mentally ill among the homeless. In Lamb H.R. (ed.) *The Homeless Mentally Ill.* APA Press, Washington.

Wacker A. (1977) Arbejdsloshed som socialisationserfaring. In Leithanser T. & Heinz W. (eds) *Production, Arbejde, Socialisation.* Medusa, Kopenhaum.

Warr P.B. (1978) A study of psychological well-being. *British Journal of Psychology* 69, 111–121.

Warr P.B. (1983) Work, jobs and unemployment. *Bulletin of the British Psychological Society* 36, 305–311.

Warr P. (1987) *Work Unemployment and Mental Health.* Clarendon Press, Oxford.

Weller B. & Weller M. (1985) Health care in a destitute population. *Psychiatric Bulletin* 10, 233–235.

Weller M., Tobiansky R., Hollander D. & Ibrahimi S. (1989) Psychosis and destitution at Christmas 1987–1988. *Lancet* ii, 1509–1511.

Whiteley J.S. (1955) Down and out in London. *Lancet* ii, 608–610.

Whitly M.D., Osborne C.H., Godfrey M.A. & Johnston K. (1985) A point-prevalence study of alcoholism and mental illness among downtown migrants. *Social Science and Medicine* 20, 579–583.

Whitman B.Y., Accardo P., Boyert M. & Kendazor R. (1990) Homelessness and cognitive performance in children: a possible link. *Social Work* 35, 516–519.

Williams S. & Allen I. (1989) *Health Care for Single Homeless People.* Policy Studies Institute, London.

Winefield, A.H. & Tiggemann M. (1990) Length of unemployment and psychological distress: longitudinal and cross-cultural data. *Social Science and Medicine* 31, 461–465.

Winefield A.H., Tiggemann M. & Goldney R.D. (1988) Psychological concomitant of satisfactory employment and unemployment in young people. *Social Psychiatry and Psychiatric Epidemiology* 23, 149–157.

Wright J. (1989) *Address Unknown: Homeless in America.* NY Aldine de Gruyter, New York.

Wunderlich F. (1934) New aspects of unemployment in Germany. *Sociological Review* 1, 97–110.

Yach D., Mathews C. & Buch E. (1990) Urbanisation and health: methodological difficulties in undertaking epidemiological research in developing countries. *Social Science and Medicine* 31, 507–514.

Zawadski B. & Lazarsfeld P. (1935) The psychological consequences of unemployment. *Journal of Social Psychology* 6, 224–251.

# PART 3
# SOCIAL CONSEQUENCES

# Chapter 22
## Attitudes towards Mental Illness

DINESH BHUGRA & ALEC BUCHANAN

## Introduction

Attitudes to mental illness are a result of several identifiable and some unidentifiable factors. Attitudes are formed by virtue of previous knowledge and experience of the topic as well as education. Nadelson & Robinowitz (1987) argue that the improvement in the status of psychiatry over the last 100 years has very little to do with the 'scientification' of psychiatry but more to do with changing attitudes and perceptions. It is difficult to ascertain which comes first. Improvement in status is bound to improve attitudes and improved attitudes are likely to add to the status. A knowledge of the public's attitudes to mental illness and its treatment is vital if one is to succeed in providing services, especially those based in the community. Positive attitudes will attract better funding and high-quality personnel to work in the specialty.

Mental illness has aroused strong feelings among the lay public as well as among medical practitioners. Seen as 'modern day witch doctors, wise and powerful and capable of great good and great harm' (Jones 1978), psychiatrists are often lampooned, made fun of and in Hollywood jargon called shrinks. Reactions of people to psychiatrists have varied from fear, guilt, shame and hostility to awe and confusion (Warner 1982).

The advent of social and community psychiatry and the development of community mental health centres and services have given an added impetus to the review of public perceptions of mental illness and the mentally ill. For community care to succeed adequate financial and personnel resources are of paramount importance. To attract both of these, attitudes have to be positive so that psychiatry is not left out. The stigma of mental illness works against the patient even within his/her social networks.

The opinions and attitudes of a community carry implications for epidemiological studies of mental disorders as well as the felt needs of the community (Prabhu et al. 1984). Epidemiological studies can also offer parameters of public knowledge, thereby identifying the lacunae that should be filled by education. In the first half of the chapter we shall look at the lay public's attitudes and possible factors influencing these attitudes. Views as discussed in the popular media and literature and views on forensic psychiatry are not dealt with here. The second half of the chapter deals with doctors' attitudes to mental illness and psychiatrists.

## Public attitudes

Deviance often produces feelings of incomprehensibility, scorn and hostility and the label of illness is often preferred to that of deviance (Horwitz 1982). A person becomes a 'patient' as soon as he/she comes in contact with psychiatric services, which then leads on to stigma. This was confirmed by Phillips (1963) who reported that the largest increase in rejection rates among his sample occurred when a person had been admitted to a mental hospital. The postulate was that these people were rejected not because they had a health problem or because they were unable to help themselves, but because contact with a psychiatrist or mental hospital (often) defined them as mentally ill. However, on most occasions it is the community members who first realize that someone is behaving 'oddly' and that there are various ways of explaining such behaviour – one of which may be illness. As noted in Chapter 5, a vast majority of illnesses are dealt with in the individual's own circle. It is only after this that professional help may be sought. The move in help-seeking from the individual to the professional sector is vital for early detection and management of illness. This distinction between the community's perception and the medical/psychiatric model often gets blurred and can lead to confusion, rejection and hostility. Thus, psychiatrists need to be aware of the way the community perceives such behaviour. This distinction is even more important in the case of individuals from other cultures which will be discussed further in Chapter 29.

An attitude is composed of three basic components – cognitive, affective and behavioural (Triandis 1971). In other words response consistencies in thinking, feeling and acting towards an attitude object suggest the existence of an attitude. The cognitive component that is central in importance to the individual is more difficult to change. The affective component is said to be derived from association of the attitude-object with previous pleasant or unpleasant states in classical conditioning theory. The behavioural component, however, is influenced by the norms of the culture and peer group to which the individual belongs. When one of the components of an attitude changes, the other two may or may not change. The degree to which the three are interrelated is not certain but there have been examples (Vassilou *et al.* 1968) where in spite of new learning the affective component has remained unaltered. It is possible that indirect experiences may leave the affective component untouched whereas direct experiences may affect all three components. The studies on attitudes need to be followed bearing in mind the above caveat.

Attitudes towards mental illness and the mentally ill are multifaceted, highly complex, and difficult to evaluate (Neumann *et al.* 1984). The results of many studies that analyse the public's attitudes are often a mixture of the positive and the negative. The occasional areas of congruency among various studies have been argued to be due to a decrease in defeatism about the prospects of treating the mentally ill (Halpert 1955). In addition there are the conceptual and methodological problems. Concepts like facts, knowledge, information, image, ideas, thinking, belief, notion, opinions, attitude, stereotype, prejudice and stigma are often confused (Prabhu *et al.* 1984). Furthermore, the attitudes to various illnesses are different but are often lumped together. Of necessity the studies conducted have been restricted to limited geographical areas each of which has its own sociocultural milieu. The personality attributes of the respondents like dogmatism, authoritarianism and locus of control influence their attitudes towards mental illness and the mentally ill. Sociodemographic factors are well known to influence attitudes. As Prabhu *et al.* (1984) go on to argue, at a macro level, political structure and climate of society and the general political orientation of the society are also important factors. Thus cross-national and cross-cultural comparisons may not always be valid.

### American attitudes

The largest number of studies on attitudes to mental illness comes from North America. Earlier studies often demonstrated that there was a general feeling of mistrust, fear and anxiety about the mentally ill. In a classic study, Cumming & Cumming (1957) tested the residents of a small town before and six months after an educational campaign about mental illness. The educators emphasized in their discussions that the range of normal behaviour is a wide one and that normal and abnormal behaviours are on a single continuum. This last proposition meant that anyone could become mentally ill and Cumming & Cumming found that because of this the whole educational programme was rejected. As Rabkin (1974) emphasized, 'Upon their return home, (ex-mental patients) often find that being an ex-mental patient is more of a liability than being an ex-criminal in the pursuit of housing, jobs and friends.' Mental patients' handicaps are often attributable to public attitudes of rejection and avoidance.

Ramsey & Seipp's (1948a,b) studies revealed that respondents with higher educational and occupational levels were less apt to view mental illness as punishment for sin or the outcome of poor living conditions, were less pessimistic about outcome and were also less likely to believe in the deleterious effects of associating with the mentally ill. These studies are worth noting because of their sound methodological background.

Nunnally's (1961) 6-year survey of 400 respondents (who were a nationally representative sample) revealed that the mentally ill were regarded with fear, distrust and dislike. Interestingly these 'bad' attitudes were not held because of misinformation but because of lack of information. Using the same scale some 20 years later, Ahmed & Vishwanathan (1984) demonstrated that attitudes had shifted only slightly which they explained was due to the historical context. The Joint Commission on Mental Illness and Health (1961) reported that there existed a major lack of recognition of mental illness as illness and a predominant tendency to reject the mentally ill as well as their therapists.

Using a social distance scale, Whatley (1958–59) was able to demonstrate that only 15% of 2001 respondents would hire as their babysitter someone who had been seeing a psychiatrist. In general, Whatley found that tendencies to restrict social contact were most likely to arise in situations of closeness. The study, however, did not reflect all the factors in the social environment to which recuperating people were exposed. Hollingshead & Redlich (1958) reported that members of the lowest social class almost never actively sought psychiatric help for themselves or their relatives. Those who were in treatment were usually doing so by orders of authorities in the community. Link *et al.* (1987) in their study demonstrated that the label of 'previous hospitalization' fostered high social distance amongst those who perceived mental patients to be dangerous and low social distance amongst those who did not see patients as a threat. They concluded that the effects of labelling are fairly strong ones.

In the 1950s and 1960s, in North America, the studies were described as either optimistic or pessimistic (Rabkin 1974). Psychiatrically oriented workers favoured the mental health movement's efforts to publicize the medical model of mental illness, while those adhering to psychosocial models viewed these efforts as a moral crusade. This dichotomy, needless to say, must have affected the attitudes as well as the way these were elicited. Subsequent studies have often reported that an increasing proportion of the public believes that mental illness is an illness like any other and that social distance from the ex-mentally ill appeared to be declining. Rabkin (1974) argues that those investigators who believe in the psychosocial model also believe that social stigma remains and such a stigma is a consequence of deviance. This discrepancy between believers in two different models has not been completely resolved.

Star case vignettes (originally described by S. Star 1955, cited in Rabkin 1974) were increasingly being used to assess the public's attitudes and the public's knowledge of mental illness. Crocetti *et al.* (1963, 1971, 1972) in different studies demonstrated that their respondents from low social class and those who were poor were not negative in their attitudes. Dunham (1963) criticized Crocetti *et al.* for equating attitudes with behaviour and Phillips (1964) pointed out that Crocetti *et al.* were concentrating on formerly mentally ill patients and not those who were currently ill. Subsequently Phillips (1966) demonstrated that rejection was based on deviation from customary role expectations. This was also related to higher visibility of the mentally ill. Interestingly, Gurin *et al.* (1960) reported that 42% of their subjects would seek out a clergyman for support, with only 18% contacting a psychologist or a psychiatrist. Clergymen also scored highest in recognizing the seriousness of mental illness (Dohrenwend *et al.* 1961). Thus, not surprisingly most people would choose friends, family physicians or clergyman before resorting to psychiatry (Woodward 1951). The reasons for this may be to do with familiarity, provision of unconditional support and/or negative image of psychiatry along with stigma of mental illness and being seen by a psychiatrist. It may also reflect Kleinman's (1980) observation that Explanatory Models are of paramount importance in help-seeking behaviours and that a majority of illnesses are treated in the folk/personal sector (see Chapter 5).

The label of mental illness has been recognized as stigmatizing (Farina *et al.* 1965, 1971). In a study that had methodological problems, Meyer (1964) noted that only 44% of his sample could imagine falling in love with a mentally ill person, whereas 75% were prepared to work with such an individual. Sarbin & Mancuso (1970) argued that the public was more tolerant of deviant conduct when it was not described using mental illness labels. Thus the person in the street needs to collaborate with the mental health worker in identifying and setting some sort of marker for deviant or perplexing conduct. Cumming & Cumming (1965) consider that stigma associated with hospitalization for mental illness is a form of ego damage – the loss of a valued attribute. However, this loss is reversible. They argue that stigma acquires its meaning through the emotion it generates within the person bearing it and the feeling and behaviour toward him of those affirming it. A vicious cycle may be set up in which the patient feels ashamed because of hospitalization and, therefore, his/her actions may induce others to respond in a way that compounds the feelings of the patient. Thus, stigma is generated and reinforced in interaction.

Some illnesses produce more stigma than others and the role that is taken up by the individuals following discharge is important in reversing the loss of reputation caused by hospitalization. Families' perceptions of mental illness have an important role to play in Expressed Emotion towards the patient. Such perceptions have been altered by using educational techniques (Leff *et al.* 1982). People who have a personal knowledge of the mentally ill are knowledgeable about their illness.

Age (Johnson & Beditz 1981), education (Clark & Binks 1966, Wright & Klein 1966), social class (Hollingshead & Redlich 1958), severity of illness and presence of a diagnostic label, as well as the availability of alternative roles (Nierdzik & Cochrane 1985), are important factors in the formation of attitudes. Sex of the respondents is also an important factor. It could be argued that women who care for the mentally ill are also more likely to be seen as mentally ill so that their cooperation is of paramount importance if any of the therapeutic endeavours are to succeed (Bhugra 1989).

Since the community mental health movement started to gain ground in the USA in the 1970s there have been several attempts to identify the variety of factors responsible for negative attitudes (see Halpert 1965, 1969). Placing people who have spent long periods in hospital back into the community without adequate preparation of the person and the community will risk subjecting these patients to negative attitudes. Furthermore, a distinction needs to be made between those who are ex-mentally ill and those who are falling ill and are beginning to look for services. Not only are their needs different, but they are bound to have different expectations by virtue of their experiences. The success of community mental health schemes depends very much upon the involvement of the local community, an area often neglected. For a recent example of successful placement of patients in the community, see Chapter 32. The 'import' of medical and para-medical personnel from other areas who may not be aware of local issues is likely to alienate the community further. Segal (1978) emphasizes that with moving of the mentally ill into the community, an educated contact with the mentally ill has proved beneficial in enabling the public to reduce the social distance, even though the basic concepts of mental illness as a serious unpredictable, dangerous disorder remain unchanged. Formal and informal attempts have often been made to exclude mentally ill patients from the community by using city ordinances, zoning codes and police arrests (Aviram & Segal 1973).

One way out of this dilemma is the use of 'demythologizing' seminars as described by Morrison (1980), who suggests using educational programmes and Client Attitude Questionnaires. He considers the latter to be a vital component in demythologizing primary prevention, thereby preparing the community and avoiding an excessive dependence on professionals. As part of preparing the community, its leaders – political, social and religious – need to be approached and made aware of various issues. McGuire (1968) proposed five stages in the attitude-change process

– attention, comprehension, yielding, retention and action. Thus of those who yield, few will remember it long enough, and of these, even fewer will act on the information. Klapper (1967) argued that mass communication may create attitudes where none exist but rarely changes the direction of existing attitudes. The media may not always play a constructive role (Linter 1979). Bentz & Edgerton (1970) noted that their leader groups were more likely to reserve judgement on a given issue and were also less able to be categorical than the general public. As noted in Chapter 5, beliefs in certain aetiological factors are bound to affect help seeking, as well as provisions of support.

### The UK/Europe

The attitudes of the public in the UK were often affected by church teachings. Men of power and the church influenced public opinion, which identified the attitudes and behaviour of marginal social elements that could then be dubbed disturbed and, hence, alien. The apparent divide between those who set and met the norms and those who did not was linked with the expectations imposed by the central state or the market economy. Industrialization 'produced' more lunatics who were then locked away, thereby making madness even more menacing.

One of the earliest studies was a survey conducted by the British Broadcasting Corporation audience research department (1957). The survey demonstrated that social distance was an important factor in accepting the mentally ill. Only 50% would work with someone who was or had been mentally ill and only 25% felt that such an individual should be in a position of authority over others. In an interesting study assessing the attitudes of ex-mentally ill patients to the hospital and staff who looked after them, Klein (1979) noted that more than half of 788 respondents would go back to the same hospital. Paramedical and non-medical staff were rated highly and Klein emphasized, 'By definition, patients are experts at knowing what it feels like to be a patient and their views thus carry a unique authority.' However, quite often in setting up services and providing services this maxim is forgotten. Following the introduction of the NHS reforms, clinical audit is going to take an increasingly higher profile. The attitudes of patients and their relatives not only to the illness but to the services provided are going to become important in funding the services. The role of voluntary organizations in formulating public opinion is an important factor which is discussed in Chapter 35. Cooperation between health and non-health service agencies can only improve levels of patient care.

Two surveys in the late 1960s in Northamptonshire and Nottinghamshire revealed considerable reservation about mentally ill people. With more personal contact, attitudes became less liberal (Gatherer & Reid 1963, Willcocks 1968). Even after an extensive and enthusiastic educational campaign there was no measurable indication that knowledge in the community had changed in the desired direction. An article in the *British Medical Journal* (Anon 1968) cautioned that achieving any change in personal habits or in public attitudes required understanding the forces that motivated individuals and groups in the community. The success or failure of the plans was seen to be dependent upon finances, doctors and positive attitudes (Anon 1962, Altman 1981).

Using Star case vignettes, Graves *et al.* (1971) demonstrated that even though their subjects recognized the need to help schizophrenic and alcoholic cases these conditions were not seen as mental illnesses. The anxious neurotic was less likely to be seen as mentally ill than a psychotic. More highly educated people were less likely to permit close contact with simple schizophrenics.

In Greece, Lyketsos *et al.* (1985) looked at the attitudes of a highly selected sample of visitors attending a concert at a psychiatric hospital. The younger age group, the well educated and those in social classes I and II saw mental illness as a social problem whereas older people saw it as an organic illness with its roots in disorder of the nervous system. The same group of investigators (Aritzi *et al.* 1987) subsequently found that rural Greeks were more tolerant of mental illness than their urban counterparts. Malliori *et al.* (1987) repeated the study in the same area and found little change in the negative views held.

A study of Arabs in Israel (Shurka 1983) showed that Christian and highly educated respondents expressed less negative attitudes. Cohen & Struening's Opinions on Mental Illness scale (Cohen & Struening 1963) was used to demonstrate that people in Israel hold dual, inconsistent opinions on mental illness although these were affected by education and age among other factors (Rahav *et al.* 1984). In an earlier study in New Zealand, Blizard (1968) demonstrated that respondents identified the presence of mental illness in terms of described behaviour as well as the help source the person is described as consulting.

In a small sample of general practice surgery attenders in the UK, Bhugra & Scott (1989) found that males were more likely to object to the opening of a hostel for mentally ill in their street and were also less liberal in their attitudes. An overwhelming majority (80%) agreed that mental hospitals were necessary for the treatment of the mentally ill but nearly one-third did not know whether mental hospitals were like prisons. Nearly four-fifths of the respondents read a daily or Sunday paper, thus the local and national media can influence opinions. There appeared to be a degree of confusion in the minds of the respondents about the role of the psychiatrist. The authors conclude, in addition to 'a need for education about mental illness there is an indication for educating the community about the role of each member of the multi-disciplinary team if community psychiatry is to succeed.'

### Indian studies

Prabhu *et al.* (1984) point out that not much information is readily available about socio-culturally based conceptions of mental illness and related problems. Some observers (Sethi *et al.* 1967, Bhaskaran 1970, Carstairs 1973) have noted the presence of social stigma attached to mental illness. The use of religious places and temples in treatment of the mentally ill is well documented (Dube 1970, Somasundaram 1973). Somasundaram (1973) observed that faith was a powerful factor in effecting cures when patients visit certain temples where the presiding deity is reported to have curative powers. The perceived causes of mental illness are seen to be important in management of such patients by the family and the community. In one study Satija *et al.* (1981) reported that nearly one-quarter of their sample of psychoneuroses felt better after praying at a specific temple. As in the Greek study, the rural population appeared to be more tolerant of mentally ill patients (Neki 1966).

Sathyavathi *et al.* (1971) used Nunnally's Mental Health Opinion questionnaire with 150 respondents. Losing interest in the surroundings and losing self-control were reported as the most commonly attributed symptoms of mental illness. In a subsequent study Sathyavathi & Dwarki (1972) studied 120 subjects and reported that information on mental health was neither influenced by sex nor with contact with a mentally ill person. Other workers used Nunnally's questionnaires (Rahamtulla & Sathyavathi 1977, Basumallik & Bhattacharya 1983) to find fairly similar results, but Prabhu (1983) found the questionnaires developed in the west unsatisfactory and went on to develop a 13-factor scale which referred to folk therapy, folk beliefs, psychosocial stress and organic causation among others. The first two were obviously culture specific. Subsequent research found that the over 50s were more likely to see mental illness as a hopeless condition and preferred to maintain a greater social distance. Females were more aware, although there was a general lack of awareness about available facilities to treat the mentally ill. The latter is in contrast to Bhugra's (1991) findings that among 316 Indian teenagers only 8 would not send a mentally ill person to an asylum. More than one-third would seek medical attention, with a majority seeking help from specialists. This may reflect the younger age of the respondents and better dissemination of general knowledge through the media.

Malhotra & Wig (1975) developed 14 case vignettes and some of these were used in a cross-national study (Wig *et al.* 1980). In India, the reported preferred sources for help were modern health services rather than traditional healers, though the latter were more likely to be consulted in cases of mental illness than of physical ones.

Acute psychoses were perceived as the conditions with most serious consequences. In the Indian sample strikingly pessimistic attitudes towards the social consequences of mental disorders were noted in the community.

Verghese & Beig (1974) reported that 58% of their sample of 539 adults still saw a relationship between the lunar cycle and mental illness. Such a relationship was rejected by an overwhelming majority in Bhugra's sample (1991). This could be a reflection of the younger age group in the latter sample. In both samples the majority of the respondents were broadly sympathetic towards mental patients. The general trend of Verghese & Beig's study was a positive one and this positive trend showed a correlation with higher education and income. A higher proportion of their sample were against a marital alliance with a family where there was a positive history of mental illness. The two studies differ in their methodology. Verghese & Beig's (1974) was an interview-based study, whereas Bhugra's was based on questionnaires only though the questions were derived from the former study.

Boral *et al.* (1980) studied the family perceptions of mental illness. In this study 240 relatives of psychiatric patients and 120 relatives of non-psychiatric patients were approached with a 22-item questionnaire. Less than one-third of the subjects would prefer traditional methods of treatment. However, awareness of psychotherapy as a form of treatment was absent in both the groups. Both groups would favour giving jobs to ex-mentally ill patients but were not in favour of marital alliance. All the respondents felt that excited mental patients must be hospitalized.

The general trend of attitudes reported from India parallels that of the west. However, these studies are by and large from cities with a somewhat westernized population, and whether the results can be generalized to the rest of the population is questionable.

## Attitudes of the medical profession

This section will review the attitude of the medical profession to psychiatry. To some extent the opinion of other doctors reflects that of society at large. During their training and professional careers, however, doctors gain unique experience of psychiatrists and psychiatric patients. In addition, doctors' attitudes have implications for recruitment into the specialty and for the treatment of the mentally ill, who may be encountered in any branch of medicine. For these reasons their views merit separate consideration.

A doctor's attitude to psychiatry is composed of several elements. It involves an impression of the psychiatrist himself. It involves the doctor's perception of psychiatric patients. Finally, the doctor will have an impression of psychiatry as a vocation. To a degree these elements are independent: a doctor can hold a low opinion of psychiatric patients while maintaining a high regard for his professional colleagues. For this reason these three elements will be examined separately.

### *Opinions before graduation*

The views of medical students with regard to psychiatrists were investigated by Nielsen & Eaton (1981) whose subjects reported that 'in psychiatry the biggest turn-off was the people who taught it', and that 'psychiatrists tended to over-conceptualize and were often weird'. These views do not seem to be unique. Yager *et al.* (1982) found that more American medical students agreed than disagreed with the proposition that 'psychiatrists are fuzzy thinkers', and Furnham (1986) found that medical students in London were more likely to draw this conclusion about psychiatrists than about specialists in eight other areas of medicine. Comparing students' opinions of psychiatrists with their opinions of surgeons, physicians and general practitioners, Harris (1981) found that psychiatrists were rated as 'confused thinkers' and as 'emotionally unstable'. Positive features attributed to psychiatrists include a 'deep interest in intellectual problems', a 'deep interest in people', a willingness to 'treat the whole patient' and a less dogmatic approach than that employed by other doctors (Harris 1981, Furnham 1986). Despite the relative inexperience of medical students in clinical work, some research does exist regarding their attitude to psychiatric patients. Wilkinson *et al.* (1983a) showed that half of their sample agreed that 'psychiatric patients, generally speaking, are not easy to like', a proportion which dropped to one-third after the students had completed their psychiatric clinical attachment. More extensive is the body of research concerning students' attitudes to psychiatry as a vocation. Students have been found to regard the subject as unscientific (Yager *et al.* 1982, Furnham 1986, Das & Chandrasena 1988), imprecise (Yager *et al.* 1982, Furnham 1986), ineffective (Moos & Yalom 1966, Nielsen & Eaton 1981) and, hardly surprisingly given their other views, low in status when compared with other branches of medicine (Bruhn & Parsons 1964, 1965, Moos & Yalom 1966, Fishman & Zimet 1972, Zimet & Held 1975, Matteson & Smith 1977). Some 20% of students attending medical school in Washington DC regarded going into psychiatry as a waste of a medical education (Yager *et al.* 1982).

The question of how consistent such views are has two aspects which will be examined separately. First, it is possible that students' views of psychiatry as compared with other medical specialities vary according to when and where they undertook their medical training. Secondly, it is possible that substantial changes occur in the attitudes of medical students as their clinical training progresses. With regard to the first of these questions, there is good evidence that students' attitudes to psychiatry, as reflected in their choice of career, have varied over the years (see Nielsen 1979 for a review). The opinions of students in different parts of the USA have been compared and have been found to be similar (Yager *et al.* 1982) and research in the USA and the UK has revealed few significant differences between the countries. A decline in recruitment into the speciality was noted during the 1970s on both sides of the Atlantic (Russell & Walton 1970, Nielsen 1979), but there does seem to have been a greater decline in interest in the speciality in the USA. Despite the prevalence of private practice and widely held perception among medical students that psychiatry is less lucrative, financial considerations may not be the sole cause

of this decline. Research suggests that it is students with an interest in psychiatry who are most likely to see it as less financially rewarding (Nielsen & Eaton 1981, Yager *et al.* 1982).

Considerable debate has taken place over the possibility that the opinions of medical students change during their training and the extent to which these opinions can be influenced by experience gained during psychiatric clerkship. With regard to the first of these points, there is probably a general decline in the level of interest in psychiatry as students progress through medical school (Bruhn & Parsons 1965). With regard to the second, Walton (1969) found that students' career choices were not affected by psychiatric instruction and a subsequent study by Yager *et al.* (1982) lends support to this view. O'Mahony (1979) found that students' evaluations of psychiatric patients were substantially unaltered by a training course. Several authors have found, however, that students' attitudes are affected by their clinical experience. Ghadirian & Engelsmann (1982) interviewed 168 Canadian medical students before and after their clinical training in psychiatry. The authors reported a change in the students' emotional attitude towards psychiatric patients and an increase in their interest in clinical work. The proportion of students who expected that psychiatric training would have no effect on their choice of future career fell from 58% to 32%. Burra *et al.* (1982), in another Canadian study, found that students' attitudes to psychiatry improved following their clinical training. Wilkinson *et al.* (1983a) interviewed 94 clinical medical students in London before and after their period of clinical instruction. The authors found that, following their training, more students agreed that psychiatric patients presented interesting and challenging problems and less agreed that they were difficult to like. The proportion of students considering the possibility of specializing in psychiatry rose from 6% to 17%. Other less detailed studies have also reported a general improvement in attitudes towards psychiatry following a clerkship (Lau & Offord 1976, Larson *et al.* 1980), and there is some evidence that students themselves see their clinical experience of psychiatry as important in changing their views (Nielsen & Eaton 1981). Brook (1983) stated that the enthusiasm of the teachers and the model of psychiatry put forward may have an important effect on an undergraduate's attitude towards psychiatry.

In the USA a 40% increase in recruitment was reported from those medical schools where liaison work was the main focus of teaching. Rezler (1974), however, reviewing a range of teaching programmes, concluded that the effects on student attitudes were short-lived. However, it is difficult to be certain about this as methods of teaching have changed as has the emphasis in teaching. Burra *et al.* (1982) reported that improvements in attitude gained in the third clinical year were lost by the fourth and Wilkinson *et al.* (1983b) found that, although some of the attitude changes noted after students' psychiatric clerkships persisted to graduation, these changes were not maintained at the end of the first postgraduate year (Sivakumar *et al.* 1986). Only one study has described an enduring change in medical student thinking (Miller *et al.* 1979). Psychiatric teaching may change some of the attitudes of medical students but many of these attitudes predate, and are not markedly affected by, their clinical training (see Shuval & Adler 1980). Scott (1986) reported that in her survey of 87 students, while an attachment in psychiatry did seem to improve the students' attitude towards psychiatry, it did not seem to increase the attractiveness of the specialty as a first-choice career option. This, in itself, may be a positive step simply because positive attitudes towards the subject will affect closer liaison with psychiatrists and early referral and closer working. Future generations of medical students may then become more attracted to the specialty.

### Opinions after graduation

Numerous measures have been employed in the assessment of doctors' attitudes to psychiatric patients. Various researchers have looked at whether psychiatric patients are liked, whether they are considered interesting, whether they are regarded as satisfying to treat and to what extent they elicit sympathy. Sivakumar *et al.* (1986) asked a sample of 88 junior doctors in London

to agree or disagree with the statement that 'psychiatric patients, generally speaking, are not easy to like'. They found that 56% of their sample agreed, a response which may reflect the particular experiences of junior medical staff in dealing with psychiatric patients in an emergency or 'on-call' capacity. The response also reflected a marked hardening of attitude on the part of the doctors: only 28% of the same sample had agreed with the statement when they were interviewed as medical students 2 years earlier. While psychiatric patients may not be widely liked they are seen as presenting stimulating problems. The same authors on asking their junior medical sample whether 'the problems presented by psychiatric patients are often particularly interesting and challenging' found that 65% agreed. Physicians and other specialists may also regard psychiatric patients as unsatisfying to treat (Ansel & McGee 1971, Patel 1975, Ramon & Breyter 1978), although this research concentrates on patients who have harmed themselves and there is considerable evidence that psychiatrists too experience problems in treating such patients (Mintz 1961, Tabachnick 1961, Motto 1965). Finally, some researchers have chosen to assess the degree of sympathy evident in the attitude of medical staff towards patients with various diagnoses. Barber *et al.* (1975), studying a group of junior doctors, found that of ten diagnoses those which elicited least sympathy were self-poisoning, alcoholism and juvenile delinquency, each to some extent the province of psychiatrists. Goldney & Bottrill (1980) reported similar results, finding that self-poisoning and alcoholic liver disease elicited significantly less sympathy than illnesses such as diabetes, asthma and kidney failure.

There remains the issue of whether these views are representative of doctors in general or whether substantial variation exists between different groups. The first possibility is that age and experience affect doctors' attitudes. Ghodse (1978) reported no statistically significant differences between the attitudes of 64 senior medical staff and those of 125 juniors in their attitudes to patients who had taken overdoses of drugs. Patel (1975), however, found significantly less hostility amongst senior medical staff towards the same group of patients and this finding is supported by the work of Goldney & Bottrill (1980) showing that although non-psychiatric consultants described unsympathetic attitudes towards patients who had attempted suicide, they did so less than their junior staff. The second possibility is that members of different medical specialties hold different views of psychiatric patients. It has been suggested that surgeons and obstetricians are particularly antagonistic towards psychiatric patients (Dabkowski & Laskowska-Przybylska 1980), although Sivakumar *et al.* (1986) found no differences when they compared the attitudes to psychiatry of doctors who had chosen to enter general practice with those of doctors in general.

The attitudes of other doctors to psychiatrists have not been widely studied. There is a similar lack of research into the attitudes of other doctors to psychiatry as a vocation, although Sivakumar *et al.* (1986), noting that 52% of doctors had a generally favourable attitude to psychiatry after their first postgraduate year, found that this correlated positively with a view that in psychiatric practice doctors 'try to treat the whole patient and not just the disease'.

### Attitudes after specialization in psychiatry

Little research has been conducted concerning the attitude of psychiatrists to psychiatry as a vocation or to psychiatric patients, with the exception of work already described covering the difficulties which psychiatrists encounter when treating patients who harm themselves. Psychiatric researchers have taken a considerable interest, however, in the mental health of other psychiatrists. Groesbeck & Taylor (1977) have described the psychotherapist as a 'wounded healer', one who bears the scars of psychological pain and is therefore uniquely qualified to understand it in others. Halleck & Woods (1962) have reported that many psychiatrists themselves believe that the choice of psychiatry as a specialty is determined by the presence of 'significant emotional conflict' within the doctor. Several other studies have investigated what the authors perceive as emotional problems specific to psychiatry (Ungerleider 1965, Merklin & Little 1967,

Pasnau & Bayley 1971). Waring (1974) analysed the General Health Questionnaire scores of 83 psychiatric trainees and found that 22% had scores 'in the range of a probable case of non-psychotic emotional illness'; this compared with similar scores for only 3% of non-psychiatric controls. Studies in this area have been reviewed by Murray (1970).

The suicide rate of psychiatrists has been claimed to be higher than that of other doctors. Blachly *et al.* (1968) identified cases of suicide from the obituary columns of the *Journal of the American Medical Association* and sent questionnaires to the next of kin. They reported that psychiatrists had a suicide rate double that of GPs and six times that of paediatricians. The methodology employed in this study has been discredited by Rose & Rowcow (1973) who demonstrated the poor reliability of case finding through obituary columns. Their own study, reviewing death certificates, revealed no differences in the suicide rates of different specialties and other workers have reached similar conclusions (Kelly 1973). Nevertheless, the issue has provoked considerable interest (Freeman 1967, Rich & Pitts 1980). As with the issue of psychiatrists' mental health in general, while the significance of published reports is unclear, the interest of psychiatrists in the topic is in little doubt.

The sources of these attitudes are likely to be many and varied, involving opinions formed in childhood, at school and at university, and influences encountered in preclinical and clinical training (Hill 1960). Personality has long been seen as one of the determinants of medical students' attitudes to psychiatry (Kreitman 1962, Walton *et al.* 1963, Walton 1969, Pallis & Stoffelmayr 1973, Toone *et al.* 1979), and Walton (1969) reported that students showing an interest in the subject were 'psychologically minded'. The importance of medical students' and doctors' attitudes to psychiatry lies in the claim that these attitudes influence not only recruitment, but the ability of doctors to identify, treat and refer patients with psychiatric disorders (Eaton & Goldstein 1977, Nielsen & Eaton, 1981). It would seem that attitudes to psychiatry as a vocation would be more likely to affect recruitment whereas attitudes to psychiatric patients would be more likely to affect clinical practice, but this issue has not been investigated.

## Conclusions

The interrelationship of attitudes, provision of services and subsequent acceptance of help are complex issues. If community care is to succeed, psychiatrists need to be the torch-bearers in education, dispelling myths and being realistic about what psychiatry can offer. Often disillusionment results from being promised what cannot be delivered. Prolonged treatment in some psychiatric illnesses followed by slow improvement adds to negative attitudes (Ingham 1985), and thus the psychiatrist has to educate the patient and the relatives at a realistic level in offering prognosis, treatment and variety of interventions. Adequate sensible information delivered in a practical format in a simple language accompanied by written information (including the use of computers or audiovisual means wherever necessary) should help to dispel fears and change attitudes and expectations. The work with Expressed Emotion (Leff *et al.* 1982) has shown that giving factual information alone has very little impact on attitudes. It is necessary to continue to be available to answer questions for long periods of time before attitudes begin to shift. This is not encouraging for one-off educational programmes for the public.

The educational package should be repeated as often as possible simply because for any sustained change to occur it takes more than one generation for the information to filter through. Education of medical students, other medical and paramedical professionals is an important task in leading to early referral and early treatment and acceptance of mental illness. Increased liaison and setting up of district general hospital units with psychiatric services is a step in the right direction. Future research should concentrate on varying attitudes to different kinds of mental illness and different types of therapy. The discrepancy between public education on mental health and contemporary psychiatric thinking needs to be addressed. Psychosocial factors in the aetiology of illnesses

and their impact on help seeking need to be studied. Attitudes have several components and increased knowledge may lower the affective component even if the cognitive component remains untouched. A combination of strategies needs to be developed to improve knowledge, affect and behavioural components of attitudes.

It would seem that while these attitudes of the students may be affected by experiences of psychiatric clerkships, this effect is largely temporary. Southwood (1961) believed that the true road to progress in lessening the extent and severity of mental illness in the community lay in teaching medical students to be better at psychological medicine by helping patients to be realistic and to tolerate the anxiety and frustration that are a necessary part of living.

There are gaps in the research literature, particularly with regard to doctors' attitudes to psychiatrists themselves and to psychiatry as a vocation. The evidence which does exist would suggest that psychiatrists, widely seen as being interested in people and prepared and able to question their own motivation, are also regarded by other doctors as lacking a rigorous approach to their work. It is this latter impression which psychiatrists will have to correct if they are to improve their perceived image. It is arguable whether 'scientification' would completely change people's attitudes but a rigorous scientific approach to mental illness is a step in the right direction.

## References

Ahmed S. & Vishwanathan P. (1984) Factor-analytical study of Nunnally's scale of popular concepts of mental health. *Psychological Reports* 54, 455−461.

Altman B. (1981) Studies of attitudes towards the handicapped: the need for a new direction. *Social Problems* 28, 321−337.

Anon (1962) Ten year hospital plan. *British Medical Journal* i, 238−239.

Anon (1968) Public attitudes to mental health education. *British Medical Journal* i, 69−70.

Ansel E.L. & McGee R.K. (1971) Attitudes toward suicide attempters. *Bulletin of Suicidology* 8, 22−28.

Aritzi S., Richardson C., Lyketsos C. *et al.* (1987) Opinions concerning mental illness and psychiatric care in a remote rural area in Greece. *British Journal of Clinical and Social Psychiatry* 5, 19−21.

Aviram U. & Segal S. (1973) Exclusion of the mentally ill. *Archives of General Psychiatry* 29, 126–131.

Barber J.H., Hodgkin G.K., Patel A.R. & Wilson G.M. (1975) Effect of teaching on students' attitudes to self poisoning. *British Medical Journal* 2, 431–434.

Basumallik T. & Bhattacharya K.P. (1983) Views on mental health: a cross-cultural study. *Indian Journal of Clinical Psychology* 10, 219–226.

Bentz W. & Edgerton J. (1970) Consensus on attitudes towards mental illness. *Archives of General Psychiatry* 22, 468–473.

Bhaskaran K. (1970) The unwanted patient. *Indian Journal of Psychiatry* 12, 1–12.

Bhugra D. (1989) Attitudes toward mental illness – a review of the literature. *Acta Psychiatrica Scandinavica* 80, 1–12.

Bhugra D. (1991) Indian Teenagers Attitudes Towards Mental Illness. Research Report, Institute of Psychiatry, London.

Bhugra D. & Scott J. (1989) The public image of psychiatry – a pilot study. *Psychiatric Bulletin of the Royal College of Psychiatrists* 13, 330–333.

Blachly P.H., Disher W. & Roduner G. (1968) Suicide by physicians. *Bulletin of Suicidology* December, 1–18.

Blizard P.J. (1968) Public images of the mentally ill in New Zealand. *New Zealand Medical Journal* 68, 297–303.

Boral G.C., Bagchi R. & Nandi D.N. (1980) An opinion survey about the cause and treatment of mental illness and the social acceptance of the mentally ill patients. *Indian Journal of Psychiatry* 22, 235–238.

British Broadcasting Corporation (1957) *The Hurt Mind: An Audience Research Report*. BBC, London.

Brook P. (1983) Who's for psychiatry? United Kingdom medical schools and career choice of psychiatry 1961–1975. *British Journal of Psychiatry*, 142, 361–365.

Bruhn J.G. & Parsons O.A. (1964) Medical student attitudes toward four medical specialties. *Journal of Medical Education* 39, 40–49.

Bruhn J.G. & Parsons O.A. (1965) Attitudes toward medical specialties: two follow-up studies. *Journal of Medical Education* 40, 273–380.

Burra P., Kalin R., Leichner P. *et al.* (1982) The ATP 30 – a scale for measuring medical students' attitudes to psychiatry. *Medical Education* 16, 31–38.

Carstairs G.M. (1973) Psychiatric problems of developing countries. *Indian Journal of Psychiatry* 15, 147–155.

Clark A. & Binks N. (1966) Relation of age and education to attitudes towards mental illness. *Psychological Reports* 19, 649–650.

Cohen J. & Struening E.L. (1963) Opinions about mental illness: mental hospital occupational profiles and profile clusters. *Psychological Reports* 12, 111–124.

Crocetti G. & Lemkau P. (1963) Public opinion of psychiatric home care in an urban area. *American Journal of Public Health* 53, 409–417.

Crocetti G., Spiro H., Lamkau P. *et al.* (1972) Multiple models and mental illness: a rejoinder to 'Failure of moral enterprise: attitudes of public toward mental illness' by T. Sarbin and J. Mancuso. *Journal of Consulting Clinical Psychology* 39, 1–5.

Crocetti G., Spiro H. & Siassi I. (1971) Are the ranks closed? Attitudinal social distance and mental illness. *American Journal of Psychiatry* 127, 1121–1127.

Cumming E. & Cumming J. (1957) *Closed Ranks: An Experiment in Mental Health*. Harvard University Press, Cambridge, MA.

Cumming J. & Cumming E. (1965) On the stigma of mental illness. *Community Mental Health Journal* 1, 135–143.

Dabkowski M. & Laskowska-Przybylska H. (1980) The attitudes of physicians of various specialties towards the mentally ill. *Psychiatria Polska* 14, 377–382.

Das M.P. & Chandrasena R.D. (1988) Medical students' attitude towards psychiatry. *Canadian Journal of Psychiatry* 33, 783–787.

Dohrenwend B., Bernard V. & Kolb L. (1961) The orientations of leaders in an urban area toward problems of mental illness. *American Journal of Psychiatry* 118, 683–691.

Dube K.C. (1970) A study of prevalence and biosocial variables in mental illness in a rural and urban community in Uttar Pradesh, India. *Acta Psychiatrica Scandinavica* 46, 327–359.

Dunham H. (1963) Discussion of Crocetti and Lemkau's study. *American Journal of Public Health* 53, 415–417.

Eaton J.S. & Goldstein L.S. (1977) Psychiatry in crisis. *American Journal of Psychiatry* 134, 642–645.

Farina A., Holland C. & Ring K. (1971) Role of stigma and set in interpersonal reaction. *Journal of Abnormal Psychology* 76, 421–429.

Farina A. & Ring K. (1965) The influence of perceived mental illness on interpersonal relationships. *Journal of Abnormal Psychology* 70, 47–51.

Fishman D.B. & Zimet C.N. (1972) Specialty choice and beliefs about specialties among freshman medical students. *Journal of Medical Education* 47, 524–533.

Freeman W. (1967) Psychiatrists who kill themselves: a study in suicide. *American Journal of Psychiatry* 124, 846–847.

Furnham A.F. (1986) Medical students' beliefs about nine different specialties. *British Medical Journal* 293, 1607–1610.

Gatherer A. & Reid J.J.A. (1963) *Public Attitudes and Mental Health Education: Northampton Mental Health Project*. Northampton County Council, Northampton.

Ghadirian A.M. & Engelsmann F. (1982) Medical students' attitude towards psychiatry: a ten year comparison. *Medical Education* 16, 39–43.

Ghodse A.H. (1978) The attitudes of casualty staff and ambulance personnel towards patients who take drug overdoses. *Social Science and Medicine* 12, 341–346.

Goldney R.D. & Bottrill A. (1980) Attitudes to patients who attempt suicide. *Medical Journal of Australia* 2, 717–720.

Graves G.D., Krupinski J., Stoller A. *et al.* (1971) A survey of community attitudes towards mental illness. *Australian and New Zealand Journal of Psychiatry* 5, 18–28.

Groesbeck C.J. & Taylor B. (1977) The psychiatrist as wounded physician. *American Journal of Psychoanalysis* 37, 131–139.

Gurin G., Verof J. & Field S. (1960) *Americans View their Mental Health*. Basic Books, New York.

Halleck S.L. & Woods S.M. (1962) Emotional problems of psychiatric residents. *Psychiatry* 25, 339–346.

Halpert H.P. (1955) *Public Opinions and Attitudes About Mental Health*. Public Health Service Publication, Washington.

Halpert H.P. (1965) Public relations in mental health programmes *Public Health Reports* 80, 195–200.

Halpert H.P. (1969) Public acceptance of the mentally ill. *Public Health Reports* 84, 59–64.

Harris C.M. (1981) Medical stereotypes. *British Medical Journal* 283, 1676–1677.

Hill D. (1960) Acceptance of psychiatry by the medical student. *British Medical Journal* 1, 917–918.

Hollingshead A. & Redlich F. (1958) *Social Class and Mental Illness*. John Wiley, New York.

Horwitz A. (1982) The reaction to mental illness. In Horwitz A. (ed.) *The Social Control of Mental Illness*, pp. 85–120. John Wiley, New York.

Ingham J. (1985) The public image of psychiatry. *Social Psychiatry* 20, 107–108.

Johnson P. & Beditz J. (1981) Community support systems: scaling community acceptance. *Community Mental Health Journal* 17, 153–160.

Joint Commission on Mental Illness and Health (1961) *Action for Mental Health*. Basic Books, New York.

Jones K. (1978) Society looks at the psychiatrist. *British Journal of Psychiatry* 132, 321–332.

Kelly W.A. (1973) Suicide and psychiatric education. *American Journal of Psychiatry* 130, 463–468.

Klapper J.T. (1967) Mass communication: attitude stability and change. In Sherif C.W. & Sherif M. (eds) *Attitude, Ego-involvement and Change*, pp. 297–310. Wiley, New York.

Klein R. (1979) Public opinion and the NHS. *British Medical Journal* 1, 1296–1297.

Kleinman A. (1980) *Patients and Healers in the Context of Culture*. University, of California Press, Berkeley, CA.

Kreitman N. (1962) Psychiatric orientation: a study of attitudes among psychiatrists. *Journal of Mental Science* 108, 317–328.

Larson D.B. Orleans C.S. & Houpt J.L. (1980) Evaluating a clinical psychiatry course using process and outcome measures. *Journal of Medical Education* 55, 1006–1012.

Lau A.Y.H. & Offord D.R. (1976) A study of student attitudes toward a psychiatric clerkship. *Journal of Medical Education* 51, 919–928.

Leff J.P., Kuipers L., Berkowitz R., Eberlein-Eeries R. & Sturgeon D. (1982) A controlled trial of intervention in the families of schizophrenic patients. *British Journal of Psychiatry* 141, 121–134.

Link B.G., Cullen F.T., Frank J. & Wozniak J.F. (1987) The social rejection of former mental patients: understanding why labels matter. *American Journal of Sociology* 92, 1461–1500.

Linter J.M. (1979) Reflection on the media and the mental patient. *Hospital and Community Psychiatry* 30, 415–416.

Lyketsos G., Mouyas A., Malliori M. *et al.* (1985) Opinion of public and patients about mental illness and psychiatric care in Greece. *British Journal of Clinical and Social Psychiatry* 3, 59–66.

McGuire W.J. (1968) Personality and susceptibility to social influence. In Borgatta E.F. & Lambert W.W. (eds) *Handbook of Personality, Theory and Research*, pp. 1130–1187. Rand McNally, Chicago.

Malhotra H.K. & Wig N.N. (1975) Vignettes for attitudinal research in Psychiatry. *Indian Journal of Psychiatry* 17, 195–199.

Malliori M., Kyriakakis V. & Papadatos Y. (1987) Public opinion and psychiatric care in Greece. *British Journal of Clinical and Social Psychiatry* 5, 78–83.

Matteson T. & Smith S.V. (1977) Selection of medical specialities: preferences versus choices. *Journal of Medical Education* 52, 548–554.

Merklin L. & Little R.B. (1967) Beginning psychiatry training syndrome. *American Journal of Psychiatry* 124, 193–197.

Meyer J.K. (1964) Attitudes towards mental illness in a Maryland community. *Public Health Reports* 79, 769–772.

Miller S.I., Lenkowski L.D. & Weinstein D. (1979) Enduring attitude change in medical students. *Journal of Psychiatric Education* 3, 171–179.

Mintz R.S. (1961) Psychotherapy of the suicidal patient. *American Journal of Psychotherapy* 15, 348–367.

Moos R.H. & Yalom I.D. (1966) Medical students' attitudes towards psychiatry and psychiatrists. *Mental Hygiene* 50, 246–256.

Morrison J. (1980) The public's current beliefs about mental illness: serious obstacle to effective community psychology. *American Journal of Community Psychology* 8, 697–707.

Motto J.A. (1965) Suicide attempts: a longitudinal view. *Archives of General Psychiatry* 13, 516–520.

Murray R.M. (1970) The health of doctors: a review. *Journal of the Royal College of Physicians of London* 12, 403–415.

Nadelson C.C. & Robinowitz C.B. (1987) *Training of Psychiatrists in the 1990s*. APA Press, Washington.

Neki J.S. (1966) Problems of motivation affecting the psychiatrist, the general practitioner and the public in their interactions in the field of mental health. *Indian Journal of Psychiatry* 8, 117–124.

Neumann M., Elizur A. & Bawer A. (1984) Changing medical students' attitudes and professional behaviour toward mental patients as a function of psychiatric clerkship. *Israel Journal of Psychiatry and Related Sciences* 21, 235–246.

Nielsen A.C. (1979) The magnitude of declining psychiatric career choice. *Journal of Medical Education* 54, 632–637.

Nielsen A.C. & Eaton J.S. (1981) Medical students' attitudes about psychiatry. *Archives of General Psychiatry* 38, 1144–1154.

Nierdzik K. & Cochrane R. (1985) Public attitudes towards mental illness: the effects of behaviour, role and psychiatric labels. *International Journal of Social Psychiatry* 31, 23–33.

Nunnally J. (1961) *Popular Conceptions of Mental Health: Their Development and Change*. Holt, Rinehart and Winston, New York.

O'Mahony P.D. (1979) An investigation of change in medical students' conceptualization of psychiatric patients due to a short training course in psychiatry. *Medical Education* 13, 103–110.

Pallis D.J. & Stoffelmayr B.E. (1973) Social attitudes and treatment orientation among psychiatrists. *British Journal of Medical Psychology* 46, 75–81.

Pasnau R.O. & Bayley S.J. (1971) Personality changes in the first year of psychiatric residency training. *American Journal of Psychiatry* 128, 79–84.

Patel A.R. (1975) Attitudes towards self-poisoning. *British Medical Journal* 2, 426–430.

Phillips D. (1963) Rejection: a possible consequence for seeking help for mental disorders. *American Sociological Review* 28, 963–972.

Phillips D. (1964) Rejection of the mentally ill: the influence of behaviour and sex. *American Sociological Review* 29, 679–687.

Phillips D. (1966) Public identification and acceptance of the mentally ill. *American Journal of Public Health* 56, 755–763.

Prabhu G.G. (1983) Mental illness: public attitudes and public education. *Indian Journal of Clinical Psychology* 10, 13–26.

Prabhu G.G., Raghuram A., Verma N. & Maridess A.C. (1984) Public attitudes toward mental illness: a review. *National Institute of Mental Health and Neurosciences Journal* 2, 1–14.

Rabkin J. (1974) Public attitudes towards mental illness: a review of the literature. *Schizophrenia Bulletin* 10, 9–23.

Rahamtulla F. & Sathyavathi K. (1977) Popular Concepts of a Mental Patient. Paper presented at VIII All India Conference of Clinical Psychologists, Lucknow.

Rahav M., Stuening E. & Andrews H. (1984) Opinions on mental illness in Israel. *Social Science and Medicine* 19, 1151–1158.

Ramon S. & Breyter C.E. (1978) Attitudes towards self-poisoning among British and Israeli doctors and nurses in a psychiatric hospital. *Israeli Annals of Psychiatry and Related Disciplines* 16, 206–218.

Ramsey G. & Seipp M. (1948a) Attitudes and opinions concerning mental illness. *Psychiatric Quarterly* 22, 428–444.

Ramsey G. & Seipp M. (1948b) Public opinions and information concerning mental health. *Journal of Clinical Psychology* 4, 397–406.

Rezler A.G. (1974) Attitude changes during medical school: a review of the literature. *Journal of Medical Education* 49, 1023–1030.

Rich C.L. & Pitts F.N. (1980) Suicide by psychiatrists: a study of medical specialists among 18 730 consecutive physician deaths during a five year period, 1967–1972. *Journal of Clinical Psychiatry* 41, 261–263.

Rose K.D. & Rowcow I. (1973) Physicians who kill themselves. *Archives of General Psychiatry* 29, 800–805.

Russell G. & Walton H.J. (eds) (1970) The training of psychiatrists. *British Journal of Psychiatry* Special Publication No. 5.

Sarbin T. & Mancuso J. (1970) Failure of a moral enterprise: attitudes of the public towards mental illness. *Journal of Consulting and Clinical Psychology* 35, 159–173.

Sathyavathi K. & Dwarki B.R. (1972) Views of an Educated Group on Mental Health Problems. Paper presented at III All India Conference of Clinical Psychologists, Hyderabad.

Sathyavathi K., Dwarki B.R. & Murthy H.N. (1971) Conceptions of mental health. *Transactions of All India Institute of Mental Health* 11, 37–49.

Satija D.C., Singh D., Nathawat S.S. & Sharma V. (1981) A psychiatric study of patients attending Mehandipur Balaji temple. *Indian Journal of Psychiatry* 23, 247–250.

Scott J. (1986) What puts medical students off psychiatry? *Bulletin of the Royal College of Psychiatrists* 10, 98–99.

Segal S.P. (1978) Attitudes toward the mentally ill: a review. *Social Work* 23, 211–217.

Sethi B.B., Gupta S.C. & Kumar P.A. (1967) Psychiatric study of 300 urban families. *Indian Journal of Psychiatry* 9, 280–302.

Shurka E. (1983) Attitudes of Israeli Arabs towards the mentally ill. *International Journal of Social Psychiatry* 29, 108.

Shuval J.T. & Adler I. (1980) The role of models in professional socialisation. *Social Science and Medicine* 14A, 5–14.

Sivakumar K., Wilkinson G., Toone B.K. & Greer S. (1986) Attitudes to psychiatry in doctors at the end of their first post-graduate year: two-year follow-up of cohort of medical students. *Psychological Medicine* 16, 457–460.

Somasundaram O. (1973) Religious treatment of mental illness in Tamilnadu. *Indian Journal of Psychiatry* 15, 38–48.

Southwood H.M. (1961) The psychiatrist and the public. *Medical Journal of Australia* 48, 771–775.

Star S. (1955) *The Public's Ideas About Mental Illness*. Public Health Service Publications, Washington.

Tabachnick N. (1961) Countertransference crisis in suicide attempts. *Archives of General Psychiatry* 4, 572–578.

Toone B.K., Murray R., Clare A., Creed F. & Smith A. (1979) Psychiatrists' models of mental illness and their personal backgrounds. *Psychological Medicine* 9, 165–178.

Triandis H.C. (1971) *Attitude and Attitude Change.* John Wiley, New York.

Ungerleider J.T. (1965) That most difficult year. *American Journal of Psychiatry* 122, 542–545.

Vassilou V., Triandis H.C. & Oncken G. (1968) *Intercultural Attitudes after Reading an Ethnographic Essay: An Exploratory Study.* Group Effectiveness Research Laboratory, Urbana.

Verghese A. & Beig A. (1974) Public attitudes towards mental illness: the Vellore Study. *Indian Journal of Psychiatry* 16, 8–18.

Walton H.J. (1969) Personality correlates of a career interest in psychiatry. *British Journal of Psychiatry* 115, 211–219.

Walton H.J., Drewery J. & Carstairs G.M. (1963) Interest of graduating medical students in social and emotional aspects of illness. *British Medical Journal* 2, 588–592.

Waring E.M. (1974) Emotional illness in psychiatric trainees. *British Journal of Psychiatry* 125, 10–11.

Warner S.L. (1982) What is a headshrinker? *American Journal of Psychotherapy* 36, 256–263.

Whatley C. (1958–59) Social attitudes towards discharged patients. *Social Problems* 6, 313–320.

Wig N.N., Sulliman A., Routledge R. *et al.* (1980) Community reactions to mental disorders: a key informant study in three developing countries. *Acta Psychiatrica Scandinavica* 61, 111–126.

Wilkinson D.G., Greer S. & Toone B.K. (1983a) Medical students' attitudes to psychiatry. *Psychological Medicine* 13, 185–192.

Wilkinson D.G., Toone B.K. & Greer S. (1983b) Medical students' attitudes to psychiatry at the end of the clinical curriculum. *Psychological Medicine* 13, 655–658.

Willcocks (1968) Cited in Anon (1968). *British Medical Journal* 1, 69–70.

Woodward J. (1951) Changing ideas on mental illness and its treatment. *American Sociological Review* 16, 443–454.

Wright F. & Klein R. (1966) Attitudes of hospital personnel and the community regarding mental illness. *Journal of Consulting Psychology* 13, 106–107.

Yager D., Lamotte K., Nielsen A. & Eaton J. (1982) Medical students' evaluation of psychiatry: a cross country comparison. *American Journal of Psychiatry* 139, 1003–1009.

Zimet C.N. & Held M.L. (1975) The development of views of specialties during four years of medical school. *Journal of Medical Education* 50, 157–166.

# Chapter 23
## Social Consequences of Severe and Persistent Psychiatric Disorders

### JOHN WING

## Introduction

Trying to make a clear separation between physical causes and social effects when discussing psychiatric disorders such as schizophrenia is notoriously unrewarding. Traps and pitfalls of every kind, logical and scientific, abound (Wing 1991). This chapter is concerned with reactions and attributions rather than with the specific effects of illness. It will not for example include, except in passing, a description of the social course of schizophrenia or of persistent bipolar disorders. These topics are dealt with elsewhere in this book. Instead, the term 'consequence' will be interpreted as covering two kinds of social response to mental disorders associated with severe disability, each of which has also been seen as helping to cause or exacerbate them.

One response is the immediate societal reaction to such disorders. Edwin Lemert (1951) considered them as part of a more general category of socially visible deviations within a group, community or society: 'Admiration, awe, envy, sympathy, fear, repulsion, disgust, hate and anger are felt and manifested by those confronted by departures from their sanctioned ways of behaving.'

These social responses tend to be proportional to the degree, amount and visibility of the deviation.

Lemert suggested that, if deviance is recurrent and accompanied by the accumulation of a deviant population,

> mythologies, stigma, stereotypes, patterns of exploitation, accommodation, segregation, and methods of control spring up and crystallize in the interaction between the deviants and the rest of society. The informal societal reation is extended and formalized in the routinized procedures of agents and agencies delegated with direct responsibility for penalizing or restraining or reforming the deviants. The status of the deviants is redefined, and special pariah roles may be assigned to them.

This second aspect of the societal reaction affects, in particular, the policies and practice of politicians, administrators and professional carers who are responsible for the structures and services intended to prevent, treat or try to cope with the deviations. Neither the primary nor the secondary consequence is unitary but each can be discussed in general terms.

Lemert's theories of primary and secondary deviance influenced a generation of sociologists who, in turn, exerted a powerful influence on the way that services for people with mental illness developed during the 1960s and 1970s. Erving Goffman (1961) and Thomas Scheff (1963), in particular, developed a radical version of Lemert's ideas, usually known as 'labelling theory', according to which the consequences of mental disorders were due, not to the usual kinds of factors responsible for disease, but to the social attribution or label itself. This radical theory has been analysed and rejected elsewhere (Wing 1978) and will only be pursued further here in respect of its effect on service provision. However, the moderate form of the theory generally adopted by Lemert is clearly relevant to our topic.

Throughout the chapter, the central point around which discussion turns will be the two modes of societal reaction to severe and persistent social disablement that is perceived to be associated with mental disorders.

## Components of social disablement

The World Health Organization's Illness, Disability and Handicap (IDH) classification of the consequences of disease and injury works well for many straightforward medical problems (World Health Organization 1980). The first level of the classification is concerned with a concept of 'impairment' involving loss or abnormality of function. At the second level lie 'disabilities', involving restrictions on personal activities that may be directly caused either by disease or injury, or by the resulting impairments. Impairments and disabilities usually lead to 'handicaps', which involve disadvantages in interacting with or adapting to the individual's environment. A simple example is a violinist who develops arthritis of a finger joint (disease), which results in some loss of movement (impairment), little personal restriction (disability), but a serious occupational block (handicap).

There are two kinds of problem in adapting the IDH system for use with psychiatric disorders. First, the distinction between impairment and disability is difficult to draw when the impairment is psychological. Second, the direction of cause and effect is drawn firmly from left to right. Although there is some discussion in the text of the classification as to how social factors might influence disorder, impairment and disability (right to left), no criteria are suggested and the classification, in effect, ignores these possibilities. It is of limited value, therefore, in the delineation of social consequences.

For present purposes, we need to begin, rather than end, with a concept of social disablement that includes any substantial inability to perform up to personal expectation, or to the expectations of important others, that is associated with designated psychiatric disorder or impairment. Someone who can perform to expectation, but chooses not to, would be excluded by definition. The measurement of personal or psychosocial functioning is dealt with elsewhere (Wing 1989).

Three major components can be recognized in social disablement, each of which may need its own forms of prevention, treatment or rehabilitation. Each can provoke its own social consequences. In the first place, there is intrinsic or primary impairment, recognized for example by the presence of psychological dysfunctions that persist as long-term psychomotor slowness, thought disorder, hallucinations, delusional thinking, rapid cycling of mood, or the intrusion against conscious resistance of unwanted and distressing thoughts (Lewis 1953). This concept is close to that of the WHO classification. The term 'intrinsic' means only that impairment persists in spite of all attempts, using contemporary 'state of the art' treatment and care, to prevent it. Such impairments interfere with everyday functioning and may be the chief cause of social disablement. Some 'premorbid' personality factors can also be regarded as primary impairments.

In the second place, there are 'social disadvantages', such as a lack of occupational or social skills due to poverty or lack of education, absence of social supports, and environmental stressors of many kinds. Inadequate or positively harmful treatment of illness or impairment, non-provision of enabling services, and stigmatizing social attributions, provide examples in which there is substantial scope for cultural variation. Such disadvantages are only considered as a component of social disablement if they are associated with evidence of impairment.

Each of these two factors, impairment and social disadvantage, can have an adverse effect on a third component, 'adverse self-attitude' or 'demoralization', which damages self-confidence and self-esteem and generally lowers motivation to achieve goals that are, in fact, attainable. This third component amplifies disablement arising from the other two, and can persist even when the others are no longer important.

Thus the three types of factor – impairment, disadvantage and adverse self-attitude – interact with each other and it is difficult to disentangle their separate effects. Nevertheless, from the point of view of needs assessment, secondary and tertiary prevention, the improvement of services, and understanding how to help those who live with or care for the people affected, it is necessary to try to do so, since different elements may need different remedies.

## The particular problems of persistence

The practical implications of what may appear to be a purely academic structure for analysing the problems associated with chronic or frequently relapsing disorders were illustrated by a study of 212 disabled men passing through an Industrial Rehabilitation Unit (IRU). This was in London in 1958 during a period of relatively low unemployment, but the general conclusions are as relevant now as they were then (Wing 1966). A marked characteristic of these men was a lack of confidence in their ability to obtain and hold down a suitable job. A substantial proportion improved in this respect, according to both objective and subjective measures. Those who gained in confidence (improved self-attitudes) were significantly more likely to be employed (decrease in social disablement) two months after leaving the Unit than those who remained unconfident.

The main difference between those who improved and those who did not was in initial attitude to their problems. Those who showed, at interview during the first week, a constructive approach to their difficulties, whether or not they were emotionally distressed by them, tended to do well compared with those whose motivation was passive or casual, or who showed strong but idiosyncratic and unconstructive drives.

There were marked divergencies in objectively rated confidence between men in four diagnostic groups – injuries and recovering tuberculosis, chronic physical illness, neurotic disorders, and psychoses and mental handicap. These were partly due to differences in the type, persistence and severity of impairments but, within each group, those with constructive attitudes were more likely to become employed or to join a training course, despite their impairments.

The improvement in about a third of the men at the IRU was due to several factors. One of the hypotheses under test, derived from Festinger (1950, 1955), was that mixing with individuals who were visibly severely impaired but were nevertheless realistically confident of success in gaining suitable employment or training, would help to change the attitudes of those who were motivated but lacking in confidence.

This study therefore had interesting implications for the social dynamics of rehabilitation units and what were then called 'therapeutic communities'. For present purposes, its interest lies in the problems of those entrants who came in unmotivated and unconfident (or, in some instances, overconfident) according to the initial measures. All units with any pretence to a therapeutic aim have this problem – what to do with those who do not respond to the therapy? There are three alternatives:

1 To exclude them from entry.

2 To provide longer or more intensive or alternative therapy.

3 To accept that some impairments are, for the time being at least, unresponsive (though not necessarily totally immutable), and that the appropriate course is to accept the fact and seek to provide an environment that suits the handicapped person, while providing for the possibility of later improvement.

The first of these options is often inappropriate because of difficulty in identifying precisely enough which unconfident entrants would not improve during the course. Too many at the IRU would have been incorrectly excluded. Nevertheless, it is tempting to those who feel that the principles of good rehabilitation and resettlement rule out the terminology of 'failure'. The second option is feasible but there will still be a proportion of people who 'fail' each alternative form of help that is offered. Those who continue to 'fail' require the unpopular and costly (because prolonged) third option.

Subsequent studies of therapeutic environments for people with severe and persistent mental disablement have confirmed that a proportion continue to be disabled (i.e. they still have severe and persistent 'intrinsic' impairments which are the main component of their social disablement) in spite of all the treatments that state of the art practice requires, and thus demonstrate the continuing need for sheltered environments (Wing 1960, Wing *et al.* 1964, Wing *et al.* 1972).

Before considering what a rational societal response to severe and persistent mental illness might look like, and how the services necessary could be put into place, it will be useful to consider two examples of small rural communities faced with more specifically defined physical disorders in earlier times. Because the biomedical and societal factors involved are clearer, comparison and contrast are simplified.

## Leprosy

The first example is the reaction to leprosy of people in small rural communities in medieval Finland and Sweden, which has been studied and described in detail by Peter Richards (1977). Leprosy is a protean disorder and most people infected with the bacterium show no sign of disease. However, at its most severe and disfiguring, large skin lesions disintegrate into discharging sores, the voice becomes hoarse because of infection in the throat, peripheral nerves are destroyed and blindness can occur. The fear that such a calamity induced in communities with no conception of infectious disease can be imagined.

The societal reaction was one of horror and demand for isolation: 'The convention that lepers should be separated from society runs through eight centuries of European history.'

In the Middle Ages the motive was largely religious. Leprosy was regarded as a punishment for moral failing, especially loose, wanton and lustful living. Lepers were banished to the less desirable Swedish islands, where conditions were harsh. As the chaplain to the leper hospital in Bergen (which did at least provide priestly care) wrote: 'the wretched leper ... must renounce the best of an individual's freedom and rights; happiness flees him as well as life itself, and only death's certain call can comfort and satisfy him'.

By the seventeenth century fear of infection (a relatively sophisticated concept) had become the chief reason given for separation but a plain, direct, probably instinctive revulsion from disfigurement must have underlain whatever reasons were given. Richards quotes: 'the dramatically simple yardstick of diagnosis recommended to a Swedish country parish meeting on May 9th, 1654: "Kirsten of Söderby was ordered to be inspected by the parish and to be placed under observation if they shudder at her.". . . This primitive fear was not particularly medieval, it was just human, and for that reason it lives on.' Hence the lazarets, the clapper and bell, the cry of 'unclean', even when segregation was not absolute.

Leprosy was visible, terrifying; what else could they do but segregate? In a sense it was a rational strategy. The disease was incurable until about 45 years ago. Now the key to successful management is early diagnosis and treatment. Understanding the nature, pathology and causes, and the ability to treat it, has taken leprosy out of the public eye. The element of terror has been transferred to a modern epidemic – AIDS. Perhaps stigma cannot be eradicated, in spite of the efforts of compassionate organizations, until there is an objective means of diagnosis and a cause and, best of all, an effective treatment and cure?

Nevertheless, for those afflicted, the societal reaction usually made matters worse than was necessary. Social disadvantage, through stigma, isolation, poor living conditions, demoralization, and exposure to other diseases, amplified social disablement. However, even in medieval times, there were examples of charitable care, notably in religious houses, where disablement was minimized to what could not be avoided.

There seems an inevitable tendency for misfortune to be blamed on those who suffer it. One possible source for the motivation behind such unwittingly cruel accusations is illustrated by John Milton's detractors' statements that his blindness was a punishment by God for his unorthodox religious views. His response was both moving and typical of the desperation such accusations cause:

> I call upon thee, my God, who knowest my inmost mind and all my thoughts, to witness that (although I have repeatedly examined myself on this point as earnestly as I could, and have searched all the corners of my life) I am conscious of nothing or of no deed, either recent or remote, whose wickedness could justly occasion or invite upon me this supreme misfortune.

## Hereditary deafness

The second example could not provide a more extreme contrast. It is taken from Nora Ellen Groce's book *Eveyone Here Spoke Sign Language* (Groce 1985). A form of hereditary deafness, due to a recessive gene, existed for 250 years on Martha's Vineyard, an island off the coast of Massachusetts, following the arrival in the 1690s of the first deaf settlers – probably from rural Kent, where the disorder may well have been common for a long time. By the mid 1800s, scarcely a family in 'up-island', furthest from the mainland, was unaffected. In one small neighbourhood, with about 60 people, the condition had become fully expressed, with an incidence of 1 in 4.

Ordinarily, in those times, such an impairment led to gross social disadvantage and personal despair, because those afflicted were thought to be dumb, unable to use any form of communication, and generally severely mentally retarded. The result was profound social disablement.

The early settlers to Martha's Vineyard may well have brought a form of sign language with them. At any rate, the entire community did learn to sign and there was complete and free communication between the hearing and the deaf. A reporter from the *Boston Sunday Herald*, who visited the island in 1895, wrote:

> The spoken language and the sign language will be so mingled in the conversation that you pass from one to the other, or use both at once, almost unconsciously. Half the family speak, very probably half do not, but the mutes are not uncomfortable in their deprivation; the community has adjusted itself to the situation so perfectly.

The characteristics that made it possible for people with this particular severe impairment to function more or less normally include the following:

1 Those affected were otherwise normal and non-verbal language was unaffected.
2 The impairment was common and could occur in any family.
3 Children naturally learn sign as readily as, or even more readily than, they learn spoken language.
4 Deaf and hearing alike were isolated on the island.
5 The whole community was well informed.
6 The only kind of segregation based on impairment occurred later when deaf children were sent to the Gallaudet college for specialist schooling. But they returned even better equipped to function normally.

For all these reasons, the societal reaction was precisely adapted to the impairment, providing conditions in which its manifestation was hardly perceived as such. Thus there was very little social disadvantage, and no special reason for adverse self-attitudes to develop. Social disablement was minimized. There is no evidence, however, that the societal reaction to other impairments that usually attract a degree of stigma was specially benign.

Other communities where mutant deafness is common, which share these characteristics, have been described (Sacks 1989), but only under circumstances that are rarely found in industrialized countries. As migration from the mainland became common, the community became more 'normal', and to that extent, disadvantageous. This is borne out by the subsequent history of Martha's Vineyard. It was a caring community because of the special characteristics outlined above, but it now shares most of the characteristics of the rest of industrialized New England: '. . . only a few people can remember the Island's deaf inhabitants and fewer still can speak sign language'. The community has become unable to provide the same impairment-minimizing environment, because it has become less isolated. The lesson is that, for a whole community to be structured so as to minimize the impact of a particular incurable and persistent disorder, even though that disorder is otherwise undisruptive, it has to be, to some extent, 'abnormal'. The specially protective nature of the society only lasted while it remained segregated.

There are further lessons to be learned from the social history of congenital deafness, notably from the 'rebellion' at Gallaudet (by then a university), when the students demanded and finally got a President who was himself deaf (Sacks 1989). This was the beginning of a new self-confidence, and a new pride in their own form of language, with its rich potentials not available to ordinary speakers. Perhaps most important from the point of view of societal reaction, there was a new perception that they could live in their own like-minded groups insulated from the attitudes of the wider community, but able to share its benefits.

It is also necessary to recognize that congenitally deaf people could never have achieved this position of independence for themselves. It needed more than one generation to be taught sign by those 'normal' speakers who had discovered how to unlock their capacity to develop a rich and enabling form of language.

## The societal reaction to persistent mental illness

The history of the treatment and care of people afflicted by what we should now call mental disorders is largely part of the history of those who, under the English Poor Law, were designated the 'impotent poor' – infants, the aged, invalids and lunatics. They had a claim on their parish for a minimal maintenance, administered by local magistrates and their overseers. There was much corruption. Many workhouses 'became little more than prisons presided over by inadequate or venal men' (Checkland & Checkland 1974). The insane were regarded as having a global derangement of all the faculties, which reduced them to the level of animals or below. This attribution provided some form of justification for brutish treatment.

Kathleen Jones (1972) has provided a clear and connected account of the gradual recognition that there was a group of people with severe mental disorders who needed special care. There were private madhouses of varying size, run for private profit, whose inmates, in practice, were without legal protection and at the mercy of their keepers. In addition, an unknown number were confined alone in cellars, sheds or attics, often tied or chained, in conditions of indescribable misery. The public hospitals, of which the largest was Bethlem (colloquially Bedlam), were hardly better.

Towards the end of the eighteenth century a different approach to the care of mentally ill people was put into practice. Philippe Pinel was appointed medical director of the Bicêtre Asylum in Paris in 1793 and of the Salpêtriere in 1795. He taught that most of the causes of insanity were environmental and, crucially, that it did not necessarily deprive a person of all faculty for reason. His regime was based on non-restraint, attention to diet, plenty of exercise and work. At much the same time a similar philosophy, known as 'moral treatment' was being developed in England, and put into practice by William Tuke at the York Retreat. By this name, Tuke conveyed the idea of: 'A quiet haven in which the shattered bark might find the means of reparation or of safety.' Good food, comforts such as beds instead of straw, plenty of porter, some opium, religious meetings, exercise, work, and an unfailingly courteous but firm approach were the rule.

This concept of moral treatment informed the regimes of the first small public asylums set up during the first part of the nineteenth century. They were enlightened by the standards of the times, the residents were allowed their dignity, independence was fostered, length of stay was relatively short and the outlook on the whole was optimistic. Perhaps too optimistic, because claims for cures began to be made that could not possibly be justified.

The reasons why the early promise was not fulfilled have been much debated. The social changes accompanying the industrial revolution must have had a strong influence. Andrew Scull (1989) quotes Stevenson MacGill, writing in 1810:

> . . . the circumstances of the great body of mankind are of such a nature as to render every attempt to recover insane persons in their own houses extremely difficult, and generally hopeless.

Scull argues:

> To improve the living conditions of lunatics living in the community would have entailed supplying relatively generous pension or welfare benefits to provide for their support, implying that the living standards of families with an insane member would have been raised above those of the working class generally . . . something approximating a modern social welfare system, while their brethren were subjected to the rigours of a Poor Law based on the principle of less eligibility.

Enormous resources were, in fact, put into building the County mental hospitals during the second half of the century. Whatever one thinks of the underlying attitudes, the motivation to make such provision was clearly strong. But as they became larger and more numerous they also lost their reforming nature. But the time of the Lunacy Acts at the end of the 1880s the custodial era was well under way. It lasted until after World War II.

During the late 1940s and the 1950s the foundations of the welfare state were laid in legislation that included every aspect of social life – pensions, family allowances, education, unemployment and sickness benefits, a complex of personal social services, a national health service and provisions for the disabled and the destitute. The 'community' that had looked so threatening and brutalizing, especially for vulnerable people, during the earlier stages of the industrial revolution, now seemed more welcoming.

Parallel changes, in part consciously based on the ideas of moral treatment, were made in the mental hospitals. All the techniques of rehabilitation and resettlement now accepted as good psychiatric practice were introduced or reintroduced in the best hospitals well before the introduction of reserpine and chlorpromazine. The Mental Health Act of 1960 codified in law procedures that were already being followed in many hospitals and largely did away with the remaining legal restrictions of the Lunacy Acts. The success of the new medications, the first really effective physical treatments to be introduced, reinforced the optimism of the time and made it inevitable that the structure of the mental health service must change. Perhaps the most obvious reason for this was that the acute symptoms of psychosis often abated within a few weeks of admission and, if patients wanted to leave hospital, it was their right to do so. What became known, often disparagingly, as 'the early discharge policy', leading to the 'revolving door' system of care, was at many hospitals not a policy at all but an acceptance of the inevitable.

What happened next was that the gradual change already occurring, which was resulting in many of the functions of asylum being shifted from a hospital to a community setting, was overtaken by the pressure of a new ideology. Sociologists studying poor hospitals, mostly in the USA, argued that the disability that had kept patients in hospital for so long was artificially imposed (Goffman 1961, Scheff 1963). At its most extreme, this view took the form of a denial that any element of illness had been involved at all. Many students at university during the 1960s and 1970s breathed from the air the message that mental illness was a myth, that the medical establishment was a fraud and parental authority a sham (Laing & Esterson 1964, Szasz 1971, Illich 1975). Twenty years later, therefore, these ideas would influence, though usually not consciously, the attitudes of many politicians, and senior administrators and professionals in the National Health and Social Services.

Societal acquiescence in such views, promulgated through the media, weakened the confidence of clinical staff, who previously had felt supported in their reforms by public opinion but now found themselves portrayed as gaolers. The result was an increased emphasis on the more respectable biomedical and therapeutic aspects of their work and on early discharge. People with long-term disabilities were given a lower priority. What had begun as genuine progress began to take on some of the aspects of a self-fulfilling prophesy. Eventually, a policy that had been *following* practical clinical and social advances became administratively prescriptive with the appointment of managers whose remit was to close the large hospitals.

The results for those who remain seriously impaired are far from satisfactory. Severe and persistent mental disorders have not disappeared as the hospitals have run down. The presence on the streets of uncared-for people who are clearly mentally disordered has brought the problem back into public visibility and become a matter of societal concern, albeit in a less malignant form than a century and a half earlier, because of the general improvement in social conditions.

### Comparison and contrast

It is impossible to make strict comparisons between the complex industrial society that has developed in the UK since the early eighteenth century and the small rural communities that faced the problems, described above, of leprosy and congenital deafness, but some conclusions can tentatively be drawn.

The most obvious is that, for a community (and Martha's Vineyard *was* that) to adapt itself so well that members with a severe and incurable intrinsic impairment did not develop severe social disablement, it had to be very unusual, even by the standards of similar communities in its own times. Once the unusual qualities disappeared, the protective function was lost. The 'societal reaction' was not premeditated; it grew naturally and unselfconsciously with the unusual circumstances that fostered it. It could not deliberately be created.

Another point of contrast, with schizophrenia for example, is that, although the impairment interfered with vocal communication, there was an alternative that could relatively easily be learned, particularly by children. Once established, sign was used as freely as speech. There is no equivalent way round the communication disorder in psychosis, although some individuals are better at coping with it than others.

Once sign language became established, the people affected could form their own communities if they so wished and many have opted to do so, since society generally is indifferent to their specific needs and ignorant of the rich and interesting potentialities of their mode of communication. But interaction with society more generally is still necessary for survival and so a degree of dependence remains.

Does this example help define a caring community – one where the societal reaction does not amplify social disablement? Nora Groce herself hints that she thinks it does. She writes: 'Today, when the medical, legal and social professions are heatedly arguing the advantages and disadvantages of incorporating disabled individuals into mainstream society, the situation that existed on Martha's Vineyard is of particular relevance.' But the only time that mental handicap is mentioned in her book, there is no evidence that there was any generalization from the reaction to deafness to a similarly favourable response to people with other kinds of impairment. However, the value of communities constructed specifically

for the benefit of people who share an impairment does raise an interesting point that might be generalized.

The example of leprosy is more comparable with severe mental disorders such as, for example, chronic schizophrenia. So far, no cause is certainly known and the medications, though very useful, are not a cure. Those affected express ideas that most people find strange and often frightening. Psychotic behaviours can be unpredictable, inexplicable and terrifying. There is much disability from the negative impairments, which include a difficulty in using both verbal and body language, without any outward sign to explain what the problem is. A reaction of fear and a stigmatizing societal response is comprehensible. A tendency to blame the sufferers, their relatives, their doctors and other carers, or more abstract entities such as 'modern civilization', is as likely as it was with leprosy, and still is with other feared and incomprehensible disorders.

It is hard to deny that such reactions are important in determining the priorities of politicians when allocating resources. The lobby for ring-fenced funding for severe and persistent mental disorder is relatively easy to resist in spite of strong recommendations (Griffiths 1988, Social Services Committee 1985, 1990). Similarly, compared with heart disease or cancer or childhood leukemia, mental health charities find funds infinitely hard to come by. The relatively sympathetic tone of those who respond to sample surveys carries little cash with it.

Nevertheless, although leprosy may seem closer as a model than congenital deafness, there is one respect in which – in different ways – a similar conclusion can be drawn from the response to both kinds of disorder. For optimum care, each needed specific understanding of the nature of the impairment, free from distortions due to fear and prejudice. Some people with leprosy did sometimes obtain understanding, care within the limitations of contemporary knowledge, and the companionship of others similarly afflicted, in communities that were not closed although there were restrictions on their behaviour when outside. Deaf people have recognized that they can set up their own communities if they wish, and create conditions in which they can realize their own special potentialities.

The two examples indicate that the nature of the impairment imposes conditions on how far a degree of 'shelter' (both protective and, at the same time, liberating) is necessary and the extent to which it can be achieved. But there is sufficient parallel to suggest that the model is worth exploring in the case of other kinds of impairment as well.

### The functions of asylum

The swing of the pendulum during the nineteenth century from neglect and cruelty in the community to reform in the small asylums, then on to a different kind of neglect in the large Victorian institutions, then back again during this century towards reform, then again back towards inadequate 'community care', suggests that the current swing might not have reached the end of its span.

The third option illustrated by the results of the evaluation of the rehabilitation unit discussed above still has to be provided for. The reluctance to make adequate provision for the chronically sick and disabled is not new, as Brian Abel-Smith (1964) has pointed out. St Thomas's hospital in London was set up for this purpose, but already in the seventeenth century had restricted its admissions to short-term care.

Doctors 'wanted to show results in terms of cure, and they were naturally reluctant to surround themselves with cases which showed the limitations of their professional skill. Doctors who taught particularly wanted to demonstrate successes.'

In fact, after St Thomas's had excluded incurable patients,

> one of its governors (Mr Guy) founded, with money he had made in speculation, a sister hospital specifically for incurable and mental cases. But the early decision of the governors of St Thomas's hospital to concentrate on curable cases proved to be an important precedent. It was not many years before Mr Guy's hospital began to exclude the type of patient it was founded to treat.

The Victorian institutions provided a ring-fenced investment of resources, not in competition with those for problems with a more favourable public profile. During the second era of reform, in the 1950s, the best of them were divesting themselves of the poverty, neglect, idleness, restrictiveness and isolation that had become the norm in the decades of 'custodial care'. Few districts now have anything as good as the facilities for social and occupational rehabilitation then available at the most advanced hospitals.

There were three other advantages that tend to be forgotten. A place was usually rapidly available at times of emergency, however difficult the problem. There was a simple and identifiable line of management responsibility. And there were the imponderable but surely appreciable benefits of space, trees and grass. Space and privacy, indoors and out, are precious assets, not just for people under severe stress who need tranquility but even more for those who cannot help being overactive, aggressive or seriously socially embarrassing.

The ladders from hospital to community were being created from within. Day hospitals, sheltered workshops, groups in open industry, group homes and hostels, domiciliary assessments before admission and regular after-care visits, were set up and demonstrated to be effective by staff, for example at Glenside (Bristol), Netherne (Coulsdon) and Mapperley (Nottingham). This was a time of tremendous optimism about the future development of the mental health services. Social psychiatry in the UK was widely regarded as the best in the world. Enoch Powell's famous lecture on the changes in structure needed to develop the innovations of the 1950s, which were already straining the resources of the old structure, was delivered in 1961.

A further point of crucial interest in the transition from 'institutional' to 'community' care is the extent to which informal agents can replace professionals. Abrams (1978) emphasizes the lack of reward, for example in terms of an ordinary personal relationship, offered by some severely disabled or disturbed people in return for care. Caring relatives often do find that they can cope in the way that good professionals do, but the problem is to provide them with some of the rewards of staff, including public approbation instead of stigma, financial compensation and time off. If relatives are not willing to take on onerous responsibilities, staff have to be provided to replace their functions. There is sufficient scope in the processes required for such a changeover to account for the numbers of mentally ill people who are left with only minimal care or no care at all (Leach & Wing 1980, Marshall 1989).

The question arises whether the community, as such, is an important variable, independently of the societal reaction to each particular kind of impairment, and the health and social services that the reaction allows to be provided. In a minority addendum to the Barclay Report on social work, Pinker (1982) made a trenchant attack on the contemporary assumption that the community can somehow be therapeutic in itself:

> Formal systems of social service delivery developed because the informal networks of mutual aid in local communities were manifestly incapable of meeting the kinds of personal need which arise in complex industrial societies ... The most vulnerable, disadvantaged and stigmatized clients will be at greatest risk in the community-based models of social work since they give greatest offence to local norms of behaviour and are often rejected by their local communities.

A system of services that could minimize social disablement without the structure of the Victorian hospitals must be founded on an understanding of the nature of the impairments that give rise to the needs, and the social and personal factors that amplify their effects. Within a comprehensive, geographically based service the functions of asylum must still be carried out.

The first function includes protection from cruelty, exploitation, competition (e.g. if unable to compete for housing or work on the open market, or unable to use ordinary amenities for recreation), pauperism (insufficiency of food, light, heat, clothing and basic personal possessions), and social isolation. The second function, reparation, includes identification of the causes of social disablement, by skilled diagnosis and social assessment; treatment, within the limits of contemporary medical knowledge; and provision, within the limits of local social attitudes and facilities, of the means of rehabilitation and resettlement.

These functions need to be carried out within the context of a comprehensive service that contains sufficient structures and skilled personnel to allow people affected by persistent impairments to use all their faculties to best advantage, and thus to find a way of living that minimizes social disablement. The elements of such a service have been set out elsewhere (Wing & Furlong 1986, Wing 1990).

## Summary and conclusions

The concept of social disablement has been analysed into three components. The starting point for this chapter has been the intrinsic impairments affecting people with severe and persisting mental disorders. The effect of these on social functioning can be amplified by social disadvantages and adverse personal attitudes. Objective studies of the value of treatment and rehabilitation have universally described a group that remains socially disabled, in spite of the best 'state of the art' care.

The question of whether the societal reaction to such mental illnesses (including the structure and functioning of services set up to help cope with them) has any influence on the degree of social disablement that results, is considered in comparison with two other conditions, in which the physical causes of the impairments are now known with considerable accuracy: leprosy and congenital deafness.

In the case of leprosy, the reaction of small close-knit rural communities before the cause was known and effective treatments introduced, was typically one of horror, stigma and segregation. More recently, leprosy has become just another treatable infectious disease.

In the case of hereditary deafness, the result was also usually severe social disablement, but this was largely due to the ignorant societal reaction. One very unusual community is described, where social disablement was minimal. The circumstances in which this occurred (isolation of the community, a common occurrence of the impairment, and an easily learned means of compensating for it) are rare; when the circumstances changed the protective nature of the community was lost. However, people with the impairment can now themselves learn how to cope with it without severe social disablement.

The history of the societal reaction to severe and persistent mental illness, and of the services that have been set up, suggests that the pattern of leprosy is more relevant than that of congenital deafness. Until effective means of prevention are found, the major responsibility for care will lie with ring-fenced services that do not depend on a spontaneous community response. The positive model provided by the newly discovered independence of those with congenital deafness may, however, suggest lessons and opportunities for living with mental illness. A structure of services with such facilities as a foundation, and ladders of opportunity leading to fully competent domestic, occupational and personal functioning, would be a proper replacement for the former system based on large hospitals.

In order to create such a system, at least as much effort and resources have to be put in by statutory authorities as was the case when the large hospitals were being built, during the latter half of the nineteenth century.

## References

Abel-Smith B. (1964) *The Hospitals, 1800–1948. A Study in Social Administration in England and Wales.* Heinemann, London.

Abrams P. (1978) Community care. Some research problems and priorities. In Barnes J. & Connelly C. (eds) *Social Care Research.* Bedford Square Press, London.

Checkland S.G. & Checkland A.O. (eds) (1974) *The Poor Law Report of 1834.* Penguin, Harmondsworth.

Festinger L. (1950) Informal social communication. *Psychological Review* 57, 271.

Festinger L. (1955) Social psychology and group processes. *Annual Review of Psychology* 6, 187.

Goffman E. (1961) *Asylums. Essays on the Social Situation of Mental Patients and Other Inmates.* Penguin, Harmondsworth.

Griffiths R. (1988) *Community Care. Agenda for Action.* HMSO, London.

Groce N.E. (1985) *Everyone Here Spoke Sign Language. Hereditary Deafness on Martha's Vineyard.* Harvard University Press, Cambridge, Massachusetts.

Illich I. (1975) *Medical Nemesis.* Calder and Boyars, London.

Jones K. (1972) *A History of the Mental Health Services.* Routledge London.

Laing R. & Esterson A. (1964) *Sanity, Madness and the Family.* Tavistock, London.

Leach J. & Wing J.K. (1980) *Helping Destitute Men.* Tavistock, London.

Lemert E.M. (1951) *Social Pathology*, p. 54. McGraw-Hill, New York.

Lewis A.J. (1953) Health as a social concept. *British Journal of Sociology* 4, 109–124.

Marshall M. (1989) Collected and neglected. Are Oxford hostels for the homeless filling up with disabled psychiatric patients? *British Medical Journal* 299, 706–709.

Pinker R.A. (1982) An alternative view. In Barclay P. (chairman) *Social Workers. Their Role and Tasks.* Appendix B, pp. 236–262. Bedford Square Press, London.

Richards P. (1977) *The Medieval Leper.* Brewer, Cambridge.

Sacks O. (1989) *Seeing Voices.* University of California Press, Berkeley.

Scheff T.J. (1963) *Being Mentally Ill.* Aldine, Chicago.

Scull A. (1989) *Social Order/Mental Disorder. Anglo-American Psychiatry in Historical Perspective.* Routledge, London.

Social Sevices Committee, House of Commons (1985) *Community Care with Special Reference to Adult Mentally Ill and Mentally Handicapped.* HMSO, London.

Social Sevices Committee, House of Commons (1990) *Community Care. Services for People with a Mental Handicap and People with a Mental Illness.* House of Commons, London.

Szasz T. (1971) *The Manufacture of Madness.* Routledge, London.

Wing J.K. (1960) A pilot experiment on the rehabilitation of long-hospitalized male schizophrenic patients. *British Journal of Preventive and Social Medicine* 14, 173–180.

Wing J.K. (1966) Social and psychological changes in a rehabilitation unit. *Social Psychiatry* 1, 21–28.

Wing J.K. (1978) *Reasoning about Madness*, chap. 5, pp. 149–157. Oxford University Press, London.

Wing J.K. (1989) The measurement of social disablement. *Social Psychiatry and Psychiatric Epidemiology* 24, 173–178.

Wing J.K. (1990) Meeting the needs of people with psychiatric disorders. *Social Psychiatry and Psychiatric Epidemiology* 25, 2–8.

Wing J.K. (1991) Social psychiatry. In Bebbington P. (ed.) *Social Psychiatry*, pp. 3–22. Rutgers, New Jersey.

Wing J.K., Bennett D.H. & Dehnam J. (1964) *The Industrial Rehabilitation of Long-stay Schizophrenic Patients.* Medical Research Council Memorandum no. 42. HMSO, London.

Wing J.K. & Furlong R. (1986) A haven for the severely

disabled within the context of a comprehensive community psychiatric service. *British Journal of Psychiatry* 149, 449–457.

Wing L., Wing J.K., Stevens B.C. & Griffiths D. (1972) An epidemiological and experimental evaluation of industrial rehabilitation of chronic psychotic patients in the community. In Wing J.K. & Hailey A.M. (eds) *Evaluating a Community Psychiatric Service. The Camberwell Register, 1964–1971.* Oxford University Press, London.

World Health Organization (1980) *International Classification of Impairments, Disabilities and Handicaps.* WHO, Geneva.

# Chapter 24
# Case Management for the Long-term Mentally Ill

## GRAHAM THORNICROFT

## Introduction

The imprecision of the term and the reputed clinical benefits of its use have ensured that case management has become a widely promoted remedy. In this chapter, by reviewing the relevant recent literature, the lineage, conceptual basis and current use of the term case management will be clarified. In doing this the range of core tasks performed by case managers will be identified, a typology of case management along 12 axes will be established and examples given of case management in routine clinical practice. Finally, the empirical evidence emerging from studies which evaluate case management for the long-term mentally ill will be summarized and interpreted. In this way the important opportunities offered by the case management approach to the care and treatment of the long-term mentally ill can be indicated, and the need for specificity in describing the forms of case management interventions most effective for particular groups of patients can be emphasized.

## Defining case management

Case management is a strategy for distributing and coordinating services on behalf of patients (Modrcin *et al.* 1985). It is a generic term that encompasses the following functions: the coordination, integration, and allocation of individualized care within limited resources. Many more precise definitions have been put forward which emphasize aspects of this range of activities, and which reflect the various levels at which case management is intended to operate.

At the individual level, for example, case management has been defined as the coordination of care for patients who require a multiplicity of services (Clifford *et al.* 1988). At the project level, case management has been used to describe a method of organizing the delivery of care for a defined patient group, which clarifies and allocates the responsibilities of the staff team. At the programme level, case management has been characterized as an approach that provides services on the basis of need, which avoids duplication of effort between agencies, and which seeks to offer an adequate range of services to target groups of patients, such as those with diagnoses both of psychosis and substance abuse (Fariello & Scheidt 1989). This third level may be more accurately called care (or system) management.

Three points arise. The definitions of case management more often refer to treatment principles (see below) than to treatment practices (Modrcin *et al.* 1985). Secondly, most accounts of case management are generalized elaborations of such principles and are not precisely defined (Bachrach 1989). Thirdly, descriptions of case management programmes for long-term mental illness refer to a very wide range of practices (Robinson & Bergman 1989). It is clear therefore that descriptions of 'case management' programmes should specifically set out their structure and working methods to allow useful comparison with other similar projects.

## The development of the case manager concept

The roots of case management lie in social case work (Robinson & Bergman 1989). This has long stressed the value of interventions with distressed individuals which encourage the development of self-reliance and adaptation (Lee & Kenworthy 1929). Within the mental health services the coordination function was first formally recognized in the USA by the Community Mental Health Centers Act (1963), and its 1975 amendments explicitly required the centres to link with other agencies providing care for long-term patients. There has, however, been an increasing recognition in the USA over the last 25 years that community-based services for long-term mental illness were still too often fragmented (Braun *et al.* 1981, Kiesler 1982, Mechanic & Aiken 1987, Thornicroft & Bebbington 1989). Methods of drawing together the health and social service care components were developed, especially in federally funded initiatives such as the Community Support Program (Tessler & Goldman 1982). These models were rapidly disseminated. In 1981, for example, no Medicaid-supported case management programmes were operating in the USA. By 1986, 19 states had more than 651 000 patients enrolled in such programmes (Spitz 1987). A parallel development in Britain has been the rapid expansion of community mental health centres (many of which include case-managed care for long-term patients), of which 87 had opened by 1987 (Sayce *et al.* 1991).

## The principles of case management

The many practices of case management share a common set of underlying principles. Their point of departure is that vulnerable patients with long-term psychiatric disorders need therapeutic interventions which optimize their adjustment and minimize their functional disabilities. The care-giver is put in facilitating relationship with a patient where the common goal is assumed to maximize the patient's level of independence (Intagliata 1982, Bachrach 1984, Kanter 1989).

In practice, case management for the long-term mentally ill has developed into a range of techniques, which aim to ensure that patients with long-term psychiatric disorders receive consistent and continuing services for as long as they are required (Torrey 1986), and that services do not inappropriately focus on patients with less severe conditions (Levine 1981). The direct care-giver variants of case management emphasize the staff–patient relationship as the key component through which effective care is channelled, in the tradition

of social case work. Brokerage models, however, have not developed a conceptual framework to link case work principles with a practice that de-emphasizes personal contact (Modrcin *et al.* 1985).

The principles most often described at the root of the case management concept are outlined in Table 24.1. Continuity refers both cross-sectionally to a comprehensive range of services for long-term mental illness (Santiago *et al.* 1985) and longitudinally to emphasize the need for enduring the possibly indefinite care for a substantial proportion of this group (Anthony *et al.* 1988).

More recent developments of case management both in Britain and in the USA have further stressed the following points: providing services on the basis of need, ensuring they are accessible, optimizing desired outcomes within given resource limitations and clarifying authority and responsibility to ensure that care-providers can be held accountable for their actions (Challis & Davies 1986, Challis 1989, Knapp *et al.* 1990).

## The core tasks of case management

There is considerable consensus about the range of tasks that case management can offer at the individual level, and these are summarized in Table 24.2 (Modrcin *et al.* 1985, Renshaw 1987b, Charnley & Davies 1987, Knapp *et al.* 1990).

Patient identification requires first the definition of the target group for the case management service. This may be clearly established from current contact with services, or may include, for example, forms of outreach to identify patients with no previous or current contact who nevertheless require psychiatric care (Charnley & Davies 1987).

**Table 24.1** Principles of case management

Continuity of care
Accessible services
Staff–patient relationship
Titrating support to need
Facilitating independence
Patient advocacy
Advocacy for services

**Table 24.2** Core tasks of case management

Identify patients (case finding)
Assess needs
Design care package
Coordinate service delivery
Monitor service delivery
Evaluate effectiveness of services
Modify care package
Repeat cycle unless services no longer needed

**Table 24.3** Twelve axes to define case management in practice

  1  Individual/team case management
  2  Direct care/brokerage
  3  Intensity of interventions
  4  Degree of budgetary control
  5  Health/social service function
  6  Status of case manager
  7  Specialization of case manager
  8  Staff : patient ratio
  9  Patient participation
 10  Point of contact
 11  Level of intervention
 12  Target population

The next stage is to assess the social, clinical, vocational, physical health, and residential needs of each patient (Brewin *et al.* 1987, Worley *et al.* 1990). This may require interviews with several members of the care team to establish the extent of disability in each domain. On the basis of this thorough assessment of need, the case manager decides, within the resources available, which services should be offered, how often, where and

by whom. Where interventions are distributed across agencies, the details of each agreed service may be set out in joint care plans, or may be itemized in formal contract specifications (House of Commons 1990). Whether the case manager acts as service broker or direct carer, the effectiveness of care next needs to be evaluated, formally or informally. Where quality standards have been included in the service contract, the process of care may be set against agreed expectations. Patient satisfaction with care is increasingly used as an important indicator of the adequacy of interventions. It is often preferable, in addition, to use outcome measures of clinical and social function to establish the effectiveness of care (Hall 1979).

## Twelve axes to define case management in practice

It may be said with some justification that there are as many ways to implement the principles of case management as there are case management programmes. Several authors have attempted to bring order to this disarray by developing contrasting models of case management (Bachrach 1980, Lamb 1980, Hargreaves *et al.* 1984, Renshaw 1987a, Schwab *et al.* 1988). For example, these commonly distinguish between direct care and service broker applications of case management, and one illustration of this typology is given in Fig. 24.1. It may be more useful, however, to consider each programme in terms of 12 axes that, together, precisely define the characteristics of its practice (Table 24.3).

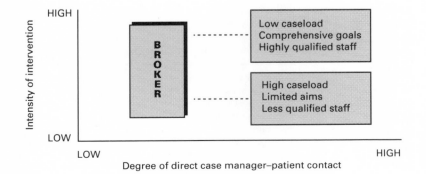

**Fig. 24.1** Classification of case management systems according to degree of patient contact and intensity of interventions.

## Axis 1: individual–team case management

Most case management programmes give clear responsibility for a given patient group either to an individual (Breakey 1989) or to a team of staff (Intagliata 1982). Test (1979) has described four advantages to team case management: continuous coverage, continuity in the absence of individuals, better quality planning, and better support between care-givers. Individual case loads may intensify the staff–patient relationship and provide better continuity of care (Renshaw *et al.* 1988), but can act at the expense of effective delegation to the most appropriate worker.

## Axis 2: direct care–service brokerage

At one extreme of this axis lie brokerage models in which the case manager may have little or no direct continuing contact with the patient, but whose primary role is to ensure that a range of other care staff provide the necessary level of care (Lamb 1980, Schwartz *et al.* 1982, Schwab *et al.* 1988). In contrast, direct care staff gain a personal understanding of the patient and family, but may undertake tasks which conflict with or which fall outside their competence or expertise, and which can produce boundary disputes about the proper therapeutic tasks for each speciality.

## Axis 3: intensity of interventions

The frequency of case management contacts may vary from at least daily to less than monthly (Robinson & Bergman 1989). The intensity of the therapeutic, material and social support that can be offered to the patient is importantly constrained by the frequency of contact, and this in turn is closely associated with the target group served and the caseload.

## Axis 4: degree of budgetary control

The effectiveness of case managers for long-term mental illness is often closely associated with the degree of control they exercise over the budget for patient services (Challis 1985). Where such decentralized control exists, case managers may

have flexibility for care substitution, the better to match resources to patients' needs. Financial autonomy may ensure accountability and encourage creativity (Davies 1987). Conversely, budgetary control at the level of the case manager can introduce inequitable resource allocation, and may produce inconsistent decisions on expenditure between practitioners, and unless closely supervised, may encourage overspending. It can operate best where patients have detailed individual treatment plans and budgets (Knapp *et al.* 1990). In the USA, for example, considerable advantages have been described from a capitation system of payments to the case manager who has wide discretion about which services to purchase (Goldman & Taube 1988), and conversely case managers with clinical responsibility but little financial discretion may be unable to act fully in the patient's interests.

## Axis 5: health or social service staff

Case management teams may be established within health or social service settings, and may contain staff from either or both of these agencies (Clifford *et al.* 1988). Alternatively, staff with a range of professional training may be employed by an independent agency such as a locally based mental health consortium or housing partnership. There is some evidence that a predominantly social work orientation is associated with more and more frequent contacts with patients with neurotic rather than psychotic disorders (Levine 1981), and clinical practice in British community mental health centres (CMHCs) also suggests that this tendency is reinforced by poor managerial direction, and individual discretion by case managers about which referrals to accept (Sayce *et al.* 1991). The clear implication here is that clear lines of managerial accountability are required, preferably with agreed guidelines about the mix of diagnoses within individual case loads.

## Axis 6: status of case manager

Case managers with professional qualifications may offer long-term psychiatric patients greater expertise in assessment and psychological intervention, and are themselves more costly to employ, but may be unwilling to do more mundane tasks, such as negotiate social welfare benefit entitlements. For these reasons, and especially within the context of psychiatric hospital closure, new 'community carers' or care assistants (Griffiths 1988), with relatively little formal training and professional status, are increasingly being used to provide direct care to the long-term mentally ill.

### Axis 7: specialization of the case manager

Case management teams show considerable variation in how far staff work as generic case managers or as specialists. As non-specialists, case managers may be allocated irrespective of their formal training and offer a common core service. In contrast, patients who need help with regular medication, for example, may be allocated to psychiatric nurses in the team, while patients on no medication but with substantial debts may be allocated to a social work colleague. The issue of specialization is likely to become increasingly important because of the distinction drawn between health care and social care in the National Health Service and Community Care Act (1990).

### Axis 8: staff to patient ratio

Sustained quality in case management services to the long-term mentally ill depends on a relatively restricted caseload. Direct care models usually operate within a range of 10–25 patients per staff member, but ratios of more than 1:15 run the risk of rapidly diminishing benefits (Harris & Bergman 1988). The broker model of indirect care may allow the ratio to extend to 1:40 (Robinson & Bergman 1989).

### Axis 9: degree of patient participation

Case management teams show great variation in the emphasis given to patient participation. One pole of the axis includes programmes which aim to establish treatment and care targets jointly with the patient, while at the other extreme lie approaches in which patients' needs are defined by third parties, and in which outcome includes no reference to the patients' satisfaction with services.

### Axis 10: the point of contact

Case management programmes may make contact with patients in a wide range of settings, including their family homes (Breakey 1989), in hotel rooms (Bond 1984), in the team offices (Stein & Diamond 1985), or in primary care facilities. Contact can be established at the point of first referral (Marks *et al.* 1988) or after discharge from hospital (Wasylenki *et al.* 1985).

### Axis 11: level of intervention

Case management interventions may take place at the individual, network, or systems level (Ross 1979). Individual care includes those activities referred to as core tasks above, including for example advocacy services for individual patients (Freddolino *et al.* 1989). At the network level, services can be offered to other formal carers, to family and other natural supports, or to specialized groups such as those fostering self-help. In systems terms, the case manager may offer public education on mental disorders or advocate for resource allocation to the long-term mentally ill.

### Axis 12: the target population

While case management is conceptually well suited to the continuing service needs of the long-term mentally ill, case managers may in fact spend much of their time with people suffering from more brief or intermittent forms of mental disorder. More specifically, where CMHCs aiming to offer a comprehensive service to the catchment population have no formal priority for defined patient groups, then patients with the more severe conditions are selectively undertreated (Levine 1981). Indeed, Stein & Diamond (1985) have described the characteristics most likely to benefit from 'assertive' case management: those who are unwilling to attend hospital-based services, who show poor medication compliance, and poor ability to monitor themselves, and who have frequent crises.

## The National Health Service and Community Care Act (1990)

With Britain case management has become more widely discussed since the House of Commons Social Services Committee (1985). In 1988 Sir Roy Griffiths published his review of how to implement British policy on community care most efficiently, and identified the need for 'care managers' to devise 'packages of care' for the recipients of community services. He proposed that social services departments (SSDs) should take prime responsibility for fulfilling the case management function, within a 'mixed economy' in which services were bought from the statutory, private and voluntary sectors (Murphy 1987, 1988, Thornicroft 1990a). Case management has been substantially adopted in principle by the White Paper 'Caring for People' (1989) and within the subsequent National Health Service and Community Care Act (1990). It is now likely that British health and social services will jointly need to introduce case management systems by 1993.

This Act puts on the statute book a requirement for SSDs to use case managers to target resources and plan services to meet the specific needs of individual patients, so that each service user has a named single point of contact. The Act does not prescribe the style of case management to be used locally as long as a clearly identified worker is designated for each component of the 'care package', nor does it indicate the severity of disability which needs to be present for individual patients to fall within the responsibility of local case management services. The Act also indicates the advantages of devolved budgets for case managers. The background speciality of the case manager is also left open to interpretation and allows for social workers, community nurses and care assistants to take the case management role (Beardshaw & Towell 1990).

There are a number of issues that, soon after their enactment, suggest that these measures may fall short of their intent. First, division made within the Act between social care and health care, for example, may serve to undermine the very integration of service provision that case management aims to overcome. Second, the designation of SSDs as the 'lead agencies' in providing community care does not acknowledge that in many areas of England and Wales the level of services they provide for psychiatric patients is extremely poor. One survey in England and Wales, for example, found that in 9% of health districts the local SSDs provided no day centre places (Thornicroft 1990a).

Third, the mechanism established by the Act to encourage joint local planning between health and social services is the provision of an annual, centrally funded mental health-specific grant. This is sent to SSDs if the local mental health service plan, jointly formulated with health authorities, conforms to national standards and priorities. The grant, however, is only for 70% of the proposed service costs, and evidence is accumulating that some local government authorities will not apply for such extra mental health service funds in order to save their own costs of 30%. Should this become a widespread reaction it will combine with the delay in the full implementation of the community care part of the Act until 1993 to stifle the flexibility that would allow case management to develop.

## Examples of case management in practice

### The COSTAR programme in Baltimore

Established in 1985, the Community Support Treatment and Rehabilitation programme (COSTAR) is a mobile multidisciplinary assertive community treatment service of the Johns Hopkins Community Psychiatry Program in East Baltimore. The catchment population of about 73 000 is over 80% black, and the area is characterized by high indices of social deprivation. The mobile clinical team includes six nurses, three social workers, one counsellor, two clerical staff and two part-time psychiatrists (9.5 whole-time-equivalent staff). Serving 97 patients, the team's staff to patient ratio is between 1:10 and 1:15. The typical patient is poor, black, single, about 40 years old and has not remained in contact with hospital-based outpatient services between admissions (Breakey 1989).

The primary characteristics of the form of case management employed by the COSTAR team are given in Table 24.4. Each patient is assigned to a psychiatrist and a non-medical 'primary clinician' (nurse or social worker), who are jointly responsible for all aspects of the patient's assessment and treatment. The treatment team accepts potentially indefinite care for its patients. Each clinician offers direct care to patients and acts as broker between them and other agencies. The primary clinician continues contact with each patient during periods of hospital admission or imprisonment.

Contact with the 97 patients takes place predominantly outside the programme offices: at the patients' homes, in local cafes, in visits to local shops, or at social service agencies. The frequency of contact varies from daily to less that once a month, with a mean of three contacts per week. An on-call clinician provides an out-of-hours service to patients, and can consult or refer to one of the programme psychiatrists. Urgent treatment is available at the Psychiatric Emergency Service of Johns Hopkins Hospital. The programme is closely linked with Changing Directions, a local psychiatric rehabilitation centre (Breakey 1989).

A recent extension of the COSTAR work is the provision of an emergency outreach service which offers short-term intensive support at home, either as a bridge between inpatient and outpatient status, or as an alternative to admission. The service is under evaluation, and a pilot study suggests that such intensive home-based treatment can substantially improve the social networks of such long-term patients (Thornicroft & Breakey 1992), while a randomized controlled trial of this form of care is in progress.

### The South Verona Community Psychiatric Service

The South Verona area consists of three suburban districts and three rural communities, with a total population of about 75 000, comprising a stable mix of working and middle class neighbourhoods (Mosher & Burti 1989). The South Verona

**Table 24.4** The case management characteristics of the COSTAR and South Verona psychiatric services

|  | COSTAR programme | South Verona service |
|---|---|---|
| Individual/team case loads | Individual case loads with most patients well known to all staff | Core team of two to three staff allocated to each patient |
| Direct/indirect care | Direct care predominates with a minor brokerage role | Direct care model, staff–patient relationship central |
| Intensity | Up to two contacts daily (average nine contacts per month) | Varies with need, can exceed daily contact in crises |
| Budgetary control | With director of programme | With director of service |
| Health/social service balance | A part of Johns Hopkins Hospital Community Psychiatry Program | Within local administration of national health service (USL) |
| Status of case managers | Most are trained and experienced psychiatric nurses and social workers | Trained psychiatric nurses and social workers |
| Specialization | Act as generic case managers except that nurses administer depot medication | Act as generic case managers |
| Staff:patient ratio | Between 1:10 and 1:15 | Varies according to the case-mix of patients treated |
| Patient participation | Patients actively collaborate in identifying treatment goals | Patients' groups take place at the community mental health centre (CMHC) |
| Point of contact | Largely at patients' homes and other community sites | Largely at CMHC, home or outpatient department |
| Level of intervention | Primarily individual and family with some system-level advocacy | Individual and systemic family therapeutic interventions |
| Target population | Long-term psychiatric patients not treated by traditional hospital service | All psychiatric patients within each catchment area |

Community Mental Health Service, established in 1978, includes the following components: a community mental health centre, a 15-bedded inpatient unit in a nearby general hospital, an outpatients service, home visits, a liaison service with other hospital departments, a hospital-based emergency on-call doctor, and an expanding network of residential facilities.

The service emphasizes psychosocial interventions, integrating medication, family support and rehabilitation (Tansella 1989). The staff team includes 9 full-time psychiatrists, 24 psychiatric nurses, 3 social workers and 13 unpaid trainee psychiatrists. Ten of the nurses are dedicated to the inpatient ward, and all the remaining staff work both in hospital and community settings, organized into three subsector teams, each serving areas with populations between 18 500 and 28 500. Within each subsector the staff use a team caseload method, with 2–3 staff allocated to each patient to ensure continuity in the absence of any individual member of staff. The team is committed to evaluating the service it provides, especially through the use of a local case register (Tansella & Williams 1987, Ballestrieri *et al.* 1989).

### Evaluations of case management

The use of case management for long-term mental illness has increased rapidly in the USA over the last 25 years, and most published accounts that describe process and outcome evaluations are American, though few are methodologically rigorous (Hargreaves & Shumway 1989). The federally funded Community Support Program (CSP), for example, established and evaluated case management programmes at 18 demonstration sites for 1471 patients (Tessler & Goldman 1982). The patient group was in many ways typical of the long-term mentally ill usually targeted by case management programmes. The mean age of patients was 42, with an average 18 years of psychiatric contact including three previous admissions. Their most frequent problems were with transport, money management, taking prescribed medications, getting meals, and finding companionship.

The size of the staff–patient ratio has crucial implications for the range and quality of services that can be provided. A study in New York State which evaluated changes as this ratio increased from 1:15 to 1:50 found that services progressively became more reactive rather than proactive; spent less time assessing needs; acted for patients rather than assisting patients to act on their own behalf; and focused on documentation rather than direct patient contact (Baker & Intagliata 1984).

Evidence is now accumulating that outcome within home-based case management services is usually no worse and often better than traditional outpatient contact (Braun *et al.* 1981, Kiesler 1982). Randomized controlled trials of the case manager model for long-term psychiatric patients have been described in Madison (Stein & Test 1980), Sydney (Hoult 1986), Montreal (Fenton *et al.* 1982) and London (Marks *et al.* 1988, Onyett *et al.* 1990). The positive results from these demonstration programmes, which show improvements in patients' social integration, use of inpatient and outpatient services, and satisfaction with services (Goering *et al.* 1988), must be treated with caution.

In a further randomized controlled trial of a case manager programme at a community mental health centre, for example, Franklin *et al.* (1987) randomly assigned 417 stable psychiatric patients who had at least 2 admissions in the previous 26 months. The control group received the usual forms of care, which included an 'assertive' aftercare programme. The experimental group received this and in addition attached case managers who spent 59% of their time in direct contact with patients and a further 39% in brokering activities for the patients. Although the control group does not seem either typical of standard follow-up services, or very different from the experimental condition, the results are of interest. At one-year follow-up the experimental group were receiving more services, but did not show improvement in their quality of life. The favourable findings from the randomized controlled trials elsewhere, therefore, may offer a misleadingly positive picture.

Cost–benefit studies have shown that outreach

teams may cost more (Weisbrod *et al.* 1980), less (Bond 1984, Bond *et al.* 1988), or the same as traditional treatment (Borland *et al.* 1989), but that when patients' earnings are taken into account, the balance is in favour of the benefits of case management programmes. Overall, the published evaluations of model case management programmes for long-term mental illness have produced favourable findings in relation to a wide range of clinical, social and economic variables.

## Conclusions

The contribution that the case management approach can make to the welfare of the long-term mental illness must be put in context. Approximately 1% of the population suffer from chronic mental illness (Goldman *et al.* 1981). Over half of these people have a diagnosis of schizophrenia (Bebbington *et al.* 1981), only about 10% are now psychiatric inpatients (Goldman *et al.* 1983), and an estimated 8% of patients seen in primary care suffer from chronic mental disorders (Wilkinson *et al.* 1985). These patients are frequently undemanding of services (Talbott 1978), and are a considerable strain to their families (Creer & Wing 1974, Intagliata *et al.* 1986), who are equally unlikely to complain (Johnstone *et al.* 1984). Geographically mobile (Caton & Goldstein 1984), their physical disorders are undertreated (Schwab *et al.* 1988), many are lost to psychiatric follow-up (Tantam & Klerman 1979), and some lapse into homelessness (Fischer & Breakey 1986, Lamb & Talbott 1986). With the continuing rundown in psychiatric hospitals, former long-term inpatients and younger chronic patients are both at risk of neglect by fragmented and dispersed services (David 1988).

Within this context, the wide range of practices which constitute case management have an important role to play. First, they may ensure that patients with long-term mental illness do maintain contact with services, especially for rehabilitation. Indeed evidence is emerging that case managers may be a necessary but not sufficient component of adequate continuing care, and that vocational training is particularly important in influencing the long-term outcome of younger severely disabled psychiatric patients (Solomon *et al*, 1984). Secondly, they may offer an array of interventions which the patient may value and benefit from, and which the patient collaborates in choosing. Thirdly, they may avoid both gaps and redundancy in services provision. Finally, they may determine, through continuing regular review, when services should be varied or discontinued. Case management is a unifying concept which promises to represent a patient group where there has been neglect, to integrate services where there has been fragmentation, and to offer care shaped by the needs of the patients rather than of service-providers. Careful evaluation will allow us to judge how far these opportunities can be realized.

## References

Anthony W., Cohen M., Farkas M. *et al.* (1988) The chronically mentally ill and case management — more than a response to a dysfunctional system. *Community Mental Health Journal* 24, 21–28.

Bachrach L. (1980) Overview: model programs for chronic patients. *American Journal of Psychiatry* 137, 1023–1031.

Bachrach L. (1984) Asylum and chronically ill psychiatric patients. *American Journal of Psychiatry* 141, 975–978.

Bachrach L. (1989) Case management: towards a shared definition. *Hospital and Community Psychiatry* 40, 883–884.

Baker F. & Intagliata L. (1984) The New York State community support system. *Hospital and Community Psychiatry* 35, 39–44.

Ballestrieri M., Systema S., Gavioli I. & Miciolo R. (1989) Patterns of psychiatric care in South-Verona and Groningen. A case-register follow-up study. *Acta Psychiatrica Scandinavica* 80, 437–444.

Beardshaw V. & Towell D. (1990) *Assessment and Case Management.* King's Fund, London.

Bebbington P., Hurry L., Tennant C. *et al.* (1981) Epidemiology of mental disorders in Camberwell. *Psychological Medicine* 11, 561–579.

Bond G. (1984) An economic analysis of psychosocial rehabilitation. *Hospital and Community Psychiatry* 35, 356–362.

Bond G., Miller L., Krumwied R. & Ward R. (1988) Assertive case management in three CMHCs: a controlled study. *Hospital and Community Psychiatry* 39, 411–418.

Borland A., McRae J. & Lycan C. (1989) Outcomes after five years of intensive case management. *Hospital and Community Psychiatry* 40, 369–376.

Braun P., Kochansky G., Shapiro R. *et al.* (1981) Overview: deinstitutionalisation of psychiatric patients, a critical review of outcome studies. *American Journal of Psychiatry* 138, 736–774.

Breakey W. (1989) Integrating training and research with clinical services in a community setting. *Hospital and Community Psychiatry* 40, 1175–1179.

Brewin C., Wing J., Mangen S., Brugha T. & MacCarthy B. (1987) Principles and practice of measuring needs in the long-term mentally ill, the Medical Research Council Needs for Care assessment. *Psychological Medicine* 17, 971–981.

Caton C. & Goldstein J. (1984) Housing change of chronic schizophrenic patients: a consequence of the revolving door. *Social Science and Medicine* 1, 758–764.

Challis D. (1985) *Case Management of Consumer Choice: The Community Care Scheme. Personal Social Services Research Unit Discussion Paper No. 396.* University of Kent, Canterbury.

Challis D. (1989) *Case Management: Problems and Possibilities.* PSSRU, University of Kent, Canterbury.

Challis D. & Davies B. (1986) *Case Management in Community Care.* Gower, Aldershot.

Charnley H. & Davies B. (1987) *Blockages and the Performance of the Core Tasks of Case Management. Personal Social Services Research Unit Discussion Paper No. 473.* University of Kent, Canterbury.

Clifford P., Craig T. & Sayce L. (1988) *Towards Co-ordinated Care for People with Long-term, Severe Mental Illness.* National Unit for Psychiatric Research and Development, London.

Creer C. & Wing J. (1974) *Schizophrenia at Home.* National Schizophrenia Fellowship, Surbiton.

David A. (1988) On the streets in America. *British Medical Journal* 296, 1016.

Davies B. (1987) Review article: making a reality of community care. *British Journal of Social Work* 18, 173–186.

Fariello D. & Scheidt S. (1989) Clinical case management of the dually diagnosed patient. *Hospital and Community Psychiatry* 40, 1065–1067.

Fenton F., Tessier L., Struening E. *et al.* (1982). *Home and Hospital Psychiatric Treatment.* Croom Helm, London.

Fischer P. & Breakey W. (1986) Homelessness and mental health: an overview. *International Journal of Mental Health* 14, 6–41.

Franklin J., Solovitz B., Mason M., Clemons J. & Miller G. (1987) An evaluation of case management. *American Journal of Public Health* 77, 674–678.

Freddolino O., Moxley D. & Fleishman J. (1989) An advocacy model for people with long-term psychiatric disabilities. *Hospital and Community Psychiatry* 40, 1169–1174.

Goering P., Wasylenski D., Farkas M., Lancee W. & Ballantyne R. (1988) What difference does case management make? *Hospital and Community Psychiatry* 39, 272–276.

Goldman H., Adams H. & Taube C. (1983) Deinstitu-

tionalisation: the data demythologised. *Hospital and Community Psychiatry* 34, 12–13.

Goldman H., Gatzionni A. & Taube C. (1981) Defining and counting the chronically mentally ill. *Hospital and Community Psychiatry* 32, 21–27.

Goldman H. & Taube C. (1988) High users of outpatients mental health services, II implications for practice and policy. *American Journal of Psychiatry* 145, 24–28.

Griffiths R. (1988) *Community Care: An Agenda for Action.* HMSO, London.

Hall J. (1979) Assessment procedures used in studies on long-stay patients. *British Journal of Psychiatry* 135, 330–335.

Hargreaves W., Shaw R., Shadoan R., Walker E., Surber R. & Gaynor J. (1984) Measuring case management activity. *Journal of Nervous and Mental Diseases* 172, 296–300.

Hargreaves W. & Shumway M. (1989) Effectiveness of services for the severely mentally ill. In Taube C., Mechanic D. & Hohmann A. (eds) *The Future of Mental Health Services Research.* NIMH, Rockville.

Harris M. & Bergman H. (1988) Misconceptions about use of case management services by the chronic mentally ill: a utilisation analysis. *Hospital and Community Psychiatry* 39, 1276–1280.

Hoult J. (1986) Community care of the acutely mentally ill. *British Journal of Psychiatry* 14, 137–144.

House of Commons (1990) *The National Health Service and Community Care Act.* HMSO, London.

House of Commons Social Services Committee, 1984/85 Session (1985) *Second Report. Community Care with Special Reference to Adult Mentally Ill and Mentally Handicapped People.* HMSO, London.

Intagliata J. (1982) Improving the quality of care for the chronic mentally disabled: the role of case management. *Schizophrenia Bulletin* 8, 655–674.

Intagliata J., Willer B. & Egri G. (1986) Role of the family in case management of the mentally ill. *Schizophrenia Bulletin* 12, 699–708.

Johnstone E., Owens D., Gold A. *et al.* (1984) Schizophrenic patients discharged from hospital – a follow-up study. *British Journal of Psychiatry* 145, 586–590.

Kanter J. (1989) Clinical case management: definition, principles, components. *Hospital and Community Psychiatry* 40, 361–368.

Kiesler C. (1982) Mental hospitals and alternative care. *American Psychologist* 4, 354–360.

Knapp M., Cambridge P., Thomsaon C., Beecham J., Allen C. & Darton R. (1990) *Care in the Community Newsletter No. 9.* PSSRU, University of Kent, Canterbury.

Lamb R. (1980) Therapist-case managers: more than brokers of services. *Hospital and Community Psychiatry* 31, 762–764.

Lamb R. & Talbott J. (1986) The homeless mentally ill. The perspective of the American Psychiatric Association. *Journal of the American Medical Association* 256, 498–501.

Lee P. & Kenworthy M. (1929) *Mental Hygiene and Social*

*Work*. The Commonwealth Fund, New York.

Levine M. (1981) *The History and Politics of Community Mental Health*. Oxford University Press, Oxford.

Marks I., Connolly J. & Muijen M. (1988) The Maudsley Daily Living Programme. *Bulletin of the Royal College of Psychiatrists* 12, 22–24.

Mechanic D. & Aiken L. (1987) Improving the care of patients with chronic mental illness. *New England Journal of Medicine* 317, 634–638.

Modrcin M., Rapp C. & Chamberlain R. (1985) *Case Management with Psychiatrically Disabled Individuals: Curriculum and Training Programme*. University of Kansas School of Social Work, Lawrence, Kansas.

Mosher L. & Burti L. (1989) *Community Mental Health*. Norton, New York.

Murphy E. (1987) Community care: I problems. *British Medical Journal* 295, 1505–1508.

Murphy E. (1988) Community care: II possible solutions. *British Medical Journal* 296, 6–8.

National Health Service and Community Care Act (1990) HMSO, London.

Onyett S., Tyrer P., Connolly J. *et al.* (1990) The early intervention service: the first 18 months of an inner London demonstration project. *Psychiatric Bulletin* 14, 267–269.

Renshaw J. (1987a) *Individual Care Planning and Case Management. Personal Social Services Research Unit Discussion Paper No. 478.* University of Kent, Canterbury.

Renshaw J. (1987b) Care planning and case management. *British Journal of Social Work* 18, 79–105.

Renshaw J., Hampson R, Thomsaon C. *et al.* (1988) *Care in the Community: The First Steps*. Gower, Aldershot.

Robinson G. & Bergman G. (1989) *Choices in Case Management*. Policy Resources Incorporated, Washington DC.

Ross H. (1979) *Proceedings of the Conference on the Evaluation of Case Management Programs*. Volunteers for Services to Older Persons, Los Angeles.

Santiago J., McCall-Perez F. & Bachrach L. (1985) Integrated services for chronic mental patients: theoretical perspectives and experimental results. *General Hospital Psychiatry* 7, 309–315.

Sayce L., Craig T. & Boardman A. (1991) The development of community mental health centres in the UK. *Social Psychiatry and Psychiatric Epidemiology* 26, 14–20.

Schwab D., Drake R. & Burghardt E. (1988) Health care of the chronically mentally ill: the culture broker model. *Community Mental Health Journal* 24, 174–184.

Schwartz S., Goldman H. & Churgin S. (1982) Case management for the chronic mentally ill: models and dimensions. *Hospital and Community Psychiatry* 33, 1006–1009.

Secretaries of State for Health, Social Security, Wales and Scotland (1989) *Caring for People. Community Care in the Next Decade and Beyond* (Cmnd 849). HMSO, London.

Secretaries of State for Health, Wales, Northern Ireland and Scotland (1989) *Working for Patients* (Cmnd 555). HMSO, London.

Solomon P., Davis J. & Gordon B. (1984) Discharged state hospital patients' characteristics and use of aftercare: effects on community tenure. *American Journal of Psychiatry* 141, 1566–1570.

Spitz B. (1987) A national survey of Medicaid case management programs. *Health Affairs* Spring, 61–86.

Stein L. & Diamond R. (1985) A programme for difficult to treat patients. *New Directions in Mental Health Services* 26, 29–39.

Stein L. & Test M. (1980) Alternative to mental hospital treatment. I Conceptual model, treatment program and clinical evaluation. *Archives of General Psychiatry* 37, 392–397.

Talbott J. (1978) *The Death of the Asylum*. Grune & Stratton, New York.

Tansella M. (1989) Evaluating community psychiatric services. In Williams P., Wilkinson G. & Rawnsley K. (eds) *The Scope of Epidemiological Psychiatry*, pp. 386–403. Routledge, London.

Tansella M. & Williams P. (1987) The Italian experience and its implications. *Psychological Medicine* 17, 283–289.

Tantam D. & Klerman G. (1979) Patient transfer from one clinician to another and dropping out of out-patients treatment. *Social Psychiatry* 14, 107–113.

Tessler R. & Goldman H. (1982) *The Chronic Mentally Ill, Assessing the Community Support Program*. Ballinger, Cambridge, Massachussetts.

Test M. (1979) Continuity of care in community treatment. *New Directions for Mental Health Services* 1, 15–23.

Thornicroft G. (1990a) Are England's psychiatric services for schizophrenia improving? *Hospital and Community Psychiatry* 41, 1073–1075.

Thornicroft G. (1990b) Case managers for the mentally ill. *Social Psychiatry and Psychiatric Epidemiology* 25, 141–143.

Thornicroft G. & Bebbington P. (1989) Deinstitutionalisation: from hospital closure to service development: a review of the literature. *British Journal of Psychiatry* 155, 739–753.

Thornicroft G. & Breakey W. (1992) The COSTAR programme (1). Improving the social networks of the long-term mentally ill. *British Journal of Psychiatry* 158, 475–484.

Torrey F. (1986) Continuous treatment teams in the care of the chronic mentally ill. *Hospital and Community Psychiatry* 37, 1243–1247.

Wasylenki D., Goeing P., Lancee W., Balantyne R. & Farkas M. (1985) Impact of a case manager program on psychiatric aftercare. *Journal of Nervous and Mental Disease* 173, 303–308.

Weisbrod B., Test M. & Stein L. (1980) Alternative to mental hospital treatment. *Archives of General Psychiatry* 37, 400–405.

Wilkinson G., Falloon I. & Sen B. (1985) Chronic mental disorders in general practice. *British Medical Journal* 291, 1302–1304.

Worley N., Drago L. & Hadley T. (1990) Improving the physical health–mental health interface for the chronically mentally ill: could nurse case managers make a difference? *Archives of Psychiatric Nursing* 2, 108–113.

# Chapter 25
# Social Factors in the Genesis and Management of Postnatal Psychiatric Disorders

## DINESH BHUGRA & ALAIN GREGOIRE

Childbirth is an event of profound personal significance. It forms part of the most significant transitional process in a person's life. From the psychiatric standpoint, the time-period surrounding childbirth has long been considered a time of risk for minor and major psychiatric disturbances. Such an association has been described by Hippocrates (Hamilton 1962), as well as in the traditional Indian medical texts (Bhugra 1992).

A large body of literature has accumulated on the psychological and social processes which surround the transition to parenthood in normal populations of different cultures (see below). This is not surprising, given the individual, social, political and economic implications of childbirth. All this literature points to the crucial importance of childbirth in the life of the individual woman, as well as to the place of women generally in what is still throughout the world a largely androcentric society (Oakley 1980). It is, therefore, not surprising that this transition is associated with the full range of human emotions, cognitions and behaviours. In a somewhat arbitrary and, many might say, blinkered way, psychiatry has come to focus on this process, bringing with it the labels on which this branch of medicine largely depends. We are aware of the argument for and against the concept of discrete psychiatric disorders, as opposed to the concept of continua in distress and symptomatology. But as this debate is beyond the scope of this chapter, we will, for present purposes, conform with the current categorization of puerperal psychiatric disorders (Brockington & Cox-Roper 1988).

## Motherhood and madness

The history of the psychiatric treatment of women, much of which has concentrated on their sexual and reproductive lives, is one of neglect and institutionalized cruelty (Ripa 1990). In Victorian times cases of puerperal insanity seemed to violate all of Victorian culture's most deeply cherished ideals of feminine propriety and maternal love (Showalter 1987). In particular, if such a patient committed infanticide, she became the worst criminal in a society that exalted maternity. The prevalent medical attitudes and theory struggled to account for infanticide in a way that maintained the mythology of motherhood and the maternal instinct, and it was branded as an unfortunate product of woman's 'nature'.

Thus, it is clear that our current concepts of puerperal mental disorders are inextricably linked to both the current state of psychiatric thinking and sociocultural attitudes towards women and the state of motherhood. It is only relatively recently that a contribution has been made by scientific research. Although this research has contributed to a growing interest in the area from mental health professionals, it has also underlined our confusion as much as extending our knowledge. Three main disorders are commonly considered in the psychiatric literature: puerperal psychosis, postnatal depression and postnatal blues. We will be considering each of these in turn, with particular reference to their interaction with psychosocial factors. Before doing so, we will first consider the significance of childbirth as a life event, and, secondly, the transcultural issues which surround the transition to parenthood. Finally, we will consider briefly the psychosocial aspects of management which are of special relevance to postnatal disorders.

## Childbirth as a life event

Studies of the relationship between life events and affective disorder following childbirth have been plagued by conceptual and methodological problems which have led to considerable confusion in attempts to understand their findings. The methodological problems associated with life event research are discussed in Chapter 10. Some of the conceptual problems specific to life event research with postnatal disorders have been reviewed by Elliot (1990). One of these is the simplistic assumption that the life event at birth is a negative one which therefore puts women at risk of depression. This concept may have arisen from a false and reverse logic which assumes that the apparent increase in affective disorder following childbirth indicates that childbirth is the cause, and that therefore childbirth is a negative event. Although no one would deny that childbirth can be a negative event for some women because of the physical or psychological experiences associated with it, there is little doubt that it can also be an extremely positive experience (albeit *in spite* of the unpleasant and sometimes humiliating experiences that women so frequently describe). The concept of childbirth as a positive life event for some or indeed most women would suggest a protective effect against depression, which is borne out by the results of several studies (Rees & Lutkins 1971, Elliott *et al.* 1983, Pitt 1968, O'Hara & Zekoski, 1988). However, it is still not enough to accept that the life event of childbirth may have a positive or a negative significance, we must also acknowledge that for any individual woman the event may have both *a negative and a positive impact*. Furthermore, whatever the impact of childbirth as a life event *per se*, its occurrence can have significant effects in modulating the impact of other chronic or acute stressors, for example, marital disharmony or the death of the woman's mother. Such an effect has been suggested by Cooper *et al.* (1988).

Given these theoretical uncertainties, it is hardly surprising that the life event literature in relation to childbirth is inconclusive. This has led Brown (1989) to conclude that we should no longer 'talk about life events at all, unless we also deal with the context that tells something about the concerns and plans involved'. It may be that the currently held views of childbirth in our society are providing researchers and clinicians with a false perception of childbirth as an event rather than an important phase in a much longer lasting transitional process in which many other experiences and stresses can have equally important negative or positive effects on a woman's health.

## Cross-cultural factors

The study of the cultural norms surrounding childbirth and the transition to parenthood in other contemporary societies, coupled with knowledge about postpartum disorders in these cultures, should increase our understanding of the social factors involved in these disorders. However, the study of both these areas is difficult for methodological and conceptual reasons, and there is, therefore, a substantial risk of arriving at false conclusions because of the inadequate understanding of the cultural norms or the occurrence of postpartum disorders in the societies under study. Given the confusion which, despite numerous studies, still persists about these issues in western society, the obstacles to be overcome in transcultural research cannot be overestimated. At the same time as acknowledging the value of the results of such studies, and of anthropological observations, we feel it is essential to emphasize the hypothetical nature of any conclusions derived from such work.

### *Birth and puerperium in different cultures*

A society's customs, in relation to childbirth and the postnatal period, reflect that society's view of women and children, and determine the role of the mother in the community. The wide range of traditional rituals and customs surrounding pregnancy, birth and the puerperium in different cultures is beyond the scope of this chapter (see the reviews by Mead & Newton 1967, Homans 1982, Stern & Kruckman 1983). During the postpartum period, the rituals and customs commonly involve a number of the following components, occurring in one form or another:

*Isolation/seclusion of the mother.* For example, Jamaican women are secluded for 9 nights following delivery, and then relatively isolated for 31 nights following that (Kitzinger 1982), or the longer period of 2–3 months during which Nigerian mothers and babies are kept in a special hut described by Kelly (1967). The Ayurvedic texts recommend that the mother should not be left alone for 10–12 days after childbirth, in order to prevent exogenous illnesses influencing her. Clear instructions are laid down for the decoration and the availability of the delivery room so as not to make the mother more vulnerable to illnesses after delivery, since during the process of childbirth her body has been 'depleted and broken up by the demand made on it for the growth of the foetus and since the body is drained of vitality by the delivery throes and by the loss of fluids and of blood' (Caraka Samhita 1943).

*Practical help and support.* In most traditional cultures the isolation described above is accompanied by intensive caring and support, often by specific individuals, such as the woman's mother or grandmother.

*Behavioural proscriptions.* For example, Pillsbury (1978) has described the complex rules to be obeyed by the mother in Chinese society, which cover most of her day-to-day activities, such as eating, washing, physical activity, sexual intercourse and rest.

*Suspended social roles and protection from previous demands.* In many cultures the isolation, provision of help and prescribed rest are accompanied by a release from the woman's normal social roles and the demands made on her so that she can concentrate on herself and her new baby. This suspension of her previous social roles can be seen as part of a rite of passage. In many societies such rites of passage mark the transition of individuals in society from one important phase in their lives to another, at such times as puberty, marriage and childbirth. Rites of passage can be considered in three stages. First, the separation from the previous role. Secondly, an intermediatory or 'liminal' period (a sort of social

no man's land). And, finally, incorporation into the new role. Seel (1986), in considering western customs surrounding the transition to parenthood, has commented on the absence of any rituals or customs marking a rite of incorporation. Indeed, women postnatally frequently complain of the sense of abandonment by both professional services and friends and family as the intense period of interest in the pregnancy and the birth is followed by a transfer of attention to the child and a perceived loss of interest in the mother.

The time-period during which these various components are applied varies from a few days to several months. In a review of 202 traditional societies, Jimenez & Newton (1979) describe half of them expecting women to return to full duties within 2 weeks of the birth. It is difficult to know how this limit has been determined. Observations of a variety of procedures relating to pregnancy and childbirth have highlighted both essential biological similarities of births wherever they occur and the vast range of practices, particularly diverse in the west where policy may differ even within one district or between consultants in the same hospital. Nevertheless, societal attitudes are reflected in the array of choices available (Raphael-Leff 1991). Childbearing practices dictate allocation of resources as well as attitudes towards bodies, babies and paternal roles. Folk models of bodily function and specific imagery of the human body can be seen to underpin cultural management of the birth process itself. As Raphael-Leff (1991) goes on to emphasize, labour and birth patterns vary around the world but the cultural beliefs and values shape and influence the individual's experience of this universal biological process. These beliefs also affect the attitudes towards the baby and illness which may be seen as secondary to childbirth.

### Postnatal mental illness in different cultures

The studies by Assael *et al.* (1972) and Cox (1979a, 1983) clearly demonstrate the higher than expected rate of depression in pregnant women in

Uganda. Follow-up of Cox's sample postnatally revealed a 10% prevalence of depressive illness. This figure in a semirural African group is remarkably similar to the findings of studies in western societies.

The findings regarding the occurrence of puerperal psychosis in Africa appear to consistently reflect the higher rates of physical complications in the puerperium, in that a higher proportion of women have organic psychoses than would be expected in western countries (Ebie 1972, Swift 1972, Ifabumuyi & Akindele 1985, for a review see Cox 1988).

### Puerperal psychosis

This category of postpartum psychiatric disturbance is defined more in terms of severity of the disorder and its timing in relation to childbirth, rather than the more usual criteria of symptomatology. Thus, it contains a mixture of schizophrenic, unipolar depressive, manic-depressive and organic psychoses. This apparently heterogeneous diagnostic category appears out of step with current concepts of the classification of psychiatric disorders and, indeed, is not used in the World Health Organization's International Classification of Diseases or DSM-III-R. However, Brockington & Cox-Roper (1988) present good arguments in favour of retaining this category. One of the main reasons they suggest for doing so is the importance of the temporal association between these psychotic disorders and the event of childbirth. They suggest that since this is of aetiological significance, such information should not be eliminated from classificatory systems. Furthermore, they point to the often confusing mixture of symptoms which occurs in such patients, and of which current classificatory systems fail to take adequate account. They argue that puerperal schizophreniform states are in fact a variant of mania, and that it would be misleading to classify them as schizophrenic illnesses. The view that puerperal psychoses are essentially a variant of manic-depressive illnesses and unrelated to schizophrenia, is supported by the findings of Kendell *et al.* (1987). There is little doubt that the term puerperal provides a con-

siderable amount of information about the circumstances, course and management of these disorders, and that the absence of such critical information from any classificatory system is unacceptable.

The incidence of puerperal psychosis is generally considered to be 1 admission per 1000 births (Sim 1963), although much higher rates of 6.8 per 1000 have been reported (Jansson 1964). Meltzer & Kumar (1985) reported an overall rate of 1.6 per 1000 live births. Other studies have offered rates from 0.8 to 2.5 cases per 1000 deliveries (see Thomas & Gordon 1959 for a review of earlier studies).

In the great majority of patients, the onset of puerperal psychoses occurs in the first week after delivery, with the incidence rates dropping sharply over the subsequent one or two weeks (Dean & Kendell 1981, Brockington *et al.* 1982, Meltzer & Kumar 1985).

Prior to the arrival of modern treatment methods, the duration of puerperal psychosis appears to have been in the order of six months (Esquirol 1845, Menzies 1893). The prognosis with modern treatments is generally good and, indeed, tends to be better than for matched women suffering from non-puerperal psychoses (Platz & Kendell 1988). Some women recover completely within weeks of the onset. The risk of relapse in a subsequent pregnancy is in the order of 20%, and approximately 50% of women will experience a non-puerperal relapse of psychosis on long-term follow-up (Protheroe 1969).

### *Psychosocial correlates of puerperal psychosis*

The existence of a hereditary predisposition to puerperal psychosis was recognized by Esquirol (1845). His view has been consistently confirmed by more recent studies demonstrating an increased family history of mental illness in women with puerperal psychosis (Protheroe 1969). Whalley *et al.* (1982) demonstrated that the family histories of affective disorder in first-degree relatives are the same in women with puerperal and non-puerperal psychosis. It is also clear that a history of previous affective psychosis, puerperal or non-puerperal, substantially increases the risk of puerperal psychosis from 1 in 500 to approximately 1 in 5 (Protheroe 1969, Reich & Winokur 1970, Paffenbarger 1982). Taken together, the genetic evidence suggests that although there is clearly an inherited risk of psychotic illness in general, there appears to be no specific inherited predisposition to puerperal illness. As Brockington *et al.* (1982) point out, this suggests that other factors, be they psychosocial or physical, are precipitating the postnatal illness in *at-risk* women. Unfortunately, despite extensive research into both types of factors, we still know little about what precipitates puerperal psychotic illness.

Although a number of studies have been carried out examining the psychosocial correlates of puerperal psychosis, their results are conflicting and subject to methodological criticism, such as the absence of control groups. Comparisons between these studies are also made difficult by major methodological differences including the use of diverse definitions of disorders and timings of the assessments. Despite these difficulties, a number of factors emerge with enough consistency to allow one to presume an association with the occurrence of puerperal psychosis. Probably the most consistent of these factors is the increased risk in primiparous women (Thomas & Gordon 1959, Protheroe 1969). Paffenbarger (1982) calculated the relative risk to be 2.04. Kendell *et al.* (1981) obtained a similar figure and were able to rule out the possibility that this difference was secondary to either an age-related effect or the avoidance of further pregnancies by women who had experienced puerperal psychosis. Brockington *et al.* (1982) have argued that such an association with first pregnancy might be construed as favouring a psychological aetiology, because the arrival of the first baby involves the transition to parenthood, which revolutionizes a woman's way of life. However, as they rightly point out, organic disorders such as eclampsia and pre-eclampsia are also associated with first pregnancies. Furthermore, one might expect the rate for psychosis to be increased in first-time fathers, but this does not appear to be the case. Two recent control studies have examined life events in relation to the recurrence of postpartum

psychosis in at-risk women but have failed to find any significant association (Dowlatshahi & Paykel 1990, Marks *et al.* 1991).

Other psychosocial factors which might conceivably be involved in the precipitation of puerperal psychosis have been examined but with inconsistent results.

Puerperal psychosis has been linked with single motherhood (Tetlow 1955, Kendell *et al.* 1981), dystocia and prematurity (see Brockington *et al.* 1982 for review) and caesarean sections (Kendell *et al.* 1981). McNeil (1986, 1987), in a prospective study, looked at 88 'high risk' women who had a history of puerperal or non-puerperal functional psychosis and who became pregnant. The results showed that there was no difference in demographic characteristics between those who developed psychosis and those who did not. However, division of the cases into early- or late-onset groups yielded evidence that the former were more likely to be younger and primiparous and the latter more likely to be older, unmarried and multiparous in comparison to non-psychotic cases. In the study by Marks *et al.* (1991) the only social factor to emerge as significantly associated with psychotic relapse in at-risk women was a poor marital relationship. Another powerful effect to emerge from this study was the significant protective effect of communicative spouses in decreasing the risk of both psychotic and non-psychotic relapse in this group.

## Postnatal depression

Estimates of the incidence of postnatal depression vary between 10% and 15% (Pitt 1968, Paykel *et al.* 1980, Cox *et al.* 1982, Kumar & Robson 1984). Given the major differences in criteria and methodology between studies, the incidence figures are surprisingly consistent. However, the lack of consistency in defining symptomatology, time of onset, duration and course of the disorder, naturally creates difficulties when one is trying to describe these parameters. Pitt (1968) defined puerperal depression as the development of depressive symptoms following childbirth which are unusual in severity, are disabling, and persist for more than a fortnight. He argued that puerperal depression was atypical because it was mild to moderate in severity, and did not have typical endogenous features or suicidal ideation. In his random sample of 305 women, 10.8% developed puerperal depression but only one had classical symptoms of major depression. However, Kendell (1985) argues that in most respects such depressions are in fact typical depressive illnesses. In general, postnatal depression is conceptualized as a depressive disorder with an onset in the first few weeks postpartum. Although the vagueness of this definition seems somewhat unsatisfactory, it is debatable whether a more precise universal definition should be adopted, in view of the currently inadequate information on the nature and aetiology of this disorder. Indeed, it is probable that postnatal depression is in fact a heterogeneous group of apparently similar disorders which differ in aetiology and, possibly, course and onset. It should be recognized that another area of debate surrounds the very existence of postnatal depression as a separate entity from depression at any other time. Cooper *et al.* (1988) and O'Hara (1989), in their controlled prospective studies of postnatal women, found a similar prevalence in depression in the puerperal and non-puerperal women. Before leaping to the conclusion that postnatal depression is not specific, two important points should be considered. Although the *prevalence* may be similar for the two groups, the *incidence* in the early weeks postpartum does appear to be increased. Secondly, the influence of the very positive nature of the life event on many women's mood is often ignored. It is clear, for example from Pitt's (1968) findings, that the majority of women in fact show lower scores on anxiety and depression in the postpartum period than during the pregnancy. It is likely that childbirth can exert a protective effect on some women which may balance out the increased risk of depression it produces in others. Finally, and possibly most importantly for the clinician, whatever the arguments regarding the specific nature of postnatal depression, there is little doubt that a woman experiencing depression at this critical and very special time of her life requires special care and attention.

### Psychosocial correlates of postnatal depression

Despite much research, the importance of psychosocial factors in the genesis of postnatal depression remains unclear. Neither social class nor parity appear to influence the incidence of postnatal depression (Pitt 1968, Nilsson & Almgren 1970, Kumar & Robson 1978, Hayworth *et al.* 1980, Paykel *et al.* 1980). Contradictory results emerge from the study of the association with stressful life events. Paykel *et al.* (1980), Cutrona (1983) and O'Hara *et al.* (1984), all found significant associations between negative life events and the occurrence of postnatal depression. However, in the studies by Kumar & Robson (1984), Hopkins *et al.* (1987), Martin *et al.* (1989) and Brockington *et al.* (1990), no such association was found. The latter two studies, however, did demonstrate a significant association between psychosocial stressors and the occurrence of *antenatal* depression. This difference between antenatal and postnatal depression confirms suggestions made by other authors (Cox *et al.* 1982, Kumar & Robson 1984). Their observations suggest that the women who experience depression antenatally are different from those who become postnatally depressed. There does, however, appear to be an association between anxiety during pregnancy and the occurrence of depression postnatally. Such an association was described by Tod in 1964, and has subsequently been replicated by Watson *et al.* (1984) and Bridge *et al.* (1985).

Similar inconsistencies between studies are found when one examines the literature on all the other measures which have been investigated. Commonsense would suggest that one important potential stressor at this time would be the experience of the birth itself and any accompanying obstetric complications or interventions. This factor has been examined in most of the studies in this area, and the majority have failed to identify any significant association (Martin 1977, Cox *et al.* 1982, O'Hara 1986). Indeed, three studies have demonstrated that a significant decrease in postnatal depression followed the occurrence of obstetric complications (Pitt 1968, Paykel *et al.* 1980, O'Hara *et al.* 1982). Two social factors, however, have emerged with relatively greater consistency as being associated with an increased incidence of depression postnatally. These are poor quality of marital relationship and inadequate social support. Several authors have been able to demonstrate the association with poor marital relationship in a prospective manner, examining the state of the marital relationship during pregnancy and, therefore, prior to the onset of the postnatal depressive symptoms (Kumar & Robson 1984, Watson *et al.* 1984, O'Hara 1986).

In their review of postpartum depression, Hopkins *et al.* (1984) conclude that social support appears to protect women against postpartum depression. Not long after, the same authors conclude from their own study that: 'Contrary to expectation . . . social support was not related to postpartum depression'. However, most of the other studies examining this factor have demonstrated a significant association (Paykel *et al.* 1980, O'Hara *et al.* 1983, Cutrona 1983, O'Hara 1986). It is important, however, to note that these studies are measuring the mother's *perceptions* of social support, rather that actual social support. It is clear that depression colours the subject's perception of levels and quality of support that they receive (Monroe *et al.* 1983). Studies which had adequately controlled for this in a prospective manner are still needed. Gottlieb & Pancer (1988) point to the need for more detailed process-orientated research into social support. Investigation of not only how much support but also who from and, more importantly, what type of support, is likely to yield more useful, albeit more complex, information. Scales now exist which attempt to meet these demands, for example, the social provision scale (Russell *et al.* 1984), and the Significant Other Scale (SOS; Power *et al.* 1988) (also see Chapter 30).

The confusion which still exists over the influence of psychosocial and other variables can be explained in terms of methodological inadequacies and differences between studies. However, in doing so, we risk dismissing the important possibility that these inconsistent results represent very real differences between subgroups of women with postnatal depression.

Unravelling the complex interactions of multiple aetiological factors in such a heterogeneous disorder requires the frequent and prospective application of more sophisticated measures than have hitherto been used.

## Maternity 'blues'

The 'blues' is characterized by transient mood disturbances usually lasting one to two days during the first ten days postpartum (Cox *et al.* 1982, York 1990). The incidence has been found to peak fairly consistently at about five days postpartum, irrespective of culture or 'lying in' practices (Kendell *et al.* 1981, Iles *et al.* 1989, Cox 1979b, York 1990). Bell & Katona (1989) found a prevalence of 15–80% in the studies they reviewed – the majority ranging between 50% and 70%. Kennerley & Gath (1989) reported that the most frequent cluster of symptoms included tearfulness, tiredness, anxiety, lability of mood, feeling overemotional, low spirited and muddled in thinking. Iles *et al.* (1989), using a specially developed blues scale in a sample of postnatal women and a control sample of postoperative gynaecology patients, found the pattern of these mood changes to be characteristic of the puerperium.

A number of factors suggest biological causes for this disorder, including the nature and timing of the blues, findings of the relationship with premenstrual syndrome (Nott *et al.* 1976, Kennerley & Gath 1989) and the absence of consistent findings on the effects of social class, life events, and chronic stressors (Davidson 1972, Pitt 1973, Paykel *et al.* 1980, Stein 1980). Furthermore, obstetric factors seem to have little influence on the occurrence of the 'blues' (Pitt 1973, Stein 1980, Kennerley & Gath 1989), although Pitt (1973) did find a relationship with breast-feeding problems. The only social factor which has emerged with any consistency is the association between the blues and social relationships primarily with family or spouse. Such an association was described by Nilsson (1972), Ballinger *et al.* (1979), Katona (1982) and Kennerley & Gath (1989). It is interesting to note that this psychosocial factor is also the only one which emerges consistently in studies of puerperal psychosis and postnatal depression (see above). This leads one to speculate on the considerable importance of this factor, not so much for any specific postpartum psychiatric disorder, but for postpartum *mental health* generally. The specific way in which individual women respond to in-adequacies in social or marital relationships and support may thus depend on other (possibly biological) factors. If indeed this finding continues to be replicated, it would have preventive im-plications and also identify single parents as more at risk.

### Biological theories for puerperal disorders

The possibility of biological causes for puerperal mental disorders has long been recognized (Marcé 1858). The main focus of attention in contem-porary literature on biological aspects of these disorders has centred on hormonal changes. Despite extensive research, no clear or consistent associations have emerged between postpartum disorders and either hormone levels postpartum, or changes in levels associated with childbirth. The hormones which have been investigated include the ovarian steroids oestradiol, pro-gesterone, LH and FSH, gonadotrophin releasing hormone (GnRH), endogenous opioid peptides, prolactin, and thyroid hormones. A review of these studies is beyond the scope of this chapter but has recently been carried out by Wieck (1989). The most promising findings to emerge from this research include the evidence of an association between postnatal depression and thyroid dys-function in some women. Wieck *et al.* (1991) reported that in a study of women with a previous history of bipolar affective illness, those who had relapsed showed an enhanced growth hormone response to apomorphine four days postpartum (before the onset of the relapse). It is conceivable that this is due to D2 receptor hypersensitivity, which would be consistent with the dopaminergic theory of psychosis and may be related to the effects of oestrogen withdrawal on the function of dopaminergic systems. Preliminary results from a double-blind placebo-controlled study of oestradiol therapy for postnatal depression

indicate a significant improvement in women in the active group compared to controls after one month of treatment, maintained at three months (Gregoire *et al.* 1991, Henderson *et al.* 1991).

Thus it seems likely that biological factors have a significant influence in predisposing and pre-cipitating puerperal disorders. If this is so, the consideration most relevant in the present con-text, given the frequency of these disorders at such a critical time for the reproduction of the human species, must be to question what possible evolutionary advantage might have allowed the high risk of such disorders to persist. It is con-ceivable that the outward signs of distress in a mother caring for a newborn child might at some stage in human evolutionary history have led to caring and protective behaviour in the individuals around her. Experiencing and exhibiting such distress would then be particularly advantageous to women receiving inadequate levels of care and protection, and thus increase her and her off-spring's chances of survival. The consistent findings of an association between poor levels of social support and the blues, postnatal depression and puerperal psychosis would support such a hypothesis. Furthermore, it is often noted with some surprise that the occurrence of these dis-orders, except in the most severe of cases, does not impair the survival of the child (although there is some evidence that subtle effects on their development may occur). Unfortunately, in modern society such a care and protection 're-sponse' to postnatal expressions of distress is limited by a number of factors, including the elimination of close-knit communities and ex-tended families, leaving women largely isolated in the postnatal period, the medicalization of distress making it 'an illness' that needs 'treatment' by professionals, and the institutionalization of care.

### Social factors in management

The management of these disorders is based on the same principles as applied to psychotic or neurotic disorders generally. Some aspects of these are discussed elsewhere in this book (see Chapters 24 and 28). However, the critical additional consideration with puerperal disorders is of course their occurrence at such an important transitional period for the individual, the family and society. This consideration demands modifications and additions to these general principles in all areas of management.

### Detection

The first step in providing help for sufferers is to identify those in need of it. Until recently, this has relied principally upon presentation, a system which operates reasonably well in the case of puerperal psychosis as the severity of the disorder usually provides a clear signal of the need for professional help. With maternity blues, the increased popular awareness of the disorder, and the fact that most women are in contact with professional services at this early stage, ensure that symptoms in most women will be correctly identified, if only by the woman herself. However, the situation for postnatal depression is very different. It is well established that the incidence for depression in community samples is considerably higher than the numbers presenting either to primary care or mental health care professionals. This applies equally, and possibly even more so, to postnatal depression. The postpartum period is associated with powerful and sometimes contradictory popular expectations of the mother, which tend towards a denial of her negative feelings. She is expected to be happy and uplifted about her situation, and may thus make great efforts to hide her suffering and negative thoughts. Her superficially cheerful outward appearance is then accepted without question by all around her and any hints of her distress are denied or ignored. Conversely, if she openly displays her suffering, she is frequently told that 'it's not surprising', 'what do you expect when you have got a new baby', 'it's because you are not getting enough sleep', and so on. Such explanations provide little to help the mother, but release those around her from having to deal with her feelings. What brings women to seek help with postnatal depression has never been formally studied, but it is clear from the experiences of clinicians working in the field, and of self-help groups, that one key factor is simply knowing that there are services available.

The growing awareness that so many women with postnatal depression go undetected and unhelped has led to the development of a brief, simple, ten-item self-rating scale, specifically designed for the identification of postnatal depression (Edinburgh Post-natal Depression Scale, EPDS; Cox *et al.* 1987). This scale has been standardized and validated and is currently in use in primary care, hospital and research settings throughout the world. Its high level of acceptability to women who are asked to complete it and to health visitors, midwives and other health care professionals ensure that we now have a way to detect postnatal depression, even though the will may sometimes be lacking and the provision of treatment services is woefully inadequate.

### Treatment

Most women who present with puerperal psychosis are admitted to a hospital, although the types of facility available vary greatly. Specialized joint facilities for mother and baby may not be generally available in some countries (e.g. the USA), and in those countries where they are available, such as the UK, the quality and level of provision varies enormously between areas (Prettyman & Friedman 1991). Fortunately, there is a growing awareness of the need to provide specialist care in dedicated units, avoiding the separation of mother and baby. However, models for caring for psychotic women in their homes are also being developed (Oates 1988). The special needs for this group of women are, of course, not restricted to the relationship with their babies but include the whole family, and planning of care and aftercare should, of course, take this into account. It is thus in combination with an observance of these needs that the more traditional physical, psychological and social interventions are implemented.

Women with non-psychotic depressions only rarely require admission. Again, the traditional, physical, psychological and social interventions can be applied with due consideration to the mother's situation. For example, less sedative tricyclic antidepressants should be selected (these can even be given if the mother is breast feeding, Loudon 1987). Cognitive approaches (Brierley

1988) and supportive counselling (Holden *et al.* 1989) are appropriate psychological interventions, although the effort and time required of the mother in attending, and child-care needs, should be addressed by the service providers if they wish to have a therapeutic impact rather than producing additional strain. Furthermore, the possibility should be considered that particular types of support may be countertherapeutic for some women (e.g. taking the baby 'off her hands for a bit').

The evidence discussed above for an association between postnatal depression and social support strongly suggests a role for increasing social support in any intervention programme. The usefulness and importance of social networks to mothers both depressed and not depressed is emphasized in the review by Gottlieb & Pancer (1988). A number of models have been described for improving social support networks at this time (e.g. McGuire & Gottlieb 1979, Pound & Mills 1985, Elliot *et al.* 1988; also see Chapter 30). The following sources of support for the mother should be considered:
• Close friends, family and partner, if she has one. (The partner's need for support should also be considered.)
• Self-help organizations. (For example, in the UK the Association for Post-natal Illness and the Meet-a-Mum Association.)
• Health visitor.
• Community psychiatric nurse.
• General practitioner.
• Social worker.
• Psychologist.
• Psychiatrist.
As Gottlieb & Pancer (1988) have pointed out, it is important to consider the interplay between the professional services that are offered and the mother's social network, as destructive conflicts may be produced where harmony might otherwise have produced considerable benefit.

The need for intervention with the *blues* is limited by the very nature of this brief and transient disorder. The two considerations are, firstly, the provision of reassurance and support for both mother and family during the disorder and, secondly, assessment on follow-up that the mother has indeed fully recovered. This provision should be within the realms and training of midwives and health visitors, who will normally come into contact with all women in the first few days or weeks postnatally.

## Current developments and future prospects

The field of reproductive psychiatry is a relatively new one which is rapidly developing into an independent subspecialty. It is clear that the needs of psychiatrically ill parents have long been neglected and given the impact of parental disorder on children and society an expansion of services in this area is long overdue. At present, the majority of women with puerperal disorders receive inadequate help or none at all. Self-help groups such as the Association for Post-natal Illness, the Meet-a-Mum Association, and projects such as NEWPIN (Pound & Mills 1985; also see Chapter 30) are partially compensating for this neglect by providing much needed support and information services. We are beginning to develop a crude understanding of the extraordinarily complex interaction of psychological, social and physical factors which contribute to these disorders. Although more investigations into the basic nature and aetiology of these disorders are still needed, research has now progressed into the evaluation of different forms of interventions. Encouraging findings from methodologically sound studies of both psychosocial (Holden *et al.* 1989) and physical interventions (Gregoire *et al.* 1991) are now emerging. It is likely that in time, effective treatment and even prophylaxis will be available for postpartum mental illness. However, improvement in postpartum *mental health* will require social and political changes which can only be brought about through a re-evaluation of the position of both women and children in our society.

## References

Assael M.I., Namboze J.M., German G.A. & Bennett F.J. (1972) Psychiatric disturbances during pregnancy in a rural group of African women. *Social Science and Medicine* 6, 387–395.

Ballinger C.B., Buckley D.E., Naylor G.J. & Stansfeld D.A. (1979) Emotional disturbance following childbirth: clinical findings and urinary excretion of cyclic AMP.

*Psychological Medicine* 9, 293–300

Bell G.T. & Katona C.L.E. (1989) Disorders associated with menstruation, pregnancy and the puerperium. In Prasad A. (ed.) *The Biological Basis of Neuroses*, pp. 159–185, CRC Press, Roca Raton.

Bhugra D. (1992) Psychopathology in ancient Indian text. *History of Psychiatry* iii, 167–186.

Bridge L.R., Little B.C., Hayworth J., Dewhurst J. & Priest R.G. (1985) Psychometric antenatal predictors of postnatal depressed mood. *Journal of Psychosomatic Reseach* 29, 325–531.

Brierley E.A. (1988) A cognitive-behavioural approach to the treatment of postnatal distress. *Marcé Society Bulletin*. Summer, 27–39.

Brockington I.F. & Cox-Roper A. (1988) Nosology of puerperal illness. In Brockington I.F. & Kumar R. (eds) *Motherhood and Mental Illness 2: Causes and Consequences*, pp. 1–16, Wright, London.

Brockington I.F., Martin C., Brown G.W., Goldberg D. & Margison F. (1990) Stress and puerperal psychosis. *British Journal of Psychiatry* 157, 331–334.

Brockington I.F., Winokur G. & Dean C. (1982) Motherhood and mental illness. In Brockington I.F. & Kumar R. (eds) *Puerperal Psychosis*, pp. 37–69. Academic, London.

Brown G. (1989) Discussion. In Cox J.L., Paykel E.S. & Page M.L. (eds) *Childbirth as a Life Event*, p. 94. Duphar Medical Relations, Southampton.

Caraka Samhita (1943) Vol. V. Sri Gulab Kunerba Vedic Society, Jammagar, India.

Cooper P.J., Campbell E.A., Day A., Kennerley H. & Bond A. (1988) Non-psychotic psychiatric disorder after childbirth: a prospective study of prevalence, incidence, course and nature. *British Journal of Psychiatry* 152, 799–806.

Cox J.L. (1979a) Amakiro: a Ugandan puerperal psychosis. *Social Psychiatry* 14, 49–52.

Cox J.L. (1979b) Psychiatric morbidity and pregnancy: a controlled study of 263 semi-rural Ugandan women. *British Journal of Psychiatry* 134, 401–405.

Cox J.L. (1983) Postnatal depression: a comparison of African and Scottish women. *Social Psychiatry* 18, 25–28.

Cox J.L. (1988) The life event of childbirth: sociocultural aspects of postnatal depression. In Kumar R. & Brockington I.F. (eds) *Motherhood and Mental Illness 2: Causes and Consequences*, pp. 64–77. Wright, London.

Cox J.L., Connor Y. & Kendell R.E. (1982) Prospective study of the psychiatric disorders of childbirth. *British Journal of Psychiatry* 140, 111–117.

Cox J.L., Holden J.M. & Sagovsky R. (1987) Detection of postnatal depression: development of the 10-item Edinburgh Postnatal Depression Scale. *British Journal of Psychiatry* 150, 782–786.

Cutrona C.E. (1983) Causal attributions and perinatal depression. *Journal of Abnormal Psychology* 92, 161–172.

Davidson J.R.T. (1972) Postpartum mood changes in Jamaican women. *British Journal of Psychiatry* 121, 659–663.

Dean C. & Kendell R. (1981) The symptomatology of puerperal illness. *British Journal of Psychiatry* 139, 128–133.

Dowlatshahi D. & Paykel E.S. (1990) Life events and social stress in puerperal psychoses: absence of effect. *Psychological Medicine* 20, 655–662.

Ebie J.C. (1972) Psychiatric illness in the puerperium among Nigerians. *Tropical and Geographical Medicine* 24, 253–256.

Elliott S.A. (1990) Commentary on 'Childbirth as a Life Event'. *Journal of Reproductive and Infant Psychology* 8, 147–159.

Elliott S.A., Rugg A.J., Watson J.P. & Brough D.I. (1983) Mood changes during pregnancy and after the birth of a child. *British Journal of Clinical Psychology* 22, 295–308.

Elliott S.A., Sanjack M. & Leverton T.J. (1988) Parents groups in pregnancy. In Gottlieb B.H. (ed.) *Marshalling Social Support: Formats, Processes, and Effects*, vol. 3, pp. 87–110. Sage, Newbury Park.

Esquirol E. (1845) *Mental Maladies: A Treatise on Insanity* (translated by Hunt E.K.). Lea and Blanchard, Philadelphia.

Gottlieb B.H. & Pancer S.M. (1988) Social networks and the transition to parenthood. In Michales G.Y. & Goldberg W.A. (eds) *The Transition to Parenthood*, pp. 235–269. Cambridge University Press, Cambridge.

Gregoire A., Kumar R., Henderson A. & Studd J. (1991) The role of oestrogens in the treatment of postnatal depression. *Biological Psychiatry* 29, 11S, 130S.

Hamilton J.A. (1962) *Post Partum Psychiatric Problems*. C.V. Mosby, St Louis.

Hayworth J., Little B.D., Bonham Carter S., Raptopoulos P., Priest R.G. & Sandler M.A. (1980) A predictive study of postpartum depression: some predisposing characteristics. *British Journal of Medical Psychology* 53, 161–167.

Henderson A.F., Gregoire A.J.P., Kumar R. & Studd J.W.W. (1991) Treatment of severe postnatal depression with oestradiol skin patches. *Lancet* 338, 816–817.

Holden J.M., Sagovsky R. & Cox J.L. (1989) Counselling in a general practice: controlled study of health visitors intervention in treatment of post natal depression. *British Medical Journal* 298, 223–226.

Homans H. (1982) Pregnancy and birth as rites of passage. In MacCormack C.P. (ed.) *Ethnography of Fertility and Birth*, pp. 269–290. Academic Press, London.

Hopkins J., Campbell S.B. & Marcus M. (1987) Role of infant-related stressors in postpartum depression. *Journal of Abnormal Psychology* 96, 237–241.

Hopkins J., Marcus M. & Campbell S.B. (1984) Postpartum depression: a critical review. *Psychological Bulletin* 95, 498–515.

Ifabumuyi O.I. & Akindele M.O. (1985) Postpartum mental illnesses in Northern Nigeria. *Acta Psychiatrica Scandinavica* 2, 63–68.

Iles S., Gath D. & Kennerley H. (1989) Maternity blues. II A comparison between post-operative women and post-natal women. *British Journal of Psychiatry* 155, 363–366.

Jansson B. (1964) Psychic insufficiencies associated with child bearing. *Acta Psychiatrica Scandinavica* 39, (suppl. 172).

Jimenez M. & Newton N. (1979) Activity and work serving pregnancy and the postpartum period: a cross-cultural study of 202 societies. *American Journal of Obstetrics and Gynecology* 135, 171–176.

Katona C. (1982) Puerperal mental illness: comparisons with non-puerperal controls. *British Journal of Psychiatry* 141, 447–452.

Kelly J.V. (1967) The influence of native customs on obstetrics in Nigeria. *Obstetrics and Gynaecology* 30, 608–612.

Kendell R.E. (1985) Emotional and physical factors in the genesis of puerperal mental disorders. *Journal of Psychosomatic Research* 29, 3–11.

Kendell R.E., Chalmers J.C. & Platz C. (1987) Epidemiology of puerperal psychoses. *British Journal of Psychiatry* 150, 662–673.

Kendell R.E., Rennie D., Clause J.A. & Dean C. (1981) The social and obstetric correlates of psychiatric admission in the puerperium. *Psychological Medicine* 11, 341–350.

Kennerley H. & Gath D. (1989) Maternity blues III. Associations with obstetric, psychological and psychiatric factors. *British Journal of Psychiatry* 155, 367–373.

Kitzinger S. (1982) Social context of birth: some comparisons between child birth in Jamaica and Britian. In MacCormack C.P. (ed.) *Ethnography of Fertility and Birth*, pp. 181–203. Academic, London.

Kumar R. & Robson K. (1978) Neurotic disturbance during pregnancy and the puerperium. In: Sandler M.J. (ed.) *Mental Illness in Pregnancy and the Puerperium*, pp. 40–51. Oxford University Press, Oxford.

Kumar R. & Robson K. (1984) A prospective study of emotional disorders in child bearing women. *British Journal of Psychiatry* 144, 35–47.

Loudon J.B. (1987) Prescribing in pregnancy: psychotropic drugs. *British Medical Journal* 294, 167–169.

McGuire J. & Gottlieb B.H. (1979) Social support groups among new parents: an experimental study in primary prevention. *Journal of Clinical and Child Psychology* 8, 111–116.

McNeil T.F. (1986) A prospective study of post partum psychoses in a high risk group: clinical characteristics of the current post partum episodes. *Acta Psychiatrica Scandinavica* 74, 205–216.

McNeil T.F. (1987) A prospective study of post partum psychoses in a high risk group: relationships to demographic and psychiatric history characteristics. *Acta Psychiatrica Scandinavica* 75, 35–43.

Marcé L.V. (1858) *Traite de la Folie des Femmes Enceintes, des Nouvelles Accouchees et des Nourrices*. Baillère, Paris.

Marks M.N., Wieck A., Checkley S.A. & Kumar R. (1991) Life stress and post-partum psychosis: a preliminary report. *British Journal of Psychiatry* 158, 45–49.

Martin C.J., Brown G.W., Goldberg D.P. & Brockington J.F. (1989) Psychosocial stress and puerperal depression. *Journal of Affective Disorders* 16, 283–293.

Martin M.E. (1977) A maternity hospital study of psychiatric illness associated with childbirth. *Irish Journal of Medical Science* 146, 239–244.

Mead M. & Newton N. (1967) Cultural patterning of perinatal behaviour. In Richardson S.A. & Guttmacher A.F. (eds) *Childbearing: Its Social and Psychological Aspects*, pp. 142–243. Williams and Wilkins, Baltimore.

Meltzer E.S. & Kumar R. (1985) Puerperal mental illness; clinical features and classification: a study of 142 mother and baby admissions. *British Journal of Psychiatry* 147, 647–654.

Menzies W.F. (1893) Puerperal insanity. An analysis of 140 consecutive cases. *American Journal of Insanity* 50, 148–185.

Monroe S.M., Imhoff D.F., Wise B.D. & Harris J.E. (1983) Prediction of psychological symptoms under high risk psychosocial circumstances; life events, social support, symptom specificity. *Journal of Abnormal Psychology* 92, 338–350.

Nilsson A. (1972) Paranatal emotional adjustment. In: Morris N. (ed.) *Psychosomatic Medicine in Obstetrics and Gynaecology*, pp. 157–160. Karger, Basel.

Nilsson A. & Almgren P.E. (1970) Paranatal emotional adjustment. A prospective investigation of 165 women. II. The influence of background factors, psychiatric history, parental relations and personality characteristics. *Acta Psychiatrica Scandinavica* Suppl. 220, 65–141.

Nott P., Franklin M., Armitage C. & Gelder M.G. (1976) Hormonal changes and mood in the puerperium. *British Journal of Psychiatry* 128, 379–383.

Oakley A. (1980) *Women Confined – Towards a Sociology of Childbirth*. Martin Robertson, Oxford.

Oates M. (1988) The development for an integrated community orientated service for severe post-natal mental illness. In Kumar R. & Brockington I.F. (eds) *Motherhood and Mental Illness 2: Causes and Consequences*, pp. 133–158. Wright, London.

O'Hara M.W. (1986) Social support, life events and depression during pregnancy and puerperium. *Archives of General Psychiatry* 43, 569–573.

O'Hara M.W. (1989) The Iowa study: childbirth as a life event: effects on mood and social adjustment. In Cox J.L., Paykel E.S. & Page M.L. (eds) *Childbirth as a Life Event*, pp. 46–56. Duphar, Southampton.

O'Hara M.W., Neunaber D.J. & Zekowski E.M. (1984) A prospective study of postpartum depression: prevalence, course and predictive factors. *Journal of Abnormal Psychology* 93, 158–171.

O'Hara M.W., Rehm L.P. & Campbell S.B. (1982) Predicting depressive symptomatology: cognitive and behavioural models and postpartum depression. *Journal of Abnormal Psychology* 91, 245–254.

O'Hara M.W., Rehm, L.P. & Campbell S.B. (1983) Post-partum depression: a rule for social network and life stress variables. *Journal of Nervous and Mental Disease* 171, 336–341.

O'Hara M.W. & Zekoski E.M. (1988) Post partum depression: a comprehensive review. In Kumar R. & Brockington I.F. (eds) *Motherhood and Mental Illness 2: Causes and Consequences*, pp. 17–63. Wright, London.

Paffenbarger R.S. (1982) Epidemiological aspects of mental illness associated with childbearing. In Brockington I.F. & Kumar R. (eds) *Motherhood and Mental Illness*, pp. 19–36. Academic, London.

Paykel E.S. Emms E.M., Fletcher J. & Rassaby E.S (1980) Response to phenelzine and amitriptyline in sub-types of neurotic depression. *Archives of General Psychiatry* 39, 1041–1049.

Pillsbury B.L. (1978) Doing the 'month': confinement and convalescence of Chinese women after childbirth. *Social Science and Medicine* 12, 11–22.

Pitt B. (1968) Atypical depression following childbirth. *British Journal of Psychiatry* 114, 1325–1335.

Pitt B. (1973) Maternity blues. *British Journal of Psychiatry* 122, 431–432.

Platz C. & Kendell R.E. (1988) A matched control follow up and family study of puerperal psychoses. *British Journal of Psychiatry* 153, 90–94.

Pound A. & Mills M. (1985) A pilot evaluating of NEWPIN home visiting and befriending scheme in South London. *Association of Child Psychiatry and Psychology Newsletter* 7, 13–15.

Power M.J., Champion L.A. & Aris S.J. (1988) The development of the measure of social support: the Significant Others Scales (SOS). *British Journal of Clinical Psychology* 27, 349–358.

Prettyman R.J. & Friedman T. (1991) Care of women with puerperal psychiatric disorders in England and Wales. *British Medical Journal* 302, 1245–1246.

Protheroe C. (1969) Puerperal psychosis: a longterm study. *British Journal of Psychiatry* 115, 9–30.

Raphael-Leff J. (1991) Childbearing Practices across the Continents – Reflections of Cultural Metaphor and Pregnant Fantasies. Paper presented at the Society for Reproductive and Infant Psychology Annual Conference, Durham.

Rees W.D. & Lutkins S.G. (1971) Parental depression before and after childbirth. *Journal of the Royal College of General Practitioners* 21, 26–31.

Reich T. & Winokur G. (1970) Postpartum psychoses in patients with manic depressive disease. *Journal of Nervous and Mental Disease* 151, 60–68.

Ripa Y. (1990) *Women and Madness. The Incarceration of Women in Nineteenth Century France*. Polity Press, Cambridge.

Russell D., Cutrona C.E., Rose J. & Yurko K. (1984) Social and emotional loneliness: an examination of Weiss' typology of loneliness. *Journal of Personality and Social Psychology* 46, 1313–1321.

Seel R.M. (1986) Birth rite. *Health Visitor* 59, 182–184.

Showalter E. (1987) *The Female Malady: Women, Madness and English Culture*. Virago, London.

Sim M. (1963) Abortion and the psychiatrist. *British Medical Journal* 2, 145.

Stein G.S. (1980) The pattern of mental change and body weight change in the first postpartum week. *Journal of Psychosomatic Research* 24, 165–171.

Stern G. & Kruckman L. (1983) Multi-disciplinary perspectives on postpartum depression: an anthropological critique. *Social Science and Medicine* 17, 1027–1041.

Swift C.R. (1972) Psychosis during the puerperium among Tanzanians. *East African Medical Journal* 49, 651–657.

Tetlow C. (1955) Psychosis of childbearing. *Journal of Mental Sciences* 101, 629–639.

Thomas C.L. & Gordon J.E. (1959) Psychosis after childbirth: ecological aspects of a single impact stress. *American Journal of the Medical Sciences* 238, 363–368.

Tod E.M. (1964) Puerperal depression: a prospective epidemiological study. *Lancet* ii, 1264–1266.

Watson J.P. Elliott S.A., Rugg A.J. & Brough D.I. (1984) Psychiatric disorder in pregnancy and the first postnatal year. *British Journal of Psychiatry* 144, 453–462.

Whalley L.J., Roberts D.F., Wentzel J. & Wright A.F. (1982) Genetic factors in puerperal affective psychoses. *Acta Psychiatrica Scandinavica* 65, 180–193.

Wieck A. (1989) Endocrine aspects of postnatal mental disorders. In Oates M. (ed.) *Psychological Aspects of Obstetrics and Gynaecology*, pp. 857–877. Baillière, Tindall, London.

Wieck A., Kumar R., Hirst A.D., Marks M.N., Campbell I.C. & Checkley S.A. (1991) Increased sensitivity of dopamine receptors and recurrence of affective psychosis after childbirth. *British Medical Journal* 303, 613–616.

York R. (1990) Pattern of postpartum blues. *Journal of Reproductive and Infant Psychology* 8, 67–73.

# Chapter 26
# What Happens to Autistic Children
# when they Grow Up?

LORNA WING

Autism was first recognized and named by Leo Kanner approximately 50 years ago. Kanner (1943) wrote about the manifestations in early life and, for many years, interest was focused on autistic children. There are a few publications giving results of follow-ups into adolescence or the first half of adult life (Rutter 1970, DeMyer *et al.* 1973, Kanner 1973, Wing 1988), but there is little information concerning middle-aged and elderly people with autism. The information to be given in this chapter is derived from the published follow-up studies, from the findings of an evaluation, carried out by members of the MRC Social Psychiatry Unit, of the effects of the closure of Darenth Park mental handicap hospital (Shah *et al.* 1982, Rawlings 1985a,b, Wing 1989a) and from the clinical experience of the author (Wing 1989c) and others (Schopler & Mesibov 1983).

Autism is a developmental disorder almost always present from birth or early childhood but having life-long effects. It is characterized by severe impairment of the normally innate capacity to interact, empathize and communicate with other human beings and to make sense of experiences by weaving them into a coherent story (Shah & Wing 1986, Frith 1989). Creative imagination is markedly limited or absent (Gould 1986) and the pattern of activities is dominated by repetitive stereotyped routines. Wing & Gould (1979) considered this triad of impairments of social interaction, communication and imagination to be essential to diagnosis but other abnormalities are often found in association. They include language delay and deviance, poor gross motor coordination, odd responses to sensory stimuli, rapid inexplicable changes of mood and a wide range of non-specific behaviour problems including aggression, destructiveness, screaming, wandering and self-injury (now euphemistically termed 'challenging' behaviour). In the majority of cases, but by no means all, there are varying degrees of general mental retardation (Rutter 1970, Wing & Gould 1979).

Autism results from any one of a variety of biological, including genetic, causes (Coleman & Gillberg 1985, Schopler & Mesibov 1987, Gillberg 1988, Waterhouse *et al.* 1989, Wing 1989a).

Kanner believed the pattern he described was a specific, unique syndrome, different from other childhood conditions, but it is now clear that it overlaps with other developmental disorders. One autistic-like condition that has received much attention recently is Asperger's syndrome (Asperger 1944, 1979, Gillberg & Gillberg 1989, Tantam 1988, Wing 1981a, Frith 1991), characterized by social naivety and inappropriateness, long-winded repetitive speech but impaired verbal and non-verbal communication, repetitive circumscribed interests, poor motor coordination and general lack of commonsense. The concept that best fits the research and clinical data is that Kanner's autism is part of a continuum of conditions, all characterized by the triad of impairments of social interaction, communication and imagination (Wing & Gould 1979, Gillberg *et al.* 1986).

Wing & Gould (1979) calculated that the prevalence in children of disorders in the whole continuum was around 21 in 10000, that is four to five times the rate for typical Kanner's syndrome. There are possibly 60000 adults with autistic disorders in the UK, of whom perhaps 15000 would have Kanner's autism.

This chapter will discuss people with any of the disorders within the autistic continuum.

## Outcome in adult life

The behaviour patterns, life-styles and needs for services of individuals with autistic disorders vary widely. This section considers subgroups divided according to overall level of ability, since this is very significantly correlated with outcome (Rutter 1970, DeMyer *et al.* 1974, Wing 1988). Specialized education throughout childhood has been shown to encourage the development of useful skills and to reduce behaviour problems (Bartak & Rutter 1973, Rutter & Bartak 1973). But, helpful though education is, it does not affect the basic impairments underlying autistic disorders and its effect is strictly limited by the cognitive potential of the individual concerned. No psychological or physical treatments have, to date, been found that cure autism or make any real difference to the level of severity of the handicaps, despite the many different methods that have been tried.

The typical, though not universal, profile on cognitive testing is markedly uneven, with visuospatial better than language-dependent skills (Gould 1977, Lockyer & Rutter 1969, Shah & Frith 1983, Shah 1988). The subgrouping used here is based on visuospatial abilities.

### *Autism and severe mental retardation*

This subgroup comprises those with visuospatial IQs under 50 and includes people who are profoundly mentally retarded (IQ under 20). In the epidemiological study of Camberwell children aged under 15, Wing & Gould (1979) found that 62% of those with autistic disorders had visuospatial IQ scores in the severely retarded range. No similar study has been published concerning adults but it seems likely that this subgroup will be the largest among those with autistic disorders aged over 15, as it is for the children.

THE CLINICAL PICTURE

Individuals in this subgroup generally have poor self-care and practical skills and even poorer language and communication. As children, most were aloof and indifferent to others and rejected attempts at social contact. Most remain aloof even in adult life (Wing 1988). Stereotypies are a marked feature. These are usually of a simple kind such as hand flapping, jumping, flicking objects, repetitive vocalizations, or self-injuring, including head banging, lip chewing or eye poking. They are highly resistant to behaviour-modification techniques. Major behaviour problems of the kind mentioned above are common and often persist into early adult life. Exacerbation of such problems tends to occur during adolescence (Favell 1983, Wing 1983, Gillberg & Schaumann 1989). However, although no follow-up studies into later adult life have been published, the general impression among carers is that challenging behaviour becomes less evident with increasing age after the early adult years have passed. Cross-sectional data from the study of the closure of Darenth Park mental handicap hospital (Wing 1989b) provided some evidence for this. Among the 893 people in the hospital at the beginning of the study, 348 (39%) had autistic conditions. Of these, 216 were aloof in social interaction, most of whom were severely retarded. Out of this group, 65% had at least one type of severe behaviour problem, but there was a steady drop in the proportions so rated within succeeding age bands. Thus, 77% of those aged under 35 had one or more severe behaviour problems, compared with 55% aged 35–69 and 22% of those who were 70 and over. Such data must be viewed with caution, first, because the Darenth residents were not a random sample, tending to be those with the most difficult behaviour and, secondly, the findings were not based on the follow-up of individuals.

The general impression from personal experience is that the basic impairments of social interaction, communication and imagination and the repetitive, stereotyped activities remain but tend to change in their manifestations. From middle age onwards, such changes, though minor, improve the quality of life for the individuals concerned and those who care for them.

SERVICE PLACEMENTS

Some adults in this subgroup live at home with ageing parents. Some of these attend day centres for people with mental handicaps run by social services, but this type of placement is prone to break down because, in most cases, no special provision is made for people with autism. The National and Local Autistic Societies (voluntary bodies concerned with the welfare of autistic people) have set up a small number of day centres but these, at present, provide only about 50 places in the whole of the country.

Until the movement to provide residential care for people with mental handicaps in small homes outside hospital began to be effective, most severely retarded people with autism were sooner or later admitted to mental handicap hospitals where they became long-stay residents. This used to be almost the only type of residential care available to families, apart from a very few voluntary or private homes.

National and local autistic societies have opened some small residential communities for adults. However, comparatively few of the most severely retarded people with autistic disorders have benefited directly because the overall number of places available (about 400) is low in relation to the numbers needing residential care and there is a tendency to accept the somewhat more able people when there is a choice among applicants for places. There are also various voluntary and private bodies that have set up homes in which people with autistic disorders are accepted. More of these have been opened in recent years and some will take those with severe or profound handicaps.

The move to reduce in size or close mental handicap hospitals and to move the residents to small living units in the local authority districts from which they were admitted has involved at least some people in this subgroup. During the course of the Darenth Park closure, the residents with autistic disorders, being on the whole less able, more difficult to care for and more likely to have 'challenging' behaviour, were discharged at a slower rate than the sociable residents. In the early years of the run down to closure, many people were moved to existing hostels, private homes or other hospitals. In the later years, purpose-built or adapted accommodation was provided. These were either small houses scattered in ordinary streets, or campuses with several small living units on one site together with day care and administrative services. There was a tendency for the people with autistic disorders and severe or profound mental retardation to be placed in campuses when these were available. Data are still being collected and results analysed but some general findings can be given.

While living in Darenth, the severely handicapped residents with autism had very significantly worse skills, behaviour and life-styles than the sociable residents. After moving, the autistic group experienced improvements in personal privacy, use of community services, and level of independence within the living units, including opportunities for using domestic equipment with help from staff. There was no improvement in freedom outside the living units, most of which were on or near roads with traffic, nor in challenging behaviour, level of language development (though more use was made of the language available), stereotypies, or social impairment. In short, improvements were related to the amenities that money could buy, such as more staff, small living units, nice furnishings, more equipment. No improvements occurred in aspects of life that could not be bought, namely large, outdoor, traffic-free space surrounding living units in towns and cures for the biological handicaps underlying the pattern of skills and behaviour.

The changes that did occur for the group as a whole were clearly worthwhile and were much appreciated by the relatives who visited. Examination of the experiences of individual residents was needed to show more precisely the advantages and disadvantages. The majority of those in the subgroup under discussion appeared to have settled down in their new living units when seen one year after moving, though they had insufficient language to express an opinion. Some had had a period of disturbance but then improved. However, approximately one-quarter were causing great problems because of their aggressiveness to others, destructiveness or self-injury. A few of these went to private hospitals where there were high security and high staff ratios. A small number of others were cared for in houses or flats on their own with a high level of staffing. The rest were in campuses or small houses with other residents. Such mixing tended to distress the more amenable residents exposed to the challenging behaviour.

Looking at the country as a whole, the provision made for people with autistic disorders, severe mental retardation and extremely challenging behaviour is diverse and mainly dependent on chance. There are some who still live at home with parents who are determined to care for their son or daughter as long as they can. Such parents may have no help at all and no chance of respite care for the person with autism. In these circumstances the families live lives that are grossly abnormal, stressful and isolated from the rest of the world.

### Autism and mild mental retardation

This subgroup comprises those who have visuo-spatial IQs in the range 50–69. In the study of Camberwell children, referred to above, 23% of those with autistic disorders had IQ scores in this range. Again, no comparable figures are available for adults.

THE CLINICAL PICTURE

Adults in this subgroup have a range of practical skills and, though some are mute, more have varying degrees of language comprehension and use, albeit with characteristic oddities such as immediate and delayed echolalia and idiosyncratic use of words or phrases. A minority have superior skills in isolated areas (see later in this chapter). Even as adults they tend to need supervision in the skills of everyday living, despite their competence in specific areas. They may choose to wear clothes that are inappropriate and to put them on back to front. Their behaviour in public may elicit disapproval from strangers because they ignore other people and, for example, barge straight through them and allow doors to swing in people's faces. They may never learn to cross the road safely. They may be able to memorize and carry out the formula 'look right, look left, then look right again' but then step into the road even if a car is coming because they cannot grasp the meaning of the ritual they have performed so precisely.

Although many were aloof and indifferent in early childhood, there is, later on, a tendency for a change to passive or active but odd social interaction lasting into adult life.

No precise statistics are available concerning the outcome for older adults in this group. The Darenth Park study provides some cross-sectional data but this has to be viewed with caution for the same reasons as mentioned above. It was found that around one-half of this subgroup had at least one type of severe behaviour problem compared with two-thirds of those with severe retardation. Again, there was a tendency for the proportion with such problems to decrease with increasing age; the rates were 64% under age 35, 41% from 35 to 69 years, and 33% at age 70 and above.

This subgroup tends to have more elaborate organized repetitive behaviour than those who are severely retarded. Examples include making long lines of objects, insisting on a complex bedtime routine, following the exact same route to the shops every day, or amassing vast numbers of particular objects for no apparent purpose. Simple stereotypies are often present as well. Among those who can talk are a number whose speech is plentiful but monotonously repetitive, and who demand stereotyped replies from the person addressed.

SERVICE PLACEMENTS

The range of possible placements is wider for this subgroup. Some live at home with their parents and some of these attend day centres for people with mental handicaps. As noted previously, this type of day provision may not prove satisfactory because autistic behaviour is not understood or catered for. The national and local autistic societies' day centres cater for a small number of those in need of day placements. The quality of life of those living at home and that of their carers depends upon the amount of challenging behaviour and the degree of rigidity of the individual's pattern of activities but, however mild the handicap, an autistic person in the house always means some restrictions in the life of the family. Even something as trivial sounding as repetitive questioning with a demand for answers can, when continued day in day out, be a source of great stress.

As with the severely retarded subgroup, many were admitted to mental handicap hospitals in the past, when little choice was available (Rutter 1966). As the hospitals are gradually run down to closure, these residents are being moved into campuses or small houses.

The residential homes run by the national or local autistic societies are particularly suitable for people in this subgroup. As yet, there are only some 400 places of this kind, but it is hoped that more will be opened in the future. As mentioned previously, there is a range of homes run by voluntary or private bodies that are willing to accept as residents people with autistic disorders.

A small minority of the mildly retarded group stand out from the rest in being extremely aggressive, destructive, or self-injurious. The same variety of placements have been used for these people as for the similar group among those with severe mental retardation.

### Autism without mental retardation

This subgroup comprises people with visuospatial IQs of 70 or above. They include most of those who could be diagnosed as having Asperger's syndrome, others who are the most able among those with Kanner's autism and yet others who fit no named clinical picture, but have the triad of impairments. They represented 15% of all the children with autistic disorders in the Camberwell study. It is difficult to calculate the true prevalence in childhood and even more difficult in adult life since an unknown number do not make contact with psychiatric or social services. Others do make such contacts but are never diagnosed as having an autistic disorder. Gillberg & Gillberg (1989) on the basis of population studies in Goteborg, Sweden, have cautiously suggested that the prevalence of Asperger's syndrome among people of normal intelligence may be within the range of 10–26 per 10 000 – that is at least twice as common as the usual estimate for Kanner's classic autism.

THE CLINICAL PICTURE

In this subgroup, social interaction tends to be passive or active but naive and inappropriate. Very few remain aloof to others. Those who have made the most progress have a subtle form of social impairment that can best be described as a stilted, formal, over-polite and pedantic manner.

Behaviour problems may have been present in childhood but do tend to improve greatly with age. Nevertheless, there is still a vulnerability to any kind of stress, which can precipitate childish temper tantrums.

Repetitive behaviour tends to take the form of absorption in a limited range of topics, such as railway time tables, types of owls, the characters in a soap opera, facts about the British weather, the listing of prime numbers ad infinitum and so on. In most cases, the interest is in the amassing of facts on these subjects rather than any possible application of the knowledge.

The profile on cognitive testing may be uneven and show the superiority of visuospatial skills commonly found in the other subgroups but in some people verbal scores may be similar to or even higher than those on non-verbal tests (Wing 1981a). The main value of IQ testing is to reveal the strategies for problem solving, which tend to be rigid and idiosyncratic.

Grammar and vocabulary are usually good but are used for monologues on the special interests rather than for two-way communication with others. Non-verbal communication is either minimal or inappropriate in form, for example the voice may be monotonous, or speech may be accompanied by wild flailing of the arms that signify nothing. There may have been a history of learning difficulties in some school subjects but much better performance in others. Memory for facts is typically better than comprehension of the wider meaning.

The basis of self-care is achieved but even the most able in this group may choose inappropriate clothes, ignore the need to change them when they are dirty, and forget to brush the back of their hair or to tuck shirts in at the back.

Some find a social group that accepts them but most tend to have little or no social life. This suits some individuals though others feel lonely but do not know how to make friends.

SERVICE PLACEMENTS

Among those in contact with services, there are some who live at home with their parents or, rarely, with other relatives. Things go reasonably well if the person concerned has some regular occupation, either sheltered or in open employment. Problems arise if they are not employed and are bored and restless because they have to stay at home all day. A source of stress for the carers is the stubbornness and rigidity of thought and action and the insistence on preserving sameness in tiny details of the daily routine. Inappropriate social behaviour can also be a problem with someone able enough to go out on their own. Parents describe feeling constantly anxious in case their son or daughter becomes embroiled in some embarrassing, even dangerous situation because of their naivety and innocence of the world and its wiles.

There are particular difficulties in finding suitable leisure activities, unless a special interest, such as chess or train spotting, is catered for in a specialist club.

Some are found places in the sheltered communities run by the national or local autistic societies. If they can accept the idea of living with a group of residents of widely varying ability, some being very handicapped, there is a good chance that such a placement will be successful. But some autistic adults who are not themselves mentally retarded do not want to be placed together with people of low ability. A small group home with autistic residents of similar cognitive levels can work well, given skilled staff. The occasional autistic person of normal intelligence can be found in many different kinds of homes and hostels. Success and failure depend upon the staff and other residents. Some can be found in hospitals or homes for adults with mental illnesses.

OUTCOME IN PEOPLE NEVER IN CONTACT WITH SERVICES

As emphasized earlier, it is impossible to give prevalence figures for adults in the present sub-group who have never been diagnosed officially and never been in touch with the special education, health or social services. Some are known because of contacts made by concerned relatives. There are certainly some who are using their skills in paid work, who have their own homes and even some who have married and have children. Success is most likely in work that is mainly routine and which does not involve much spontaneous social interaction. Marriage is a more difficult area of life. The non-autistic spouse, mostly the wife because of the high male to female ratio among autistic people of high ability (Wing 1981b), has to be content with a partner who demands a regular routine and who gives little emotional support and is incapable of those small acts of understanding and empathy that cement a relationship. The wife also has to take almost all the responsibility for child rearing. Some wives accept and are happy with the situation, especially if their husbands are steady workers and good providers, some accept although not happy, while others find it bewildering and an intolerable strain.

There are adults with autistic disorders who live on their own in eccentric ways, having no contact with anyone, surrounded, for example, by empty jam jars, thousands of advertising circulars or toothpaste tubes collected throughout a lifetime. While some are meticulously neat and orderly others live in dirt and squalor because their rigid routine does not include cleaning.

People with undiagnosed autism can occasionally be found among the homeless. One young man in a Salvation Army hostel insisted his name was Clapham North. His only interest was riding on the London Underground all day and his only conversation was describing, in meticulous detail, routes from one station to another.

*Individuals with special skills*

In all of the subgroups there are some people with outstanding skills in certain areas. These are almost always in the fields of music, drawing, model making, sculpting, arithmetical calculations or feats of memory for dates, time tables, maps, soap operas or any other collections of facts. For those with overall ability in the normal range, the possession of a skill of the kind that has commercial value is one of the factors needed for success in obtaining gainful employment. Other important factors are a strong desire to become independent, determination to keep trying despite initial setbacks and a temperament that is equable enough to allow the acceptance of some changes and some stress without responding with a crisis of rage and anxiety. Temple Grandin (Grandin & Scariano 1986) is an example of someone who has successfully used her visuospatial skills and childhood fascination with cattle grids to become an expert in designing cattle handling facilities for ranches. The present author knows a man with classic autism whose absolute pitch and musical skills have enabled him to earn a good living as a tuner of concert pianos. He also composes music.

Those whose skills and interests are unwanted by the world, or who lack the drive to apply them, use their special abilities for themselves alone, finding pleasure in endless repetition.

The individuals who capture the imagination are those who are mentally retarded on conventional tests but who have one or two skills in the superior range of ability – now known as the 'savant syndrome' (Treffert 1989). Many, perhaps most, of these have disorders in the autistic continuum. Examples in the literature are the artist Nadia (Selfe 1977), and the calendar calculator twins John and Michael and the artist Jose described by Sacks (1985). Despite his autism and learning difficulties, Stephen Wiltshire's architectural drawings are becoming famous (Wiltshire 1987, 1989); with guidance and help he is producing remarkable work that sells.

O'Connor & Hermelin (1988) and O'Connor (1989) have examined such phenomena in autistic and non-autistic people with mental retardation. The proportion of people with specific skills appears to be considerably higher among those with Kanner's autism (10%) than those with mental retardation without typical autism (0.06%) (Hill 1977, O'Connor 1989).

These strangely discrepant patterns of ability have not yet been satisfactorily explained. Neither is there any explanation for the fact that some autistic-savants suddenly cease to use their skills after having practised them for years. How many do this is not known. Nor is it clear whether the

skill is lost in some or all such cases or just never used. Occasionally some reason for the change can be suggested. The twins described by Sacks ceased to show their numerical power when they were separated in the name of 'normalization'. Nadia stopped drawing her remarkable pictures as her speech developed. But, as pointed out by O'Connor (1989), there are other autistic artists whose talent has survived the development of speech.

Whatever the underlying neurology of these limited but outstanding islets of ability, their existence will continue to surprise and to fascinate us all.

## Special problems

There are some aspects of life that may present special problems for adults with autistic disorders and their carers.

### Sexual development

When their child is diagnosed as autistic, one of the questions parents often ask is 'will he or she ever marry and have children'. In most of those who make contact with psychiatric or social services, the cognitive retardation in itself prevents the achievement of independence in any sphere of adult life. The autistic handicap, with its impairment of social interaction and empathy, adds another dimension. The physical changes associated with puberty tend to occur within the usual age range (Rutter 1970). Among those who are mentally retarded, basic sexual drives are manifested in masturbation and, in some individuals, interest in the secondary sexual characteristics of other people. It is only the more able autistic people who may express a desire for a girlfriend or boyfriend. Most autistic adolescents and adults lack the social understanding necessary to associate their physiological urges with the idea of a relationship with another person.

Overtly sexual behaviour may occur in public in the more handicapped autistic people. This can cause all kinds of difficulties whether it is self or other directed. The innocence and lack of understanding that are basic to autism are rarely appreciated by the general public who see only the unacceptable outward behaviour. Autistic adolescents and adults who are able enough to want a relationship often have problems finding a partner because of their social naivety and clumsiness. They may ask for help to find a book that will set out the rules for attracting and keeping a partner, in the belief that these can be learnt by rote.

Despite all the difficulties, as mentioned previously, some very able autistic people, especially those who have never been in touch with services and who have gone through mainstream school and are in regular employment, do marry and have children.

An approach to sex education for adolescents with autism is described by Melone & Lettick (1983).

### Delinquent or criminal behaviour

This occurs in a small minority of those with normal intelligence or mild mental retardation. They stand out from other law breakers because there is no tendency for them to come from disturbed or criminal families. They tend to be unaware of the legal implications or the social and human consequences of their behaviour (Baron-Cohen 1988). They are not motivated by gain; their actions arise from pursuit of their circumscribed interests or by responses to experiences of which they have an irrational and extreme dislike. Some aggressive acts are a response to the feeling that others are critical and mocking. This can appear to be paranoid but may be based on reality. The odd gait and manner of speech do tend to attract adverse comments from strangers.

Mawson *et al.* (1985) described a middle-aged man in Broadmoor Hospital with Asperger's variant of autism who attacked babies and dogs for making sounds that he found unpleasant. He was extremely interested in poisons and water pipes and contemplated using the former for homicide. Mawson *et al.* suggested that an unknown number of such individuals may be found in long-term institutions of various sorts.

Less dramatic conflicts with the law are more common. For example, one boy loved to touch shiny fabrics and would stroke women's clothes made of such materials. He had no interest in the women but this was not understood by those whose clothes he touched. His normal physical appearance did not make matters any easier.

### Neurological and psychiatric complications

Gillberg & Schaumann (1989) and Gillberg & Steffenburg (1987) noted that possibly the majority of individuals with autistic disorders go through adolescence without special problems and some show positive improvements at this time. Kanner *et al.* (1972) followed up 96 children and found that 11 did quite well as adults. On the other hand, Gillberg (1984) and Gillberg & Steffenburg (1987) described the problems that can occur in adolescence. They calculated, from their own and other authors' findings, that a substantial minority experienced an exacerbation of behavioural problems or the onset of psychiatric or neurological abnormalities in adolescence or early adult life.

By the time of adult life, about one-third of people with typical autism will have had one or more epileptic seizures (Rutter 1970, Gillberg & Steffenburg 1987). Some have their first fits in adolescence. Some of these have a few fits only and then no more, while others continue to have seizures in adult life. This complication can occur at any level of cognitive ability (Gillberg *et al.* 1987) but is considerably more common in those who are severely mentally retarded (Rutter 1970).

Rutter (1970) and Gillberg & Steffenburg (1987) reported a setback in skills in a small group of adolescents with autism. Rutter (1970) found that a few of the adolescents in a follow-up study developed neurological signs together with progressive deterioration of skills.

After a period of relative improvement from around 6 to 12 years of age, there may be a return of the behaviour problems seen in early childhood including aggression, temper tantrums and destructiveness. The increased physical size and strength of an adolescent make it harder for the parents, who are themselves growing older, to control the behaviour.

Affective illnesses of varying degrees of severity, usually depressive in form, may appear in adolescence or adult life and are the most frequent of the psychiatric problems that can complicate autistic disorders. These are more easily recognizable in higher functioning individuals because they can express their feelings in speech (Wing 1981a). The affective disorder is often related to an increasing awareness of difference from others, difficulty in fitting into normal life, and failure to establish a satisfactory friendship or relationship with someone of the opposite sex. Anxiety in response to changes in routine and to pressure to perform beyond their level of ability is common in autistic people. Occasionally, frank anxiety states are seen in adolescents or adults. Among those in the mildly or severely mentally retarded subgroups, some show rapid and extreme mood swings which may be related to affective disorder.

The diagnosis of schizophrenia depends absolutely upon the reporting of symptoms by the individual concerned. It can, therefore, be identified only in those autistic people with sufficient speech. The impairment of social interaction and the literal interpretation and use of language has led to misdiagnosis of schizophrenia in higher functioning individuals (Wing 1981a, Gillberg & Schaumann 1989). As pointed out by Tantam (1988), there is little evidence for the occurrence of schizophrenia in people with autistic disorders, nor in their families (Kolvin *et al.* 1971).

Some autistic adolescents and adults react to stress by becoming disturbed and bizarre in behaviour as if their inner world, limited and patchy at the best of times, had shattered into fragments. Actions and speech utterances are incoherent and unpredictable. Some seem to have hallucinations and delusional beliefs. These states are often referred to as 'psychotic' but this term adds little to the understanding of their nature.

Obsessional disorder in autism presents an interesting diagnostic dilemma. Repetitive behaviour is characteristic of autistic disorders but, as discussed by Baron-Cohen (1989), resistance to the repetitive acts, crucial to the diagnosis of obsessional disorder, do not appear to the observer to be present in autism, and few if any autistic people can describe their inner feelings. The content of the repetitive acts in autistic children differs from that in obsessional conditions but, in adolescence, some autistic people develop hand-washing and touching compulsions in appearance like those in classic obsessional disorders. The question of the relationship between these disorders remains open.

The present author has observed six young adults (five men and one woman) who in childhood had Asperger's variant of autism and were of normal intelligence. In adolescence their repetitive activities changed to more typically obsessional rituals such as hand-washing and routines associated with dressing. They gradually became slower in completing everyday tasks, apparently because of the necessity to perform the rituals without the slightest error. The end state was precisely like that of classic catatonia. The only way they could function was if someone else physically prompted them through the day's routine. Yet, at times, they moved rapidly and unexpectedly, perhaps to dash out and away for no apparent reason. Fortunately, this clinical picture is very rare. However, fragments of catatonic behaviour, such as odd hand posture, freezing during movements, repeated unsuccessful attempts to complete an action and automatic, uncomprehending imitation, are fairly common in autistic people, especially in the more severely retarded subgroups and during adolescence. Catatonia is, of course, one of the possible consequences of encephalopathy (Sacks 1982). Its presence is not a diagnostic sign of schizophrenia (Magrinat *et al.* 1983) though the two conditions can coexist.

Clinical observation has shown that the psychiatric and behavioural complications of adolescence or early adult life do tend to improve over time in some but not all (Gillberg & Schaumann 1989). The removal of a source of stress can effect dramatic improvement in affective or 'psychotic' states. No detailed and reliable information is as yet available on the reasons for the occurrence of these problems, or which people are particularly vulnerable, or the eventual prognosis.

### Helping autistic adults

The wide range of abilities and handicaps that can be associated with autistic disorders makes it difficult to give useful advice regarding children and the problem is even greater with adults, but certain general principles apply to all levels of ability and all ages. The first of these is respect for each person as an individual with their own personality and needs. However, all autistic people function better if life is structured and follows a predictable pattern. New experiences are helpful to development and can be enjoyed but only if they are carefully planned and the autistic person understands and is well prepared for such events. Parents, carers and others in contact with autistic people need to grasp the nature of the underlying impairments. They are then better able to anticipate and avoid misunderstandings due to the limitations and literalness of language comprehension. It is easier to accept the lack of overt warmth and the poverty of empathy if the autistic handicap is clearly understood.

Autistic people, like everyone else, enjoy doing things they are good at and resent being made to do tasks that are beyond their capacity or that they find boring. The trouble is that the things they can do and like doing tend to cover a very narrow range. Parents and carers have to study each individual and organize appropriate occupations and leisure activities. Pressure to perform beyond level of ability is, as stressed in this chapter, a potent cause of behaviour problems and psychiatric complications. Adults, whether handicapped or not, are less compliant than children and resent being told what to do all the time. Sympathy and tact are essential qualities for success in helping.

Some autistic people have sufficient understanding and drive to desire an independent life. This can be worrying for parents but autistic people are characteristically determined once they have their minds set on a particular course, be it acquiring an empty detergent packet or learning to drive. The rule is never to meet this determination with head-on opposition but to attempt tactful and constructive guidance and be ready to help if and when things go wrong. The opposite problem is the apparently able autistic adult who expects to remain at home and be supported by his parents all his life. Little or nothing can be done to induce more constructive aims.

Since most autistic people known to the services do not have the ability to become independent, there is a great need for appropriate day and residential provision. Many require specialist placements such as the sheltered communities run by the national or local autistic societies. Others can fit into services for those with a variety of handicaps as long as the autism is recognized and the staff are trained to understand and provide for the special needs of autistic people. Lack of such understanding is one of the major causes of breakdowns in placement.

It is inevitable in a chapter of this kind that the problems are given more prominence than the positive aspects. It should be emphasized that, in the majority of people with autism, improvement does occur over the years and problems tend to lessen with advancing age. Some of the most able cope well in adult life while those with more disabilities give pleasure and enjoyment as well as worry and sadness to their families, friends or carers. Children and adults with autism suffer much distress as a result of their lack of understanding of the world but they also experience episodes of pleasure and happiness that are all the more intense because of the inability to anticipate the future. The problems have been described because they are the facets of autism that require practical action and further research for the resolution.

## Interaction of social, psychological and biological factors

The findings described in this chapter illustrate the complex interaction of social, psychological and biological factors in conditions in the autistic continuum. This interaction has affected prevalence and theories of aetiology as well as having major implications for care and service provision.

Before the present century, autistic conditions had not been conceptualized. The story of Victor, the wild boy of Aveyron (Itard 1801, 1807, translated by Lane 1977), showed that individuals with autism did exist, but it seems likely that the higher infant mortality produced by social conditions led to a lower prevalence of severe congenital disorders of all kinds. Interest in the subtleties of classification of such disorders had to await advances in standards of living and in medicine and psychology.

When, in the last century, institutions for people with mental retardation were built, most autistic children who survived infancy were probably classified simply as 'mentally defective' and, sooner or later, were placed in institutional care. Thus, social forces conspired to render them invisible to the general community.

Authors before Kanner described the autistic behaviour pattern (see Wing & Gould 1979) but Kanner named the condition and began the process of making it visible and deserving of attention. Social conditions again played a role in forming attitudes. When Kanner (1943, 1954) first wrote on autism, he noted that the great majority of the parents of the affected children he saw were of high social, educational and occupational class. He developed the hypothesis that autism was an emotional disorder due to the distant, formal child-rearing habits of the upper class, intellectual families. Some other authors reported similar findings, but, in recent years, epidemiological studies have found no social class bias (Wing 1980). The most likely explanation is that, in Kanner's time, it was only people who had the financial means and the determination to seek an explanation of their child's strange behaviour who found their way to specialists in childhood behavioural disorders. As society's attitudes to all kinds of handicapping conditions have become more positive and knowledge of autism has spread, it has become clear that autistic conditions are not class bound. This is one finding among many that have contributed to hypotheses of the biological origins of these conditions.

Most important of all is the interaction of social, psychological and biological factors in the provision of care and services. The psychological impairments, caused by biological abnormalities, cut autistic people off from ordinary social life. They do not learn through social interaction and they are not affected by the types of social experiences that influence the behaviour of non-autistic people. However, aspects of an autistic individual's social environment can make their problems much worse and, conversely, an ap-

propriate social setting can help to make their life easier. It has already been emphasized that people with autistic conditions need a programme that is low-key, without pressure but which provides a structured, organized routine and occupation, and leisure activities appropriate for their level of development. Changes have to be introduced with care so that they are acceptable and enjoyable and not a source of confusion and fear.

Understanding the impairments, disabilities and handicaps of the autistic conditions has special relevance to the organization of residential care. Uncritical acceptance of the idea of 'normalization' is associated with a tendency to deny the existence of biological disorders underlying psychological impairments. This can lead to an assumption that these impairments have been caused entirely by psychological or social factors, for example by life in an institution. The corollary of this assumption is that moving to a small house in the community will remove the problems. The opposite misunderstanding is that of a purely biological approach, which assumes that, because the impairment is due to a biochemical abnormality or a structural pathology, it is impervious to environmental influences. Both of these extreme points of view are mistaken. In practice, most people with autistic conditions need an environment that is carefully adapted to suit them. Most cannot cope with the flexibility and unpredictability of ordinary life. They are distressed when asked to make choices in the absence of visual cues because they lack the concepts involved in choosing. They benefit from small living units, personalized care, physical comfort, good food and access to those community facilities that they can enjoy. However, some find exposure to noise, bustle and crowds painful and frightening. They need space indoors and out to be alone, to be odd in, and to wander in safety. The more able can accept and even desire contact with people outside their own family or residential group but they too need a secure retreat where they can be alone when they so wish.

The conclusion is that a wide range of types of residential accommodation is required, varying from groups of small living units in their own substantial grounds to small houses in ordinary streets. The aim should be to provide the right place for each individual so that the biological, psychological and social interaction works for their benefit and not their detriment.

## References

Asperger H. (1944) Die autistischen psychopathen im kindesalter. *Archiv fur Psychiatrie und Nervenkrankheiten* 117, 76–136.

Asperger H. (1979) Problems of infantile autism. *Communication* 13, 45–52.

Baron-Cohen S. (1988) An assessment of violence in a young man with Asperger's syndrome. *Journal of Child Psychology & Psychiatry* 29, 351–360.

Baron-Cohen S. (1989) Do autistic children have obsessions and compulsions? *British Journal of Clinical Psychology* 28, 139–200.

Bartak L. & Rutter M. (1973) Special educational treatment of autistic children: a comparative study – 1. Design of study and characteristics of units. *Journal of Child Psychology & Psychiatry* 14, 161–179.

Coleman M. & Gillberg C. (1985) *The Biology of the Autistic Syndromes*. Praeger, New York.

DeMyer M., Barton S., Alpern G. *et al.* (1974) The measured intelligence of autistic children. *Journal of Autism & Childhood Schizophrenia* 4, 42–60.

DeMyer M.K., Barton S., DeMyer W.E., Norton J.A., Allen J. & Steele R. (1973) Prognosis in autism: a follow-up study. *Journal of Autism & Childhood Schizophrenia* 3, 199–246.

Favell J.E. (1983) The management of aggressive behaviour. In Schopler E. & Mesibov G.B. (eds) *Autism in Adolescents & Adults*, pp. 187–224. Plenum, New York.

Frith U. (1989) *Autism: Explaining the Enigma*. Blackwell, Oxford.

Frith U. (1991) *Autism and Asperger Syndrome*. Cambridge University Press, Cambridge.

Gillberg C. (1984) Autistic children growing up: problems during puberty and adolescence. *Developmental Medicine and Child Neurology* 26, 125–129.

Gillberg C. (1988) The neurobiology of infantile autism. *Journal of Child Psychology & Psychiatry* 29, 257–266.

Gillberg I.C. & Gillberg C. (1989) Asperger syndrome – some epidemiological considerations: a research note. *Journal of Child Psychology & Psychiatry* 30, 631–638.

Gillberg C., Persson E., Grufman M. & Themner U. (1986) Psychiatric disorders in mildly and severely mentally retarded urban children and adolescents: epidemiological aspects. *British Journal of Psychiatry* 149, 68–74.

Gillberg C. & Schaumann H. (1989) Autism: specific problems of adolescence. In Gillberg C. (ed.) *Diagnosis and Treatment of Autism*. Plenum, New York.

Gillberg C. & Steffenburg S. (1987) Outcome and prognostic factors in infantile autism and similar conditions: a population based study of 46 cases followed through puberty. *Journal of Autism and Developmental Disorders* 17, 273–287.

Gillberg C., Steffenburg S. & Jacobson G. (1987) Neurobiological findings in 20 relatively gifted children with Kanner-type autism or Asperger Syndrome. *Developmental Medicine & Child Neurology* 29, 641–649.

Gould J. (1977) The use of the Vineland Social Maturity scale, the Merrill–Palmer scale of Mental Tests (nonverbal items) and the Reynell Developmental Language scales with children in contact with the services for severe mental retardation. *Journal of Mental Deficiency Research* 21, 213–226.

Gould J. (1986) The Lowe and Costello Symbolic Play Test in socially impaired children. *Journal of Autism and Developmental Disorder* 16, 199–214.

Grandin T. & Scariano M.M. (1986) *Emergence – Labelled Autistic*. Costello, Tunbridge Wells.

Hill A.L. (1977) Idiot-savants rates of incidence. *Perceptual & Motor Skills* 44, 161–162.

Kanner L. (1943) Autistic disturbances of affective contact. *Nervous Child* 2, 217–250.

Kanner L. (1954) To what extent is early infantile autism determined by constitutional inadequacies? *Proceedings of the Association for Research in Nervous and Mental Diseases* 33, 378–385.

Kanner L. (1973) *Childhood Psychosis: Initial Studies and New Insights*. Winston/Wiley, New York.

Kanner L., Rodrigues A. & Ashenden B. (1972) How far can autistic children go in matters of social adaption? *Journal of Autism & Childhood Schizophrenia* 2, 9–33.

Kolvin I., Ounsted C., Richardson L. & Garside R.F. (1971) The family and social background in childhood psychoses. *British Journal of Psychiatry* 118, 396–402.

Lane H (1977) *The Wild Boy of Aveyron*. Allen & Unwin, London.

Lockyer L. & Rutter M. (1969) A five to fifteen-year follow-up study of infantile psychosis; III. Psychological aspects. *British Journal of Psychiatry* 115, 865–882.

Magrinat G., Danziger J.A., Lorenzo I.C., & Flemenbaum A. (1983) A reassessment of catatonia. *Comprehensive Psychiatry* 24, 218–228.

Mawson D., Grounds A. & Tantam D. (1985) Violence and Asperger's syndrome: a case study. *British Journal of Psychiatry* 147, 566–569.

Melone M.B. & Lettick A.L. (1983) Sex education at Benhaven. In Schopler E. & Mesibov G.M. (eds) *Autism in Adolescents and Adults*, pp. 135–149. John Wiley, New York.

O'Connor N. (1989) The performance of the 'idio-savant': implicit & explicit. *British Journal of Disorders of Communication* 24, 1–20.

O'Connor N. & Hermelin B. (1988) Low intelligence and special abilities. *Journal of Child Psychology and Psychiatry* 29, 391–396.

Rawlings S. (1985a) Life-styles of severely retarded non

communicating adults in hospitals and small residential homes. *British Journal of Social Work* 15, 281–293.

Rawlings S. (1985b) Behaviour and skills of severely retarded adults in hospitals and small residential homes. *British Journal of Psychiatry* 146, 358–366.

Rutter M. (1966) Prognosis. In Wing J.K. (ed.) *Early Childhood Autism*, 1st edn. Pergamon, Oxford.

Rutter M. (1970) Autistic children: infancy to adulthood. *Seminars in Psychiatry* 2, 435–450.

Rutter M. & Bartak L. (1973) Special educational treatment of autistic children: a comparative study – 2. Follow-up findings and implications for services. *Journal of Child Psychology & Psychiatry* 14, 241–270.

Sacks O. (1982) *Awakenings*, revised edn. Picador, London.

Sacks O. (1985) *The Man Who Mistook His Wife for a Hat*, pp. 185–223. Duckworth, London.

Schopler E. & Mesibov G.M. (eds) (1983) *Autism in Adolescents and Adults*. Plenum, New York.

Schopler E. & Mesibov G.B. (1987) *Neurobiological Issues in Autism*. Plenum, New York.

Selfe L. (1977) *Nadia: A Case of Extraordinary Drawing Ability in an Autistic Child*. Academic, London.

Shah A. (1988) Visuo-spatial Islets of Abilities and Intellectual Functioning in Autism. Unpublished PhD Thesis, London.

Shah A. & Frith U. (1983) An islet of ability in autistic children. *Journal of Child Psychology and Psychiatry* 24, 613–630.

Shah A., Holmes N. & Wing L. (1982) Prevalence of autism and related conditions in adults in a mental handicap hospital. *Applied Research in Mental Retardation* 3, 303–317.

Shah A. & Wing L. (1986) Cognitive impairment affecting social behaviour in autism. In Schopler E. & Mesibov G. (eds) *Social Behaviour in Autism*. Plenum, New York.

Tantam D. (1988) Asperger's syndrome. *Journal of Child Psychology & Psychiatry* 29, 245–256.

Treffert D. (1989) *Extraordinary People*. Bantam, London.

Waterhouse L., Wing L. & Fein D. (1989) Re-evaluating the syndrome of autism in the light of empirical research. In Dawson G. (ed.) *Autism: Perspectives on Diagnosis, Nature and Treatment*. Guilford Press, Hove.

Wiltshire S. (1987) *Drawings*. Dent, London.

Wiltshire S. (1989) *Cities*. Dent, London.

Wing L. (1980) Childhood autism and social class: a question of selection. *British Journal of Psychiatry* 137, 410–417.

Wing L. (1981a) Asperger's syndrome; a clinical account. *Psychological Medicine* 11, 115–129.

Wing L. (1981b) Sex ratios in early childhood autism and related conditions. *Psychiatry Research* 5, 129–137.

Wing L. (1983) Social and interpersonal needs. In Schopler E. & Mesibov G.B. (eds) *Autism in Adolescents and Adults*. Plenum, New York.

Wing L. (1988) The continuum of autistic characteristics. In Schopler E. & Mesibov G. (eds) *Diagnosis and Assessment in Autism*. Plenum, New York.

Wing L. (1989a) *Hospital Closure and the Resettlement of Residents: The Case of Darenth Park Hospital*. Avebury, Aldershot.

Wing L. (ed.) (1989b) *Aspects of Autism: Biological Research*. Gaskell, London.

Wing L. (1989c) Autistic adults. In Gillberg C. (ed.) *Diagnosis and Treatment of Autism*, pp. 419–432. Plenum, New York.

Wing L. & Gould J. (1979) Severe impairments of social interaction and associated abnormalities in children: epidemiology and classification. *Journal of Autism and Developmental Disorders* 9, 11–29.

# Chapter 27
# Disaster and Mental Health

RUTH WILLIAMS, STEPHEN JOSEPH
& WILLIAM YULE

## Introduction

In the second half of the 1980s, the UK witnessed a catalogue of civilian disasters – the fire at the Bradford football stadium in 1985; the capsize of the *Herald of Free Enterprise* ferry at Zeebrugge in 1987; the sinking of the cruise ship *Jupiter* with 400 British schoolchildren on board near Athens in 1988; the explosion on the Piper Alpha oil rig near Aberdeen in July 1988; the M1 air crash near Kegworth in 1989; the King's Cross underground fire in November 1988; the devastation of Lockerbie when the Pan Am jumbo jet was blown up above the town in December 1988; the sinking of the pleasure boat *Marchioness* in the Thames in August 1989; the mass shootings at Hungerford in Berkshire in August 1987. Less dramatic, but no less distressing for those involved, were the rail crashes at Glasgow, Clapham, Purley and Cannon Street. The sporadic political violence in Northern Ireland continued, with only spectacular atrocities such as the Enniskillen Remembrance Day bombing grabbing the headlines. Many smaller groups of individuals faced their own tragedies in accidents at work, in the home or on the roads. Many fell victim to individual acts of violence.

Whilst any individual mental health service may go for years without having to respond to the psychosocial sequelae of a major disaster, when such a disaster happens, services are all too often ill-prepared and overwhelmed. The catalogue above demonstrates that the numbers of people affected by disasters in a five-year period are enormous. This chapter will argue that survivors of such disasters are at greatly increased risk of developing serious psychopathology. In particular, their reactions can often usefully be conceptualized as post-traumatic stress disorders,

although other major psychiatric disorders such as depression, anxiety and phobias are also very common. Given this increase in morbidity following a disaster, mental health services need to plan their crisis intervention and long-term treatment to meet the needs.

This chapter will consider current views of post-traumatic stress disorders, and present three influential models that attempt to explain the phenomenology. Fortunately, not everyone exposed to a major trauma develops a psychiatric disorder. It is, therefore, important to examine individual differences, both in susceptibility and in reaction. Such information is important in screening survivors and planning for long-term needs. In particular, in keeping with the theme of this book, the chapter will concentrate on social psychological aspects of functioning relevant to responses to disasters. Thus, the role of social support will be considered along with the intervening roles of attribution and coping styles. Finally, the implications for planning services and for intervention are considered.

## Post-traumatic stress disorder

Historically, there has been much debate about the cause of mental illness following a traumatic event, and it is only comparatively recently that the role of disasters in the onset of psychiatric disorder has been recognized. The third edition of the diagnostic and statistical manual of the American Psychiatric Association (DSM-III, American Psychiatric Association 1980) described the syndrome, post-traumatic stress disorder (PTSD), which is thought to result from severe trauma. Since DSM-III, the American Psychiatric Association has introduced a revised set of diagnostic criteria for PTSD (DSM-III-R, American

Psychiatric Association 1987). The DSM-III-R definition of PTSD includes behavioural, cognitive, social and physiological responses following exposure to a recognizable stressor of sufficient magnitude to evoke stress in almost anyone. The criteria for PTSD as defined by DSM-III-R are shown in Table 27.1.

PTSD is unusual in that it is one of only three diagnostic categories whose symptoms are linked to a definite aetiology, in this case to psychological trauma. Events within the range of 'usual human experience', such as bereavement and illness, are not in themselves considered sufficient for the development of PTSD. Events producing the dis-

order include: deliberate man-made disasters such as war, bombing and torture; accidental man-made disasters such as aeroplane crashes and large fires; and natural disasters such as floods and earthquakes (e.g. Raphael 1986). The disorder is, however, thought to be more severe and long lasting when the stressor is of human design (American Psychiatric Association 1980). A delayed PTSD diagnosis may be made where the onset of the disorder occurs at least six months after the event, although whether immediate and delayed PTSD differ in anything other than the date of onset (or rather, the date of diagnosis) is still uncertain.

**Table 27.1** PTSD as defined by DSM-III-R

---

**A** An event that is outside the range of usual human experience and that is psychologically traumatic, e.g. serious threat to one's life or personal physical integrity; serious threat or harm to one's children, spouse, or other close relatives or friends; destruction of one's home or community, or seeing another person who is mutilated, dying or dead, or the victim of physical violence.

**B** The traumatic event is persistently re-experienced in at least one of the following ways:
  1 Recurrent and intrusive distressing recollections of the event without any awareness of environmental stimuli that trigger the reaction.
  2 Recurrent distressing dreams of the event.
  3 Sudden acting or feeling as if the traumatic event were recurring (includes a sense of reliving the experience, illusions, hallucinations, and dissociative (flashback) episodes, even those that occur upon awakening or when intoxicated) (in children, repetitive play in which themes or aspects of the trauma are expressed).
  4 Intense psychological distress or exposure to events that symbolize or resemble an aspect of the traumatic event, including anniversaries of the trauma.

**C** Persistent avoidance of stimuli associated with the trauma or numbing of responsiveness (not present before the trauma), as indicated by one of the following:
  1 Deliberate efforts to avoid thoughts of feelings associated with the trauma.
  2 Deliberate efforts to avoid activities or situations that arouse recollections of the trauma.
  3 Inability to recall an important aspect of the trauma (psychogenic amnesia).
  4 Markedly diminished interest in significant activities (in young children, loss of recently acquired developmental skills, such as toilet training or language skills).
  5 Feeling of detachment or estrangement from others.
  6 Restricted range of affect, e.g. 'numbing', unable to have loving feelings.
  7 Sense of a foreshortened future, e.g. child does not expect to have a career, marriage or children, or a long life.

**D** Persistent symptoms of increased arousal (not present before the trauma) as indicated by at least two of the following:
  1 Difficulty falling or staying asleep.
  2 Irritability or outburst.
  3 Difficulty concentrating.
  4 Hypervigilance.
  5 Physiological reactivity at exposure to events that symbolize or resemble an aspect of the traumatic event (e.g. a women who was raped in an elevator breaks out in a sweat when entering any elevator).

**E** 'B', 'C', and 'D' symptoms all were present during the same six-month period of at least one month, although there may be other phases of the illness during which they do not coexist.

---

The introduction of the concept of PTSD has been of great importance in providing a common language for those involved in the study of disaster and mental health. However, March (1990) notes that the diagnosis of PTSD is often accompanied by other psychiatric diagnoses.

PTSD is classified as an anxiety disorder and DSM-III-R recognizes depression and anxiety as associated features of PTSD. At present the relationship of PTSD to the other anxiety disorders is not clear. Both 'anxiety' and 'panic' reactions are reported in PTSD. Individuals may experience a variety of physical symptoms such as headache, dizziness, gastrointestinal distress, chest discomfort, nausea, tremulousness and palpitations. Behavioural concomitants may include restlessness, nocturnal dyspnoea, irritability, fatigue, insomnia and distractibility. Depression and anxiety have been reported following a large number of disasters: floods (Bennet 1970), explosions (L. Weisaeth 1984, unpublished paper), bushfires (McFarlane 1985), the collapse of man-made structures (Wilkinson 1983), and night club fires (Lundin 1984).

### Measurement of post-traumatic stress

This overlap with other, more generally recognized anxiety and affective disorders highlights the need for specificity in PTSD measurement. Although there is some empirical evidence for the diagnostic criteria of PTSD (American Psychiatric Association 1980, Silver & Iacono 1984), many of the signs and symptoms were included on the basis of clinical practice. In order to address the need for more precise quantification of the psychological phenomena associated with trauma, several measures have been specifically developed: notably, the Mississippi scale developed by Keane and colleagues (1988). This is a 35-item self-report scale derived from the DSM-III criteria. Principal component analysis of responses from 362 male Vietnam veterans identified six factors. These included: intrusive memories and depressive symptomatology; interpersonal adjustment problems; lability of affect and memory; and sleep problems. However, one must be cautious about interviews and instruments that merely assess

DSM-III-R signs since the syndrome itself is still not fully agreed.

The most widely used instrument for the assessment of post-traumatic stress, particularly in the UK, has been the Impact of Events Scale (IES; Horowitz *et al.* 1979). The IES is a 15-item self-report measure that taps intrusively experienced ideas, images, feelings and dreams, and the avoidance of ideas, feelings or situations. The scale was based on the statements of stressed individuals and evaluated in a sample of 66 individuals admitted to an outpatient clinic for the treatment of stress response syndromes. About half the subjects had experienced bereavement, the remainder had personal injuries resulting from road accidents, violence, illness or surgery. These events are somewhat heterogeneous, and not necessarily traumatic. Although a strong relation between a DSM-III PTSD inventory and the IES has been demonstrated with Israeli combat veterans (Weisenberg *et al.* 1987), the question remains as to its relationship with the DSM-III-R criteria, and also whether it is appropriate for use with other traumatized populations. Preliminary use of the IES with survivors of the *Herald of Free Enterprise* disaster showed a similar pattern of endorsement of items as previously reported by Zilberg *et al.* (1982) and Schwarzwald *et al.* (1987). Factor analysis of the scale yielded two general factors of intrusion and avoidance, but also two further factors characterized specifically by sleep disturbance/dreams, and emotional numbing/denial (Joseph *et al.* 1992c).

### Social functioning

Clinical experience with survivors of the *Herald of Free Enterprise* has suggested to us that disaster often provokes a range of problems in social functioning. Many have experienced difficulties in their family and working lives. Problems tend to be a result of the person's emotional response to the disaster: increased irritability leading to interpersonal friction; concentration difficulties leading to problems at work.

Substance-abuse problems have been particularly reported in studies of combat veterans. For example, Keane *et al.* (1983) in a study of 40

Vietnam veterans with PTSD found that 63% reported heavy and often abusive alcohol consumption. Roth (1986) in a study of 268 Vietnam veterans found that almost half of the combat veterans with stress disorders were heavy drinkers and that over half used drugs other than alcohol. An increase in cigarette smoking and alcohol abuse, as well as other types of risk taking, has also been noted following a number of civilian disasters (Sims *et al.* 1979, Shepherd & Hodgkinson, 1990).

A major problem stems from the widely divergent estimates of impairment found within and between traumatized populations. Estimates of impairment in the first year reported by Raphael (1986) range from around 20% in survivors of Cyclone Tracy (Parker 1977) to around 50% in survivors of the Xenia Tornado (Taylor *et al.* 1976). Similarly, estimates of impairment 2–5 years later range from around 20% in survivors of a factory explosion (L. Weisaeth 1984, unpublished paper) to around 80% in survivors of a marine explosion (Leopold & Dillon 1963). The reason for these discrepancies, March (1990) suggests, is that they reflect real differences in the populations studied. Another problem is the comparison of prevalence rates when different instruments for assessing symptomatology have been employed. This stresses the need for a common methodology.

## Models of explanation

Although mental health professionals have long recognized a variety of traumatic stress reactions – from the 'railway spine' of the nineteenth century and the battle neuroses of the two World Wars – it was not until veterans of the Vietnam War began presenting with significant problems many years after the end of the conflict that a shift in understanding occurred. In the following section, we highlight different models that address the major symptoms presenting after a major trauma.

### Horowitz: a psychodynamic model of PTSD

Horowitz (1979, 1982, 1986) argues that individuals hold models of the world and themselves

which help to interpret incoming information and guide action. The experience of trauma presents information that is not compatible with the existing schemata, and it is this incongruity that gives rise to a stress response. Adaptation, then, involves revision of the schemata.

The intrusion and avoidance symptoms observed during stress responses occur as a result of opposite actions of a control system that regulates the incoming information to tolerable doses. This acts as an inhibition–facilitation feedback system modulating the flow of information required for revision of the schemata. If inhibitory control is not strong enough, intrusive symptoms such as nightmares and flashbacks emerge. When inhibitory efforts are too strong in relation to active memory, symptoms indicative of the avoidance phase occur.

Typically, avoidance and intrusion symptoms fluctuate in a way particular to the individual without causing either flooding or exhaustion. The person, then, oscillates between the states of avoidance and intrusion until a relative baseline is reached when the person is said to have worked through the experience. The numbing symptoms are thus viewed as a defence mechanism against intrusion. Horowitz suggests that the personal salience of traumatic events causes them to be held in active memory. The images and thoughts held in active memory break through into consciousness unless actively inhibited. Horowitz, then, presents phases of response to stressful events, which are shown in Table 27.2 (see Horowitz 1989).

Jones & Barlow (1990) note that although Horowitz's model accommodates the signs and symptoms characteristic of PTSD, it is limited in that it fails explicitly to incorporate perceptions of control and coping.

### Janoff-Bulman: the assumptive world

The work of Janoff-Bulman (1985) is of interest in that it focuses more specifically on the cognitive schemata that individuals hold, and thus complements the work of Horowitz. Janoff-Bulman (1985) suggests that there are common psychological experiences shared by victims who have

**Table 27.2** Phases of response

| Phases | Common states during each phase of response |
|---|---|
| EVENT OUTCRY | States are high in arousal, emotion and action |
| DENIAL | States are lower in arousal and emotion as some memories or ideational implications of the stressor event are avoided |
| INTRUSION | Intrusive ideas and images occur with pangs of intense feeling |
| WORKING THROUGH | Oscillation occurs between states like those during phases of denial and intrusion, with gradual reduction in the degree of avoidance and sense of involuntary recollection |
| COMPLETION | The person returns to states like those experienced before the stress-inducing events |

experienced a wide range of traumatic situations. It is proposed that post-traumatic stress following victimization is largely due to the shattering of basic assumptions victims hold about themselves and the world. Traumatic experience is not easily assimilated into this framework, and may shatter these assumptions, producing psychological upheaval. The number and extent of assumptions that are shattered are dependent upon the individual, but central is the belief in the individual's own personal invulnerability.

Victimization shatters our assumption of invulnerability, that bad things only happen to others, leaving a sense of helplessness against overpowering forces, and an apprehension that anything may now happen. The sense of vulnerability may manifest itself as a preoccupation with, and fear of, recurrence. The sense of vulnerability appears to be tied, Janoff-Bulman believes, to the disruption of certain core ties about the self and the world; in particular, the world as benevolent, the world as meaningful, and the self as worthy. Adjustment to disaster involves rebuilding these shattered assumptions.

## Rachman: emotional processing

Rachman's (1980) theory of emotional processing provides a useful cognitive–emotional framework for conceptualizing responses to disaster. Emotional processing is regarded as a process whereby emotional disturbances are absorbed, and decline to the extent that other experiences can proceed without disruption.

If an emotional disturbance is not absorbed satisfactorily there is a persistence or return of intrusive signs of emotional activity. Rachman describes several direct signs of incomplete processing, many of which are diagnostic criteria for PTSD. For example, obsessions, nightmares, phobias and inappropriate expressions of emotion. Indirect signs, he suggests, are an inability to concentrate, excessive restlessness and irritability. Successful processing, Rachman believes, can be gauged from the person's ability to talk about, see, listen to or be reminded of the emotional events without experiencing distress or disruptions. Thus, Rachman identifies an internal process (emotional processing), failure of which results in symptoms akin to PTSD. Moreover, disappearance of these symptoms can be seen as an indicator of the effectiveness of treatment.

Rachman identifies factors that impede emotional processing along with factors that promote it. These carry important implications for intervention. For instance, brief presentations of distressing experiences, such as may occur when retelling the event, are likely to increase distress; whereas, paradoxically, lengthy presentations that give rise to distress but permit habituation of anxiety will be more beneficial.

A parallel analysis of factors in the stressor as well as in the stressed individual likewise carry important implications for the managers of a disaster. When the disaster is sudden, unexpected, intense, gives rise to many deaths, touches on prepared fears (such as of the dark or of drowning), then one can expect a greater proportion of victims to present with psychological distress. Thus, in retrospect, when the *Herald of Free Enterprise* unexpectedly capsized in 45 seconds, tipping people into the rising, cold sea, in the dark and where half those on board perished, one should have predicted a very high rate of disorder among survivors, as indeed has been found (Williams & Yule 1988, Hodgkinson & Stewart 1991). Taking Rachman's (1980) and Weisaeth's (1983) ideas on exposure parameters and stimulus factors together should permit managers of disasters to predict more accurately the potential extent of mental health services required. In the early phase of responding to disasters, managers will not be interested in the premorbid personalities of the survivors, but these factors will be important later in planning individual therapies.

## Explaining individual differences in distress

A major question remains as to why some individuals will experience greater distress than others following a disaster. Rachman's theory provides a useful conceptual umbrella under which to consider the personal and social resources which may moderate response. As Gibbs (1989) notes, the wide range of disorders observed following disaster also indicates the importance of studying characteristics of the individual in understanding the emotional impact of disasters. In this section, we will consider factors relating to the disaster itself, factors in the individual and social factors.

### *Factors related to the disaster itself*

#### INTENSITY OF IMPACT

Rachman (1980) focuses on stimulus characteristics that lead to difficulty in subsequent emotional processing. In other studies, greater mental disturbance has been shown to be related to: bereavement (Gleser *et al.* 1981, Singh & Raphael 1981, Bolin 1982, Green *et al.* 1983, Lundin 1984); the threat of death (Parker 1977, Western & Milne 1979, Gleser *et al.* 1981, Bolin, 1982, Green *et al.* 1983, Weisaeth 1983, Lundin 1984), and injury (Western & Milne 1979, Green *et al.* 1983, Lundin 1984, McFarlane 1985).

In his study of the aftermath of a paint factory fire, Weisaeth (1983) demonstrated an exposure–response relationship. Those workers nearest the centre of the explosion suffered most post-traumatic distress; those furthest from it suffered the least. Similarly, Pynoos & Nader (1988) dem-

onstrated that following a fatal sniper shooting of children in a Californian school, children trapped in the playground had the strongest post-traumatic reactions, with those not attending school that day showing the least. Of course, even in this gradient there were individual differences with one little boy who had left school early but who had left his sister in the playground showing a severe reaction. Yule and colleagues (1990b) found that within one school that had sent a party of children on the *Jupiter* cruise, children who had wanted to go on the cruise but failed to get a place showed scores on depression and anxiety that were intermediate between controls and the victims. Thus, there is evidence that in some circumstances, the intensity of the disaster is related to the level of subsequent distress, but also there is evidence that both the objective and subjective aspects must be considered.

### *Factors in the individual: personality factors*

#### EXPLANATORY STYLE

The notion of control has been much discussed in relation to disaster response. Most work has been concerned with generalized expectancies, such as explanatory style (Peterson *et al.* 1982) and locus of control (Rotter 1966).

The Attributional Style Questionnaire (ASQ) was developed as a measure of the personality style characteristic of depression (Peterson *et al.* 1982). Based on the logic of the reformulated model of learned helplessness (Abramson *et al.* 1978) (see p. 458), Peterson *et al.* (1982) believe that, to the extent that individuals show characteristic attributional tendencies, it is appropriate to speak of an attributional style. The ASQ presents the subject with 12 different hypothetical events, half are good events and half are bad events. For each hypothetical event the subject is asked to write down what they feel would be the major cause of that event if it happened to them, and then to rate that cause along the three attributional dimensions of internality, stability and globality. Depression has been shown to be associated with a style characterized by more internal, stable and global attributions for negative outcomes, and more external, unstable and specific attributions for positive outcomes.

There is some evidence that this relationship extends to PTSD. McCormick *et al.* (1989) found measures of PTSD to be significantly related to measures of explanatory style in male veterans with alcohol dependence or pathological gambling problems. Patients with symptoms of PTSD tended to explain the causes for hypothetical negative events in ways that were more internal, global and stable than patients without PTSD, and to explain the causes for hypothetical positive events in a manner that was less internal, stable and global than patients without PTSD.

As regards locus of control (Rotter 1966), there is much evidence that external locus of control subjects show higher levels of depression than those with internal locus of control (Benassi *et al.* 1988). There is some evidence that this relationship between higher externality and greater depression may extend to PTSD.

Frye & Stockton (1982) administered a modified form of Rotters I-E (Internal-External) scale to Vietnam veterans. They found locus of control accounted for over 10% of the variance in PTSD symptoms, and that PTSD subjects had more external locus of control as well as experiencing higher levels of combat. They suggested that men with an external locus of control were more susceptible to the unpredictable and uncontrollable nature of their war experiences. However, while this may reflect a consequence of combat rather than an antecedent, it suggests that locus of control may be important in the way veterans perceived and coped with negative events after their return to civilian life, which in turn may exacerbate PTSD symptoms. Solkoff *et al.* (1986) also report Vietnam veterans suffering from PTSD to have a more external locus of control. Similarly, Solomon *et al.* (1988a) found external locus of control to be associated with PTSD in Israeli combat veterans. With regard to civilian trauma, Gibbs (1986) reported more external locus of control in victims of toxic exposure compared to control group levels. This suggests that the experience of trauma may also impact on a person's locus of control.

One of the criticisms of the locus of control research is that the measures do not always take into regard whether the outcomes are positive or negative. Brewin & Shapiro (1984) established that the Rotter scale was measuring control over positive outcomes, and that locus of control for positive outcomes should be considered distinct from locus of control for negative outcomes. Further, they note the conceptual similarity between locus of control for positive outcomes and the notion of self-efficacy. In accord with this, Murphy (1988) reported that high self-efficacy was associated with better health outcomes at one and three years following disaster.

The findings regarding locus of control are consistent, then, with the predictions of the reformulated model of learned helplessness. Our own work has employed the Brewin & Shapiro (1984) locus of control measure with adult survivors of the *Jupiter* cruise ship disaster. Findings suggest that internal locus of control for negative outcomes is related to lower self-esteem, greater self-depreciation, greater withdrawal from other people, and more emotional numbing. Internal locus of control for positive outcomes was related to less withdrawal from others, greater confiding in others, more emotional social support from the person's social network, and more satisfaction with the social support received from others (Joseph *et al.* 1992a).

COPING STYLES

Individual differences in the ways in which people cope with stressful events are thought to be important in the development and maintenance of a variety of emotional disorders. Folkman & Lazarus (1985) distinguish between problem-focused and emotional-focused coping. The former refers to acts taken to remove or mitigate the source of stress, the latter to attempts to reduce the psychological distress. Although most stressors elicit both types of coping, generally problem-focused strategies tend to predominate when something constructive can actually be done, whereas emotional-focused strategies tend to predominate when the stressor is something that must be endured.

Problem-focused     strategies     include     active

coping, that is, the process of taking active steps to try and remove a stressor, or to ameliorate its effects. Active coping involves initiating direct action, increasing one's efforts, and trying to execute a coping attempt in a stepwise fashion. There is some empirical support for the value of active coping. Gleser *et al.* (1981) reported that the best predictor of psychopathology after the Buffalo Creek flood was being able to clean and repair one's home, and give help to others.

Green and colleagues (1985) in their study of the Beverly Hills Supper Club fire grouped coping responses into one of three categories. These were denial (e.g. using drugs or turning to work), philosophical/intellectual (e.g. turning to religion) and interpersonal (e.g. talking to others). Although coping added little to the prediction of outcome, they did note a trend for people using philosophical/intellectual strategies to have lower pathology scores, and those using denial and interpersonal strategies to have higher pathology scores. Similarly, Genest *et al.* (1990) found escape and avoidant strategies to be related to higher levels of anxiety, while facing the situation was related to lower anxiety. Suls & Fletcher (1985) in a review of the health psychology literature, concluded that non-avoidant coping strategies are more adaptive than avoidant coping strategies. Solomon and colleagues (1988b) found that greater reliance on emotion-focused and distancing tactics was associated with more severe PTSD. These workers suggest that individuals who rely on emotion-focused and distancing strategies may view their distress as uncontrollable. Consequently, the use of problem-focused coping tactics is futile. Alternatively, the life events experienced by those with more severe PTSD actually are more uncontrollable and therefore less amenable to problem-focused strategies. However, it would seem that when action can be taken it is beneficial to mental health.

There is evidence that particular emotion-focused strategies are adaptive following a crisis. A study by Affleck *et al.* (1987) found that men who perceived benefits from a heart attack were less likely to have a subsequent attack, and exhibited less morbidity eight years later. Research by Pennebaker *et al.* (1987) concludes that not disclosing traumatic events is associated with increased physical health problems. Pennebaker *et al.* (1987) examined the autonomic correlates of confiding traumatic events. According to the inhibition–disease framework (Pennebaker 1985, Pennebaker & Beall 1986), the act of inhibiting or otherwise restraining ongoing behaviour, thoughts and feelings requires physiological work. There is much support for this. Derogatis *et al.* (1979) found that women who lived the longest after diagnosis of breast cancer were those who were most openly angry and depressed. Pennebaker & Beall (1986) demonstrated that written disclosure of traumatic experiences may ultimately reduce physician visits and improve health perceptions. For long-term benefits to accrue, it appears to be important for the person to disclose not only the event but also the emotions aroused by the event. Pennebaker *et al.* (1987) conclude that not disclosing traumatic events – which can be viewed as a form of inhibition – is associated with increased physical health problems. In contrast, in a study of psychiatric nurses' responses to violence from patients, Wykes & Whittington (1991) report that those nurses who did not talk about their feelings fared better in the short term, although most gave up their posts within a year, irrespective of their initial method of coping.

## PREVIOUS PSYCHOPATHOLOGY

DSM-III-R also recognizes that previous psychological disturbance may make for vulnerability to emotional dysfunction following disaster. This is difficult to determine because of the problems in obtaining predisaster measures. However, there is some evidence suggesting that self-reported prior disturbance is associated with increased impairment following some kinds of trauma such as rape (Frank *et al.* 1981, Atkeson *et al.* 1982) or exposure to a toxic chemical explosion (Markowitz & Gutterman 1986). The problem with retrospective enquiries is that present symptomatology levels may influence the perception of one's prior functioning.

McFarlane (1988) investigated the longitudinal course of post-traumatic morbidity in a sample of trained volunteer firefighters who had an intense exposure to the Australian bushfires that destroyed large areas of South Australia in 1983. The aim of his study was to compare and contrast the role of the disaster and premorbid factors in the aetiology of PTSD. His data suggested that different patterns of post-traumatic morbidity may be partially predicted by the combination of four variables: first, adversity before the event; secondly, neuroticism; thirdly, a history of treated past psychological disorder; and fourthly, the tendency to avoid thinking through unwanted or negative experiences. McFarlane found no significant differences in the experience of the disaster as measured by losses, injury, exposure and perceived threat. McFarlane believes these findings keep alive the longstanding debate about the relative importance of event and premorbid factors in the development and maintenance of PTSD, and that it raises questions about the categorization of PTSD as a separate diagnostic entity in which the event plays the central aetiological role. However, he does acknowledge that the data may have been contaminated by current symptoms. Further, other factors apart from past psychopathology are likely to determine whether a person has psychotherapy. In addition, people may be reluctant to admit to past psychological problems and, unless the sample is very large, few victims will have had prior treatment. Methodologically, it is difficult to tease out the relative contribution of premorbid factors from the effects of exposure within a single disaster, as reduced variance on key variables may distort the relationships. Thus, in the Australian bush fires, nearly all the firefighters were exposed to similar degrees of risk.

McFarlane suggests that a complex interaction may exist between the onset of PTSD and the level of exposure to danger. A relatively low threshold of exposure may be required to precipitate PTSD, but once over this threshold an increased level of exposure may lead to a more rapid development of PTSD. In accord with this, Foy and colleagues (1987) reported that a positive family history of psychiatric disorders, particularly alcoholism, plays a role in the development of PTSD in low combat exposure conditions. However, family history is less important for high combat exposure conditions.

## STRESSFUL LIFE EVENTS

There is much evidence that stressful events are associated with the onset of psychiatric symptomatology (e.g. Brown & Harris 1978; also see Chapter 10). Stressful events following disaster may serve to exacerbate symptoms. Little research has been conducted on this, and so the question remains as to whether such life events would act to exacerbate PTSD symptoms or only those related disturbances such as depression. McFarlane (1988) in his study of survivors of an Australian bushfire found that individuals with PTSD had more adverse life events both before and after the trauma.

## CAUSAL ATTRIBUTION

It has been suggested that what is important is the person's own appraisal of the stressful experience (Lazarus 1966). One way of addressing this is through the study of causal attributions. According to attribution theory people have a need to explain the events that occur in their world, particularly when anything unusual, unwanted or unexpected happens (Weiner 1985).

Abramson *et al.* (1978) put forward the reformulated model of learned helplessness where effects depend on the attribution of causality made to the outcome. According to the logic of the reformulated model, it is predicted that an individual who attributes the cause of the negative event to internal factors (as opposed to external), to stable factors (as opposed to unstable) and to global factors (as opposed to specific), will show depression. The reformulated model, then, states that the occurrence of uncontrollable negative events leads to depression via the expectancy that future outcomes are independent of one's response. Expectancies about future outcomes are influenced by the perceived stability and globality of the cause, such that more stable causes will tend to lead to more long-lasting depression, and more global causes to more generalized depressive deficits. Internal attributions are held to lead to the specific deficit of low self-esteem. In addition, the intensity of the depressive deficit is thought to depend on the strength or certainty of the expectation of uncontrollability (Peterson & Seligman

1984). There is much evidence that such attributional dimensions are related to depression (Sweeney *et al.* 1986). McCormick *et al.* (1989) notes that there is considerable conceptual overlap between PTSD and learned helplessness theory. Brewin (1985), however, suggests that important event-related cognitions may often be moral and self-evaluative rather than causal.

Much of our work has focused on this issue. Joseph and colleagues (1991) examined the relationship between causal attributions and psychiatric symptomatology. Written statements about their experiences during disaster were provided by survivors of the *Herald of Free Enterprise* disaster. Causal attributions were extracted and rated using the Leeds Attributional Coding System (Stratton *et al.* 1986). It was found that more internal and controllable attributions for negative events during the disaster were related to higher anxiety, greater depression, and more intrusion of thoughts and feelings one and two years following the capsize.

The explanation for this may lie in Weiner's (1986) cognitive theory of emotions which suggests that internal and controllable attributions for negative events are related to the emotion of guilt. Guilt is commonly reported following disaster (Raphael 1986) and is also a feature of depression (Beck 1967, DSM-III – American Psychiatric Association 1980). Further, the results are consistent with the prediction of Foa *et al.* (1989) that symptoms of PTSD would be enhanced by the perception of unexercised control. These findings have subsequently been extended to child victims (Joseph *et al.* 1992b) of the *Jupiter* cruise ship disaster.

### Factors in the social environment

SOCIAL SUPPORT

It has generally been accepted that social support is associated with psychological functioning (Cohen & Wills 1985). Disasters in themselves are often associated with a reduction in social support. This was the case, for example, in the 1972 dam collapse at Buffalo Creek. Erikson (1976) and Lifton & Olson (1976) described the social consequences of this technological disaster.

Much of the community was destroyed, and individuals often found themselves to be the lone survivors of a family.

Good social support has been shown to be associated with less post-disaster morbidity (Solomon 1986). Green and colleagues (1985) in their study of reponse to the Beverly Hills Supper Club fire reported that the availability and use of naturally occurring social supports was generally associated with lower levels of psychopathology. The role of support was, however, quite modest. Support was measured by asking subjects whether they felt supported and had someone to talk to, and by rating the sources of support (e.g. family, friends) as used or not used, and whether they had been helpful or harmful. Fleming *et al.* (1982) in their study of the Three Mile Island accident in 1979 reported a mediating influence of support on depression and anxiety. However, Murphy (1988) in her study did not find social support to be a predictor of health outcome one and three years following disaster.

Social support for Vietnam veterans with PTSD has been analysed by Keane and colleagues (1985). They studied retrospective reports of social support over the following dimensions: social network, material support, physical support, and sharing, advice, and positive social interactions. Prior to Vietnam, comparable levels of support across all dimensions were found for those with and without PTSD. After Vietnam, combat veterans with PTSD reported that qualitative and quantitative measures of support had systematically declined over time to extremely low levels. Solkoff *et al.* (1986) also report that PTSD subjects had fewer contacts with other veterans, and felt that they received little support from their families or spouses.

It has been suggested that the way in which social support works is by enhancing perceptions of control over the environment. Schulz & Decker (1982) speculate that social support reduces helplessness by fostering internal attributions, providing assurances of environmental stability, directing attention to positive features of a situation, and providing accurate information for problem solving.

Recent work by Solomon *et al.* (1988a) examined the relationship between coping, locus of control, social support and combat-related PTSD. Their sample consisted of 262 Israeli soldiers who suffered a combat stress reaction (CSR) episode during the 1982 Lebanon war. In contrast to much previous work that has set out to examine the impact of personal and social resources on the development of PTSD among CSR casualties, Solomon *et al.* (1988a) employed a longitudinal design, focusing on two points in time: two years and three years following combat. They examined, first, the relation between personal resources and social resources and PTSD at each point in time, and, secondly, the relation between changes in the course of PTSD and changes in both personal and social resources. Measures consisted of several self-report instruments: the PTSD inventory (Solomon *et al.* 1987), a shortened version of Rotter's locus of control scale (Rotter 1966), a shortened version of the ways of coping checklist (Folkman & Lazarus 1980), and a social support questionnaire devised on the basis of Mueller's (1980) social network interview. As expected, the intensity of PTSD declined between the two points of time, reflecting a process of recovery. In addition, locus of control became more internal, there was less emotion-focused coping, and more perceived social support. As hypothesized, associations were found at each point in time between PTSD intensity and personal and social resources. Both in the second and third years after the war, more intense PTSD was associated with external locus of control, emotion-focused coping style, and insufficient social support. With regard to locus of control, although correlated at both times with PTSD, the removal of the contributions of coping strategies and social support to PTSD variance cancelled out the significance of locus of control. It is suggested that this is consistent with the idea that internal locus of control is associated with the use of more task-relevant problem-focused coping strategies, and less task-irrelevant emotionally focused strategies. The findings are thus thought to point to coping strategies as mediating between locus of control and PTSD.

The study of Solomon *et al.* (1988a) is limited by several methodological problems in common with much of the disaster literature. First, since the subjects had PTSD prior to the start of the study, the findings cannot provide definitive evidence as to the direction of causality between resources and PTSD. Once established one would expect a mutually reinforcing relation between resources and PTSD. Secondly, the conceptualization of emotion-focused coping can actually be viewed as an expression of PTSD rather than as a contributing factor. Thirdly, assessments of personal and social resources are retrospective, and thus may be influenced by current psychological state.

The role of these factors in the development of PTSD has a number of implications for therapeutic intervention following disaster. For example, the relevance of attribution theory to clinical practice has been much discussed (Antaki & Brewin 1982, Brewin 1988). There may be considerable scope for identifying vulnerable individuals and for improving distress following disaster by altering people's perceptions of the causes of significant events that took place during the disaster. Attribution therapy may be beneficial in helping an individual to come to terms with guilty feelings, and thus more able to make use of available support networks (Joseph *et al.* 1991).

## Services and intervention

### Planning

The experience of a distressing number of public transportation and other kinds of disasters in the UK during the late 1980s has led to an acute awareness of the importance of planning services prior to a disaster. In the absence of such planning, problems arising from failures in communication and coordination, and competition between rival services has been seen. To facilitate an effective and efficient response to an unpredicted traumatic event, working relationships should be established well before any incident between the relevant organizations which include the emergency services and police, social services, health authorities, education authorities, voluntary agencies and religious bodies. In the UK, it has been recommended (Draft Report of the Disasters Working Party, Department of Health 1990) that local authority departments of social services should take the lead role in coordinating a response, although the determination of responsibility for the financial implications of this recommendation has not been squarely addressed and currently awaits a political decision. Some agencies have argued for a Central Disaster Fund to which local authorities could make application, perhaps along the lines of the US federal arrangements after a major disaster area is declared centrally.

In addition to the existing plans for rescue, under the responsibility of the police, protocols need to be established with the police for the provision of psychosocial care in the immediate aftermath. Training in the planning phase should include use of communication systems by administrators and for all individuals, across discipline, in the psychological effects of trauma. All workers should be prepared for the effects of massive stress on themselves in dealing with disasters. In addition, some have argued for a National Disaster Squad of expert professionals who could be held in readiness to respond immediately and to consult and supervise a response to a disaster in any particular locality.

The role of such a national squad needs very careful consideration. It would be impossible as well as undesirable for a small specialized team to take responsibility for treating all those affected by a disaster. Far better, local services should be facilitated in responding to local disasters. They would need advice on particular aspects, but they will already have many relevant skills in dealing with anxiety, depression and bereavement. The function of a specialist unit should not be inadvertently to deskill local staff. Rather, they should have an important role in disseminating information, in training, and in mounting high quality research. In Norway, armed forces mental health professionals are used to attend disasters in time of peace thereby using resources efficiently in tasks that may be relevant in times of conflict. It may well be worth other countries considering the virtues of this model of service delivery.

The following is a necessarily brief outline of services for psychosocial care, highlighting key areas. The main aims of such services are: first, the prevention of long-term disorder; secondly, the identification of vulnerable individuals; and

thirdly, the provision of specialized intervention services for individuals with more severe and chronic problems. It must be stressed that although there is a considerable amount of expertise developing and many theoretical notions about how to achieve these aims, the concrete evidence about the effectiveness of services, particularly for civilian disasters, is still very sparse.

## Immediate-impact phase

### SURVIVORS

The immediate necessity for the rescue of survivors may obscure the practical needs of individuals who may have lost all their possessions and lost contact with companions and be ignorant of the exact nature of what has happened, including loss of lives. Assigned helpers could be useful in providing information, solving practical problems, and establishing contact between those separated in the disaster. Brom & Kleber (1989), in describing a programme of preventive work, point out that the importance of practical help in the early stages is often underestimated. Individuals who are in shock may need quiet to rest and protection from the most intrusive agents of the media. When ready, survivors may benefit from talking through their experiences either individually or in groups and giving expression to the strong feelings that these generate. There is some evidence that talking through at a relatively early stage can protect individuals from a more severe later reaction, although such an intervention needs to be held off until the immediate phase of shock has passed (Hodgkinson & Stewart 1991).

### RELATIVES AND FRIENDS

To minimize the agonizing uncertainty that relatives and friends may experience as to the fate of their loved ones caught up in the disaster, adequate telephone lines for information and the support of relatives need to be established and publicized. The needs of relatives at this time emphasize the central importance of accurate, up-to-date information being available as the details of what happened and to whom become clearer over time. Staff answering information and help lines should be trained to expect to deal with high levels of anxiety and anger in stressed callers.

Space should be assigned, with relevant services, for relatives who wish to visit the site of the disaster. Helpers assigned to individual families can give support, information, and help to solve the practical problems families may have. In the case of death, a family member will be required by the police to provide identification. Distressed and worried relatives may be further stressed when asked to give the name of the missing person's dentist so that dental records may be compared. Assigned workers can assist in explaining procedures such as this, conveying information about the condition of bodies or the likelihood and time of their recovery.

Bereaved individuals may wish to view the body. It has been suggested that this can be helpful in the process of accepting the reality of a sudden, unexpected death, and in finding out how the person died, even if the body is disfigured or deterioration has occurred (Hodgkinson & Stewart 1988). Alternatively, recovered bodies are photographed as part of the procedure for the coroner's court. Relatives have the right of access to all documents and should, therefore, have access to photographs at a later stage if they so wish. Relatives are often unclear of the purposes of an inquest and will be unfamiliar with the procedures of a coroner's court. The hearing may take place many months after the disaster, and this is, sadly, often the first time the bereaved relatives have an opportunity of finding out exactly how their loved one died. It is becoming increasingly obvious that at recent large-scale disasters, the needs of relatives have not been well considered and this is another time when mental health professionals may get involved to mitigate further unnecessary distress.

## INFORMATION SYSTEMS

By their nature, disasters happen unexpectedly. There is bound to be some chaos initially, but recent experience has pointed to the singular importance of good information systems being set up as quickly as possible. Disaster plans should incorporate these. To avoid endlessly overlapping questioning by staff from different departments and the loss of vital information, standard forms should be drawn up beforehand which can then be adapted to collect information. Thought needs to be given to the storage of the information in an accessible, central system. Agreements on the access to this database and considerations on how best to protect survivors' confidentiality, should be sorted out at the planning stage. Likewise, thought should be given to the ways of accessing the database for later research and evaluative purposes.

## SUPPORT STAFF

Attention has been drawn to the importance of selecting staff who are able and willing to cope with the nature of disaster work and the stress involved. Volunteers, including volunteer professionals, should be given clear information about the work being highly stressful and arrangements made to help individuals deal with stress by, for example, being trained to deal with distressed relatives, being exposed to bodies, or being trained to break difficult news.

Many studies attest to the stressful effects of disaster work upon rescue workers and helpers (Lifton 1967, Taylor & Frazer 1982, Duckworth 1986). This may apply not only to immediate rescue workers but also to mental health workers who hear about things second hand at a later date. Some workers may demonstrate many of the symptoms of the survivors themselves and resort to strategies like increasing cigarette and alcohol consumption to cope. Dealing with a disaster can itself traumatize rescuers directly, not only by helpers identifying with the distress of the victims. Some professional groups develop a 'macho' image and deny any emotional impact of confronting human death and disfigurement. At the present time, it is not entirely clear how different coping styles affect outcome. However, it is frequently recommended that staff involved in disaster work attend a stress debriefing group (Hartsough & Myers 1985), either immediately following the work or within 24–48 hours. Mitchell (1983) described a structured group usually run by a mental health professional experienced in emergency work, in which as well as sharing factual experiences, workers are encouraged to express the feelings they experienced during and after the rescue work with a view to normalizing their appraisal of their reactions and preparing them for further symptoms and the availability of further help should the need arise. As has been recommended for the survivors themselves, it has been suggested that re-experiencing the disaster memories, thoughts and feelings to which they give rise can help in coming to terms with its occurrence or emotionally processing the event. Unfortunately, although widely recommended, the effects of such critical incident stress debriefing remain to be evaluated fully.

## LONG-TERM SUPPORT SERVICES

Building on the experiences of services after the Bradford football stadium fire, Kent Social Services quickly set up a longer-term response and support team for survivors and relatives from the *Herald of Free Enterprise* which capsized in Zeebrugge in March 1987. It has now been recommended that such a support service should be set up and financed for at least two years following a disaster, as recent experience suggests that even after that time, distressed people still present to services for the first time. That is not to say that such a support team should provide all services for survivors but that they make an initial proactive contact, assess risk factors and potential needs, and refer on to other services for more specialized therapies where appropriate.

## PROACTIVE CONTACT

Since one of the main features of PTSD is avoidance of trauma-related information, many of the most severely affected will not present themselves to the services seeking help. They are, in the main, normal people unaccustomed to seeking help for psychological problems, and many have been brought up to believe that they should be able to cope without outside help. Hence, it has been recommended that an initial contact is made to all those who have been affected to offer the opportunity to talk through their experiences with one of the support team. This initial contact provides an occasion for a 'debriefing' with the counsellor providing normalizing information about how people react to a disaster and giving a further point of contact if help is required.

Following the Australian bushfires, mental health workers developed a leaflet describing common reactions to major personal crises and indicating when to seek further help. A list of sources of help was also given. This leaflet was adapted and distributed after the Bradford fire, the capsize of the *Herald of Free Enterprise*, the King's Cross fire, and other major recent disasters (Hodgkinson & Stewart 1991). It is now entitled, 'Coping with a Personal Crisis', and is distributed by the British Red Cross. We recently completed a three and a half year follow-up of survivors from the *Herald* and found that the majority found that the response team's visit and the leaflet were helpful. However, a small minority recalled that they had been upset by these contacts and judged them to be positively harmful (Yule *et al.* 1990a). Yule & Udwin (1991) describe their experiences in meeting a group of teenage schoolgirls ten days after the cruise ship *Jupiter* sank outside Athens harbour in October 1988. Effectively, they undertook a debriefing meeting, during which the survivors completed the Horowitz Impact of Events Scale and measures of anxiety and depression. These scales identified a group of high-risk children who subsequently came forward for help. At five months, there was some evidence that girls in the school which accepted offers of help were doing better than girls in a similar school which did not arrange help (Yule 1990).

## IDENTIFICATION OF VULNERABLE INDIVIDUALS

As discussed earlier, there is, as yet, no clear agreement in the literature on how best to identify those individuals who are most vulnerable to the effects of disasters. Brom & Kleber (1989) emphasize the multiple determination of disorder with it being important to consider the characteristics of the event, the characteristics of the individual, and the post-disaster environment. Similar points were made by Rachman (1980) and elaborated earlier.

## SPECIALIZED PSYCHOTHERAPY FOR PTSD

Space precludes a full exposition of the literature on the treatment of PTSD. This has recently been reviewed by Fairbank & Nicholson (1987) and Foa *et al.* (1989) in relation to adults and by Yule (1991) in relation to children. In summary, there are two main approaches stemming from the psychodynamic and the cognitive-behavioural perspectives, although there is considerable conceptual if not procedural similarity given the importance placed upon 'confrontation' with the trauma in psychodynamic therapy and 'exposure' to the traumatic stimuli in cognitive-behavioural therapy.

Horowitz & Kaltreider (1980) describe a brief psychodynamic therapy in which, from the basis of a safe relationship, persons with a stress disorder can adjust their avoidant controls over emotion and come to reappraise the traumatic event, together with the meaning associated with it, and make adjustments to the presently existing mental models or schemata of him or herself and the world. Horowitz emphasizes the distinction between avoidant and intrusive states and of therapeutic strategies appropriate to both. Horowitz *et al.* (1984) report an uncontrolled outcome study of this type of therapy with 52 patients seeking help following a bereavement, 16 of whom met criteria for PTSD. They report significant changes on standardized measures of specific stress-related and more general symptomatology, with more modest changes on measures of work and interpersonal functioning at five months following end of therapy. Their process analysis suggested that individuals with 'a more stable and coherent self-concept' before treatment showed better outcomes, although most patients obtained symptomatic relief.

Foa *et al.* (1989) conclude from their review of the literature that there are two main elements to the cognitive-behavioural therapies as carried out largely on Vietnam veterans or victims of rape. One element is exposure with a view to habitua-

tion of anxiety to trauma-related stimuli. Lyons & Keane (1989) give a detailed account of the procedures of implosion therapy when applied to a person with PTSD. They stress the length of the sessions (two to two and a half hours each) needed to obtain anxiety decrement. This was noted by Rachman (1980), and by Saigh (1986) in his treatment of a six year old with PTSD.

In the sessions, the therapist presents 'symptom-contingent cues' initially. That is, the therapist describes environmental stimuli that depict the traumatic event or are associated with it. Then the therapist focuses attention upon 'internally elicited cues' such as affect, cognitions or somatic sensations elicited by the trauma. If symptom relief has not been achieved by these means, the therapist may go on to present 'hypothesized sequential cues' which represent cues hypothesized to be present but not reported by the subject. These may be such things as guilt, shame or fear of reprisal. Another strand of behavioural methodology present in the literature is the use of anxiety management methods. For example, Lyons & Keane (1989) also include, in addition to the prolonged imaginal exposure, training in relaxation first as a way of increasing rapport and establishing a therapeutic relationship, and secondly to enhance skill in the use of imagery. Relaxation can also be used as a method of coping with emotion without avoidance. Veronen & Kilpatrick (1983) treated 15 victims of rape using stress-inoculation training which included a package of education about anxiety and training in a variety of cognitive and behavioural coping skills. A treatment-related decrement in anxiety and depression was reported.

Keane *et al.* (1989) have reported a controlled outcome study of the use of 14–16 sessions of implosion therapy for 12 Vietnam veterans meeting criteria of PTSD in comparison with matched controls on a waiting list. The treated group showed significant improvement in the re-experiencing symptoms of PTSD, in anxiety and depression, although the 'numbing' and social avoidance features were not affected. The authors suggest that a social skills training intervention as an additional therapeutic dimension could produce more generalized benefits.

The question of the specific benefit of exposure treatment is addressed by Boudewyne & Hyer (1990), who compared either an exposure treatment or individual counselling as an adjunct to intensive group milieu treatment for Vietnam veterans. Broad psychological and social measures three months following treatment showed an advantage for the exposure group and, furthermore, individuals who showed a treatment-related decrement in physiological response to traumatic material showed a better outcome, regardless of which treatment group they came from. This would suggest that a decreased physiological response to traumatic material is an indicator of recovery but that this change could be achieved in a variety of ways of which implosion is a particularly direct method. Lyons & Keane (1989) compare the method in implosion therapy of presenting traumatic stimuli from a variety of perspectives with a cognitive conceptualization of examining and challenging maladaptive schemata. They also see parallels between their own method and the changing images that emerge during therapy with changes in dreams and images reported in psychodynamic 'working through'. As pointed out earlier, there appears to be considerable convergence in the theories underlying psychodynamic and cognitive-behavioural approaches in PTSD. Specifically one could conceptualize implosive therapy as parallel to Horowitz's confronting phase of therapy and anxiety management to his more supportive 'covering' phase of treatment.

A comparison between different psychological treatment approaches has recently been published by Brom and colleagues (1989). This study of 112 individuals, many of whom were bereaved as well as suffering from PTSD, is the largest study to date and compared a trauma desensitization procedure with hypnotherapy, psychodynamic therapy, and a waiting list control. The authors report that all treatments were more effective than the control condition, especially upon focal PTSD symptomatology. There was a suggestion that psychodynamic therapy had more impact upon avoidant symptoms and other therapies upon intrusion phenomena.

More recently, Thompson (1991) reported the preliminary findings of a controlled trial of brief psychotherapy with survivors of the King's Cross and *Marchioness* disasters. Six sessions of therapy resulted in a modest, 20% reduction in symptom severity. In contrast, Richards & Lovell (1990) and Richards & Rose (1991) describe a short-term treatment approach of up to eight long (one and a half hour) sessions of imaginal and real-life exposure, together with homework sessions, with survivors of the *Jupiter* and *Marchioness* sinkings. This resulted in over 80% reduction in symptom severity – improvements that lasted to 6- and 12-month follow-up.

## Conclusions

Recent experience of major disasters in the UK has highlighted the need for prior planning to achieve better coordination of services. Clinical services have focused especially upon immediate intervention with a view to long-term prevention, but the research literature is as yet sparse as to effectiveness. There is a suggestion that quantitative scales such as the Horowitz Impact of Events Scale may be useful in identifying most highly stressed individuals. The research literature focuses more upon intervention with individuals suffering from chronic PTSD where there is a suggestion that reducing physiological response to traumatic material may promote generalized recovery. However, it is not clear how this is best achieved although the behavioural exposure/implosion technique theoretically is most clearly directed at this goal. Furthermore, it can be argued that a change in physiological response may merely represent integration of traumatic material at a different cognitive level. It is also not clear that methods appropriate to Vietnam veterans or victims of rape can be generalized to survivors of disasters.

## References

Abramson L.Y., Seligman M.E. & Teasdale J.D. (1978) Learned helplessness in humans; critique and reformulation. *Journal of Abnormal Psychology* 87, 49–74.

Affleck G., Tennen H., Croog S. & Levine S. (1987) Causal attribution, perceived benefits, and morbidity after a heart attack: an 8-year study. *Journal of Consulting and Clinical Psychology* 55, 29–35.

American Psychiatric Association (1980) *Diagnostic and Statistical Manual of Mental Disorders*, 3rd edn. APA, Washington DC.

American Psychiatric Association (1987) *Diagnostic and Statistical Manual of Mental Disorders*, 3rd edn. revised. Washington DC.

Antaki C. & Brewin C.R. (eds) (1982) *Attributions and Psychological Change: Applications of Attributional Theories to Clinical and Educational Practice*. Academic, London.

Atkeson B.M., Calhoun K.S., Resick P.A. & Ellis E.M. (1982) Victims of rape: repeated assessment of depressive symptoms. *Journal of Consulting and Clinical Psychology* 50, 96–102.

Beck A.T. (1967) *Depression: Clinical, Experimental, and Theoretical Aspects*. Hoeber, New York.

Benassi V.A., Sweeney P.D. & Dufour C.L. (1988) Is there a relation between locus of control orientation and depression? *Journal of Abnormal Psychology* 97, 357–367.

Bennet G. (1970) Bristol floods 1968: controlled survey of effects on health of local community disaster. *British Medical Journal* 3, 454–458.

Bolin R.C. (1982) *Long-term family recovery from disaster*. Monograph No. 36. Institute of Behavioural Science, University of Colorado, Boulder.

Boudewyne P.A. & Hyer L. (1990) Physiological response to combat memories and preliminary treatment outcome in Vietnam veterans PTSD patients treated with direct therapeutic exposure. *Behavior Therapy* 21, 63–87.

Brewin C.R. (1985) Depression and causal attributions: what is their relation? *Psychological Bulletin* 98, 297–309.

Brewin C.R. (1988) *Cognitive Foundations of Clinical Psychology*. Lawrence Erlbaum Associates, Hove, East Sussex.

Brewin C.R. & Shapiro D.A. (1984) Beyond locus of control: attributions of responsibility for positive and negative outcomes. *British Journal Psychology* 75, 43–49.

Brom D. & Kleber R.J. (1989) Prevention of post-traumatic stress disorders. *Journal of Traumatic Stress* 2, 335–351.

Brom D., Kleber R.J. & Defares P.B. (1989) Brief psychotherapy for posttraumatic stress disorders. *Journal of Consulting and Clinical Psychology* 57, 607–612.

Brown G.W. & Harris T. (1978) *Social Origins of Depression*. The Free Press, New York.

Cohen S. & Wills T.A. (1985) Stress, social support, and the buffering hypothesis. *Psychological Bulletin* 2, 310–357.

Department of Health (1990) *Disasters Planning for a Caring Response. Draft Report of the Working Party on the Psychosocial Aspects of Disasters*. Department of Health, London.

Derogatis L.R., Abeloff M.D. & Melisaratos N. (1979) Psychological coping mechanisms and survival time in metastatic breast cancer. *Journal of the American Medical Association* 242, 1504–1508.

Duckworth D. (1986) Psychological problems arising from disaster work. *Stress Medicine* 2, 315–323.

Erikson K.T. (1976) *Everything in its Path*. Simon and Schuster, New York.

Fairbank J.A. & Nicholson R.A. (1987) Theoretical and empirical issues in the treatment of post-traumatic stress disorder in Vietnam veterans. *Journal of Clinical Psychology* 43, 44–55.

Fairley M. (1984) Tropical cyclone Oscar: psychological reactions of a Fijian population. Paper presented at Disaster Research Workshop, Mt. Macedon, Victoria, Australia.

Fleming R., Baum A., Gisriel M. & Gatchel R. (1982) Mediating influences of social support on stress at Three Mile Island. *Journal of Human Stress* 8, 14–22.

Foa E.B., Steketee G. & Rothbaum B.O. (1989) Behavioural/cognitive conceptualizations of post-traumatic stress disorder. *Behavior Therapy* 20, 155–176.

Folkman S. & Lazarus R.S. (1980) An analysis of coping in a middle-aged community sample. *Journal of Health and Social Behaviour* 21, 219–239.

Folkman S. & Lazarus R.S. (1985) If it changes it must be a process: study of emotion and coping during three stages of a college examination. *Journal of Personality and Social Psychology* 48, 150–170.

Foy D.W., Resnick H.S., Sipprelle R.C. & Carroll E.M. (1987) Premilitary, military, and postmilitary factors in the development of combat-related stress disorders. *Behaviour Therapist* 10, 3–9.

Frank E., Turner S.M., Stewart B.D., Jacob M. & West D. (1981) Past psychiatric symptoms and the response to sexual assault. *Comprehensive Psychiatry* 22, 479–487.

Frye J. & Stockton R.A. (1982) Discriminant analysis of posttraumatic stress disorder among a group of Vietnam veterans. *American Journal of Psychiatry* 139, 52–56.

Genest M., Bowen R.C., Dudley J. & Keegan D. (1990) Assessment of strategies for coping with anxiety: preliminary investigations. *Journal of Anxiety Disorders* 4, 1–14.

Gibbs M.S. (1986) Psychopathological consequences of exposure to toxins in the water supply. In Lebovits A.H. Baum A. & Singer J.E. (eds) *Advances in Environmental psychology. Volume 6. Exposure to Hazardous Substances: Psychological Parameters*, pp. 47–70. Erlbaum, Hillsdale, NJ.

Gibbs M.S. (1989) Factors in the victim that mediate between disaster and psychopathology: a review. *Journal of Traumatic Stress* 2, 489–514.

Gleser G.C., Green B.L. & Winget C.N. (1981) *Prolonged Psychosocial Effects of Disaster*. Academic, New York.

Green B.L., Grace M.C. & Gleser G.C. (1985) Identifying survivors at risk: long-term impairment following the Beverly Hills Supper Club fire. *Journal of Consulting and Clinical Psychology* 53, 672–678.

Green B.L., Grace M.C., Lindy J.D., Tichener J.L. & Lindy J.G. (1983) Levels of functional impairment following a civilian disaster: the Beverly Hills Supper Club Fire.

*Journal of Consulting and Clinical Psychology* 51, 573–580.

Hartsough D.M. & Myers D.G. (1985) *Disaster Work and Mental Health*: *Prevention and Control of Stress Among Workers*. NIMH, Washington DC.

Hodgkinson P.E. & Stewart M. (1988) Missing, presumed dead. *Disaster Management* 1, 11–14.

Hodgkinson P.E. & Stewart M. (1991) *Coping with Catastrophe: A Handbook of Disaster Management*. Routledge, London.

Horowitz M. (1979) Psychological response to serious life events. In Hamilton V. & Warburton D.M. (eds) *Human Stress and Cognition: An Information Processing Approach*. Wiley, Chichester.

Horowitz M. (1982) Psychological processes induced by illness, injury, and loss. In Millon T., Green C. & Meagher R. (eds), *Handbook of Clinical Health Psychology*, pp. 53–68. Plenum, New York.

Horowitz M.J. (1986) Stress-response syndromes: a review of posttraumatic and adjustment disorders. *Hospital and Community Psychiatry* 37, 241–249.

Horowitz M.J. (1989) *Intoduction to Psychodynamics: A New Synthesis*, p. 19. Routledge, London.

Horowitz M.J. & Kaltreider N.B. (1980) Brief psychotherapy of stress response syndromes. In Karasu T.B. & Bellack I. (eds) *Specialized Techniques in Individual Psychotherapy*. Brunner/Mazel, New York.

Horowitz M.J., Marmar C., Weiss D.S., DeWitt K.N. & Rosenbaum R. (1984) Brief psychotherapy of bereavement reactions: the relationship of process to outcome. *Archives of General Psychiatry* 41, 438–448.

Horowitz M., Wilner N. & Alvarez W. (1979) Impact of Event Scale: a measure of subjective stress. *Psychosomatic Medicine* 41, 209–218.

Janoff-Bulman R. (1985) The aftermath of victimisation: rebuilding shattered assumptions. In Figley C.R. (ed.) *Trauma and its Wake*, vol. 1. Brunner/Mazel, New York.

Jones J.C. & Barlow D.H. (1990) The etiology of post-traumatic stress disorder. *Clinical Psychology Review* 10, 299–328.

Joseph S., Andrews B., Williams R. & Yule W. (1992a) Crisis support and psychiatric symptomatology in adult survivors of the Jupiter cruise ship disaster. *British Journal of Clinical Psychology* 31, 63–73.

Joseph S.A., Brewin C.R., Yule W. & Williams R. (1991) Causal attributions and psychiatric symptomatology in survivors of the Herald of Free Enterprise disaster. *British Journal of Psychiatry* 159, 542–546.

Joseph S.A., Brewin C.R., Yule W. & Williams R. (1992b) Causal attributions and post-traumatic stress in adolescents. *Journal of Child Psychology and Psychiatry* (in press).

Joseph S.A., Williams R., Yule W. & Walker A. (1992c) Factor analysis of the impact of events scale with survivors of two disasters at sea. *Personality and Individual Differences* 13, 693–697.

Keane T.M., Caddell J.M., Martin B., Zimering R.T. &

Fairbank J.A. (1983) Substance abuse among vietnam veterans with posttraumatic stress disorders. *Bulletin of Psychologists and Addictive Behaviour* 2, 117–122.

Keane T.M. Caddell J.M. & Taylor K.L. (1988) Mississippi scale for combat-related posttraumatic stress disorder: three studies in reliability and validity. *Journal of Consulting and Clinical Psychology* 56, 85–90.

Keane T.M., Fairbank J.A., Caddell J.M. & Zimering R.T. (1989) Implosive (flooding) therapy reduces symptoms of PTSD in Vietnam combat veterans. *Behavior Therapy* 20, 245–260.

Keane T.M., Scott W.O., Chavoya G.A., Lamparski D.M. & Fairbank J.A. (1985) Social support in Vietnam veterans: a comparative analysis. *Journal of Consulting and Clinical Psychology* 53, 95–102.

Lazarus R.S. (1966) *Psychological Stress and the Coping Process*. McGraw-Hill, New York.

Leopold R.L. & Dillon H. (1963) Psychanatomy of a disaster: a long-term study of post-traumatic neurosis in survivors of a marine explosion. *American Journal of Psychiatry* 119, 913–921.

Lifton R.J. (1967) *Death in Life: Survivors of Hiroshima*. Random House, New York.

Lifton R.J. & Olson E. (1976) The human meaning of total disaster: the Buffalo Creek experience. *Psychiatry* 39, 1–18.

Lundin T. (1984) Disaster Reactions: A study of Survivors' Reactions Following a Major Fire Disaster. Unpublished paper, University of Uppsala, Sweden.

Lyons J.A. & Keane T.M. (1989) Implosive therapy for the treatment of combat-related PTSD. *Journal of Traumatic Stress* 2, 137–152.

McCormick R.A., Taber J.I. & Kruedelbach N. (1989) The relationship between attributional style and post traumatic stress disorder in addicted patients. *Journal of Traumatic Stress Studies* 2, 477–487.

McFarlane A.C. (1985) The Etiology of Post-traumatic Stress Disorders Following a Natural Disaster. Unpublished paper, Department of Psychiatry, The Flinders University of South Australia.

McFarlane A.C. (1988) The longitudinal course of post-traumatic morbidity: the range of outcomes and their predictors. *Journal of Nervous and Mental Disease* 176, 22–29.

March J.S. (1990) The nosology of posttraumatic stress disorder. *Journal of Anxiety Disorders* 4, 61–82.

Markowitz J.S. & Gutterman E. (1986) Predictors of psychological distress in the community following two toxic chemical incidents. In Lebovits A.H., Buam A. & Singer J.E. (eds) *Advances in Environmental Psychology* (vol. 6); *Exposure to Hazardous Substances: Psychological Parameters*, pp. 89–107. Erlbaum, Hillsdale, NJ.

Mitchell J.T. (1983) When disaster strikes.... The critical incident stress debriefing process. *Journal of Emergency Medical Services* 8, 36–39.

Mueller D.P. (1980) Social networks: a promising direction for research on the relationship of the social environment to psychiatric disorder. *Social Science and Medicine* 14, 147–161.

Murphy S.A. (1988) Mediating effects of intrapersonal and social support on mental health 1 and 3 years after a natural disaster. *Journal of Traumatic Stress* 2, 155–172.

Parker G. (1977) Cyclone Tracy and Darwin evacuees: on the restoration of the species. *British Journal of Psychiatry* 130, 548–555.

Pennebaker J.W. (1985) Traumatic experience and psychosomatic disease: exploring the roles of behavioural inhibition, obsession, and confiding. *Canadian Psychology* 26, 82–95.

Pennebaker J.W. & Beall S. (1986) Confronting a traumatic event: toward an understanding of inhibition and disease. *Journal of Abnormal Psychology* 95, 274–281.

Pennebaker J.W., Hughes C.F. & O'Heeron R.C. (1987) The psychophysiology of confession: linking inhibitory and psychosomatic processes. *Journal of Personality and Social Psychology* 52, 781–793.

Peterson C. & Seligman M.E.P. (1984) Causal explanations as a risk factor for depression: theory and evidence. *Psychological Review* 91, 347–374.

Peterson C., Semmel A., von Baeyer C., Abramson L.Y., Metalsky G.I. & Seligman M.E. (1982) The attributional style questionnaire. *Cognitive Therapy and Research* 6, 287–299.

Pynoos R.S. & Nader K. (1988) Psychological first aid and treatment approach for children exposed to community violence: research implications. *Journal of Traumatic Stress* 1, 243–267.

Rachman S. (1980) Emotional processing. *Behaviour Research and Therapy* 18, 51–60.

Raphael B (1986) *When Disaster Strikes.* Hutchinson, London.

Richards D. & Lovell K. (1990) Imaginal and In-vivo Exposure in the Treatment of PTSD. Paper read at Second European Conference on Traumatic Stress, Netherlands, September 1990.

Richards D.A. & Rose J.S. (1991) Exposure therapy for post-traumatic stress disorder: four case studies. *British Journal of Psychiatry* 158, 836–840.

Roth L.M. (1986) Substance use and mental health among Vietnam veterans. In Boulanger G. & Kadushin C. (eds) *The Vietnam Veteran Redefined*, pp. 61–78. Lawrence Erlbaum, Hillsdale, NJ.

Rotter J.B. (ed.) (1966) Generalized expectancies for internal vs. external control of reiforcement. *Psychological Monograph* 80, 1–28.

Saigh P.A. (1986) In vitro flooding in the treatment of a 6-year-old boy's post-traumatic stress disorder. *Behaviour Research and Therapy* 24, 685–688.

Schultz R. & Decker S. (1985) Long-term adjustment to physical disability: The role of social support, perceived control, and self-blame. *Journal of Personality and Social Psychology*, 48, 1162–1172.

Schwarzwald J., Solomon Z., Weisenberg M. & Mikulincer M. (1987) Validation of the impact of event scale for psychological sequelae of combat. *Journal of Consulting and Clinical Psychology* 55, 251–256.

Shepherd M. & Hodgkinson P.E. (1990) The hidden victims of disaster: helper stress. *Stress Medicine* 6, 29–35.

Silver S.M. & Iacono C.U. (1984) Factor-analytic support for DSM-III's post-traumatic stress disorder for vietnam veterans. *Journal of Clinical Psychology* 40, 5–14.

Sims A.C.P., White A.C. & Murphy T. (1979) Aftermath neurosis: psychological sequelae of the Brimingham bombings in victims not seriously injured. *Medicine, Science and the Law* 19, 78–81.

Singh B. & Raphael B. (1981) Postdisaster morbidity of the bereaved. *Journal of Nervous and Mental Disease* 169, 203–212.

Solkoff N., Gray P. & Kiell S. (1986) Which Vietnam veterans develop posttraumatic stress disorders? *Journal of Clinical Psychology* 42, 687–698.

Solomon S. (1986) Mobilizing social support networks in times of disaster. In Figley C. (ed.) *Trauma and Its Wake* (vol. 2), *Traumatic Stress Theory, Research, and Intervention*, pp. 232–263, Brunner/Mazel, New York.

Solomon Z., Mikulincer M. & Avitzur E. (1988a) Coping, locus of control, social support, and combat related posttraumatic stress disorder: a prospective study. *Journal of Personality and Social Psychology* 55, 279–285.

Solomon Z., Mikulincer M. & Flum H. (1988b) Negative life events, coping responses, and combat-related psychopathology: a prospective study. *Journal of Abnormal Psychology* 97, 302–307.

Solomon Z., Weisenberg M., Schwarzwald J. & Mikulincer M. (1987) Post-traumatic stress disorder among soldiers with combat stress reaction: the 1982 Israeli experience. *American Journal of Psychiatry* 1944, 448–454.

Stratton P., Heard D., Hanks H.G.I., Munton A.G., Brewin. C.R. & Davidson C. (1986) Coding causal beliefs in natural discourse. *British Journal of Social Psychology* 25, 299–313.

Suls J. & Fletcher B. (1985) The relative efficacy of avoidant and non-avoidant coping strategies: a meta analysis. *Health Psychology* 4, 249–288.

Sweeney P.D., Anderson K. & Bailey S. (1986) Attributional style in depression: a meta-analytic review. *Journal of Personality and Social Psychology* 50, 974–991.

Taylor A.J.W. & Frazer A.G. (1982) The stress of post-disaster body handling and victim identification work. *Journal of Human Stress* 8, (December), 4–12.

Taylor V.A., Ross G.A. & Quarantelli E.L. (1976) *Delivery of Mental Health Services in Disasters: The Xenia Tornado and Some Implications.* (Book and Monograph Series II.) Disaster Research Center, The Ohio State University, Colombus.

Thompson J. (1991) A Controlled Treatment Trial with Survivors of the King's Cross Fire. Paper presented at conference on Post Traumatic Stress Disorders, Institute of Psychiatry, London, April 1991.

Veronen L.J. & Kilpatrick D.G. (1983) Stress management

for rape victims. In Meichenbaum D. & Jarenko M.E. (eds) *Stress Reduction and Prevention*. Plenum, New York.

Weiner B. (1985) Spontaneous causal thinking. *Psychological Bulletin* 97, 74–84.

Weiner B. (1986) *An Attributional Theory of Motivation and Emotion*. Springer Verlag, New York.

Weisaeth L. (1983) The Study of a Factory Fire. Doctoral dissertation, University of Oslo.

Weisenberg M., Solomon Z., Schwarzwald J. & Mikulincer M. (1987) Assessing the severity of posttraumatic stress disorder: relation between dichotomous and continuous measures. *Journal of Consulting and Clinical Psychology* 55, 432–434.

Western J.S. & Milne G. (1979) Some social effects of a natural hazard: Darwin residents and cyclone Tracy. In Heathcote R.L., & Thom B.G. (eds) *Natural Hazards in Australia*. Australian Academy of Science, Canberra.

Wilkinson C.B. (1983) Aftermath of a disaster: the collapse of the Hyatt Regency Hotel Skywalk. *American Journal of Psychiatry* 140, 1134–1139.

Williams R. & Yule W. (1988) The assessment of 'Nervous Shock' in Compensation Litigation. Paper presented to the First European Conference on Traumatic Stress Research, Lincoln, August.

Wykes T. & Whittington R. (1991) Coping strategies used by staff following assault by a patient: an exploratory study. *Work and Stress* 5, 37–48.

Yule W. (1990) Post Traumatic Stress in Children who Survived the Jupiter Cruise Ship Disaster. Paper presented at the 1990 American Psychological Association Conference.

Yule W. (1991) Working with children following disasters. In Herbert M. (ed.) *Clinical Child Psychology: Social Learning, Development and Behaviour*, pp. 349–363. Wiley, Chichester.

Yule W., Hodgkinson P., Joseph S., Parkes C.M. & Williams R. (1990a) The Herald of Free Enterprise: 30 Months Follow-up. Paper presented at the second European Conference on Traumatic Stress, Netherlands, 23–27 September 1990.

Yule W. & Udwin O. (1991) Screening child survivors for post traumatic stress disorders: experiences from the 'Jupiter' sinking. *British Journal of Clinical Psychology* 30, 131–138.

Yule W., Udwin O. & Murdoch K. (1990b) The 'Jupiter' sinking: effects on children's fears, depression and anxiety. *Journal of Child Psychology and Psychiatry* 31, 1051–1061.

Zilberg N.J., Weiss D.S. & Horowitz M.J. (1982) Impact of Event Scale: a cross-validation study and some empirical evidence supporting a conceptual model of stress response syndromes. *Journal of Consulting and Clinical Psychology* 50, 407–414.

# PART 4
# PRINCIPLES
# OF MANAGEMENT

# Chapter 28
# The Principles of Setting Up
# Mental Health Services in the Community

GERALDINE STRATHDEE
& GRAHAM THORNICROFT

## Defining community services

Setting up community psychiatric services has been one of the foremost preoccupations of contemporary psychiatry. Reflecting the diversity of historical influences on their development, there is little agreement on what constitutes the 'community'. At its most basic, the term is used to refer to the locality of services, commonly regarded as those outside the psychiatric hospital. Sabshin's view (1966) was that the nature of the care is more important than locality, and proposed that:

> community psychiatry involves the utilisation of the techniques, methods, theories of social psychiatry and other behavioural sciences to investigate and to meet the mental health needs of a functionally or geographically defined population over a significant period of time, and the feeding back of information to modify the central body of social psychiatric and other behavioural science knowledge.

Focusing on the organizational context, Hunter & Wistow (1987) consider that two themes have underpinned the development of community services: that they should be directed to meeting individual needs rather than producing services (Ministry of Health 1963) and that this objective is best met by replacing inherited service systems dominated by large institutions with a more balanced and flexible range of alternative services. As Wing (1977, unpublished paper) has stated, 'no system of care can be understood except in relation to the underlying social and political structures of the society it serves'. Indeed the development of community services for the mentally ill is almost exclusively a product of the latter half of this century. Their evolution has been influenced by a complex interaction of factors, which we shall explore in this chapter, and which include alterations and advances in mental health treatment practices, legislation, attitudes among the public and professions, the organization and extent of decentralization in health care systems, national political movements, the extent of state and private finance burdens in the provision of health, and local geography and health service history (Mechanic 1987, Ramon 1988, Klein 1991).

## Historical perspectives

For most of the preceding two centuries psychiatric services were based on, and located almost entirely within, mental hospitals geographically remote from their catchment populations. The rising numbers of psychiatric inpatients until the mid-point of the twentieth century has been thoroughly documented (Jones 1972, Scull 1979, Morrisey & Goldman 1984, Busfield 1986). Freeman (1983) concluded that despite the early optimistic phases of moral treatment and non-restraint, the weight of chronic mental illness finally overwhelmed the mental hospitals, resulting in a rigid authoritarian pattern and a peculiar internal culture. The adverse effects of these custodial institutions have been extensively described and studied (e.g. Goffman 1961, Wing & Brown 1970).

The process of deinstitutionalization in Britain, which was paralleled in the USA, reached its peak in the 1970s (Mechanic 1987). From a maximum inpatient population of 558 900 in 1955, numbers had fallen to 132 164 by 1980 (Scull 1984). Of an estimated 1.7–2.4 million chronically mentally ill persons in the USA (Goldman *et al.* 1983), only 116000 remained within state mental hospitals by 1983 (Bachrach 1986). In Britain, the decline in numbers of psychiatric inpatients has continued at an even rate since 1954 (Thornicroft 1988), and the average number of psychiatric beds occupied each day in 1985 in England and Wales, for example, was 64800 (Audit Commission 1986).

Deinstitutionalization, although it began earlier (Scull 1979), was influenced and facilitated by the introduction of antipsychotic drugs. These were important in changing the attitudes and administrative behaviour of staff in the large institutions and their effect on symptoms gave families greater confidence that they could manage patients at home (Mechanic 1987). Therapeutic communities introduced by Jones (1952) emphasized the giving of autonomy and responsibility to patients and represented a significant change in the format of residential services.

In 1961 Enoch Powell, then the Minister of Health, announced that the mental hospital population should be halved by 1975, and that most of those psychiatric inpatients remaining would be treated in units in district general hospitals. Psychiatrists, many of whom had begun to develop district services, welcomed the trend, regarding it as an opportunity to end the traditional isolation of the mental hospitals and bring psychiatry closer to general medicine (Carse *et al.* 1958, Leyberg 1959). This directive resulted in a rapid extension of the growing trend to establish outpatient clinics at general hospitals (Gillis & Egert, 1973), polyclinics or health centres within urban areas and the development of occasional day places and hostels (Foucault 1971, Walsh 1987).

The 1960s saw a period of further attitude changes with strong ideological overtones. As with the term community care, the use of 'normalization', a term coined by Wolfensberger (1970), has played a significant role in the thinking behind the structure of many forms of community services, particularly residential ones. Wolfensberger argued that individuals should be as independent, free to move about and empowered to make meaningful choices as are typical citizens of comparable age in the community (Garety 1988). In his later social valorization philosophy he argued

that the most explicit and highest goal of normalization must be the creation, support and defence of valued social roles for people who are at risk of social devaluation (Wolfensberger 1983). This concept has influenced such policy documents as the House of Commons Social Services Committee report on Community Care (1985).

## International mental health policy trends

The USA community programmes have influenced much of the service development in Europe, despite differences in the organization of health care systems. Present US Government policy is embodied in the National Plan for the Chronically Mentally Ill, which was a consequence of a wide-ranging review of policy (General Accounting Office 1977) demonstrating that community based facilities, developed in line with plans to introduce a national network of comprehensive community mental health centres, had in fact been implemented 'in the absence of a planned, well-managed and systematic approach'.

In response to this criticism, NIMH Community Support Programs were established from 1977. Fifteen sites provided demonstration projects of services for chronic mentally ill patients. In reviewing the outcome of these initiatives, Tessler & Goldman (1982) saw this programme as 'an incomplete reform'. They found that the political trend towards shifting responsibility and costs for the chronic mentally ill from federal to state level threatened to undermine the benefit of these federal programmes.

Far-reaching policy changes have been introduced more rapidly in Italy than in Britain and the USA (Mollica 1983), and allow limited comparisons to be made. Law 180, enacted in 1978, formalized and accelerated this pre-existing trend in the care of the mentally ill (Tansella *et al.* 1987). In contrast to the policies in the USA and Britain, the major provisions set out that no new patients be admitted to the large state hospitals, nor should there be any readmissions after 1 January 1982. No new psychiatric wards or hospitals were to be built. Psychiatric wards in general hospitals were not to exceed 15 beds and must be affiliated to community mental health centres. Community-based facilities would be responsible for a specified geographical area, staffed by existing mental health personnel (Mosher 1983). In essence, the legislative reforms have reversed the previous order of priorities accorded to hospital and community forms of service provision (Tansella 1986).

In Scandinavia the dominant model in the organization of comprehensive psychiatric care has been the creation of geographically defined areas, known as sectors. A series of political, legal and organizational changes influenced the development of the services. In Sweden two factors were particularly significant. First, in 1967 the responsibility for mental health services was decentralized from federal to local government with the aim of integrating with other health care services (Goldie & Freden 1991). Secondly, in 1973 the National Board of Health and Welfare outlined a plan which gave the primary care services increased responsibility for minor psychiatric morbidity, with the psychiatric services to provide inpatient and outpatient care for the more seriously ill (Lindholm 1983). Similarly decentralization and the creation of sectors was embodied in a law passed in 1978 in Finland. There was even greater emphasis on the role of primary care with the idea that psychiatric outpatients should be treated by primary care staff in health services centres with advice and consultation available from specialists in polyclinics and hospitals.

## The levels of mental health service planning

### National planning

In Britain the 1975 Government White Paper (Department of Health & Social Security 1975) marked the first in a series of policy moves which has resulted in the evolution of the community care policies (Jones 1972, Thornicroft & Bebbington 1989). It set a target of 47 900 inpatient psychiatric beds after the completion of the programme of closure of psychiatric hospitals. On these estimates, 84% of the planned reduction in long-stay psychiatric beds towards this goal from the high point in 1954 has already happened,

and only the final sixth of long-stay patients remain to be relocated. Alongside this attrition, there has been a corresponding increase in the annual number of admissions: from 78 586 in 1955 to 185 514 in 1981 (Social Services Committee 1985).

Since this original legislation, policy has crystallized rapidly through publication of successive reports (Social Services Committee 1985, Audit Commission 1986, Murphy 1987, 1988, Griffiths 1988, Secretaries of State for Health, Wales, Northern Ireland & Scotland 1989, 1990) to the current statutory framework (Department of Health 1989a,b). These latter policies attempt to provide a framework for community care in Britain in the 1990s and beyond. The key objectives include the promotion of domiciliary, day and respite services enabling people to live in their own homes, making practical support for carers a high priority, promoting the development of an independent sector. Local authorities are given the lead responsibility for the provision of community care with the introduction of the distinction between health and social care. The most significant recent legislation is that of the National Health Service and Community Care Act (House of Commons 1990), within which it is now required of local social service and health authorities that they draw up jointly agreed community care plans which clearly indicate the local implementation of needs-based individual care plans for long-term, severe and vulnerable psychiatric patients.

### Regional planning

In Great Britain it is at regional level that most strategic planning of resources takes place, financial allocations are set and constraints on manpower determined. Seymour (1986) has defined the role of the Regional Health Authority as:

> establishing, in collaboration with the district
> health authorities, a clear strategic plan
> defining objectives, and, through the issue of
> planning guidelines giving a time-framework
> for change. An essential part of this plan is
> the development of comprehensive local
> psychiatric services where necessary, and the
> provision of alternative and more

appropriate facilities for patients residing in the large psychiatric institutions; ensuring that the revenue, capital and manpower resources necessary are available and sufficient to achieve the changes required. At a regional level there is a need to develop accessible services in addition to creating centres for education, tertiary referral and research.

Regions have the difficult task of balancing a prescriptive approach to coordinate developments throughout the area, while recognizing local initiatives and needs. Policy statements in recent years have placed emphasis on the need to develop research and service evaluation and to respond flexibly to the findings (South East Thames Regional Health Authority 1985, 1986).

### The district perspective

The district has been regarded as the fundamental building block on which to base community care provision. The development of a comprehensive district psychiatric service has been a key objective embodied in successive policy statements (Department of Health & Social Security 1971, 1974). Three main elements have been advocated: a district general hospital psychiatric unit providing inpatient, day-hospital and outpatient services; local authority community services such as social work support, homes for the elderly, hostels, group homes, day centres; and a mechanism for joint planning and operation of services, including setting up therapeutic teams. The contribution by GPs and other primary care workers and the role of the voluntary organizations has been regarded as central (Greater London Council 1984). Other less definable influences are crucial to the shape of any local services and include the local morbidity, financial strength of the organization, the attitudes and competencies of clinicians and managers.

One specific component, district general hospital units, have been described as highly acceptable to patients and relatives, and financially viable (Goldberg & Jones 1980, Goldberg 1986). More widely, the extent to which districts fulfil their role in a planned and comprehensive way has been studied by Kingdon (1989). He surveyed 192

English health authorities and found that almost half did not mention any joint planning group and still less included any contribution from the voluntary organizations; two-fifths did not state the objectives of the service; only one-quarter mentioned data collection facilities such as case registers or at-risk registers, and information on the community for whom the service was being planned was frequently not made explicit.

### The process of setting up services

The process of planning and developing community services is complex and in this section a series of steps is delineated. There is a focus on the creation of a consensus philosophy and vision, an identification of the strategic, management and organizational issues involved in the planning mechanisms and the gathering of appropriate information on which to base the developments. Throughout there is an emphasis on the development of mechanisms to facilitate implementation.

### Step 1: the philosophy and vision of the service

Fundamental to the development of any service is an agreement from the outset of who the service should serve and what its objectives should be. The creation of a mission statement by the team of senior personnel and major stake-holders including users is a powerful process in developing team cohesion and in enabling each individual and organization to recognize the inherent strengths, skills and biases of each other. This produces significant gains later at the implementation stage.

### Step 2: the principles of community psychiatric services

Based on the mission statement clinicians and planners can clarify the principles on which to develop their service. Many organizations and groups have enunciated their views of the essential principles of community services and the summary below is based on the definitions of four disparate bodies: MIND (1983); Lord Glenarthur, speaking as Government spokesman in 1985; the Royal

College of Psychiatrists in *Caring for a Community* in 1990; and in a stimulating and practical document entitled 'Towards a model plan for a comprehensive community based mental health system' produced by the National Institute of Mental Health's (1987) formulation. They consider that:

*Services should be local and accessible* and to the greatest extent possible delivered in the client's usual environment.

*Services should be comprehensive* and address the diversity of needs of individuals with mental health disorders.

*Services should be flexible* by being available whenever and for whatever duration. There should be a range of complementary models which provide individuals with choice and vary, depending on need, at any point in time.

*Services should be consumer orientated*, that is based on the needs of the client rather than those of providers. Achieving this balance is one of the major difficulties to be overcome in resource allocation. Central, highly resourced facilities, for example hospital-based units, may appear more efficient and effective in terms of easy movement of staff between wards, training, information gathering and reduction in staff isolation, but be inflexible in addressing patient's needs.

*Services should empower clients* by using and adapting treatment techniques which enable clients to enhance their self-help skills and retain the fullest possible control over their own lives. This can take place at both the individual level and at all stages in the planning and development of a service. By integrating an educational component into treatment, patients can determine the strategies in terms of medications and manipulation of social environments which enable them to take part in secondary and tertiary prevention. At the services level, clients should be actively involved in planning and policy-making decisions and be represented on all relevant committees.

*Services should be racially and culturally appropriate* (see Chapter 29). Mechanisms to ensure provision of appropriate and acceptable services include use of culturally appropriate needs assessment tools, representation on planning groups, cross-cultural training for staff, use of indigenous workers and bilingual staff, identification and provision of alternative basic facilities and evaluation of the provision against accepted indicators.

*Services should focus on strengths.* They should be built on the skills and strengths of clients and help them maintain a sense of identity, dignity and self-esteem. Patients should be discouraged from adopting the sick-role and the service from developing an environment organized around permanent illness with lowered expectations.

*Services should be normalized and incorporate natural supports* by being in the least restrictive, most natural setting possible. The natural work, education, leisure and support facilities in the community should be used in preference to specialized developments.

*Services should meet special needs* with particular attention being paid to those with physical disabilities, mental retardation, the homeless or imprisoned.

*Services should be accountable* to the consumers and carers and evaluated to ensure their continuing appropriateness and acceptability and effectiveness on agreed parameters.

### Step 3: establishing joint planning mechanisms

In planning a comprehensive service for individuals with mental health disorders a wide range of needs must be accommodated. At both the national and district level there is, therefore, a need to create joint planning mechanisms and to involve and consult with a complex network of agencies including the primary health care teams, social services and housing departments, the prison and probation services, advocacy groups, education, employment agencies and the voluntary organizations and users. In an ideal model, a common and shared set of priorities would be evolved, based on clear policies produced by intensive and committed forward-looking individuals, and having the prior benefit of substantive research demonstrating their primacy and efficacy.

## Step 4: models of service planning

A number of approaches to planning community services have been adopted, and we describe here three which are in common use. These we have termed the needs model (based on a 'bottom-up' approach), the components model (a 'top-down' approach) and the functions model.

*The needs model.* A prime example is the National Institute of Mental Health's formulation of a Model Plan for a comprehensive community-based mental health system. This attractive model first delineates the range of needs of individual patients (Fig. 28.1) and then formulates a series of steps to convert the cumulative needs of patients into the necessary elements of service.

*The components model* takes the approach of defining the necessary elements for the provision of a comprehensive service. A list of specific facilities are formulated, including inpatient beds, outpatient clinics and day hospitals (Department of Health & Social Security 1971, 1974, MIND 1983, Hirsch 1988).

*The functions model* focuses on the expected function of the service. Leff (1986) formulates a series of steps to enable the optimal facility to be devised. For example, when an acute treatment facility is needed, the requirement may be for an environment in which removal from stress is the main attribute, while in others, the presence of highly skilled staff, provision of a temporary home or containment of aggressive behaviours may be the predominant need.

## Step 5: information systems required

To set up and monitor locally based mental health services, a clear, systematic and continuing method of collecting clinical and social need and service usage data is required. The most comprehensive method to elicit, code and store these data is the case register, which is defined as a local information system that records the contacts with designated social and medical services of patients or clients from a defined geographical area (Wing 1989). Although such systems were formerly labour intensive, the recent availability of on-site micro and mini computers has made their more

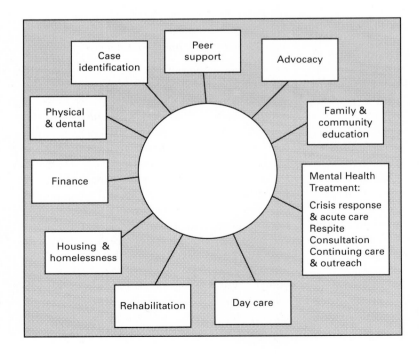

**Fig. 28.1** The range of needs of individuals with mental health disorders.

widespread use a practical option in many districts. The routine collection of clinical contact data allows aggregate data to show patterns of service with respect to patterns of diagnoses (Der & Bebbington 1987, Tansella & Williams 1989), social class (Wiersma *et al.* 1983) and geographical mobility (Lesage & Tansella 1989). Further, the use of standardized coding and diagnostic systems allows comparisons of service use within local areas (Giel & Horn 1982), within regions (Torre & Marinoni 1985) and between countries (Horn *et al.* 1986, Sytema *et al.* 1989). Such data can therefore indicate how variations in treated morbidity occur with local sociodemographic characteristics, with the nature and extent of local service provision, and with the service trends at the national level. Where one of the primary aims of developing local mental health services is to deliver services to identified priority groups of patients, then the detailed information produced by case registers will be required to ensure that the outcome of implementation is consistent with the declared aims of the service.

### Step 6: strategic and organizational issues

#### ESTABLISHING THE ORGANIZATIONAL FRAMEWORK

In planning community services the organization of services is of paramount importance. As Tansella (1989) counsels, 'what is important in community care is not only the number and characteristics of various services but the way in which they are arranged and integrated'. Mechanisms must be found which enable effective service delivery, the three principles of which have been enunciated by Paumelle, an early proponent of community care in France (Walsh 1987).

The first principle is that *continuity of care* should be ensured. This, he believed, could best be achieved by ensuring that persons and families were dealt with at all stages and at all levels of illness by the same team. In turn, this meant assigning such teams and their associated structures such as beds and clinics to populations of manageable size. Given the range of needs of individuals with mental health problems, *co-*

*ordination of care* was cited as the second fundamental principle. Only by the introduction of multidisciplinary and interagency teams could the range of treatments necessary to overcome the impairment and disability of the mentally ill be delivered. *Integration of care* was regarded as the third essential based on the premise (World Health Organization 1983) that in any community, first contact for individuals in distress is often not with the psychiatric specialist team, but rather persons in key positions of responsibility in the community such as teachers, police, public health nurses, community nurses, social workers and GPs. The specialist team must therefore integrate its efforts with those of the non-specialists, as well as taking the lead in educating and counselling non-specialists.

#### INTEGRATION WITH PRIMARY HEALTH CARE SERVICES

In Great Britain these principles must be considered in the light of two important aspects of our health care system. First, there is a uniquely strong tier of primary care. GPs play a major role in the care of those with both acute and chronic psychological disorders (Shepherd *et al.* 1966, Goldberg & Blackwell 1970, Sharpe & Morrell 1989, Paykel 1990, Strathdee 1992a). For many patients with severe, long-term disorders the GP is indeed the only source of continuing care (Murray Parkes *et al.* 1962, Pantellis *et al.* 1988, Johnstone *et al.* 1984, Brown *et al.* 1988, Lee & Murray 1988). As Jones concluded: 'unless attention is given to finding administrative solutions to the repeated official exhortations (Department of Health & Social Security 1975, 1978, 1981, Griffiths 1988) for collaboration and co-operation with GPs we will fail to provide the mix of services needed'.

#### INTERAGENCY COORDINATION

Further, although arguably receiving implicit support in recent legislation, there is an absence of a unitary core agency responsible for assuring the delivery and coordination of all services. Given the nature of the involvement of health, social and the range of non-statutory agencies, the organization of services is therefore fundamental to their ability to fulfil the principles of delivery. Joint working is a vital component of local service development and can be conceptualized at many levels, from planning and joint financing, through to management and individual clinical matters (Jeffreys 1979). Two levels are made explicit in a policy statement (Department of Health & Social Security 1986):

*At the strategic level*: to encompass health and local authority services, and the voluntary sector, in an integrated network to meet the full range of needs, to achieve jointly owned policies and to avoid unnecessary duplication of services through parallel developments. To achieve this a mental illness subgroup of the joint care planning team is needed.

*At the operational level*: to create multidisciplinary teams to integrate as far as possible professional services such as occupational therapy and community psychiatric nurses/social workers, using the case manager approach when this can improve care, to organize joint training where appropriate, and to generate ideas for the joint development of services.

CASE MANAGEMENT SYSTEMS

There should be case management, or at least care coordination systems (Strathdee 1992b) available to all individuals with multiple and continuing needs. Models of case management are described elsewhere in this volume (see Chapter 24), and it is sufficient here to indicate that whichever case manager model is used in each locality, that clear lines of responsibility be established to ensure that patients needing care receive it in appropriate form and measure (Thornicroft 1990).

ESTABLISHING A SECTORIZED SERVICE

In order to achieve the principles of effective delivery of psychiatric care as delineated above, one approach has been hailed as achieving success. Workers, both abroad (Lindholm 1983, Hansson 1989) and in Great Britain (Tyrer *et al.* 1989) consider that an essential prerequisite to the de-

velopment of effective community psychiatric services is the delineation of small, geographically defined areas or sectors as the unit of service provision. The concept of the 'psychiatrie de secteur' was first developed in France after 1947. By 1961, over 300 sectors had been established in departments across half of the country. In 1963 the Kennedy Community Mental Health Centres (CMHC) Act in the USA was introduced, and with it the concept of a catchment area for each CMHC, which by 1975 provided for 40% of the US population (Levine 1981, Goldman *et al.* 1983).

In Europe, throughout the 1970s, the organizing principle of sectorization was widely applied to areas in West Germany (sector size 250 000), The Netherlands (300 000), Denmark (60–120 000), Finland (100 000), Norway (40 000), and Sweden (25–50 000) (Lindholm 1983), and the most comprehensive implementation of the concept in Italy with sectors of in the range 50–200 000 population (Tansella *et al.* 1987). Evaluations have concentrated to a large extent on establishing whether sectorization would facilitate the development of community alternatives to inpatient hospital treatment. A number of advantages have been claimed for sectorized services (Tyrer 1985, Hansson 1989), and these are summarized in Table 28.1.

**Table 28.1** Reported advantages of sectorization

1 Defined responsibility for each patient requiring a service
2 Economies of small scale: close working local links between agencies
3 Clarity of functions of local teams
4 Manageable scale for local needs assessments
5 Minimizes patients lost to follow-up
6 Allows comparative research and evaluation between different service models across sectors
7 Improves identity of staff with locality
8 Greater budgetary clarity
9 Potential for improved primary care liaison
10 Allows interagency assessment, treatment and care
11 Enables integration of health, social and voluntary services
12 Facilitates home treatment and day care services
13 Preferred by patients and families

## Components of a comprehensive community mental health service

A comprehensive community care system must address the wide range of needs of individuals with mental health disorders (Fig. 28.1). Using the 'components' and 'functions' distinction outlined above, this section focuses on some of the main components of community services and outlines some of the 'functions' considered to be of importance. The categories delineated are not mutually exclusive, and as in any local settings, the organization and form of such services should ideally be constructed on the basis of the results of the local data available.

### Crisis response and acute care

One of the fundamental aims of mental health treatment must be the practice of secondary and tertiary prevention (Newton 1989). There is a body of literature which indicates that adequate treatment, associated with client, family and staff education and training, can prevent the onset of many crises (Falloon *et al.* 1984, Birchwood *et al.* 1989). Because of the episodic nature of the illness, however, there will be instances that require acute care and rapid response crisis stabilization services. The aim of the services should be to enable the client, family members, and others to cope with the emergency while maintaining the client's status as a functioning community member to the greatest extent. The services should be available on a 24-hour basis and be known to providers, families, clients and the community. Immediate psychiatric consultation should be available for rapid evaluation, diagnosis, and chemotherapeutic interventions as indicated.

The traditional provision of crisis intervention has been through consultation at the local GPs surgery (Murray Parkes *et al.* 1962), domiciliary consultation (Littlejohns 1986, Fry & Sandler 1988, K. Sutherby *et al.* 1991, unpublished report) and in many districts accident and emergency departments of general hospitals. With the development of community services this has been extended by a range of options which include: 24-hour telephone helpline; walk-in emergency clinics (Lim 1983, Haw & Lanceley 1987); community mental health centre facilities and mobile outreach crisis intervention teams (Boardman 1987); community crisis residential beds for temporary respite care outside the normal residential environment when needed; and inpatient beds in a variety of settings such as the psychiatric units of a district general hospital. In reviewing the community care experience of the USA, Bachrach (1984) has cautioned that the decrease in beds has led to excessive use of emergency services by young psychotic patients who use no other facilities. The system of open access of British primary care services may result in primary care teams having an increasing role to play in this regard (Kendrick *et al.* 1991).

Acute treatment facilities should be available in a range of residential settings to provide assessment by a multidisciplinary team: investigation facilities to exclude an organic basis for a mental health disorder; supportive counselling and psychotherapeutic treatment; and mechanisms for the provision and monitoring of medication and to ensure maximum therapeutic effectiveness.

The location of such services has been the subject of major debate. Particular attention has been paid to the question of the role of the hospital and the appropriateness of alternative facilities including hospital hostels, home-based teams and pre-admission facilities. Tyrer (1985), in proposing his 'Hive' model, advocates that the hospital base should form the core of a system with closely coordinated subunits of care such as day hospitals, community clinics, or mental health centres located in areas of greatest morbidity.

### Continuing care and outreach

Since the early 1960s a number of studies have compared home-based care with hospital care (Test & Stein 1980, Hoult & Reynolds 1984, Marks *et al.* 1988, Dean & Gadd 1990). Despite differences in the models and evaluative methodologies used, these studies confirm a decrease in hospital admissions, improvement in clinical outcome and social functioning and greater patient satisfaction from acute home-orientated care. The outreach model of service delivery to the seriously mentally ill assumes that such patients require the following elements to avoid frequent rehospitalization: material resources (such as food, shelter and clothing), coping skills, motivation, freedom from pathologically dependent relationships, community support and education, and assertive home-based psychiatric treatment (Stein & Test 1980, Tessler & Goldman 1982). Replication of this model in Sydney (Hoult 1986) and Montreal (Fenton *et al.* 1982) has demonstrated that the approach can be successfully adapted, and an application of case management in inner city Chicago has been shown to be cost effective (Bond 1984). Patient outcome from these outreach programmes is in no published case worse than standard hospital treatment, and is often better (Kiesler 1982).

### Consultation and liaison services

Until the past few decades the majority of consultation services were conducted in hospital outpatient settings. Evaluation of the services indicates dissatisfaction with communication patterns (Pullen & Yellowlees 1988), clinical and referrer outcome (Kaeser & Cooper 1971, Strathdee 1990). The appropriateness of psychiatry's uncritical emulation of the model of general medicine, particularly for those with long-term disorders, has been questioned (Todd 1984).

Two innovations in community provisions have begun to redress the deficiencies. First, there has been an evolution of outpatient clinics from hospital sites and the establishment of consultation clinics in primary care settings; 19% of all consultant general adult psychiatrists in England and Wales (Strathdee & Williams 1984) and half the Scottish psychiatrists (Pullen & Yellowlees 1988) work in this way. The evidence indicates that the clinics enhance continuity of care, particularly when the psychiatric team works in an integrated manner with their primary care colleagues. Additional advantages cited are that patients prefer the accessibility and non-stigmatizing setting of their local surgery; the GPs enhance their knowledge of psychiatric disorders and treatment techniques; and the psychiatric team

have increased access to community resources and are better placed to intervene at an earlier stage in the development of illness and relapse (Tyrer 1984, Mitchell 1985, Hansen 1987, Brown *et al.* 1988, Creed & Marks 1989, Joseph *et al.* 1990).

Secondly, a growing number of community mental health centres have been established. Kingdon's survey (1989) indicates that they have been developed in 18% of districts, with plans afoot in another 40%. The American community mental health centres attempted to provide five services: inpatient, outpatient, partial hospitalization, emergency services, consultation and education. In the UK those described have functioned more as a resource for crisis intervention, coordinating multidisciplinary teams and as consultation services (Tufnell *et al.* 1985, Patmore & Weaver 1991).

### Day care

Day care facilities vary enormously in their range and remit. In a comprehensive review Holloway (1988) defines five possible functions of the day hospital: an alternative to admission for the acutely ill; provision of support, supervision and monitoring in the transition between hospital and home; source of long-term structure and support for those with chronic handicaps; site for brief intensive therapy for those with personality difficulties, severe neurotic disorders and those who require short-term focused rehabilitation; an information, training and communication resource. The development of day centres by local authorities has progressed in parallel to the provisions by health authorities (Vaughan 1986).

### Respite

The practices covered by the term 'respite care' are of increasing importance in mental health service provision. Such respite care provides relatively brief planned periods of residential care, usually of between one week and one month, during which the patient may be fully reassessed, treatment can be modified, the family can benefit from relief of the burden of care, and the patient may be given temporary sanctuary from the demands of everyday life, which may include an emotionally charged atmosphere at home. To date, respite care has been most fully developed for people with learning difficulties (Gerard 1990), with physical disabilities (Robinson 1984) and for the elderly (Harper 1988). While there is evidence of substantial benefits for patients and their carers, within mental illness services, respite services are as yet poorly developed and await full evaluation.

## Health and dental care

Patients treated in the community are often the most severely ill and vulnerable who have significant requirements for physical, as well as psychiatric care (Eastwood & Trevelyan 1972, Brugha *et al.* 1989). In a study of 145 long-term users of hospital and social services day psychiatric facilities, Brugha *et al.* (1989) found that 41% suffered medical problems potentially requiring care. Therefore it is important to liaise with the providers of medical care, most often the primary care doctors. This aspect of need is advantaged when services are located in the general hospital.

## Housing

Carling & Ridgeway (1985) have asserted that individuals have a basic right to affordable, acceptable housing available in the normal housing arrangements typically used in the community. Garety (1988), in a comprehensive review, examines the range of provisions currently evolving. These include sheltered accommodation, hostels or foster family care schemes. To the greatest extent possible, the individual should exercise choice and control over his/her living environment. The skills, training, supports and services needed to enable clients to reside successfully in their own homes in normal community settings should be available and accessible regardless of where the individuals are living. There should also be a small number of supervised, structured settings for extremely dysfunctional individuals.

To ensure the success of community housing provisions, liaison with community members and caring agencies is essential. Horder (1990) has defined practical guidelines for the functioning of community hostels. She states that they should be within easy access of shops, sports facilities, cinemas, day centres, workshops and pubs; a clear plan for medical cover should be formulated before the admission of residents; there should be detailed discussion with all staff members, especially GPs, if they are to be involved, and agreement about spheres of responsibility, emergency work, prescribing and communication needs to be reached. Aside from permanent housing, homeless individuals who are mentally ill will require additional living situations with varying degrees of supervision and structure including emergency shelters (Fisher & Breakey 1986).

Studies suggest that mental illness rates in the homeless range from 41% to 93%, alcohol dependency occurs in over 60%, and chronic medical and dental problems in over 40% of this group (Morrisey & Levine 1987, Bassuk 1984, Kroll *et al.* 1986) (see also Chapter 21). These individuals characteristically have restricted social support networks, little contact with psychiatric services, lower readmission rates than their domiciled counterparts, and little likelihood of referral to long-term care facilities (Appleby & Desai 1985). Local psychiatric facilities clearly do not serve these homeless mentally ill at all adequately (Lamb 1984).

There is, by comparison, relatively scant British psychiatric literature on the homeless mentally ill and this has focused on people living in lodging houses (Priest 1986), reception centres, and those in prison or hospital who are of no fixed abode (Herzberg 1987). The American Psychiatric Association Task Force on the Homeless Mentally Ill (Lamb & Talbott 1986) recommended the establishment of a wide range of local supervised housing options, a greater provision of general medical care, peripatetic psychiatric services and crisis intervention, together with a secure and simplified source of income. It further recommended that the mental health services should become more integrated, based upon the case manager model, and that asylum should be provided for the small proportion of patients who continued to need sanctuary (Lamb & Talbott 1986).

## Advocacy

The importance of advocacy and user involvement at all levels within services has been increasingly acknowledged (Brandon & Brandon 1987, World Psychiatric Association 1990). Bassett *et al.* (1991) define four categories of involvement. At the individual clinical level, active participation can include having access to documentation and involvement in goal setting and reviews. Involvement of users at all stages of the planning process may facilitate alliances between professionals and their clients and ensure more effective implementation of the services. User participation in the monitoring and management of the service and in training and education are also important areas. Users' charters emphasize the rights of patients to privacy, consultation, information and choice (Beeforth *et al.* 1991). Mechanisms to inform individuals and their families of their legal rights are the responsibility of the services.

## Family and community education and support

Many persons with severe, disabling mental illness reside with their families, with consequences which must be addressed. The process of daily care for relatives who have severe social and behavioural disturbance takes place at the cost of disruption to family routine, resulting physical and psychological morbidity to the health of the other family members, and costs to the economic viability of the family unit. There should be assistance to families that provides education on the nature of the illness, consultation and supportive counselling on handling daily problems and intermittent crisis situations, appropriate involvement in the treatment planning process, respite care and referrals to family support groups and advocacy organizations such as the national or local mental health associations. In addition, in order to facilitate community integration and acceptance, practical support and education should be available to landlords, employers, educationalists, community agencies and others.

A number of approaches are in common use and although they have different names have very similar components (Leff 1985). These include work conducted in Pittsburgh and originally described as 'social therapy', now superseded by 'psycho-educational programmes', focusing on the transfer of useful knowledge about schizophrenia and the teaching of communication and problem-solving skills (Anderson *et al.* 1986). Falloon *et al.* (1984) and Falloon (1989) have developed an effective, family-based treatment package for schizophrenia. The patient-orientated management combines optimal neuroleptic drug therapy, rehabilitation, counselling, problem-solving psychotherapy, crisis intervention, and practical assistance with problems such as finances and housing. Other approaches employ more eclectic methods in family meetings with the aim of reducing expressed emotion (Leff *et al.* 1990). The main problem is the dissemination of the techniques to teams in ordinary clinical settings, and a number of programmes have been established with this aim.

## Rehabilitation and resettlement services

Rehabilitation services are critical for most individuals living in the community. The functions of rehabilitation include: enabling the individual to acquire or regain the practical skills needed to live and socialize in the community; teaching clients how to cope with their disabilities; assistance in developing social skills, interests and leisure-time activities that provide a sense of participation and personal worth and that include opportunities for age-appropriate, culturally appropriate daytime and evening activities; and activities occurring to the extent possible in the natural setting where the client lives, works, learns and socializes, that teach daily and community living skills such as diet, personal hygiene, cooking, shopping, budgeting, housekeeping and use of transportation and other community resources. There should be a range of vocational services and employment opportunities available to assist in preparation for obtaining and maintaining employment. These could include vocational assessment and counselling, on-the-job training, job sharing, transitional employment, job development with local employers, and innovative approaches to using recovering consumers as mental health workers (Bennett 1983).

Interesting outcome data are now appearing from the study of the Team for the Assessment of Psychiatric Services (TAPS) at Friern and Claybury which to date has examined the clinical and social outcome of 278 long-stay patients one year after they have left hospital. The model of this team is further described in Chapters 24 and 32. Compared to hospital, this group of patients preferred their community homes, where they found a much less restrictive environment. In addition, there were no significant clinical or social differences when compared with the matched group who remained in hospital. The results support the view that community care cannot be provided cheaply, but for the former long-stay hospital patients discharged so far, the costs of community care are slightly less than for hospital treatment. It does not appear to be the case from these results that community care needs to be very expensive, and indeed it appears that reasonably good quality community care can continue to be provided for future cohorts of leavers without requiring major additional funds over and above the amounts eventually released from the closure of long-stay hospitals, and that this will be clearly preferred by patients.

### Peer support

The NIMH guidelines advocate consumer self-help groups and consumer-operated services in each locality, which are self defined and consumer controlled. These services are voluntary and based on choice, shared power, and people's needs for survival, friendship and a sense of community. The services generally supplement the formal mental health system and meet a variety of social and life support needs through: peer-support groups that meet regularly to share ideas, information and provide mutual support; drop-in centres or social clubs for individuals to socialize and build a support network; independent-living programmes that provide services such as assisting individuals to obtain financial benefits, housing, counselling and referral, independent living skills, training; job counselling and employment;

consumer-run housing, businesses, respite care or crisis assistance services and community education on mental illness and the potential of individuals with mental illness to lead productive, satisfying lives and to contribute to the communities in which they live.

### Conclusion

The approach to setting up a community psychiatric service described above is an attempt to make rational a process which is seldom so in the furious pace of change in psychiatric services in present-day Britain. In practice, service developments are frequently determined by expediency and lack any theoretical basis (Leff 1986). In addition to fluctuations in local financial resources, plans are vulnerable to political and policy changes (Holloway 1990, Murphy 1991). Despite the complexity of the task, establishing services will be facilitated if joint strategic objectives are agreed from the outset, priorities are determined and the professionals, users and others involved are committed to audit and evaluation, with a genuine willingness to alter the service in the light of the results.

### References

Anderson C., Hogarty G. & Reiss D. (1986) Family treatment of adult schizophrenic patients: a psycho-educational approach. *Schizophrenia Bulletin* 6, 490–505.

Appleby L. & Desai P. (1985) Documenting the relationship between homelessness and psychiatric hospitalisation. *Hospital and Community Psychiatry* 36, 732–736.

Audit Commission (1986) *Making a Reality of Community Care*. HMSO, London.

Bachrach L.L. (1984) The young adult chronic psychiatric patient in an era of deinstitutionalisation. *American Journal of Public Health* 74, 382–4.

Bachrach L. (1986) Deinstitutionalisation: what do the numbers mean? *Hospital and Community Psychiatry* 37, 118–121.

Bassett T., Braisby D., Edwards S. & Newbiggin K. (1991) Involving service users in community mental health services. In Echlin R. (ed.) *Community Mental Health Centres/Teams*. Good Practices in Mental Health, London.

Bassuk E. (1984) The homelessness problem. *Scientific American* 251, 40–46.

Beeforth M., Conlon E., Field V., Hoser B. & Sayce L. (eds) (1991) *Whose Service is it Anyway?* Research & Development for Psychiatry, London.

Bennett D. (1983) The historical development of rehabilitation services. In Watts F. & Bennett D. (eds) *The Theory and Practice of Psychiatric Rehabilitation*, pp. 15–42. Wiley, Chichester.

Birchwood M., Smith J., Macmillan F. *et al.* (1989) Predicting relapse in schizophrenia: the development and implementation of an early signs monitoring system using patients and families as observers, a preliminary investigation. *Psychological Medicine* 18, 649–656.

Boardman J. (1987) *The Mental Health Advice Centre in Lewisham. Service Usage: Trends from 1978–1984. Research Report No. 3*. The National Unit for Psychiatric Research and Development, Lewisham.

Bond G. (1984) An economic analysis of psychosocial rehabilitation. *Hospital and Community Psychiatry* 35, 356–362.

Brandon D. & Brandon A. (1987) Consumers as colleagues. In *Power in strange places: user involvement in mental health services*. Good Practices in Mental Health, London.

Brown R., Strathdee G., Christie-Brown J. & Robinson P. (1988) A comparison of referrals to primary care and hospital outpatient clinics. *British Journal of Psychiatry* 153, 168–173.

Brugha T.S., Wing J.K. & Smith B.L. (1989) Physical ill-health of the long-term mentally ill in the community. Is there an unmet need? *British Journal of Psychiatry* 155, 777–782.

Busfield J. (1986) *Managing Madness: Changing Ideas and Practice*. Hutchinson, London.

Carling P. & Ridgeway P. (1985) Community residential rehabilitation: an emerging approach to meeting housing needs. In Carling P. & Rideway P. (eds) *Providing Housing and Supports for People with Psychiatric Disabilities*, pp. 1–28. NIMH, Rockville, MD.

Carse J., Panton N. & Watt A. (1958) A district mental health service. The Worthing Experiment. *Lancet* i, 39–41.

Creed F. & Marks B. (1989) Liaison psychiatry in general practice: a comparison of the liaison-attachment scheme and the shifted outpatient clinic models. *Journal of the Royal College of General Practitioners* 39, 514–517.

Dean C. & Gadd E.M. (1990) Home treatment for acute psychiatric illness. *British Medical Journal* 301, 1021–1024.

Department of Health & Social Security (1971) *Hospital Services for the Mentally Ill*. HMSO, London.

Department of Health & Social Security (1975) *Better Services for the Mentally Ill*. HMSO, London.

Department of Health & Social Security (1978) *Collaboration in Community Care. Central Health Services Council*. HMSO, London.

Department of Health & Social Security (1981) *Care in Action*. HMSO, London.

Department of Health & Social Security (1986) DHSS Background Policy Papers. In Wilkinson G. & Freeman H. (eds) *The Provision of Mental Health Services in Britain: The Way Ahead*. Royal College of Psychiatrists, Gaskell, London.

Department of Health (1989a) *Caring for People*. HMSO, London.

Department of Health (1989b) *Working for Patients*. HMSO, London.

Der G. & Bebbington P. (1987) Depression in inner London. A register study. *Social Psychiatry* 22, 73–84.

Eastwood M.R. & Trevelyan M.H. (1972) Relationship between physical and psychiatric disorder. *Psychological Medicine* 2, 363–372.

Falloon I.R.H. (1989) Behavioural approaches in schizophrenia. In Williams P., Wilkinson G. & Rawnsley K. (eds) *Scientific Approaches on Epidemiological and Social Psychiatry. Essays in Honour of Michael Shepherd*. Routledge, London.

Falloon, I., Boyd J.L. & McGill C.W. (1984) *Family Care of Schizophrenia*, pp. 355–375. Guildford Press, New York.

Fenton F., Tessier L., Struening E., Smith F. & Benoit C. (1982) *Home and Hospital Psychiatric Treatment*. Croom Helm, London.

Fisher P. & Breakey W. (1986) Homelessness and mental health: an overview. *International Journal of Mental Health* 14, 6–41.

Foucault M. (1971) *Madness and Civilisation*. Tavistock, London.

Freeman H. (1983) Concepts of community psychiatry. *British Journal of Hospital Medicine* 30, 90–96.

Fry J. & Sandler G. (1988) Domiciliary consultations: some fact and questions. *British Medical Journal* 297, 337–338.

Garety P. (1988) Housing. In Lavender A. & Holloway F. (eds) *Community Care in Practice*, pp. 143–161. Wiley, Chichester.

General Accounting Office (1977) *Returning the Mentally Disordered to the Community: The Government Needs to Do More*. Government Printing Office, Washington, DC.

Gerard K. (1990) Determining the contribution of residential care to the quality of life of children with severe learning difficulties. *Child Care Health and Development* 16, 177–188.

Giel R. & Horn ten G. (1982) Patterns of mental health care in a Dutch register area. *Social Psychiatry* 17, 117–123.

Gillis L. & Egert S. (1973) *The Psychiatric Outpatient: Clinical and Organisational Aspects*. Faber & Faber, London.

Goffman E. (1961). *Asylums*. Pelican, Harmondsworth.

Goldberg D. (1986) Implementation of mental health policies in the North West of England. In Wilkinson G. & Freeman H. (eds) *The Provision of Mental Health Services in Britain: The Way Ahead*. Royal College of Psychiatrists, Gaskell, London.

Goldberg D.P. & Blackwell B. (1970) Psychiatric illness in general practice: a detailed study using a new method of case identification. *British Medical Journal* 2, 439–443.

Goldberg D. & Jones R. (1980) The costs and benefits of psychiatric care. In Robins L. (ed.) *The Social Consequence of Psychiatric Illness*. Brunner-Mazel, New York.

Goldie N. & Freden L. (1991) A crisis of closure and openness: the present state of Swedish mental health system in the light of a policy of sectorisation. *Social Science and Medicine* 32, 499–506.

Goldman H., Adams N. & Taube C. (1983). Deinstitutionalisation: the data demythologised. *Hospital and Community Psychiatry* 32, 21–27.

Greater London Council (1984) *Mental Health Services in London*. GLC, London.

Griffiths R. (1988) *Community Care: An Agenda for Action*. HMSO, London.

Hansen V. (1987) Psychiatric service within primary care. Mode of organisation and influence on admission rates to a mental hospital. *Acta Psychiatrica Scandinavica* 76, 121–128.

Hansson L. (1989) Utilisation of psychiatric in-patient care. *Acta Psychiatrica Scandinavica* 79, 571–578.

Harper N. (1988) Planned short-stay admission to a geriatric unit: one aspect of respite care. *Age and Aging* 17, 199–204.

Haw C. & Lanceley C. (1987) Patients at a psychiatric walk-in clinic: who, how, why and when. *Bulletin of the Royal College of Psychiatrists* 11, 329–332.

Herzberg J. (1987) No fixed abode. *British Journal of Psychiatry* 150, 621–627.

Hirsch S. (1988) *Psychiatric Beds and Resources: Factors Influencing Bed Use and Service Planning*. Royal College of Psychiatrists, Gaskell, London.

Holloway F. (1988) Day Care and Community Support. In Lavender A. & Holloway F. (eds) *Community Care in Practice*. Wiley, Chichester.

Holloway F. (1990) Caring for people: a critical review of British Government policy for the community care of the mentally ill. *Psychiatric Bulletin* 14, 641–645.

Horder E. (1990) Medical care in three psychiatric hostels in Hampstead and Bloomsbury District Health Authority. Hampstead and South Barnet GP Forum and the Hampstead Department of Community Medicine, London.

Hornten G., Giel R., Gulbinat W. & Henderson J. (eds) (1986) *Psychiatric Case Registers in Public Health. A Worldwide Inventory, 1960–1985*. Elsevier, Amsterdam.

Hoult J. (1986) Community care of the acutely mentally ill. *British Journal of Psychiatry* 149, 137–144.

Hoult J. & Reynolds I. (1984) Community orientated treatment compared to hospital orientated psychiatric treatment. *Social Science and Medicine* 18, 1005–10.

House of Commons (1985) *Second Report from the Social Services Committee, Session 1984–85, Community Care*. HMSO, London.

House of Commons (1990) *National Health Service and Community Care Act*. HMSO, London.

Hunter D. & Wistow G. (1987) Mapping the organisational context. 1. Central departments, boundaries and responsibilities In *Community Care in Britain: Variations on a Theme*, pp. 18–46. King Edward's Hospital Fund for London.

Jeffreys P. (1979) Joint approaches to community care. In Meacher M. (ed.) *New Methods of Mental Health Care*, pp. 15–33. Mental Health Foundation, London.

Johnstone E.C., Owens D.G.C., Gold A., Crow T.J. & MacMillan J.F. (1984) Schizophrenic patients discharged from hospital – a follow-up study. *British Journal of Psychiatry* 145, 586–590.

Jones K. (1972) *A History of the Mental Health Services*. Routledge and Kegan Paul, London.

Jones M. (1952) *Social Psychiatry*. London, Tavistock.

Joseph P., Bridgewater J.A., Ramsden S.S. & El Kabir D.J. (1990) A psychiatric clinic for the single homeless in a primary care setting in inner London. *Psychiatric Bulletin* 14, 270–271.

Kaeser A.C. & Cooper B. (1971) The psychiatric out-patient, the general practitioner and the out-patient clinic; an operational study: a review. *Psychological Medicine* 1, 312–325.

Kendrick A., Sibbald B., Burns T. & Freeling P. (1991) Role of general practitioners in care of long term mentally ill patients. *British Medical Journal* 302, 508–511.

Kiesler C. (1982) Mental hospitals and alternative care. *American Psychologist* 37, 349–360.

Kingdon D. (1989) Mental health services: results of a survey of English district plans. *Psychiatric Bulletin* 13, 77–78.

Klein R. (1991) The politics of change. *British Medical Journal* 320, 1102–1103.

Kroll J., Carey K., Hagedorn D., Dog P. & Benavides, E. (1986). A survey of homeless adults in urban shelters. *Hospital and Community Psychiatry* 37, 283–286.

Lamb H. (1984) Deinstitutionalisation and the homeless mentally ill. *Hospital and Community Psychiatry* 35, 899–907.

Lamb R. & Talbott J. (1986) The homeless mentally ill. *Journal of the American Medical Association* 156, 498–501.

Lee A.S. & Murray R.M. (1988) The long-term outcome of Maudsley depressives. *British Journal of Psychiatry* 153, 741–751.

Leff J. (1985) Family treatment of schizophrenia. In Granville-Grossman K. (ed.) *Recent Advances in Clinical Psychiatry* 5, pp. 49–61. Churchill Livingstone, London.

Leff J. (1986) Planning a community psychiatric service: from theory to practice. In Wilkinson G. & Freeman H. (eds) *The Provision of Mental Health Services in Britain: The Way Ahead*. Royal College of Psychiatrists, Gaskell, London.

Leff J., Berkowitz R., Shavit N., Strachan A., Glass I. &

Vaughn C. (1990) A trial of family therapy versus a relatives' group for schizophrenia. Two year follow-up. *British Journal of Psychiatry* 157, 571–577.

Lesage A. & Tansella M. (1989) Mobility of schizophrenic patients, non-psychotic patients and the general population in a case register area. *Social Psychiatry and Psychiatric Epidemiology* 24, 271–274.

Levine M. (1981) *The History and Politics of Community Mental Health.* Oxford University Press, London.

Leyberg J.T. (1959) A district psychiatric service. The Bolton pattern. *Lancet* i, 282–284.

Lim M.H. (1983) A psychiatric emergency clinic; a study of attendances over six months. *British Journal of Psychiatry* 143, 480–466.

Lindholm H. (1983) Sectorised psychiatry. *Acta Psychiatrica Scandinavica* 67, supplement 304.

Littlejohns P. (1986) Domiciliary consultations – who benefits? *Journal of the Royal College of General Practitioners* 36, 313–315.

Lord Glenarthur (1986) Introduction and current developments. In Wilkinson G. & Freeman H. (eds) *The Provision of Mental Health Services in Britain: The Way Ahead,* pp. 1–5. Gaskell, London.

Marks I.M., Connolly J. & Muijen M. (1988) The Maudsley Daily Living Programme. *Psychiatric Bulletin of the Royal College of Psychiatrists* 12, 22–23.

Mechanic D. (1987) Correcting misconceptions in mental health policy: strategies for improved care of the seriously mentally ill. *The Millbank Quarterly* 65, 203–230.

MIND (1983) *Common Concern.* MIND Publications, London.

Ministry of Health (1963) *Health and Welfare: The Development of Community Care. Plans for the Health and Welfare Services of the Local Authorities in England and Wales.* Cmnd 1973. HMSO, London.

Mitchell A.R.K. (1985) Psychiatrists in primary health care settings. *British Journal of Psychiatry* 147, 371–370.

Mollica R. (1983) From asylum to community. *New England Journal of Medicine* 308, 367–373.

Morrisey J. & Goldman H. (1984) Cycles of reform in the care of the chronically mentally ill. *Hospital and Community Psychiatry* 35, 785–793.

Morrisey J. & Levine I. (1987) Researchers discuss latest findings, examine needs of homeless mentally ill persons. *Hospital and Community Psychiatry* 38, 811–812.

Mosher L. (1983) Alternatives to psychiatric hospitalisation. *New England Journal of Medicine* 309, 1579–1580.

Murphy E. (1987) Community care: I problems. *British Medical Journal* 295, 1505–1508.

Murphy E. (1988) Community care: II possible solutions. *British Medical Journal* 296, 6–8.

Murphy E. (1991) Delaying community care. *British Medical Journal* 302, 361–362.

Murray Parkes C., Brown G.W. & Monck E.M. (1962) The general practitioner and the schizophrenic patient. *British Medical Journal* 1, 972–976.

National Institute of Mental Health (1987) *Towards a Model for a Comprehensive Community-based Mental Health System.* NIMH, Washington DC.

Newton J. (1989) *The Prevention of Mental Illness.* Routledge & Kegan Paul, London.

Pantellis C., Taylor J. & Campbell P. (1988) The South Camden schizophrenia survey. *Psychiatric Bulletin* 12, 98–101.

Patmore C. & Weaver T. (1991) *Community Mental Health Teams: Lessons for Planners and Managers,* pp. 165–184. Good Practices in Mental Health, London.

Paykel E. (1990) Innovations in mental health in the primary care system. In Marks I. & Scott R. (eds) *Mental Health Service Evaluation.* Cambridge Univeristy Press, Cambridge.

Priest R. (1986) Hospital beds for psychiatric patients. *Bulletin of the Royal College of Psychiatrists* 10, 322–323.

Pullen I. & Yellowlees A. (1988) Scottish psychiatrists in primary health care settings: a silent majority. *British Journal of Psychiatry* 153, 633–636.

Ramon S. (1988) Community care in Britain. In Lavender A. & Holloway F. (eds) *Community Care in Practice.* Wiley, Chichester.

Robinson A. (1984) *Respite Care Services for Families with a Handicapped Child.* National Children's Bureau, London.

Royal College of Psychiatrists (1990) *Caring for a Community: 1. The Model Mental Health Service.* Gaskell, London.

Sabshin M. (1966) Theoretical models in community and social psychiatry. In Roberts L., Halbeck S. & Loeb M. (eds) *Community Psychiatry.* University of Wisconsin Press, Madison.

Scull A. (1979) *Museums of Madness.* Allen Lane, London.

Scull A. (1984) *Decarceration.* Polity, Cambridge.

Secretaries of State for Health, Wales, Northern Ireland and Scotland (1989) *Working for Patients.* HMSO, London.

Secretaries of State for Health, Wales, Northern Ireland and Scotland. Medical Audit (1990) *Caring for People.* HMSO, London.

Seymour F. (1986) Regional perspectives on planning mental health services. In Wilkinson G. & Freeman H. (eds) *The Provision of Mental Health Services in Britain: The Way Ahead,* pp. 6–63. Gaskell, London.

Sharpe D. & Morrell D. (1989) The psychiatry of general practice. In Williams P., Wilkinson G. & Rawnsley K. (eds) *Scientific Approaches on Epidemiological and Social Psychiatry. Essays in Honour of Michael Shepherd,* pp. 404–420. Routledge, London.

Shepherd M., Cooper B., Brown A. & Kalton G. (1966) *Psychiatric Illness in General Practice.* Oxford University Press, Oxford.

Social Services Committee 1984/85 Session, Second Report, (1985) *Community Care with Special Reference to Adult Mentally Ill and Mentally Handicapped People.* HMSO, London.

South East Thames Regional Health Authority (1985) *Regional Mental Health Strategy 1985–1994*. SETRHA.

South East Thames Regional Health Authority (1986) *A Policy for Mental Health Services*. SETRHA.

Stein L. & Test M. (1980) Alternative to mental hospital treatment. I Conceptual model, treatment program and clinical evaluation. *Archives of General Psychiatry* 37, 392–397.

Strathdee G. (1990) The delivery of psychiatric care. *Journal of the Royal Society of Medicine* 83, 222–225.

Strathdee G. (1992a) The role of primary care in the development of community psychiatric services. In Weller M. & Muijens M. (eds) *Community Psychiatric Services*. Ballière, Tindall, London (in press).

Strathdee G. (1992b) The interface between psychiatry and primary care in the management of schizophrenic patients in the community. In Jenkins R., Field V. & Young R. (eds) *The Primary Care of Schizophrenia*, pp. 59–68. HMSO, London.

Strathdee G. & Williams P. (1984) A survey of psychiatrists in primary care: the silent growth of a new service. *Journal of the Royal College of General Practitioners* 34, 615–618.

Sytema S., Balestrieri M., Geil R., Horn ten G., & Tansella M. (1989) Use of mental health services in South-Verona and Groningen. *Acta Psychiatrica Scandinavica* 79, 153–162.

Tansella M. (1986) Community psychiatry without mental hospitals – the Italian experience: a review. *Journal of the Royal Society of Medicine* 79, 664–669.

Tansella M. (1989) Evaluating community psychiatric services. In Williams P., Wilkinson G. & Rawnsley K. (eds) *Scientific Approaches on Epidemiological and Social Psychiatry. Essays in Honour of Michael Shepherd*. Routledge, London.

Tansella M., de Salvia D. & Williams P. (1987) The Italian psychiatric reform: some quantitative evidence. *Social Psychiatry* 22, 37–48.

Tansella M. & Williams P. (1989) The spectrum of psychiatric morbidity in a defined geographical area. *Psychological Medicine* 19, 765–770.

TAPS (Team for the Assessment of Psychiatric Services) (1990) *Better Out than In?* North East Thames Regional Health Authority, London.

Tessler R. & Goldman H. (1982) *The Chronic Mentally Ill, Asessing the Community Support Program*. Ballinger, Cambridge.

Test M.A. & Stein L.J. (1980) Alternative to mental hospital treatment. 3, Social cost. *Archives of General Psychiatry* 37, 409–412.

Thornicroft G. (1988) Progress towards DHSS targets for community care. *British Journal of Psychiatry* 153, 257–258.

Thornicroft G. (1990) Case management for the severely mentally ill. *Social Psychiatry and Psychiatric Epidemiology* 25, 141–143.

Thornicroft G. & Bebbington P. (1989) Deinstitutionalisation: from hospital closure to service development. *British Journal of Psychiatry* 155, 739–753.

Todd J.W. (1984) Wasted resources. Referral to hospital. *Lancet* ii: 1089.

Torre E. & Marinoni A. (1985) Register studies: data from four areas in Northern Italy. *Acta Psychiatrica Scandinavica* Supplement 136, 87–94.

Tufnell G., Borras N., Watson J.P. & Brough D.I. (1985) Home assessment and treatment in community psychiatric service. *Acta Psychiatrica Scandinavica* 72, 20–28.

Tyrer P. (1984) Psychiatric clinics in general practice: an extension of community care. *British Journal of Psychiatry* 145, 9–14.

Tyrer P. (1985) The 'hive' system: a model for a psychiatric service. *British Journal of Psychiatry* 146, 571–575.

Tyrer P., Turner R. & Johnson A. (1989) Integrated hospital and community psychiatric services and use of inpatient beds. *British Medical Journal* 299, 298–300.

Vaughan P.J.C. (1986) A question of balance. *Health Service Journal* 96, 1260–1261.

Walsh D. (1987) Mental health service models in Europe. In *Mental Health Services in Pilot Study Areas: Report on a European Study*. WHO, Copenhagen.

Wiersma D., Giel R., de Jong A. & Slooff C. (1983) Social class and schizophrenia in a Dutch cohort. *Psychological Medicine* 13, 141–150.

Wing J. (1989) *Health Services Planning and Research*. Royal College of Psychiatrists, Gaskell, London.

Wing J. & Brown G. (1970) *Institutionalism and Schizophrenia*. Cambridge University Press, Cambridge.

Wolfensberger W. (1970) The principle of normalisation and its implications to psychiatric services. *American Journal of Psychiatry* 127, 291–297.

Wolfensberger W. (1983) Social role valorisation: a proposed new term for the principle of normalisation. *Mental Retardation* 21, 234–239.

World Health Organization (1983) *First Contact Mental Health Care*. WHO Regional Office for Europe, Copenhagen.

World Psychiatric Association (1990) WPA statement and viewpoints on the rights and legal safeguards of the mentally ill. *WPA Bulletin*. 1, 32–33.

# Chapter 29
## Setting Up Services for Ethnic Minorities

PARIMALA MOODLEY

Ethnic minorities or racial minorities in the UK comprise about 4% of the population, some two and a quarter million people, the largest proportion being of South Asian origin: people from India, Pakistan, Bangladesh and Sri Lanka. People of Afro-Caribbean origin constitute the next largest group accounting for about one million people. There are also significant numbers of people from Africa, South-East Asia and the Mediterranean. Ethnic minorities therefore are not one homogeneous group but extremely diverse with a bewildering mix of cultures, traditions, languages and experiences of migration and resettlement. People originating from one continent or geographical region may have very little in common, for example, Somalis and Zambians, Southern Indian Tamils and Punjabi Sikhs.

This chapter presents principles of service provision for ethnic minorities whilst acknowledging their diversity. It has tended to concentrate on the most visible of the minority groups and those who are represented in the largest concentrations. The principles however remain the same for all.

The language used in this chapter varies considerably both in terms of describing people of ethnic minority origin and when describing those we serve. There is no consensus on whether the people we serve should be known as patients, clients, customers, survivors, users or recipients. Similarly there is no single satisfactory term to describe those who are not white. Black is a political term which many South Asians and South-East Asians find unacceptable. It does, however, bring together those of us who have as their one commonality discrimination on the basis of colour.

Given that racial minorities constitute such a small percentage of the general population, why is there a need to discuss services for them separately? There is a growing recognition that ethnic minority communities are being inadequately served by the psychiatric services. According to Davies (1990), 'In many boroughs (of London) the mental health needs of the black and ethnic communities are not met.' This is despite the fact that in many inner city areas the racial minority communities may represent between 20% and 30% of the population. There is now increasing evidence that psychiatric services are operating differently for blacks and whites and services may be differentially disadvantaging blacks (Moodley & Perkins (1991).

According to Connelly (1988), there are five reasons why race aspects need to be considered:
1 *Common humanity*. People with mental health problems are vulnerable; ignoring their diversities will add to their problems instead of alleviating them.
2 *Social justice*. Black people are taxpayers and community charge payers. As such they are entitled to expect services as a matter of routine and not as an afterthought.
3 *Professional integrity*. Competence in dealing with diversity should be a matter of professional integrity.
4 *Statutory obligations*. All providers of services are required by the 1976 Race Relations Act to ensure that there is no direct or indirect discrimination occurring.
5 *Utilization of resources*. There are many potential sources of support and care within the community which can be used to improve care.

Equal access and equal treatment are not occurring automatically. They require critical attention at the earliest stages of planning. Failure to do so will result in inadequate planning, inadequate resources and inevitably inadequate services.

## Philosophy and principles

A shared philosophy of care is the bedrock of any service. *The aim must be to provide equitable services for all users*, but equitable does not mean equal in the sense of the *same* service, rather a service equally appropriate to the needs of all. If for example my staple diet is curry and rice then I should be able to receive that as regularly as you would expect to get your meat and two vegetables if that is your staple diet.

Agreement should be reached at the outset by all the shareholders – health, social services, voluntary services, housing, education, the community and the users – concerning who shall be served and what the aims and objective should be.

Appropriate services for ethnic minority users should be clearly enunciated in the mission statement and in all other documentation relating to the philosophy and principle. In the previous chapter we described the principles as described by Paumelle (continuity, coordination and integration) and the National Institute of Mental Health (consumer-centred, client empowerment, racial and cultural appropriateness, flexibility, focused on strengths, normalization and the use of natural supports, meeting special needs, accountability, and coordination).

There are three additional principles that are fundamental to the provision of services to ethnic minorities:

### 1 SERVICES SHOULD BE APPROPRIATE

Services are seen to be too heavy handed in their responses at times, whilst on other occasions there is no response when people are in desparate need (Francis *et al.* 1989). Heavy handedness may be a result of negative stereotyping, as may be neglect, and this can affect both the type and the amount of care. For example:

> A young body builder who had his third hypomanic episode and threatened to kill himself if he was dragged into hospital where his previous admission lasted more than 3 months, was viewed by the GP as potentially dangerous to other people (although there was no evidence of violence to people) and as

requiring immediate admission under a Section of the Mental Health Act. The large and very caring family, having had previous experience of the police requiring to manhandle him to get him to the hospital where he required high doses of medication, preferred him to be admitted voluntarily. He refused but agreed to accept medication at home and was 'specialled' by his family. His mental state improved with home care over the next 48 to 72 hours.

Clearly this was a particular set of circumstances which enabled this form of management. A young man in very similar circumstances, who had no visible family or social network, was surrounded by hostile neighbours and was refusing to accept any form of treatment, did require admission under the Mental Health Act. Decisions have to be made on the basis of the person's situation and the resources or lack of them in the person's community. Appropriateness needs to be considered in all aspects of assessment and delivery of care. Recognition of the need to assess appropriately is crucial; for example, an occupational therapy report on a 21-year-old Nigerian man stated that he needed training in activities of daily living, including cooking because he was unable to use the baking class. This was despite the comment within the report that he was able to prepare a Nigerian dish without the benefit of a recipe.

### 2 SERVICES SHOULD BE ACCESSIBLE

Services should not be just geographically accessible but, more importantly, they should be accessible in terms of language, culture and racial identity. Accessibility is thus not synonymous with being located in the community but rather that wherever the location of the service it is more 'user friendly'. The users should be aware that interpreters will be available should there be difficulties in communicating. Acknowledgement of the different festivals that people celebrate, for example, Eid and Diwali, and facilitating their celebration would make a service more user friendly.

## 3 SERVICES SHOULD BE ACCEPTABLE

Services should be acceptable to the community we are serving. There are many elements which make up an acceptable service. The employment of staff from similar backgrounds in positions other than that of the most menial is a convincing demonstration of 'positivity'. A good staff mix in terms of gender as well as ethnic origin, and staff who demonstrate their understanding of, or willingness to learn about, cultural and racial issues help to make a service acceptable. The facilities which are provided in terms of physical structure of buildings should be appropriate, for instance, the provision of washing facilities in the toilet areas for those people who traditionally use water to cleanse themselves rather than toilet paper.

The preceding chapter has described the constituents of a good service, whether they are based on the needs of the users or the functional components. Services to ethnic minorities have to have additional components:

## 1 INTERPRETATION AND TRANSLATION SERVICES

Communication is a vital aspect of psychiatric assessment and management and of service provision. All relevant documentation pertaining to users' rights should be translated into the languages spoken by the local community. A bank of well-trained interpreters should be available in the local area for all the commonly spoken languages. Access to interpreters for those languages which are required less frequently should be available. All staff should be aware of the necessity to use the interpreter service if there is any doubt about communication. Failure to do so will disadvantage the patient and could be seen as discriminatory. Family members should only be used as interpreters *in extremis*. It is unfair to both patients and families for many reasons, including embarrassment and vested interests in the outcome.

Interpreters should be trained for the purpose of conducting psychiatric interviews. This is a highly skilled exercise. Common errors that occur include omission, addition, condensation, substitution and role exchange (Vasquez & Javier 1991). Staff need to be trained to use interpreters. Both interpreters and those using them should be trained to separate 'data' from 'judgement' or 'opinion'. A good interpreter tells you what the person says, including the neologisms, the swear words, the references to ghosts and spirits and the flight of ideas, with no embarrassment. The interpreter should be asked to give an opinion on the utterances, the general demeanour and presentation at a different point in the interview. This process, made explicit before the interview begins, will facilitate the separation of data from judgement. Staff should be enabled to practise interviewing with the aid of an interpreter.

## 2 SENSITIVITY TO RACIAL ASPECTS

No practitioner can do justice to the people they serve if they do not understand the 'culture' of their discipline and the broader context, i.e. social climate, of the society they belong to.

It is important to understand the extremely negative position that many black people find themselves in and the consequential judgement that all white authority figures are likely to persecute them or do them harm in some way. Thus confrontation by a white social worker and a white doctor for the purposes of an assessment for detention under the Mental Health Act may exacerbate an already tense situation. Racial minorities may live in areas where they are frequently the targets of racist attacks on the streets, in their schools and even in their homes. Black people may be isolated in the workplace with overt or covert racism. They have difficulties in gaining employment, as evidenced by the very high unemployment rates. All assessments must take into account these aspects of people's lives. Treatment plans which ignore these are not likely to succeed. Rehabilitation must take into account the fact that blacks are less likely to succeed in the job market. Day-care facilities where there are no other blacks may serve to increase the sense of isolation, and this has been seen particularly in the black elderly. Racial abuse and racial harassment which people may experience from other users of services and from the general public as they make their way to and from services is something which all service providers should be aware of. These are not issues which are easily brought to professional carers, and especially if they are white.

Fernando (1988) argues very cogently that psychiatry as a discipline has always been and continues to be imbued with racism. According to Sashidharan (1986), the transcultural approach which emphasizes the cultural dependence of clinical problems ignores 'the political and structural dimensions of contemporary racism . . . and the model for welfare/treatment provisions is isolated from the day to day struggles of black people in this country'. Whilst most psychiatrists will avow that they do look at the patient in context, few can honestly say that they examine the race aspects. It is too emotive a topic and it may go away if we ignore it. Unfortunately it does not go away but festers like a sore which erupts periodically. As a 27-year-old man with hypomania said:

> Man, you don't know what its like to be black in South London; you're just a nigger. You don't know what school I went to. They used to have National Front meetings. The teacher told me everything black was bad – blackmail, dirt, . . . .

He had left school 11 years ago. During his previous admission his school history had been recorded as 'uneventful'.

### 3 SENSITIVITY TO CULTURAL AND RELIGIOUS ISSUES

Recognition and acknowledgement of the diversity of culture and lifestyles of those around us is essential. People may have different eating habits, for example, many Indians eat with their fingers rather than with cutlery. This may make them the object of ridicule. Some people would never immerse their bodies in 'dirty water' as in a bath and would prefer to have a bucket from which they would scoop and pour the water over themselves if there were no shower available. These and other practices need to be remembered when assessing individuals.

Religious and cultural practices frequently interrelate and it may be difficult to separate them. Most people who practice religion pray more when they are distressed. Some practices entail loud chanting and this can be very disturbing to those unfamiliar with the practice. Observation of strict religious/moral codes such as no premarital sex may be seen as pathological or interpreted as latent homosexuality. Many psychiatric practitioners are non-believers and find the religious preoccupations of some of their clients pathological.

### 4 APPRECIATION OF THE MENTAL HEALTH CONSTRUCTS OF THE PEOPLE WE SERVE

There are several ways of understanding the causation of mental health problems within western psychiatric tradition. Crudely this could be described as nature, nurture or a bit of both. Within certain other traditions there may be different explanatory models and failure to acknowledge this and seek a compromise between the two models may result in the complete breakdown of the therapeutic relationship. For instance, there may be a much larger component of spiritualism in a particular individual's belief system. Failure to appease the spirits of the ancestors may have a very powerful negating effect on whatever treatment we offer. Some philosophical traditions may not subscribe to the separation of the soma and the psyche (see below). This may become very confusing when we attempt to separate into somatopsychic and psychosomatic.

### Translating theory into practice

#### Demographic information, both quantitative and qualitative

A prerequisite to planning and providing good services is a sound information base. Basic demographic information is collected by a number of sources and should be available in planning offices of health and local authorities. The 1991 Census has just been completed and should be useful in establishing some baseline information on the distribution of the various minority communities. It is widely acknowledged that the 1981 census underestimated the racial minority communities. The same situation may arise on this occasion because of the concerns that some groups have expressed over the data collection. Labour Force Surveys have been considered as more informative than previous census data, as have been local surveys like the Docklands Development Survey.

Detailed information bases should be set up in each district jointly by health and local authorities and constantly updated. The information that should be available should include age and sex distribution as well as ethnic profile and physical and psychiatric morbidity as predicted from norms and as actually determined by attendance at primary care and secondary and tertiary facilities. This information can only be gathered over time, but a database system can be set up to do it. Many services already have computerized data collection which could be utilized for these purposes.

The exact distribution in the catchment area of the racial minority families and communities in terms of their location in more or less affluent areas, concentrations in run-down estates, etc. should be ascertained, as should the numbers of families of any one origin in an area. This may reveal potential sources of support or social isolation: whether there is communication with the neighbours or whether the particular area has a concentration of elderly people who are having difficulty coping with the rather diffent lifestyle of the young Rasta in their midst and are consequently very hostile.

In addition to the basic demographic information it is essential to gather information about the history and development of our clients if we are going to provide a good service. In psychiatry we make judgements about people on the basis of how they present themselves – how they look, what they say and what they do. We make certain assumptions on the basis of their dress, tone of voice, the language used, where they went to school, for example, Dulwich College, Cheltenham Ladies College or Peckham Manor and so on. The judgement we make of their symptoms is set against a background of which we

have some knowledge. What can we recognize of a Loretta College in Darjeeling or Ooty?

It is not possible for clinicians to acquaint themselves with the historical background of all of their patients. However, it is possible to diminish our failings by attempting to find out what people have experienced in a more general way. This is usually easier where a substantial percentage of the community come from a particular geographical region. Whilst people are scattered across the country there are still pockets or areas where people have tended to concentrate, for example East African South Asians in Wembley, Bangladeshis in Tower Hamlets, Jamaicans in South London. People have come to the UK for many reasons (Rack 1982, Hiro 1991). Many were invited to come to supplement the labour force. Others have migrated in search of better living conditions and better prospects for their children. Yet others are refugees who may have suffered enormously and may continue to suffer because they live in fear of their persecutors.

Questions to be considered include the experiences of any community before, during and after getting here. Men may have brought wives over to join them a long time after their own immigration. Families may have been separated for long periods whilst their papers were being processed by the authorities. Parents may have come separately from children and subsequently sent for them. Children may have been sent back to be cared for by grandparents. The early migrants may have intended to go back, and that may still remain a dream for many. Their offspring however, may have no other experience except the British one and the country of origin of their parents may be considered a spiritual home, a country to be feared and despised because of the treatment of their parents, a holiday venue or something completely irrelevant.

The languages spoken; levels of literacy; prevailing family structures and support systems; patterns of family growth and development; religious practices and various other rituals, for example marriages, funerals; styles of greeting; formal and informal networks within the community, are some of the factors that need to be assessed prior to the setting up of any services.

Information can be gathered both formally and informally.

## Prevalence of psychiatric disorder in different communities

Perceived rates of mental illness in any community are bound to influence the services that are designed for that community.

Reports of hospital admission data for people of different ethnic origins are difficult to interpret because of different techniques of age and sex standardization, ethnic classification and methods of determining diagnosis (Hemsi 1967, Pinto 1970, Hitch 1975, Cochrane 1977). However, most studies have shown higher rates of diagnosis of schizophrenia in people of Afro-Caribbean and South Asian origin (Carpenter & Brockington 1980, Dean *et al.* 1981, Shaikh 1985, Cochrane & Bal 1987a). For people of Afro-Caribbean origin these rates are even higher in people born or brought up in the UK (McGovern & Cope 1987b, Harrison *et al.* 1988). To date there are no similar studies of second-generation South Asians. Varying rates of alcoholism have been reported for Afro-Caribbeans and Asians (Burke 1984, Cochrane & Bal 1987b).

## Use of services

Ethnic differences in general practice consultation rates have been demonstrated in several recent studies (Murray & Williams 1986, Balarajan *et al.* 1989, Gillam *et al.* 1989). Higher consultation rates were found for Asian men in all these studies, with increased rates for Afro-Caribbean men in the general household survey of Balarajan *et al.* (1989). However, the study by Gillam *et al.* (1989) which looked at reasons for consultation found that consultation rates for mental disorder were reduced in all ethnic minority groups. This underusage of GPs had been noted in previous studies of admissions of Afro-Caribbeans to inpatient psychiatric care in the inner cities (Rwegellera 1980, Ineichin *et al.* 1984, Harrison *et al.* 1984, 1988, 1989, Moodley & Perkins 1991). Underutilization of GPs for mental health

problems by South Asians has been attributed to less psychological morbidity and/or fear of stigmatization. Fenton & Poonia (1989) in their study of South Asian women in Bristol, found that these women talk freely of their emotional problems and where there was a clear connection between life circumstances and ill-health the doctors' powers of intervention were considered to be very limited. Similarly, Beliappa (1991) found in her study of South Asians living in inner London that the emotional difficulties which were recognized as linked to their life situation were not categorized as 'illness' and GPs were not consulted.

Somatization theory has assumed that people from different cultures use the western construct of mind and body. A redefinition may conclude that those societies, in which a cultural definition of self, personhood, social roles and identities is more holistic, are more aware of the interconnectedness of psychological and physical problems. It is possible that when there is a greater awareness of the limitations of medical intervention to alleviate life problems, only those physical symptoms that may be alleviated by medical intervention are brought to services. Difficulties with a mother-in-law, for instance, may be causing sadness and worry but the doctor cannot get rid of her. However, he probably could do something about the headaches that this is causing. Other possibilities are that people are simply unaware that relief for their psychological symptoms may be obtained from their GPs. This obviously has implications for the development of services as well as the delivery of care to any particular individual.

Given the underutilization of GP services but similar or slightly higher admission rates for most of the racial minority groups that have been studied, it would appear that emergency services are used excessively. Within the inner cities there is a high level of police involvement in the admissions of Afro-Caribbean patients (Rwegellera 1980, Rogers & Faulkner 1987, Harrison *et al.* 1984, 1988, 1989, Dunn & Fahy 1990). Studies in Leicester and Bradford have suggested that the same may not be true for South Asians (Hitch & Clegg 1980, Rack 1982).

## Treatment

Ethnic minority patients are believed to receive a different spectrum of care from the indigenous population. Evidence for this is found in excessive use of the Mental Health Act, physical treatments and decreased use of the 'talking therapies' and aftercare services.

Littlewood & Lipsedge (1977), Rwegellera (1970), Ineichin *et al.* (1984), McGovern & Cope (1987a) and Moodley & Perkins (1991) have reported an excess of compulsory detentions among Afro-Caribbeans. Noble & Rodger (1989) in their study of violence by psychiatric inpatients found that in the non-violent control group, over 50% of the Afro-Caribbeans were formally detained or detained in a locked ward, compared with only about 15% of the whites. Most studies have concluded that this excess is related to the excess in diagnosis of schizophrenia. Moodley & Perkins (1991) have shown that it was ethnic status rather than diagnostic category that accounted for the higher rates of compulsory detention of Afro-Caribbean people. Pinto (1970) reported an excess of compulsory detention amongst Asians, while McGovern & Cope (1987) found no significant differences in the detention rate for Asians compared with whites.

Black outpatients are more likely to receive major tranquillizers and ECT than native patients (Littlewood & Cross 1980). Shaikh (1985) reported an excess of ECT amongst Asians with the diagnosis of schizophrenia compared to indigenous patients with the same diagnosis.

Littlewood & Cross (1980) also reported that black patients were more likely to receive intramuscular medication. Glover & Malcolm (1988) in a prevalence study of depot neuroleptic treatment among Afro-Caribbeans and Asians found a high prevalence for Afro-Caribbean women of all ages, young Afro-Caribbean men and older Asian women. It was not possible to determine whether these groups received treatment for longer periods or whether more of them receive treatment. Lloyd & Moodley (1990) found that without matching for diagnosis, more black patients than white patients received oral and depot antipsychotic drugs, and blacks also received higher doses of oral and depot antipsychotic preparations. Whilst white patients who had been involved in a violent incident or were formally admitted received significantly higher doses of medication than white patients who had not been in such incidents, black patients received similar doses whether formal or informal, violent or not. Chen *et al.* (1991) whilst finding few differences in oral neuroleptic medication between Afro-Caribbeans and whites found that many more Afro-Caribbeans were on more than 2000 mg of chlorpromazine equivalent than white psychotic patients. They also found that more than half the patients were initiated on depot neuroleptics during the first episode of illness compared to less than one-fifth of the non-Afro-Caribbeans.

Some racial and ethnic differences have been reported in response to psychotropic medication similar to differences in non-psychotropic medication (Lawson 1986, Kalow 1982, Lin *et al.* 1986). South-East Asians and South Asians demonstrate clinical response at lower average levels of neuroleptics compared to Americans and Europeans (Allen *et al.* 1977, Lewis *et al.* 1980, Lin & Finder 1983). Peak plasma levels with tricyclic antidepressants were reported to be achieved earlier in South-East Asians compared to Caucasians (Rudorfer *et al.* 1984), and the studies by Allen *et al.* (1977) and Lewis *et al.* (1980) reported higher plasma levels for South Asians compared to native English at fixed intervals after the administration of clomipramine. Several studies have shown that South-East Asian bipolar patients respond clinically to lower levels of lithium compared to Caucasians (Lin *et al.* 1986). To what extent these variations are clinically significant is unclear. This is clearly an area that needs further investigation if we are to ensure that our patients are not overmedicated or undermedicated.

## Local knowledge of psychiatric services and local views on mental illness

There is very little information available about local knowledge of psychiatry and psychiatric services. It has been assumed by some that most people know about the services and choose not to use them. Beliappa (1991) has reported that one third of their sample of South Asians were not aware of any statutory services. Of those who do know about services, anecdotal evidence suggests that some people regard us with the greatest suspicion because they believe that we remove people on very trivial grounds and incarcerate them and experiment on them. This is clearly an area which needs further exploration if we are to provide acceptable services (also see Chapter 22).

### Use of alternative therapies

Within some communities there is continued use of traditional healers and alternative therapies. The extent to which this occurs is unclear. Certainly among South Asian communities, various *vaids* and *hakims* conduct 'therapeutic tours', going around various cities every few months. There is little data available that looks at the type of cases that attend these practitioners and more importantly the type of treatment and response rates. In order to plan and provide services appropriately we need to know whether alternative facilities are used concurrently with orthodox services or whether they are thought to be in conflict.

The reality is that it is not possible to acquire all or even most of the information required before services have to be developed. Therefore *planning* and *implementation* of the service necessitates:

1 Knowing what psychiatry and the psychiatric services are currently offering to the various ethnic groups in the local area.
2 Knowing the possible deficiencies in psychiatric practice currently, the prevalence of mental illness in the local community and the differences in terms of treatments offered, treatment taken up and rates of response to any form of treatment.
3 Knowing what is available in terms of organizational and financial constraints.
4 Knowing the community we are attempting to serve as far as possible.
5 Allowing sufficient flexibility in the plans to enable further development as new information arises and new insights are gained.

Planning of services has already been dealt with in some detail in the preceding chapter.

Two absolute minimum requirements that are prerequisites to setting up the service are:

1 Basic demography in order to know what the service requirements are likely to be.
2 Adequate representation of ethnic monority members of the community and users at the highest levels of planning.

Particular issues of relevance here are where and how basic information is going to be collected, what formal and informal channels are already available to collect the data, and what needs to be commissioned.

### Implementation

#### RECRUITMENT AND TRAINING OF STAFF

Staff have to be recruited with the right mix of professional expertise, race, gender and knowledge of languages being spoken in the community. Particular attention needs to be paid to the recruitment process in order to facilitate the entry of the appropriate staff. Existing institutional practice should be examined to ensure that people are not being excluded by a subtle process of institutional racism. Training of staff to work in multicultural and multiethnic settings is essential. Education of all service providers to recognize and deal with their preconceptions is crucial. Staff should be aware that how threatened they feel is not necessarily based on any rational thought, and could well be on the basis of negative stereotypes established through the media, experiences of friends or relatives, etc., and they should be encouraged and enabled to discuss their difficulties, fears and lack of knowledge. Staff training should be aimed at developing and maintaining a shared valued system.

#### COMMUNICATION WITH THE COMMUNITY

To enable the optimal development of the service there should be wide networking of every possible agency in the community. This should involve all statutory and voluntary agencies including the police, local clergy and other religious leaders. There is usually a very extensive informal network, particularly on the housing estates. Statutory workers seldom gain access to this network but as credibility is established there is at least a limited access.

## INFORMING POTENTIAL USERS

It would appear that some of our potential users are ignorant about the existence of services and the purposes of services. Information should be disseminated as widely as possible, using local radio and press, mail-shots to all community agencies, notices in GPs' surgeries, etc. These should be in the appropriate languages. Additionally information could be made availiable on videotapes and played in outpatient departments in general hospitals, doctors' waiting rooms as well as at community venues.

## EXCHANGE OF INFORMATION

It is vital that there is ongoing dialogue with the community to exchange views about mental health and the services available. Discussion groups could be set up, with the aid of the local council for voluntary agencies, Community Relations Council, Community Health Council or with voluntary and community agencies directly. Initial meetings may be fraught with difficulties because of the suspicion and hostility towards services. Persistence and acceptance of some of the hostility leads ultimately to a position where both sides can listen to each other sufficiently to see each other's point of view, even if they do not accept it fully.

## FLEXIBILITY OF SERVICE PROVISION

There should be a range of service provision which allows the provision of flexible services. This should be flexible in terms of place and time of appointments as well as the type, quantity and quality of service. Anecdotal evidence suggests that some of the difficulties experienced in management and the high doses of medication required in situations of acute crisis are because patients are so frightened of losing control that they resist the effects of medication. The provision of non-medicalized crisis houses may abort a long admission to hospital by allowing people to 'chill out' in a non-threatening environment. Another example of flexibility of service provision is in terms of medication. Many patients titrate their medication according to their symptoms. Acknowledgement of this actually allows staff to discover more details about the nature of symptoms and when they are perceived by patients to be more threatening. Care should be provided regardless of patients' refusal to accept medication if they are seen to need it. As trust develops between the provider and the recipient, people will sometimes ask for medication, even if it is 'just for help with sleeping'.

## LOBBYING OPINION WITHIN AND OUTWITH THE PROFESSION

The development of a service which attempts to provide equitably may not be seen as such by many and may actually be seen as favouring the undeserving. At a time of diminishing resources it is crucial the support be maximized.

### Elements of a service that works

The basic elements are:
1 The staff are seen to have a high level of professional competence.
2 There is consultation with the community on an ongoing basis.
3 The staff team and the organization have street credibility.
4 The service operates on the basis of a value system which is seen to accord people respect.
5 There is sensitivity to racial aspects of peoples' lives.
6 There is acceptance of cultural aspects of peoples' lives.

### An ideal service for ethnic minorities

This is one which the majority will use voluntarily because it is a place they can trust to provide them with care when they need it. It will have a racial and cultural mix of staff which will enable them to feel understood (not black staff in inferior positions). If the languages they speak are not spoken by the staff, interpreters will be easily available. Assessment of their difficulties will be carried out free of negative stereotypes and taking account of cultural variations in expressions of distress. As they express less satisfaction with explanations given to them about their conditions and the treatment offered to them, particular attention will be paid to providing information in language that is easily understood by all users. Goals of management will be set jointly with users, enabling them to take greater control of their lives. In this process there will be capitalization of their strengths which may have become buried under feelings of inferiority in society and compounded by a mental illness label.

## SEPARATE SERVICES OR SENSITIVE SERVICES?

Separate facilities have arisen mainly from the voluntary sector to cater for the needs of distressed minority groups. They see themselves as filling the gap left by statutory services. There is pressure to provide more of these facilities and for statutory services to provide resources for them. With the current changes and the purchasing of care separated from the provision, it is likely that some black agencies will be commissioned to provide care for 'their own'. This is an attractive idea which may be a trap for the unwary. Projects which are inadequately costed or funded or supported are likely to founder quite quickly, thus confirming the majority view that minority groups are not capable of managing responsibly anyway.

Separatism which may be crucial in the short or medium term for some groups, because of language difficulties or because of a need to affirm their worth in a society that constantly devalues them, may be totally counterproductive in the long term. Marginalization and a pernicious system of apartheid which would be seen as self-inflicted is all too easy to envisage.

On the other hand, sensitive services may be a myth. Providing sensitive services usually means a major change in the culture of an organization. The will to make major changes in mainstream services has to exist at the top of any organization.

This has got to be backed by resources. Unfortunately many institutions still act in a 'colour blind' way. Whilst many health authorities talk about equitable provision of care, equal opportunities policies have been implemented by few. This has to be indicative of the priority accorded to this particular aspect of service development. Equal opportunities officers seem to be struggling with the might of psychiatry and unfortunately sometimes appear to be giving up the ghost.

Nevertheless the ultimate goal of all mainstream providers of care must remain the provision of an integrated and flexible service which takes account of the diversity of the population and its needs, and provides sensitive and appropriate care which is acceptable.

## References

Allen J.J., Rack P.H. & Vaddadi K.S. (1977) Differences in the effects of clomipramine on English and Asian volunteers: preliminary report on a pilot study. *Postgraduate Medical Journal* 53, supplement 4, 79–86.

Balarajan R., Yuen P. & Soni Raleigh V. (1989) Ethnic differences in general practitioner consultations. *British Medical Journal* 299, 958–960.

Beliappa J. (1991) *Illness or Distress? Alternative Models of Mental Health.* Roger Booth Associates, Newcastle Upon Tyne.

Burke A.W. (1984) Cultural aspects of drinking behaviour among migrant West Indians and related groups. In Krasner N., Madden J.S. & Walker R.J. (eds) *Alcohol Related Problems*, pp. 197–205. John Wiley, Chichester.

Carpenter L. & Brockington I.F. (1980) A study of mental illness in Asians, West Indians and Africans living in Manchester. *British Journal of Psychiatry* 137, 201–205.

Chen E.Y.H., Harrison G. & Standen P.J. (1991) Management of first episode psychotic illness in Afro-Caribbean patients. *British Journal of Psychiatry* 158, 517–522.

Cochrane R. (1977) Mental illness in immigrants to England and Wales: an analysis of mental hospital admissions 1971. *Social Psychiatry* 12, 25.

Cochrane R. & Bal S.S. (1987a) Migration and schizophrenia: An examination of five hypotheses. *Social Psychiatry* 22, 181–191.

Cochrane R. & Bal S.S. (1987b) The Epidemiology of Mental Illness among Immigrants. Paper read at Royal College of Psychiatrists, Spring Quarterly Meeting, Aberdeen.

Connelly N. (1988) *Care in the Multiracial Community.* Policy Studies Institute, London.

Davies R. (1990) *Directory of Black and Ethnic Community*

*Mental Health Services in London: 1990*. MIND South East, London.

Dean G., Walsh D., Downing H. & Shelley E. (1981) First admissions of native-born and immigrants to psychiatric hospitals in South-East England 1976. *British Journal of Psychiatry* 139, 506–512.

Dunn J. & Fahy T.A. (1990) Police admissions to a psychiatric hospital. Demographic and clinical differences between ethnic groups. *British Journal of Psychiatry* 156, 373–378.

Fenton S. & Poonia K. (1989) Paper presented at the University of Bristol inaugural conference on social change, minority groups and mental health.

Fernando S. (1988) *Race and Culture in Psychiatry*. Croom Helm, London.

Francis E., David J., Johnson N. & Sashidharan S.P. (1989) Black people and psychiatry in the UK: an alternative to institutional care. *Psychiatric Bulletin* 13, 482–485.

Gillam S.J., Jarman B., White P. & Law R. (1989) Ethnic differences in consultation rates in urban general practice. *British Medical Journal* 299, 953–957.

Glover G. & Malcolm G. (1988) The prevalence of depot neuroleptic treatment among West Indians and Asians in the London Borough of Newham. *Social Psychiatry and Psychiatric Epidemiology* 23, 281–284.

Harrison G., Holton A., Neilson D. *et al.* (1989) Severe mental disorder in Afro-Carribbean patients: some social, demographic and service factors. *Psychological Medicine* 19, 683–696.

Harrison G., Ineichen B., Smith J. & Morgan H.G. (1984) Psychiatric hospital admissions in Bristol, II. Social and clinical aspects of compulsory admission. *British Journal of Psychiatry* 145, 605–611.

Harrison G., Owens D., Holton A., Neilson D. & Boot D. (1988) A prospective study of severe mental disorder in Afro-Caribbean patients. *Psychological Medicine* 18, 643–657.

Hemsi L. (1967) Psychiatric morbidity of West Indian immigrants. *Social Psychiatry* 2, 95–100.

Hiro D. (1991) *Black British, White British, A History of Race Relations in Britain*. Grafton Books, London.

Hitch P.J. (1975) Migration and Mental Illness in a Northern City. Unpublished PhD Thesis, Bradford University.

Hitch P.J. & Clegg P. (1980) Modes of referral of overseas immigrant and native-born first admissions to psychiatric hospital. *Social Science and Medicine* 14A, 369–374.

Ineichin B., Harrison G. & Morgan H.G. (1984) Psychiatric hospital admissions in Bristol. I. Geographical and ethnic factors. *British Journal of Psychiatry* 145, 600–604.

Kalow W. (1982) Ethnic differences in drug metabolism. *Clinical Pharmacokinetics* 7, 373–400.

Kleinman A. (1980) *Patients and Healers in the Context of Culture. An Exploration of the Border Between Anthropology, Medicine and Psychiatry*. University of California Press, Berkeley.

Lawson W.B. (1986) Racial and ethnic factors in psychiatric research. *Hospital and Community Psychiatry* 37, 50–54.

Lewis P., Vaddadi K.S., Rack P.H. & Allen J.J. (1980) Ethnic differences in drugs response. *Postgraduate Medical Journal* 56, supplement 1, 46–49.

Lin K.M. & Finder E.J. (1983) Neuroleptic dosage in Asians. *American Journal of Psychiatry* 140, 490–491.

Lin K.M., Poland R.E. & Lesser M. (1986) Ethnicity and psychopharmacology. *Culture, Medicine and Psychiatry* 10, 151–165.

Littlewood R. & Cross S. (1980) Ethnic minorities and psychiatric services. *Sociology of Health and Illness* 2, (21), 194–201.

Littlewood R. & Lipsedge M. (1977) Compulsory Hospitalisation and Minority Status. 5th Biennial Meeting of the Caribbean Psychiatric Association.

Lloyd K. & Moodley P. (1990) Psychiatry and ethnic groups. *British Journal of Psychiatry* 156, 907.

McGovern D. & Cope R. (1987a) The compulsory detention of males of different ethnic groups, with special references to offender patients. *British Journal of Psychiatry* 150, 505–512.

McGovern D. & Cope R. (1987b) First psychiatric admission rates of first and second generation Afro Caribbeans. *Social Psychiatry* 22, 139–149.

Moodley P. & Perkins R. (1991) Routes to psychiatric inpatient care in an Inner London Borough. *Social Psychiatry and Psychiatric Epidemiology* 26, 47–51.

Murray J. & Williams P. (1986) Self-reported illness in general practice consultation in Asian-born and British-born residents of West London. *Social Psychiatry* 21, 139–145.

Noble P. & Rodger S. (1989) Violence by psychiatric inpatients. *British Journal of Psychiatry* 155, 384–390.

Perkins R.E. & Rowlands L. (1986) Planning Community Services for People with Major Long Term Needs: The Maudsley Experience. Paper presented at national MIND: Maudsley joint conferences, Institute of Psychiatry, London.

Pinto R.T. (1970) A Study of Psychiatric Illness among Asians in the Camberwell Area. MPhil Thesis, University of London.

Rack P. (1982) *Race, Culture and Mental Disorder*. Tavistock, London.

Rogers A. & Faulkner A. (1987) *A Place of Safety; MIND'S Research into Police Referrals to the Psychiatric Services*. MIND publications, London.

Rudorfer M.V., Lane E.A., Chang W.-H., Zhang M. & Potter W.Z. (1984) Desipramine pharmacokinetics in Chinese and Caucasian volunteers. *British Journal of Clinical Pharmacology* 17, 433–440.

Rwegellera G.G.C. (1970) Mental Illness in Africans and West Indians of African Origins Living in London. MPhil thesis, University of London.

Rwegellera G.G.C. (1980) Differential use of psychiatric services by West Indians, West Africans and English in

London. *British Journal of Psychiatry* 137, 428–423.

Sashidharan S.P. (1986) Ideology and politics in transcultural psychiatry. In Cox J.L. (ed.) *Transcultual Psychiatry*, pp. 158–168. Croom Helm, London.

Shaikh A. (1985) Cross-cultural comparison psychiatric admission of Asian and indigenous patients in Leciester. *International Journal of Social Psychiatry* 31, 3–11.

Vasquez C. & Javier R.A. (1991) The problem with interpreters; communication with Spanish speaking patients. *Hospital and Community Psychiatry* 42, 163–165.

# Chapter 30
## Social Support Networks

TRAOLACH S.BRUGHA

## Introduction

There is growing evidence that social support is important for physical and psychological health as well as for survival (House *et al.* 1988, Brugha 1991a). Unfortunately there have been very few clinical trials to evaluate the effects on illness or survival of enhancing personal social support networks. Therefore, there is a pressing need for a critical, experimental and evaluative approach to the topic at this time. Although in some ways premature, an attempt is made in this chapter to set out some of the recommended principles of psychosocial management to be considered by practitioners and others concerned specifically with the health problems of those who suffer from psychiatric disorder. Existing and partly evaluated intervention and treatment methods that may have a close and relevant relationship to the topic of social support networks will be referred to. These include environmental, social, interpersonal and cognitive techniques.

Two principles of management will be emphasized: psychosocial and multimodal. According to the best evidence available it is likely that deficiencies in social support networks are the result of a combination (or a system) involving both environmental and intrapersonal causes, operating over long periods of time (Brugha 1990, 1991a). Intervention is therefore, perhaps, more likely to succeed where both the person and his or her social network are the targets of intervention. A second and equally important principle is the multimodal clinical approach to management (Nurcombe & Gallagher 1986), in which the combined use of other physical and psychological aspects of treatment should be considered, when developing a treatment plan.

Table 30.1 provides an outline of the structure

of this chapter. Readers who are not already familiar with the scientific evidence concerning the relationship between social support networks and psychiatric disorder would be well advised to consult a detailed and up-to-date review of the literature (Brugha 1991a).

## Broad and narrow definitions of support and support networks

Partly because of the wide range of interest in the topic, the concept of social support is liable to be extremely nebulous unless clearly defined. Part of this difficulty lies in the use of the word 'support', because it presupposes unquestioningly both its existence and its benefits. Elsewhere I have defined social support as 'those aspects of social relationships thought to confer a beneficial effect on physical and psychological health' (Brugha 1988a). To this must be added that it is not so much the 'wide variety of material needs that reach individuals through the action of others' that may be important, but it is rather the 'specific "personal" provisions of social relationships and particularly their more subjective components, e.g. confiding, intensity, and reciprocity of interaction and reassurance of worth' that particularly merit study (Brugha 1988a). Thus the definition has a hypothetical status, leaving it open to validation by future work.

## Principles of management

Several conclusions can be drawn at present from the available research on social support in relation to psychiatric disorder. Social support is a heterogeneous concept (Cassel 1976, Cobb 1976), therefore specific definitions of support must be used in research and in clinical practice to

**Table 30.1** Social support networks: overview of management principles

facilitate measurement reliability (Brugha *et al.* 1987b). Amongst the psychologically or psychiatrically unwell, measurement may well be contaminated by symptoms (Brugha 1988b). Social networks and social support appear to be influenced by a variety of environmental and constitutional factors including, perhaps, genetically inherited temperamental characteristics such as sociability (Monroe & Steiner 1986), developmental factors such as extreme and early social disruption and deprivation (Rutter & Quinton 1984), as well as by such environmental factors as 'where you work' (Repetti 1987) and who you end up with as your 'life partner', along with family and friends (Cutrona 1989). Compared with these factors, cultural differences appear to be of relatively minor importance (Brugha 1988a).

Deficits in social support are associated with an increased risk of developing symptoms that can be described as psychological dysfunction or 'neurotic' (Henderson *et al.* 1981). Personality factors (Brewin *et al.* 1989) are also likely to play a significant part in the development of these disorders, although the case for this was probably overstated in earlier studies (Duncan-Jones *et al.* 1990). Recovery from psychiatric disorder such as clinical depression is also significantly predicted by levels of social support assessed during illness (Brugha *et al.* 1987a). It is also quite possible that different aspects of support are important at different times and for different groups of people (Brugha *et al.* 1990). For example, onset factors may differ from factors that influence recovery (Goldberg *et al.* 1990). Whilst perceived deficits in social support are particularly associated with a negative course, it appears that other aspects of social relationships that are not necessarily perceived as deficient have a significant influence on future levels of clinically significant symptoms (Brugha *et al.* 1990).

### The principles of psychosocial management

Although the overall role of social factors in the aetiology of psychiatric disorder remains 'unproven', it is now clear that deficits in social support (Brugha *et al.* 1987a) and stressful life events (Bebbington *et al.* 1988) play a significant role in the aetiology and pathogenesis of clinical depression (also see Chapters 7 and 10). Their aetiological importance does not seem to be significantly affected by whether or not a particular episode of depression includes 'biological symptoms' (Brugha *et al.* 1987a, Bebbington *et al.* 1988). Perhaps the most important principle to bring home to patients and their relatives is that conditions like depression are probably influenced by a multiplicity of factors, *both physical and psychosocial*, which when added together lead to illness, and therefore that successful treatment will frequently depend on a combined physical (biological) *and* a psychosocial approach (Brugha 1991b).

It is regrettable that the clinical value of this *multimodal* approach (Nurcombe & Gallagher 1986) has been relatively neglected outside social psychiatry; this more eclectic approach ought to be emphasized more widely. In this regard, social psychiatrists often make use of a combination of drug treatments, psychotherapy *and* socio-environmental 'manipulation', in dealing with a case that might not otherwise yield to just one of these approaches.

A similar difficulty may arise in trying to apply both a *social and a personal* approach. A traditional psychotherapeutic approach may well require that the therapist and patient deal only with what the patient or client brings to the therapy setting, never meeting outside it. Similarly, a strict social approach might require that the therapist meet only with the patient/client *and* their partner, family or (very rarely indeed) their extensive social network, the therapist refusing to see the patient on their own. However, the lesson that seems to have emerged from research is that both the person and their social environment may require exploration and modification at the same time (Brugha 1991b).

It could be argued that giving the patient too many different kinds of experiences and instructions might lead to confusion. For example, giving a patient a social skills training package at the same time as conducting an intervention at the level of that patient's family, may leave the patient confused as to where exactly the problem exists. On the other hand, there is a surprising lack of evidence that different treatment methods produce detectable differences in their effects in relation to depressive disorders (Beckham 1990). This may well be due to common components of all psychotherapies, including the experience of a warm, positive and supportive personal relationship. Thus there is no reason why helping a patient to improve their sources of support cannot be combined with a stress management package. Equally, in order to 'win over' the patient to the value of support from people who have previously been perceived to be disinterested, a cognitive strategy that challenges such negative beliefs and results in a positive perception of the value of such an attitude may also be effective.

The treatment strategy must of course be with the full consent of the patient, whose confidentiality must always be fully respected. In their network therapy, Speck & Ruevni (1969) made it clear from the beginning of sessions that secrets, confidences and collusions were not allowed and that confidences would be broken routinely. Whichever policy is chosen, it must be clear what the policy is before sessions begin.

Before discussing the use of personal and environmental approaches to support enhancement, it is important to consider the objective of such interventions.

## WHICH SOCIAL SUPPORT VARIABLES SHOULD BE CHANGED?

When beginning any intervention, it is essential to be clear about the problems to be worked on and the objectives to be aimed for. Similarly, although the psychological precursors of adult mental illness may already be partly laid down in childhood (Rutter & Quinton 1984, Andreasson *et al.* 1987), there is no scope here for discussing the implications of such evidence for primary prevention (see Chapters 13 and 14).

The importance of perceived satisfaction with social support is common to most observational studies (Brugha 1991a). Thus people who complain of being unsupported are more likely to be psychologically unwell concurrently and in the short-term future. Satisfaction or dissatisfaction with support presupposes a recognition that one needs support. It may well be that seeking support is in itself a bad prognostic indicator, irrespective of whether or not it is obtained. Equally, it may be argued that not being aware of its possible value may 'turn off' the supporters. This is a complex area for which there can be no simple prescriptions at the present time.

However, feeling that others are not helpful may well go along with being socially isolated. Social integration – not relying too heavily on just one or two individuals at a high level of intensity – also appears to be important. Social ties are relatively easy to ask about, and would seem to be a much more straightforward topic for a patient to focus on. However, as we have already seen, patients with small social networks are not only less likely to recover from depression but may also be unaware of their affiliative needs (Brugha *et al.* 1990). Patients who have found close social ties unsatisfactory in the past may resent the suggestion that changes need to be made in this respect.

The needs of men and of women may differ, and possibly on quite traditional, even 'sexist' lines (Brugha *et al.* 1990). For example, it may be very important to men to have casual social contact, in informal ways, with other men to whom they can relate easily, preferably outside the competitive setting of the workplace (or indeed the home). However, some men may find it difficult to seek and make use of such opportunities for informal contact. It is notable also that men seem to suffer more than women when an intimate social relationship breaks down. Some women seem to be better off when retaining independence in their social lives, beyond a specific intimate relationship, thus allowing them the freedom to maintain a number of supportive relationships with close relatives and good friends.

The quality of day to day interaction is as important as is its quantity. The importance of listening skills is fundamental to all psychotherapeutic and counselling social relationships. People vary in the extent to which they are able to do this, but equally, as individuals, we are better at listening to some people than at listening to others. Clearly this is an important issue to identify and try to work on both at the level of the person and sometimes at the wider social level. A patient's ability to listen to others and show appropriate concern will be particularly apparent in group settings and group work may be used to encourage and facilitate the use of such skills.

Just being in the presence of people can be as important as sharing specific confidences and other personal transactions. Certain individuals may not welcome a more personal interest being taken in them by others. We do not yet know enough to be able to say whether it is best to accept such people as they are or to encourage more active social participation. However, it would be a mistake to think that such 'silent company' represents an indication that a minimal degree of social contact is not welcome. Indeed, there is a danger in getting worried about silence, and in the training of social care workers it is important to point out that silence is not necessarily a sign of hostility or anger. Clearly, however, an introverted style is bound to work against greater social integration and adaptation. Such individuals may be harbouring increasingly irrational concerns and fears about their role in their social world. In order to help them to develop better support from others, such people probably should be encouraged to make particular efforts to show others their appreciation for the company they are offered.

Practical or instrumental support may be important but so too is equity – an equal exchange of favours (Schafer & Keith 1980) – and so too is the symbolic importance of 'what giving or receiving *really* tells me about what the other person feels about me'. There is also another important distinction to be made here. One should distinguish between rescuing someone who is 'helpless' and in genuine hardship on the one hand, and on the other hand, doing something for someone who themselves has the means to obtain what is being offered, and thus running the danger of fostering dependence. This is a particularly important issue for supporters, including those of us with professional responsibility for the care of others.

The needs of natural supporters (usually female members of the patient's family) are often neglected and ought properly to be provided for also (Fadden *et al.* 1987, MacCarthy *et al.* 1989). Often the unmet needs of relatives are material, for example for welfare assistance, for respite care (a break from a chronically ill or dependent patient) or for information and advice. However, contact with staff and emotional burden are also important targets of assistance (MacCarthy *et al.* 1989).

Issues of power and control should be monitored; both for the patient and for the natural supporter, cooperation and freedom to choose what is wanted should not be overlooked. This is a relatively unresearched area (Gilbert 1989), which has implications for growth through a psychotherapeutic relationship as much as for wider social issues of control in society, the workplace and the home. A marked tendency towards competitiveness and dominance will often be apparent in group settings, but the competitive person may be unaware of the danger of isolating himself or herself from the support of others (i.e. the 'losers'). Issues of control may also be important in high Expressed Emotion families.

THE NEED FOR EXPERIMENTAL STUDIES

The somewhat unpredictable nature of any attempts to help people by enhancing or in some way modifying their support systems must be acknowledged. The lack of formal experimental research makes what is being set out here extremely tentative in nature. Only two formal trials have been fully reported to date (Parker & Barnett 1986, Dalgard *et al.* 1986, Benum *et al.* 1987). Laboratory experimental studies have also shown that support can be manipulated with a positive effect on psychological performance (Kiecolt-Glaser & Greenberg 1984, Sarason & Sarason 1986) and on affect (Bowers & Gesten 1986, Lakey & Heller 1988). The difficulties are all the more compounded by the fact that so often one cannot know the underlying reason for clinical improvement in episodic psychiatric disorders. It is particularly important to be open to questioning what one is achieving and of course to fully support any formal attempts to evaluate more rigorously the effectiveness of such interventions.

*Personal interventions:*
*the psychotherapeutic approach*

Psychotherapeutic approaches, that is interventions directed at the patient rather than at supporters, can be of several kinds. A cognitive psychotherapeutic approach may be designed to alter dysfunctional attitudes and beliefs about the value of close personal relationships with others. A social skills training package may be designed to overcome skills deficits that may be restricting a patient from developing or making effective use of more supportive relationships. Interpersonal psychotherapy, by providing the patient with a social relationship that is safe to learn within, may also lead to enhanced skills in obtaining

additional sources of support from others. These three kinds of strategies have also been discussed in relation to helping the lonely and socially isolated (Rook 1984).

For example, Interpersonal PsychoTherapy of depression (IPT; Klerman *et al.* 1984) is conducted in a one-to-one, psychotherapeutic setting, with timetabled sessions, in which exploratory and interpretive rather than prescriptive (as in cognitive and behavioural therapies) techniques are employed. Thus it is closely based on traditional psychotherapy, which emphasizes the importance of the client–therapist relationship, or transference. The subject matter of IPT is of particular relevance also. The initial assessment focuses on frequency and quality of social interaction, personal expectations of key social relationships, areas of dissatisfaction and finally on what the patient wants from each social relationship. Many of these variables are covered in standard social network inventories (Brugha *et al.* 1987b, Brugha 1988b). Grief and loss, disputes, changes in roles and deficits such as loneliness are also examined. Formal training for IPT has been developed and its evaluation has been made more feasible by the development of a treatment manual (Klerman *et al.* 1984).

IPT has been evaluated in a series of clinical trials and in many cases has been shown to produce significant clinical improvement in depression (Gelder 1990). The use of interpretive rather than prescriptive techniques in IPT has not in itself been systematically evaluated. The IPT process has been shown to overlap very little with *cognitive methods* (Elkin *et al.* 1989), but there do not appear to be significant differences in their relative effects on outcome (Beckham 1990).

The content of cognitive psychotherapy for depression does focus frequently on cognitions about the self, in relation to other key persons. Classic examples of faulty cognitions are rating oneself as less able than others in the absence of confirmatory evidence, and for example thinking that '*they* wouldn't be interested in me or *they* wouldn't like me anyway'. Again, it does not appear that any work has ever been carried out to disaggregate the effects of countering such 'social cognitions' from other kinds of negative cognitions and so we cannot say to what extent their inclusion in cognitive therapy contributes to its effectiveness in the treatment of depression. However, given the evidence that individuals' perceptions of their social world may play a key role in determining levels of social support, these techniques may be worth incorporating in treatment. An excellent exposition of the possible use of cognitive behavioural therapy (CBT) in addressing problems in social support has been provided recently by Parry (1988). In addition to identifying and challenging cognitions that may lead to support from others being devalued, unused or abused, this form of CBT focuses specifically on teaching new skills in eliciting and making use of support from others.

### Environmental interventions

Community-based alternatives to traditional institutional care for the mentally ill will be the focus of a separate discussion in the next section of this chapter. The implication of the term 'environmental intervention' is that treatment should be targeted on others (the family, the wider social network, the community). As in the previous section, emphasis will be placed on using existing therapeutic techniques but with the new and specific purpose of achieving and monitoring enhancements in the number and quality of social relationships with others and in the level of social support being received by the patient.

Most studies on social support focus particularly closely on sexual or marital relationships (Brown *et al.* 1986), and some emphasize the wider range of family social relationships also. In *marital psychotherapy*, a range of interpretive and prescriptive methods have been described and evaluated (Crowe 1976, Hahlweg *et al.* 1984). The frequency and quality of interaction and attention are central issues in counselling a couple with sexual dysfunction. In *family therapy*, issues of control and the freedom to engage in age-appropriate social relationships outside the family can also be key matters for discussion and for change within the maturing family.

*Social network intervention* has also been discussed in the journal *Family Process* by several workers (Speck & Ruevni 1969, Erickson 1984). Erickson's paper is a useful source of additional reference material, helpfully discussed. The paper by Speck & Ruevni is essentially a detailed description of the problems and the therapeutic sessions that took place with a 'schizophrenic family' [*sic*]. Apart from the family, extended kin, neighbours and friends of the family were invited to participate. The aim of therapy was to strengthen the wider network of social relationships and loosen the 'double binds in significant dyads or triads' within the existing (i.e. family) network. According to those who participated in the first six sessions, the 26-year-old 'schizophrenic' daughter changed for the better in a number of ways: she would talk more in front of people, she was encouraged to and succeeded in going out of the family home to a job, she enjoyed more being with people and discovered that she had many friends. Whether therapy sessions should incorporate others in this way is debatable, but until tested and evaluated should not be quickly dismissed. The emphasis on 'doing something' rather than just on 'talking about' social isolation and withdrawal (or for some enmeshment), may also be important and worth more deliberate consideration. A particularly positive aspect of this approach may lie in the more positive expectations and understanding of the network towards the disabled individual: a truly supportive community.

Others have also discussed therapy beyond the dyad or family (Pattison *et al.* 1975, Pattison 1977, Rook 1984, Heller 1990). Pattison *et al.* (1975) argued that most American families were based on an extended psychosocial kinship system and that the separate nuclear family was something of a rarity. They argued that family therapy should extend beyond the nuclear family because the extended psychosocial kinship system was a normal source of help and support to families facing stress and challenge. Pattison (1977) then provided a more elaborated formulation of social-system therapy taking into account the structure of the psychosocial kinship system, with different kinds of intervention depending on the level or type of the system at which intervention seemed to be needed. The aim of any therapy was to 'achieve communication and congruence of goals among all the people with whom the patient may have contact'. Thus the patient would be better able to utilize the resources available in the system. More recently, Halevy-Martini and colleagues (1984) have emphasized that an important final stage in network therapy is the shifting of the locus of control from the therapeutic team to the network itself.

Group psychotherapy (Yalom 1975) represents an interesting bridge between personal and environmental approaches. Closed groups, in which interaction outside therapy sessions is strongly disapproved of, clearly belong in the former category, and yet are partly based on the premise that insight and learning comes best through an open sharing with others and the support, understanding and listening that they provide in the group setting. On the other hand, in open groups, such as those in therapeutic communities and more particularly support groups for cancer patients (Spiegel *et al.* 1981, 1989), there is little or no reason to discourage the development of social relationships that may have begun within the group, provided confidentiality is respected. The subject of self-help groups will be touched on again in the next section on community support systems.

### Community support systems

The use of the term 'community' may be misleading, because the objective of such 'support systems', or services, is to identify and solve medical, psychological and social problems, which are then managed at an individual or family level. In contrast to this, intervention with problem communities at a community or macrosocial level (e.g. through welfare legislation based on developments in social policy) is discussed briefly in the next section.

The President's Commission on Mental Health (1978) in the USA promoted a policy to foster natural support systems in the wider community. The topic takes us into a much more general aspect of community and social psychiatry, discussed elsewhere (Morris & Bennett 1983). This topic is also covered in other chapters in this book (in particular see Chapters 28 and 29 on psychiatric services), and will be referred to only briefly here. The term 'system' is intended to denote the principle that the provision of physical, social and psychological needs to individuals who are ill or disabled, and therefore at risk of being unable to fend for themselves, is well organized, managed and coordinated.

In order that such services or systems function effectively the specific medical, psychological, social and welfare (material) needs of patients and their carers in the community must be assessed (Brewin *et al.* 1987, 1988, Brugha *et al.* 1988, MacCarthy *et al.* 1989, Wing 1990) and any needs identified met. In the presence of clinically significant mental illness, problems in functioning that could contribute to social isolation, such as an inability to initiate, form and maintain social interaction, lack of use of public and recreational amenities and observed slowness and underactivity should be identified. Such disabilities should be remedied and a variety of interventions may be helpful. Such interventions include social stimulation, training in social interaction skills, guided practice in the use of public and recreational amenities, befriending schemes (Kingdon *et al.* 1989) or a sheltered environment with appropriate social contact (particularly where training or prompting to exercise skills has failed). Support and advice for relatives and carers is also an important additional ingredient of such a support system.

Another important principle is that the *location* at which care is provided should also be determined, where practicable, by the ability and capacity for independence of the patient. In essence, help should only be brought *to* patients who for good reason are unable to make their own way to a service at which it could be provided at less cost and more efficiency. Thus the provision of day and outreach services should be based on the promotion and maintenance of independence (and the discouragement of dependence) in service users, with the additional advantage that attendance at the service can bring the user into contact with a wider range of potential companionship and mutual support. According to Holloway (in Wainwright *et al.*

1988) users of day-care services mentioned social contact as the most important and valued aspect of such services for them.

Recognizing the social dimension from the point of view of individual service users is important but difficult. Preliminary data (unpublished) gathered by the present author and colleagues, in order to test the validity of a social network inventory in such a setting, revealed some interesting difficulties. As part of the Camberwell High Contact Survey (Brugha *et al.* 1988), staff were asked to identify important social relationships between a named patient and other patients or indeed with staff. Patients were also routinely asked such questions about themselves, by means of questions derived from the Interview Measure of Social Relationships (IMSR; Brugha *et al.* 1987b). It became quite apparent that staff were frequently identifying social relationships that did not exist (in the view of the patient). Leff and his colleagues have reported similar findings (1990). The principal lesson to be derived at the moment is that the *patient's own perceptions* and views should be sought. This is a particularly important issue where the transfer of one or a group of patients to a different service facility is being decided upon.

*Self-help groups* have been with us for many decades but without serious attempts to evaluate their effectiveness (Galanter 1988). Two controlled studies incorporating the concept of self help have appeared in the literature (Galanter 1988, Spiegel *et al.* 1981). However, only the study by Spiegel used acceptable randomization procedures. Although each group included therapists in this study, members were encouraged to support one another both within and between meetings. Members were women with advanced breast cancer and death was a major theme of the meetings. Social isolation, problems of communication with physicians and the impact on the marriage and family were also important themes. Countering isolation was one of the important aims of the group. Psychological outcome, including improved mood, was significantly better in the intervention cases as compared to the controls (Spiegel *et al.* 1981) (although mortality was initially slightly higher in the intervention

group). A long-term follow-up analysis showed that the group members had significantly enhanced survival (Spiegel *et al.* 1989).

Shannon & Morrison (1990) have recently described the origins and development of GROW, which they describe as 'a voluntary association of people who know they are inadequate or maladjusted to life; who earnestly desire to improve, and who are helping one another to grow in mental health or personal maturity'. A great deal more work is needed on the effectiveness of self-help groups, particularly in view of their widespread use and popularity (Galanter 1988). Similarly, a number of other descriptions of informal and voluntary support systems for the chronically mentally ill living in the community have also been described by Mitchell & Birley (1983) and by Cutler & Beigel (1978).

*Support for the supporters* has already been recommended above. The methods to be used will include many already mentioned, including individual and group work. However, advice, education about the illness and practical assistance with material and welfare problems may also greatly relieve the burden on a supporter and thus indirectly benefit the patient. The interventions that have been developed for the families of high Expressed Emotion patients, with schizophrenia, incorporate a number of these methods and have been shown to be of consistent benefit to the patients of these families in clinical trials (Kuipers & Bebbington 1988).

### Community-based interventions

An attempt to appraise the effectiveness of case-level (client-centred) and community-level social care has been provided in a recent review of the social work literature by Matilda Goldberg (1987). Whilst it was possible to identify an example of a case-level evaluation that showed measurable improvements in outcome for identifiable individuals (community survival), it proved more difficult to find such evidence in community-oriented practice, although the latter may have the advantage of influencing earlier referral of individuals at risk (presumably an analogue of population screening). A guide to the application of network techniques for use by social workers has recently been produced by Seed (1990).

Elsewhere Rook (1984) has discussed ways in which the *community environment* and the structure of the working environment can be modified so as to enhance and facilitate more social interaction for the lonely. Similarly, 'unintentional network building' can follow from projects that give people who are isolated in the community a task that can only be carried out by cooperation, sharing and thus meeting in the form of new social groups, as in groups with charitable and voluntary tasks (Rook 1984).

The role of the 'community worker', acting in a specific neighbourhood (or a cluster of physically related residential units) is also discussed by Parry (1988), who also contrasts such formal interventions with the potential contribution to community functioning of 'natural helpers' such as bartenders and hairdressers. Recently Milne & Mullin (1987) have reported on a successful structured training programme in which hairdressers were trained in the provision of social support to their customers. The programme was evaluated experimentally and its success was indicated by enhanced experimental group customers' ratings of the perceived helpfulness of their hairdressers. Mother to mother befriender schemes in Leicester (Homestart) and more recently in South London (NEWPIN) have also been described by Van der Eyken & Pound *et al.* (in Newton & Craig 1991) and by Cox *et al.* (1991).

In another important review article on social and *community intervention*, Heller (1990) makes the point that certain social contexts and community structures may enhance support, giving as an example providing unemployed men paid work, which may be viewed as far more 'supportive' than providing a 'support group'. This article is also important for arguing that enhancing individual skills and competencies may not be of value because, so often, strong adverse cultural norms or adverse social conditions serve to maintain undesirable behaviour. This particularly seems to apply to those who because of their gender, ethnic status, age or low socio-economic group status are prevented from using what would otherwise be more effective interpersonal strategies. This then leads to a call for research (and in due course interventions and new government-backed social policies) at the macrocommunity level rather than at the micropersonal level. The methodological problems, not to mention the implications for true community-based interventions, are considerable.

It is hard to know whether such community-based interventions and policies could be demonstrated to be of value to those seen in psychiatric clinical practice. An attempt to evaluate their introduction might at best provide indirect evidence for their effectiveness, possibly by monitoring case register prevalence rates for psychiatric disorder and other outcome indicators (Jenkins 1990) during the period of intervention. By implication, it would be necessary to show that certain community characteristics were damaging to mental health (e.g. stigma against the mentally ill, famine, war or other physical and social environmental problems (Freeman 1984)) and that specific community-level interventions were health enhancing for community members. In relation to physical health, cigarette smoking is a good example because of the importance of changing the values and beliefs of a society (and thus also of politicians) before such an epidemic can be eradicated. Nevertheless, improvements to the community and social environment arguably are worthwhile in themselves and should not have to await proof of their clinical value.

In the next section, the clinical approach to assessment and management is discussed and the chapter ends with a further plea for evaluation and for an audit of existing methods of practice.

### The clinical approach

Clinical and psychosocial assessment can and should be conducted together. Within psychiatry, our knowledge of the biological, developmental and psychosocial basis of *psychopathological* disorders makes it easier for us to adapt our style of social assessment to individuals who, for any of these underlying reasons, may respond in extremely unusual ways to enquiries about their social support systems. For example, symptoms such as pathological guilt, subjective retardation, irritability, simple ideas of self-reference and magical thinking, which may be elements of the clinical picture, may significantly affect the quality and quantity of social interaction between a patient and his or her social network, as well as significantly distorting the record of these events that the patient can provide. Equally, this principle may also extend to other members of the network who are distressed or have problems in psychological functioning. Although such clinical problems may distort the quality of information obtainable concerning a patient's support system, this in no way reduces the importance of pursuing such information with care and attempting to act on it in a positive way.

A second important issue that must be considered, in relation to possible intervention strategies, is the extent to which a patient's vulnerability to stress or the nature of his psychopathology may contraindicate any significant attempts to increase social stimulation (with its inevitable demands) from others. Some examples of this might include patients suffering from acute exacerbations of symptoms with a persecutory content, or those with fundamental social handicaps that greatly limit their capacity to interact with others, as for example occurs in cases of Asperger's syndrome (or schizoid personality disorder) (Wing 1981). Outlined here is a procedure for eliciting the psychosocial variables that indicate lack of social support during the clinical assessment of each patient. It is based on experience of research interviews with patients and with symptom-free subjects together with experience gained in clinical practice.

*Description of the social support system* can begin by adding to information already gathered about the family – focusing on the location of members, their frequency of contact, and the kinds of transactions that occur, and then moving on to a consideration of the strength of social relationships in terms of 'felt attachment', the ability and tendency to confide, and the degree to which these qualities appear to be reciprocated. Where the patient is married or has a close sexual relationship, particular attention is given to the

social relationship with this partner under these headings. (It may also be worthwhile to interview such a confidant and establish whether the illness has had a negative impact on their own sources of support.)

The enquiry then moves out towards the wider social network of close friends, neighbours and work associates (particularly if they are also regarded as 'friends', 'acquaintances', 'mates', etc.). Again, it seems useful to enquire about recent social interaction, its nature and context, and in particular whether there have been planned social events involving these others which are not a necessary part of work, or routine events in the community (e.g. church attendance). Where, as is often the case, a major significant life event has occurred recently, the transmission of information between other members of the network concerning such events can also be enquired about.

There are two elements to the enquiry about social support: the first concerns itself with action taken by the patient (help and support eliciting, where this seems to be appropriate) and the second concerns the behaviour and action of others. With reference to material aid (tangible support), it can be particularly revealing to enquire about the degree to which transactions of this kind have actually occurred in both directions (sometimes termed 'equity' in a dyadic social relationship). In trying to achieve a judgement about the quality of emotional support, it is important to ask questions that reveal something of the capacity of those involved to identify sources of distress, to tolerate unpleasant news and the feelings that go with it, and to empathize with the person who is distressed. A variety of both open and closed questions should be employed, the latter being used to focus, on the one hand, on how easy or difficult it is for the patient to listen to someone else who has something distressing to discuss, and on the other hand to ask whether one felt that the other person was really listening and was interested in something important that one wished to discuss.

Examples of interaction should always be asked for. When the questions focus on what actually happened during a recent crisis, they may reveal a great deal about other potentially important elements such as coping style, personality and the degree to which elements of an individual's psychopathology directly impinge on social interaction. The belief that one is not being listened to or that one's ideas and feelings are not being acknowledged may also be associated with conflict. It may be easier to identify negative interaction by approaching it with questions about the 'listening qualities' of others, in addition to questions about the extent to which others try to exert social control over oneself. Not surprisingly conflict and a tendency for competitiveness may go hand in hand.

The nature of the enquiry into current social relationships detailed here differs from traditional social enquiries and 'clinical histories' in one important and perhaps obvious way: the absence of a historical and biographical perspective. This emphasis on the 'here and now' is not unintentional. The first justification for it is that most of the available evidence concerning associations between social relationship deficits and psychiatric disorder are based on this kind of 'present state' enquiry (although contextual information used in rating the threat of life events would appear to be an exception). Secondly, this emphasis on the 'present state' of social relationships frees the patient and therapist to look at new ways of increasing the number and quality of available supportive relationships *now* and in the near future. In contrast, an excessive emphasis on the historical and biographical background to relationships, which may inevitably bring to light painful negative interpersonal experiences in the past, may serve to emphasize and reinforce powerful arguments and beliefs in the patient that go against the possibility of change.

### CLARIFYING TARGETS OF INTERVENTION

Based on this kind of information about the patient's own current social network and supports and clinical condition, it should be possible to produce a 'social formulation' that summarizes their difficulties and possible routes for action. A clearly listed set of manageable objectives, with a realistic time-frame in which to review their outcome, should be recorded at this stage. The

implementation of such a planned intervention is discussed in the next section.

### DEVELOPING AND IMPLEMENTING A PLAN OF INTERVENTION

A set of aims both for the patient's social functioning and for those in the wider social network should be recorded. Common to all such plans is the aim of bringing about an improvement in the patient's own perception of the quality of transactions with others, particularly those with whom it is appropriate to share information about feelings, worries and hopes. In addition, not only does the quality of confiding social relationships appear to matter, but an extension of the range of different kinds of social relationships and their functions (sometimes referred to as multiplex relationships) should be aimed for, as these also appear to be indicative of a better level of functioning.

Specific methods should be set out that are designed to try to achieve these aims (bearing in mind the need to consider both the short-term and long-term effects on the course of the psychiatric disturbance). The methods used will be familiar to those working in the field of rehabilitation: training and skill enhancement, monitoring of goals and making use of feedback from others. For those who do not or cannot respond to these learning strategies, sheltered social amenities and the use of visual and verbal reminders and cues by staff or relatives should be provided, possibly on a long-term basis.

The clinician (or social worker, psychologist, occupational therapist, nurse) must be open to the potential value of changing both the patient's social perceptions and behaviour, and also to the value of modifying the behaviour and perceptions of others in the network. Examples of the kind of action to be taken can range from a relatively brief set of guidelines to the patient on how to make better use of potential social resources in their existing network now, to a more detailed series of counselling sessions, incorporating both insight building and specific directions on social behaviour and social interaction with others. Such a series of counselling sessions will also provide the important opportunity both for monitoring the results of directive advice and the possibility of modifying it, in order to increase the patient's effectiveness in transactions with others. There may, of course, be some parallels between this approach and that of social skills and problem-solving training, although the important distinction between them lies in the way the approach is tailored specifically to the particular social relationships that the patient is developing with others in their network. There is evidence that patients with depression are to a small extent less socially skilled than normal controls but, interestingly, normals tend to greatly overestimate their own personal skills whereas depressives tend to provide a more accurate account of themselves in this respect (Lewinsohn *et al.* 1980). Therefore it may be unwise to emphasize the question of social interaction skills in therapy, except perhaps to reassure depressed patients that they have a tendency to be over-pessimistic about their difficulties in this respect.

It may be necessary also to intervene directly through others by working with a couple, a family, key members of a community, or others at the place of work. An example of the latter is the way in which social isolation due to the stigma of being labelled a psychiatric patient can be overcome by making direct links with employers, key figures in personnel departments, or employee organizations. Where these strategies are effective, they may lead others in the social network to change their ideas (or perhaps more specifically their own expectations) about the patient's personality. The adoption of a more realistic and also a less negative set of attitudes may well be highly therapeutic, as shown in the experimental work of Leff & Vaughn (1982) on Expressed Emotion.

EVALUATING AND MAINTAINING OUTCOMES

Information acquired initially about the social support system should be rechecked regularly, possibly as often as each meeting, with the therapist. This provides important information about achieving targets and also serves to remind the patient about what they need to be concen-

trating their own efforts on. Progress achieved will also be a source of encouragement to the patient. At present there is no published evidence of significant positive changes in social support levels, resulting from psychotherapeutic or environmental interventions, although in a study by Parker & Barnett (1987) an attempt to improve social support did lead to significant symptom reduction.

This curious finding of a significantly enhanced outcome, in the absence of consistent evidence of an alteration in the supposed aetiological variable, is also true of cognitively based psychotherapies (Beckham 1990). Thus it appears that whilst there are significant changes in the targeted aetiological variable for only some patients, the therapeutic intervention itself is of more significant benefit to the wider group of patients, including, apparently, many of those who have not significantly altered their support system or cognitions. The implication for clinical practice is that one should not give up just because the patient does not seem to be reaching the psychosocial targets that have been set at the start of therapy. Perhaps the intense, supportive relationship with the therapist is, for many patients, a sufficient remedy in itself, regardless of what technique has been used (Cross *et al.* 1982).

Obviously clinical outcome must also be assessed. It may be that any benefits of support enhancement are long term, and for this and other reasons it is important to establish some system, perhaps through collaboration with a primary health care practitioner, for monitoring long-term clinical outcome, over the subsequent months and years after treatment has ended.

Outcome indicators in clinical practice have yet to be systematically developed and evaluated but their use is bound to increase with the growing emphasis in health care systems on the need for evidence of quality and 'value for money' (Jenkins 1990). This topic will now be considered in more detail.

### Developing and evaluating services

Given the dearth of evidence concerning the possible effectiveness of support enhancement on clinical course and outcome, those providing any service that aims to carry out such work must give serious attention to the evaluation of that service. Standardized measures, both of symptoms and other aspects of psychopathology, should be used in conjunction with social support inventories of known psychometric properties (Brugha 1988b). Ideally, the data gathered should be aggregated and analysed statistically. A great deal can also be learnt from a detailed longitudinal case-study analysis of individual patients.

*Clinical trials* must also be carried out as there can be no substitute for what is learnt from randomized experiments. This area is ripe for such work; there are no major ethical dilemmas, as the interventions involved are unlikely to be significantly harmful and we genuinely do not know what the outcome of further trials will be.

*Quality assurance and audit* is particularly important. The processes involved in intervention must be closely monitored in order to assure that practice conforms to good models of care. Both patients and therapists can be asked to complete questionnaires and forms that provide accounts of the content of sessions and of what appear to be the effects of the intervention at the end of each session. Therapists working with this model should also discuss their work and share these data regularly. Audiotape or audiovisual recordings of sessions may be a very helpful addition to the audit process. However, one should be careful to avoid becoming overwhelmed by the wealth of data collected in this way.

## Conclusions and future prospects

This chapter began with a highly selective and all too brief reference to the evidence concerning the relationship between social support and the onset, course and outcome of clinical psychiatric disorders, and of psychological dysfunction in general. The nature of support and the factors that appear to influence it make up a complex system that involves environmental as well as personal components. A distinction was made between the value of emotional support provided by personal social relationships and the practical support that long-term and socially disadvantaged psychiatric

patients need from formal 'social support systems' that are typically community based, in the present era.

The main aim of this chapter was to discuss clinical and psychosocial management, a neglected topic from the research point of view, although one that is implicit in the work and functioning of many clinical and social agencies of human care. Thus the present chapter aims to provide some background to the work of such services. A series of principles and guidelines that emphasize a self-questioning and self-critical approach are set out. The need for evaluation of support-enhancing interventions has been emphasized throughout the chapter.

It must be clear from this that the future use and development of the concept of social support will depend on a more equitable balance between observational studies and experimental research. Both kinds of research have their advantages as well as their limitations. However, without a new effort devoted to the experimental evaluation of the social support hypothesis, the future development of this promising subject must be awaited in an atmosphere of uncertainty.

## References

Andreasson S., Allbeck P., Engstrom A. & Rydberg U. (1987) Cannabis and schizophrenia. *Lancet* ii 1483–1485.

Bebbington P.E., Brugha T., MacCarthy B. *et al.* (1988) The Camberwell collaborative depression study. I. Depressed probands: adversity and the form of depression. *British Journal of Psychiatry* 152, 754–765.

Beckham E.D. (1990) Psychotherapy of depression research at a crossroads: directions for the 1990s. *Clinical Psychology Review* 10, 207–228.

Benum K., Anstorp T., Dalgard O.S. & Sorenson T. (1987) Social network stimulation. Health promotion in a high risk group of middle-aged women. *Acta Psychiatrica Scandinavica* 76, Supplement 337, 33–41.

Bowers C.A. & Gesten E.L. (1986) Social support as a buffer of anxiety: an experimental analogue. *American Journal of Community Psychology* 14, 447–451.

Brewin C.R., MacCarthy B. & Furnham A. (1989) Social support in the face of adversity: the role of cognitive appraisal. *Journal of Research in Personality* 23, 354–372.

Brewin C., Wing J., Mangen S., Brugha T. & MacCarthy B. (1987) Principles and practice of measuring needs in the long-term mentally ill. *Psychological Medicine* 17, 971–981.

Brewin C., Wing J., Mangen S., Brugha T., MacCarthy B. & Lesage A. (1988) Needs for care among the long-term mentally ill: a report from the Camberwell High Contact Survey. *Psychological Medicine* 18, 457–468.

Brown G.W., Andrews B., Harris T., Adler Z. & Bridge L. (1986) Social support, self-esteem and depression. *Psychological Medicine* 16, 813–831.

Brugha T. (1988a) Social support. *Current Opinion in Psychiatry* 1, 206–211.

Brugha T. (1988b) Social psychiatry. In Thompson C. (ed.) *The Instruments of Psychiatric Research*. John Wiley, Chichester.

Brugha T. (1990) Social networks and support. *Current Opinion in Psychiatry* 3, 264–268.

Brugha T.S. (1991a) Support and personal relationships. In Bennett D. & Freeman H. (eds) *Community Psychiatry: The Principles*, pp. 115–161. Churchill Livingstone, London.

Brugha T. (1991b) Human ethology. *Current Opinion in Psychiatry* 4, 313–319.

Brugha T., Bebbington P., MacCarthy B., Potter J., Sturt E. & Wykes T. (1987a) Social networks social support and the type of depressive illness. *Acta Psychiatrica Scandinavica* 76, 664–673.

Brugha T.S., Bebbington P.E., MacCarthy B., Sturt E., Wykes T. & Potter J. (1990) Gender, social support and recovery from depressive disorders: a prospective clinical study. *Psychological Medicine* 20, 147–156.

Brugha T., Sturt E., MacCarthy B., Potter J., Wykes T. & Bebbington P. (1987b) The Interview measure of social relationships: the description and evaluation of a survey instrument for assessing personal social resources. *Social Psychiatry* 22, 123–128.

Brugha T., Wing J., Brewin C., MacCarthy B., Lesage A. & Mumford J. (1988) The problems of people in long-term psychiatric day care: an introduction to the Camberwell High Contact Survey. *Psychological Medicine* 18, 443–456.

Cassel J. (1976) The contribution of the social environment to host resistance. *American Journal of Epidemiology* 104, 107–123.

Cobb S. (1976) Social support as a moderator of life stress. *Psychosomatic Medicine* 38, 300–314.

Cox A.D., Pound A., Mills M., Puckering C. & Owen A.L. (1991) Evaluation of a home visiting and befriending scheme for young mothers: NEWPIN. *Journal of the Royal Society of Medicine* 84, 217–220.

Cross D.G., Sheehan P.W. & Khan J.A. (1982) Short- and long-term follow-up of clients receiving insight-oriented therapy and behaviour therapy. *Journal of Consulting and Clinical Psychology* 50, 103–112.

Crowe M. (1976) Behavioural treatments in psychiatry. In Granville-Grossman K. (ed.) *Recent Advances In Clinical Psychiatry*, Vol. 2. Churchill Livingstone, London.

Cutler D.L. & Beigel A. (1978) A church-based program of community activities for chronic patients. *Hospital &*

Community Psychiatry 29, 497–501.

Cutrona C.E. (1989) Ratings of social support by adolescents and adult informants: degree of correspondence and prediction of depressive symptoms. *Journal of Personality and Social Psychology* 57, 723–730.

Dalgard O.S., Anstoup T., Benum K., Sorensen T. & Moum T. (1986) Social Psychiatric Field Studies in Oslo. Some Preliminary Results. Paper read at Second International Kurt Lewin Conference, Philadelphia.

Duncan-Jones P., Fergusson D.M., Ormel J. & Horwood L.J. (1990) A model of stability and change in minor psychiatric symptoms: results from three longitudinal studies. *Psychological Medicine. Monograph Supplement* 18, 1–28.

Elkin I., Shea T., Watkins J.T. *et al.* (1989) National Institute of Mental Health Treatment of Depression Collaborative Research Program. General effectiveness of treatments. *Archives of General Psychiatry* 46, 971–982.

Erickson G. (1984) A framework and themes for social network intervention. *Family Process* 23, 187–198.

Fadden G., Bebbington P. & Kuipers L. (1987) Caring and its burdens: a study of the spouses of depressed patients. *British Journal of Psychiatry* 151, 660–667.

Freeman H. (1984) *Mental Health and The Environment*. Churchill Livingstone, Edinburgh.

Galanter M. (1988) Zealous self-help groups as adjuncts to psychiatric treatment: a study of recovery. *American Journal of Psychiatry* 145, 1248–1453.

Gelder M.G. (1990) Psychological treatment for depressive disorder. *British Medical Journal* 300, 1087–1088.

Gilbert P. (1989) *Human Nature and Suffering*. Lawrence Erlbaum, London.

Goldberg D., Bridges K., Cook D., Evans B. & Grayson D. (1990) The influence of social factors on common mental disorders: destabilisation and restitution. *British Journal of Psychiatry* 156, 704–713.

Goldberg E.M. (1987) The effectiveness of social care. A selective exploration. *British Journal of Social Work* 17, 595–614.

Hahlweg K., Revenstorf D. & Schindler L. (1984) The effects of behavioural marital therapy on couples communication and problem solving skills. *Journal of Consulting and Clinical Psychology* 52, 553–566.

Halevy-Martini J., Hemley-Van-Der-Velden E.M., Ruhf L. & Schoenfeld P. (1984) Process and strategy in network therapy. *Family Process* 23, 521–533.

Heller K. (1990) Social and community intervention. *Annual Review of Psychology* 41, 141–168.

Henderson A.S., Byrne D.G. & Duncan-Jones P. (1981) *Neurosis and The Social Environment*. Academic, Sydney.

House J.S., Landis K.R. & Umberson D. (1988) Social relationship and health. *Science* 241, 540–545.

Jenkins R. (1990) Towards a system of outcome indicators for mental health care. *British Journal of Psychiatry* 157, 500–514.

Kiecolt-Glaser J.K. & Greenberg B. (1984) Social support as moderator of the after effect of items in female psychiatric inpatients. *Journal of Abnormal Psychology* 93, 192–199.

Kingdon D.G., Turkington D., Collis J. & Judd M. (1989) Befriending: cost-effective community care. *Psychiatric Bulletin* 13, 350–351.

Klerman G.L., Weissman M.M., Rounsaville B.J. & Chevron E.S. (1984) *Interpersonal Psychotherapy of Depression*. Basic Books, New York.

Kuipers L. & Bebbington P. (1988) Expressed emotion research in schizophrenia: theoretical and clinical implications. *Psychological Medicine* 18, 893–909.

Lakey B. & Heller K. (1988) Social support from a friend, perceived support, and social problem solving. *American Journal of Community Psychology* 16, 811–824.

Leff J., O'Driscoll C., Dayson D., Wills W. & Anderson J. (1990) The TAPS Project 5: the structure of social network data obtained from long-stay patients. *British Journal of Psychiatry* 157, 848–852.

Leff J. & Vaughn C. (1982) Patterns of response and style of coping in high EE and low EE relatives of psychiatric patients. In Leff J. & Vaughn C. (eds) *Expressed Emotion in Families, Its Significance for Mental Illness*. Guilford Press, New York.

Lewinsohn P.M., Mischel W., Chaplin W. & Barton R. (1980) Social competence and depression: the role of illusory self perceptions. *Journal of Abnormal Psychology* 89, 203–212.

MacCarthy B., LeSage A., Brewin C.R., Brugha T.S., Mangen S. & Wing J.K. (1989) Needs for care among the relatives of long-term users of day care: a report from the Camberwell High contact survey. *Psychological Medicine* 19, 725–736.

Milne D. & Mullin M. (1987) Is a problem shared a problem shaved? An evaluation of hairdressers and social support. *British Journal of Clinical Psychology* 26, 69–70.

Mitchell S.F. & Birley J.L.T. (1983) The use of ward support by psychiatric patients in the community. *British Journal of Psychiatry* 142, 9–15.

Monroe S.M. & Steiner S.C. (1986) Social support and psychopathology: interrelations with pre-existing disorder, stress and personality. *Journal of Abnormal Psychology* 95, 29–39.

Morris I. & Bennett D. (1983) Support and rehabilitation. In Watts F.N. & Bennett D.H. (eds) *Theory and Practice of Rehabilitation*. John Wiley, Chichester.

Newton J. & Craig T.K.J. (1991) Prevention. In Bennett D.H. & Freeman H.L. (eds) *Community Psychiatry*, pp. 488–516. Churchill Livingstone, Edinburgh.

Nurcombe B. & Gallagher R.M. (1986) The clinical process in psychiatry: diagnosis and management planning. In Nurcombe B. & Gallagher R.M. (eds) *The Clinical Process in Psychiatry*, pp. 321–332. Cambridge University Press, Cambridge.

Parker G. & Barnett B. (1987) A test of the social support hypothesis. *British Journal of Psychiatry* 150, 72–77.

Parry G. (1988) Mobilizing social support. In Watts F.N. (ed.) *New Developments in Clinical Psychology* vol. II,

pp. 83–104. John Wiley, Cambridge.

Pattison E.M. (1977) A theoretical-empirical base for social system therapy. In Feulks E.F., Wintrob R.M., Westenmayer J. & Favazza A.R. (eds) *Current Perspectives in Cultural Psychiatry*, pp. 217–253. Spectrum Publications, New York.

Pattison E.M., De Francisco D., Wood P., Frazer H. & Crowden J. (1975) A psychosocial kinship model for family therapy. *American Journal of Psychiatry* 132, 1246–1251.

President's Commission on Mental Health. Task Panel on Community Support Systems (1978) Report of the Task Panel on Community Support Systems. In *Task Panel Reports*; submitted to the President's Commission on Mental Health. Washington DC.: US Government Printing Office.

Repetti R. (1987) Individual and common components of the social environment at work and psychological well-being. *Journal of Personality and Social Psychology* 52, 710–720.

Rook K. (1984) Promoting social bonding: strategies for helping the lonely and socially isolated. *American Psychologist* 39, 1389–1407. Rutter M. & Quinton D. (1984) Long-term follow-up of women institutionalized in childhood: factors promoting good functioning in adult life. *British Journal of Developmental Psychology* 2, 191–204.

Sarason I.G. & Sarason B.R. (1986) Experimentally provided social support. *Journal of Personality and Social Psychology* 50, 1222–1225.

Schafer R. & Keith P.M. (1980) Equity and depression among married couples. *Social Psychology Quarterly* 43, 430–435.

Seed D. (1990) *Introducing Network Analysis in Social Work*. Jessica Kingsley, London.

Shannon P.J. & Morrison D.L. (1990) Who goes to GROW? *Australian and New Zealand Journal of Psychiatry* 24, 96–102.

Speck R.V. & Ruevni U. (1969) Network therapy – a developing concept. *Family Process* 8, 182–191.

Spiegel D., Bloom J.R., Kraemer H. & Gottheil E. (1989) Effect of psychosocial treatment on survival of patients with metastatic breast cancer. *Lancet* ii, 889–891.

Spiegel D., Bloom J.R. & Yalom I. (1981) Group support for patients with metastatic cancer. *Archives of General Psychiatry* 38, 527–533.

Wainwright T., Holloway F. & Brugha T. (1988) Day care in an inner city. In Lavender A. & Holloway A. (eds) *Community Care in Practice*, pp. 231–256. John Wiley, Chichester.

Wing J.K. (1990) Meeting the needs of people with psychiatric disorders. *Social Psychiatry and Psychiatric Epidemiology* 25, 2–8.

Wing L. (1981) Asperger's syndrome: a clinical account. *Psychological Medicine* 11, 115–129.

Yalom I.D. (1975) *The Theory and Practice of Group Psychotherapy*. Basic Books, New York.

# Chapter 31
# Changing Approaches to Determining Mental Health Service Resource Needs

STEVEN HIRSCH & BRIAN JARMAN

## Introduction

Wherever health services are not provided on a strictly demand-led basis, but are organized in order to provide a fair level of care for the population, health planners and those who dispense the health care budget must answer the question, 'How much money should we spend on the Mental Health Service?' In this chapter we shall examine how this has been done in the past 30 years in Great Britain and seek to provide a modern approach, which makes use of our knowledge of the relationship between socio-demographic factors and the use of psychiatric services.

Historically, mental health care provision in the UK was financed according to the number of mental hospital beds under a regional health authority, adjusted as the number of beds increased or decreased. As psychiatric care began to be dealt with by district general hospitals and district health authorities, first with outpatient services and later with the provision of inpatient services for acute psychiatry, hospitals were provided with the resources necessary to staff psychiatric wards. Gradually during the 1970s, day hospital services were established and funds flowed from regional health authority to districts to finance these developments on a piecemeal basis. Political pressure demanded changes in health care allocation with a shift of finance from the acute medical services to what were then known as the Cinderella services – for the mentally ill, mentally handicapped and elderly. However, with the trend in the past ten years to relocate psychiatric services wholly within the remit of district health authorities and an increasing emphasis on providing services outside the hospital, a piecemeal method of funding psychiatric services became increasingly inappropriate.

As acute psychiatric services were being located on district general hospital sites, the number of psychiatric beds, particularly for the longer-stay patients, decreased and in the UK 0.5 acute psychiatric beds per 1000 population was recommended as a guideline by the Department of Health & Social Security, 'Hospital Services for the Mentally Ill Circular' (HM(71)97), and in the 1975 White Paper, 'Better Services for the Mentally Ill'. As finances tightened and local psychiatric services improved, administrators noticed that some districts were managing with less than 0.2 acute beds per 1000 population, while others required more than five times this.

## Findings of the working party on bed norms and resources

Hirsch set up a working party under the Social and Community Psychiatry Group of the Royal College of Psychiatry to study the causes for the variation in bed provision. He believed that the remarkable variation in psychiatric bed rates from one district to another was partly due to differences in demand for psychiatric care between different population groups; for example, rural versus urban, and not just differences in how the services were delivered.

By 1982, the 13 regional health authorities in England varied by a factor of 2 in the number of acute psychiatric beds per head provided, from 0.35 beds per 1000 in Oxford to 0.76 beds per 1000 in Mersey. At the district health authority level the variation was at least 6-fold. Examination of data from 8 psychiatric case registers in England and Scotland revealed an average bed usage of 0.39 beds per 1000 for the 15–64-year-old group but 0.73 beds per 1000 for all ages above 65; the over 65 age group occupied over 46% of psychiatric beds. This indicates the importance of accounting for the proportion of the population who are elderly when determining the need for psychiatric beds. Variation in bed use was not however determined by whether the service was located in a district general hospital or a mental hospital.

### Evidence of a relationship between social demographic factors and the need for psychiatric services

Reviewing the literature, the Royal College Working Party (Hirsch 1988) found a number of studies suggesting that the prevalence of psychiatric disorder correlated with various social and demographic variables (Odegard 1932, Faris & Dunham 1939, Buglass *et al.* 1980, Goodman *et al.* 1983, Richman *et al.* 1984). The majority of research supports a strong relationship between the prevalence of specific disorders such as schizophrenia (Shepherd 1957, Cooper *et al.* 1987), alcoholism (Goodman *et al.* 1983), suicide (Durkheim 1952, Sainsbury 1955), parasuicide (Burke 1976, Platt & Kreitman 1985) and a variety of sociodemographic factors. However, the working party also identified one published study (Miller *et al.* 1986) and five studies, then unpublished, which showed a relationship between admission rates and rural or urban status of the population served, as well as poverty, isolation, ethnicity, unemployment and unoccupied housing.

Thus a number of findings of the Royal College report pointed to an association between sociodemographic characteristics of a population and the use of psychiatric services.

In order to study the factors influencing the variation in bed provision further, the working party carried out their enquiry by visiting 20 district general hospital-based psychiatric units covering all the regional health authorities of England. The hospitals were chosen as a stratified sample representing district general hospital-based units with, respectively, high, medium and low bed-turnover rates. This is the number of patients treated per psychiatric bed per year and is

inversely proportional to the average length of stay. The survey noted that the proportion of patients who stay three months or longer disproportionately influences bed-turnover rates and average stay. For example reducing by one the number of patients who stay in a bed for a whole year has the same effect as halving the length of stay from 2 weeks to 1 week for 52 patients. Thus a district's policy in dealing with the new and old long stay can be the most important factor in influencing the need for psychiatric beds (Hirsch 1983). In their main report the working party noted that a high proportion of unmarried patients was a factor associated with greater lengths of stay – another clue to the importance of sociodemographic influences. But it could find no confirmation of the hypothesis that services were able to operate on fewer beds per population by providing a community-based service. Rather, the impression was that the services with the most beds had the most community-based services and vice versa. However, services were chosen on the basis of their size, location, and bed turnover so they were representative rather than model services. It could be that community care was not sufficiently developed in any of the hospitals to have had a strong impact. None the less, whether the unit had an active domiciliary service, a walk-in outpatient facility, day hospitals, high or low ratios of community psychiatric nurses (CPNs), high levels of outpatients, or good teamwork was not associated with high or low bed provision for the population served (Hirsch 1988).

### Social demographic factors and psychiatric admission rates

The working party examined closely the relationship between social deprivation and psychiatric admission rates. Admission rates from each of the electoral wards in South Hammersmith Health District were obtained and correlated with the Under Privileged Area (UPA) score of Jarman (Jarman 1983, 1984). The product–moment correlation (Pearson) was high and significant, 0.67, and explained 45% of the variation in admission rates between population groups (Hirsch 1988). This was particularly interesting because correlations held up within each of the three social service sectors of the health district, each of which was served by its own psychiatric and social work team. Thus service factors in terms of the day hospital facilities, social work team, and medical teams were held constant in each sector.

To try to confirm this result, the admission rates for each of the health districts in the North West Thames Regional Health Authority were correlated with the Jarman UPA score for each health district: the product–moment correlation was 0.76. The UPA score is a weighted composite index of eight census variables including the percentages of elderly living alone, under fives, one-parent families, unskilled workers, unemployed, overcrowded homes, people recently having moved house, and of ethnic minorities.

Perhaps this finding should not be a surprise because the Resource Allocation Working Party (RAWP) reported in 1976 (Department of Health & Social Security 1976) similar findings between sociodemographic indices and admission rates to medical and surgical units in England and Wales. In the RAWP review (Department of Health & Social Security 1988) the Jarman UPA score was found to be a robust indicator of hospital usage. The task of the RAWP was to determine a way of more fairly distributing health service finance according to the needs of the population. The Standardized Mortality Rate (SMR) was used as a proxy for the need for health care in the 1976 report on the assumption that variations between population groups, such as their mortality rate, will reflect the variation in their need for health services. Commonsense would also suggest that people who live alone, or who are poor or elderly, have a greater need for health care and need to be looked after.

### Health surveys as a way of determining need

Perhaps the most obvious and direct way to establish need for a population would be to determine the prevalence of psychiatric illness in the population by a population survey (see Chapters 3 and 4 for a fuller discussion). However, the needs of different populations vary and one would have to survey each and every population group in order to determine its respective psy-

chiatric morbidity, from which needs stem. This would be an impossibly large project as one would have to cover the whole population of the UK, requiring an army of skilled and trained interviewers, as well as money which would probably be better spent on the service itself. Given the changing characteristics of most populations over time, such surveys would have to be repeated periodically. Moreover diagnosis is not directly linked to disability and disability itself might need to be assessed as case findings vary according to the criteria used. There is said to be a six- or seven-fold difference between the prevalence of psychiatric morbidity in the community and the provision of inpatient treatment (Goldberg & Huxley 1980). Predictions from a community survey might therefore be as inaccurate and require as many assumptions as predictions of psychiatric morbidity which are based on more indirect measures, for example on sociodemographic indices or admission rates. Moreover, the need for admission depends not only on the nature of the case but also on the availability of support at home and community tolerance. An estimation of need for services based simply on identified case rates is likely to be inaccurate. Thus using direct surveys of mental health service needs for every community would be a highly impractical way of determining how resources for health care should be distributed.

The RAWP review team decided that use of hospital services in terms of admission rates could be used as an available proxy for need. Admissions are a measure of the met demand and have the advantage that they are fairly accurately recorded: information about admissions is easily available, and admissions usually reflect the utilization of services by the clinically most severe group. Psychiatric outpatient visits make up about a tenth of the overall cost of psychiatric hospital care provision. Day hospital provision is similar.*

---

* Figures derived from the Hospital Costing Returns 1988/89 (Department of Health and Social Security) show that the percentage of the total costs of hospital and community health services accounted for by mental illness inpatient costs were 10.14%, outpatients costs were 0.54%, and day-patient costs were 0.86%, total 11.54%. Thus inpatient costs account for 88% of mental health service expenditure.

Patients who are admitted to hospital are the group with the highest disclosure rate and the most rapid passage from presence in the community to treatment in hospital. In the UK the admission rates for psychiatric illness increased from 1983 to 1985 by 9%, although the number of occupied beds fell by 9% (Department of Health & Social Security 1990) This decrease in bed usage was due to an 18% decrease in the length of stay of patients. Thus the changing factor, as community services improve, is a decrease in length of stay but an increase in admissions, and the latter continue to be a relevant indicator of service activity and take up.

Services may vary (in terms of volume and cost) in comparison to the average national provision, so that a method needs to be developed which can predict service need for a population based on a national standard. Whether the district then decides to provide a higher or lower level of service is an evaluative decision which each district must make, but one which is best made in the light of comparison with some kind of standard.

### Our recent study: the relationship of social demographic, health and service variables with admission rates in England

Recently, we have carried out a survey of all psychiatric admissions in England excluding mental handicap and psychogeriatrics using the Mental Health Enquiry (MHE) data for 1986 (DHSS 1986), which is the most complete mental health data set available. A more detailed description of the study is published elsewhere (Jarman *et al.* 1992). Data from 186 of 191 health districts in England were entered into the analysis, omitting those districts where the MHE data were inconsistent with data from two other sources and which also give admission rates for the district of residence, SH3 and NHS performance indicator MI3. National admission rates were calculated by age, sex and marital status and then applied to the age, sex and marital status proportions of the population of each district to calculate the numbers of admissions in each district which would be *expected* if the national rates had

applied. The number of *actual* admissions of the residents of each district divided by the expected number of admissions $\times$ 100 gave a Standardized Psychiatric Admission Ratio (SPAR). This was calculated for age and sex ($SPAR_{as}$) and for age, sex and marital status ($SPAR_{asms}$). Using $SPAR_{asms}$ as a dependent variable, regression analyses were then carried out using as independent or explanatory variables about 150 social, health status and health service provision factors. We utilized all available factors thought to be of possible relevance to the use of psychiatric services; these included service supply and availability indices including measures of the supply of community and hospital psychiatric, medical and nursing staff and the number and availability of psychiatric beds. A stepwise regression analysis was used to determine which of these independent variables best explained the variation in the standardized psychiatric admission rates between districts. In addition, product–moment correlation coefficients were calculated between standardized psychiatric admission ratios and the independent variables.

### Results

As Figs 31.1 and 31.2 demonstrate, admission rates are only slightly influenced by sex (Fig. 31.1), but vary markedly by age and marital status (Fig. 31.2). Admission rates for females are about one-third greater than males in the 45–70-year age group, but the unmarried in both sexes have much higher psychiatric admission rates up to the age of 75. The biggest difference is between unmarried males and married males where the unmarried rate is about 6 times the married rate for the 40–44-year-old group.

Thus we found the expected psychiatric admission rate calculated using age, sex and marital status structure in the district varied by up to 30% from the admission rates expected on the basis of age and sex alone. The correlation between the actual and the expected admissions for 186 districts in England is 0.76 based on population size alone, 0.77 based on age and sex, and 0.81 based on age, sex and marital status.

Variables showing the highest correlation with

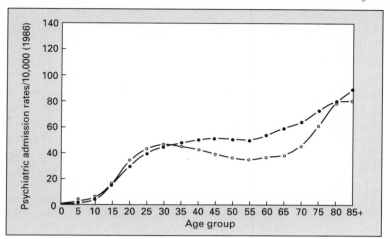

**Fig. 31.1** Psychiatric admission rates by age and sex (source: Mental Health Enquiry 1986). (●—●) Females, (○—○) males.

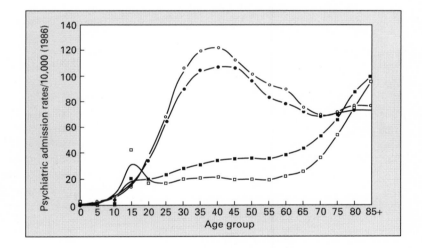

**Fig. 31.2** Psychiatric admission rates by age, sex and marital status (source: Mental Health Enquiry 1986). (●—●) Unmarried females, (■—■) married females, (○—○) unmarried males, (□—□) married males.

admission rates standardized for population size alone (SPAR$_{popn}$) were (correlation coefficients given in brackets):

1 Indicators of isolation: the percentage unmarried, single-person households and old people living alone (0.59−0.56); non-owner occupier households (0.39).

2 Illegitimacy (0.57).

3 Composite measures of social deprivation: the DOE index, UPA score and the Townsend index (0.55−0.49) (Department of Environment 1983, Townsend *et al.* 1986 respectively).

4 Indicators of poverty: personal service workers

– socioeconomic group 7, households lacking a car, unskilled workers – socioeconomic group 11 (0.57−0.44); unemployment (0.37).

5 First and total notifications of drug addiction in 1988 (0.53 and 0.51).

6 The availability of non-psychiatric hospital services: non-psychiatric bed availability, total consultants (and consultants plus junior doctors) per head of the population (0.50−0.46) (the availability of psychiatric beds was not significant).

7 Levels of mortality and morbidity: SMR to age 65 and the proportion temporarily sick (0.48 and 0.45).

**8** High population density: population density and overcrowding of households (0.47 and 0.39).

The highest correlation of $SPAR_{popn}$ was with the percentage unmarried (0.59). This illustrates the importance of controlling for marital status by calculating the age, sex and marital status standardized psychiatric admission ratios – $SPAR_{asms}$. When values of $SPAR_{asms}$ were correlated with the wide range of variables, the highest correlations were with illegitimacy (0.51) and SMR to age 65 (0.50).

In all cases the correlation coefficients were highly significant ($P < 0.0001$).

In order to determine which of these variables and others best explain the variation in psychiatric admission ratio between districts, the standardized psychiatric admission rate adjusted for population and the standardized psychiatric admission rate adjusted for age, sex and marital status for 186 districts in England and Wales were taken as dependent variables in a stepwise regression analysis.

| Dependent variables: | Explanatory variables significant at $P < 0.001$ level in stepwise regression analysis: |
|---|---|
| $SPAR_{popn}$ | % unmarried 1986 |
| | % born in UK |
| | % socioeconomic group 7 – personal service workers |
| $SPAR_{asms}$ | % illegitimacy 1986 |
| | rate of 1st notifications drug addiction 1988 |
| | SMR 1986 |

The regression equation best explaining $SPAR_{asms}$ is $SPAR_{asms} = 12 + 0.66 \times$ Drug 1st $+ 0.82 \times$ SMR (IHD), where Drug 1st is the rate per 100 000 resident population of first notification drug misuse in 1988 in the district and SMR (IHD) is the average standardized mortality rate for 1981–85 for ischaemic heart disease. This model was then used to generate the values of $SPAR_{asms}$ for each district as predicted from the regression equation. The predicted numbers of psychiatric admissions were then calculated and plotted to show the relationship between the actual number of admissions for each of 186 districts and the predicted number. This is shown in Fig. 31.3.

Table 31.1 shows the ratio ($\times 100$) for the actual number of admissions for each of the regions in England to the predicted number of psychiatric admissions using this model. Also shown are the ratios of actual admissions for the regions of England and the expected number of admissions based on age, sex and marital status. This illustrates the way the admission rate for each region is affected by using this more powerful model which more accurately predicts the number of admissions per region.

With some of the models the proportion of mental illness nurses working in the community was also significant at the $P < 0.05$ level – the higher the proportion of mental illness nurses working in the community, the lower the admission rates after allowing for other factors included in the model. However, this only contributed a small amount to the explanation of the variance, about 1%.

For subpopulations at the electoral ward level within districts for England, UPA scores are a more readily available source of information than standardized rates for age, sex and marital status. A regression analysis was also carried out using crude psychiatric admission rates for 186 districts (per 1000 resident population) as the dependent variable and the UPA scores as the independent variable. The correlation coefficient between the number of admission rates predicted by this method and the actual number per district is 0.84.

## Comment

Our recent survey is the first total survey of psychiatric admission rates for a national population (England) examined to determine the relationship between the health, social, demographic and service provision indices and psychiatric admission rates over a period of one year. Obviously the biggest source of variation between different populations in the need for psychiatric services is the size of the population itself. The importance of marital status for psychiatric admission rates has been shown. RAWP (Department of Health &

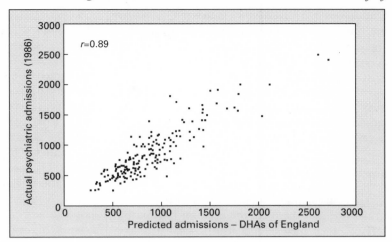

**Fig. 31.3** Actual *v.* predicted psychiatry admissions using SPAR$_{asms}$ and recommended model 1986.

**Table 31.1** Actual/expected or actual/predicted admissions ×100

| Region | Actual divided by admissions expected from age/sex/ marital status structures and national rates ×100 (SPAR$_{asms}$) | Actual divided by predicted admissions using the full model ×100 |
|---|---|---|
| Northern | 113 | 100 |
| Yorkshire | 120 | 107 |
| Trent | 89 | 91 |
| E Anglia | 89 | 101 |
| NW Thames | 92 | 98 |
| NE Thames | 94 | 93 |
| SE Thames | 104 | 116 |
| SW Thames | 106 | 121 |
| Wessex | 100 | 111 |
| Oxford | 75 | 90 |
| S Western | 87 | 96 |
| W Midland | 93 | 94 |
| Mersey | 125 | 99 |
| N Western | 116 | 95 |

Social Security 1976) recommended that marital status be used for calculating the allocation for psychiatric resources and these recommendations were followed. This paper provides support for the wisdom of this judgement and, in addition, suggests that the number of psychiatric admissions for a district can be predicted using a regression model which standardizes for the effects of age, sex and marital status and makes an allowance for illegitimacy, drug notifications and

SMR. In the regression analysis, the only service supply variable to significantly add to the explained variance of psychiatric admissions was the proportion of mental illness nurses working in the community. It should be noted from Table 31.1 that Mersey and Yorkshire regions have higher admission rates than expected from the age, sex and marital status structure of the population, and Oxford lower than expected. If an allowance is made for the levels of illegitimacy, drug notifications and SMR in the regression analysis, the predicted admissions for Mersey region approximate more closely to the actual number of admissions (that is the ratio of Predicted to Actual × 100 approaches 1.00).

This approach also highlights certain factors such as illegitimacy and drug use which may be important in influencing higher rates of admission in certain populations.

## Validity of the model

If, as we argue, these models are valid predictors of the use, and therefore the need for psychiatric services, then they should also be related to the underlying prevalence of psychiatric morbidity in different communities. Pantelis *et al.* (personal communication 1991) have carried out detailed prevalence studies of schizophrenia in four population groups using case-register information and interviews of hostels and voluntary lodgings, etc., to determine the true prevalence of schizophrenia in these populations. The correlation between the prevalence of schizophrenia in these populations and their UPA scores was 0.82.

Thornicroft (1989, 1991a) carried out a detailed study related to the findings of the Royal College Working Party (Hirsch 1988) in which he tested the ability of multiple regression models to account for the variation between health districts in the South East Thames Regional Health Authority and to identify meaningful components which predict admission rates. His paper gives an extensive review of the relationship between individual and combination variables and psychiatric morbidity and service utilization. His results support the validity of our general approach. He carried out a principal component analysis which showed that census and population factors representing deprivation accounted for 0.59% of the explained variance, while a second component reflecting isolation and chronic illness predicted 0.26% of the variance. The third component which was primarily loaded with factors indicating availability of psychiatric services accounted for less than 1% of the variance.

Thornicroft (1991b) has carried out a further study supporting the validity of our approach. In the context of an assessment of psychiatric services and a long-term follow-up of patients discharged from psychiatric hospitals, Thornicroft was able to identify the number of new long-stay patients accumulated during each of 4 consecutive years, from 1985 to 1989, totalling 303 in number. The annual accumulation rate of new long-stay patients from 7 health districts was determined. The mean was approximately 6 new long-stay patients a year with a variation across the 7 health districts of 2.5–11 patients per 100000 population per year. A product–moment correlation of 0.74 was found between the UPA score for these districts and the accumulation rates of new long-stay patients. Individual 1981 Census variables for these populations were in some cases more highly correlated with accumulation of the long-stay patients. Thus the percentage of population born outside the UK (ethnic group) was a relatively poor predictor ($r = 0.47$), while overcrowding, unemployment and social class V correlated respectively 0.81, 0.90 and 0.92. The Jarman UPA score correlated 0.74. Thus this approach appears a valid predictor of psychiatric morbidity in so far as it not only predicts admission rates but also correlates highly with the prevalence of schizophrenia as determined by community surveys and the number and rate of accumulation of new long-stay patients.

## Implications for resource allocation

For the UK in the 1990s district health authorities have become purchasing health authorities who need to determine what proportion of their budget will be spent to purchase mental health services. In so doing we would suggest that they are guided not by actual numbers of admissions to their district or by a flat rate per head of population regardless of the population need for services or current demand. The best predictor of the underlying psychiatric morbidity and likely demand for services is the adjusted predicted admission rate derived from national census data, as we have done in the study presented in this paper. For detailed calculations see Appendices 3 and 4 of the Royal College of Psychiatrists' Working Party Report (Hirsch 1988).

## References

Buglass D., Duffy K. & Kreitman N. (1980) *A Register of Social and Medical Indices by Local Government Area in Edinburgh and Lothians.* Scottish Office Central Research Papers, Edinburgh.

Burke A. (1976) Attempted suicide among the Irish born population of Birmingham. *British Journal of Psychiatry* 128, 534–537.

Cooper J.E., Goodhead D., Craig T., Harris M., Howat J. & Korer J. (1987) The incidence of schizophrenia in Nottingham. *British Journal of Psychiatry* 151, 619–626.

Department of Environment (1983) *Urban Deprivation. Information note No 2.* Inner Cities Directorate, London.

Department of Health (1975) *Better Services for the Mentally Ill* (BSMI) (Cmmd 6223). HMSO, London.

Department of Health & Social Security (1976) *Sharing Resources for Health in England. Report of the Resource Allocation Working Party.* HMSO, London.

Department of Health & Social Security (1986) *In-patient Statistics from the Mental Health Enquiry for England.* HMSO, London.

Department of Health & Social Security (1988) *Review of the Resource Allocation Working Party Formula. Final Report by the NHS Management Board.* Department of Health and Social Security, London.

Department of Health & Social Security (1990) *Health and Personal Social Services Statistics for England 1990 edn.* HMSO, London.

Durkheim E. (1952) *Suicide* (first published 1897 translated 1952). Routledge and Kegan Paul, London.

Faris R.E.L. & Dunham H.W. (1939) *Mental Disorders in Urban Areas.* Hafner, Chicago.

Goldberg D. & Huxley P. (1980) *Mental Illness in the Community. The Pathway to Psychiatric Care.* Tavistock, London.

Goodman A.B., Siegal C., Craig T. & Shang P. (1983) The relationship between socio-economic class and prevalence of schizophrenia, alcoholism and affective disorders treated by inpatient care in a suburban area. *American Journal of Psychiatry* 140, 166–170.

Hirsch S.R. (1983) Bed requirements for acute psychiatry

units, the concept of a norm. *Bulletin of the Royal College of Psychiatrists* 7, 118–122.

Hirsch S.R. (1988) *Psychiatric Beds and Resources; Factors Influencing Bed Use and Service Planning. Report of a Working Party of the Section for Social and Community Psychiatry, Royal College of Psychiatry.* Gaskell, London.

Jarman B. (1983) Identification of underprivileged areas. *British Medical Journal* 286, 1705–1709.

Jarman B. (1984) Validation and distribution of scores. *British Medical Journal* 289, 1587–1592.

Jarman B., Hirsch S.R., White P. & Driscoll R. (1992) Predicting psychiatric admission rates. *British Medical Journal* 304, 1146–1151.

Miller G.H., Dear M. & Streiner D.L. (1986) A model for predicting the utilisation of psychiatric facilities. *Canadian Journal of Psychiatry* 31, 424–430.

Odegard O. (1932) Emigration and insanity: a study of mental disease among Norwegian born population in Minnesota. *Acta Psychiatrica Neurologica Scandinavica Supplementum* 4.

Platt S. & Kreitman N. (1985) Parasuicide and unemployment among men in Edinburgh 1968–82. *Psychological Medicine* 15, 113–123.

Richman A., Boutilier C. & Harris P. (1984) The relevance of sociodemographic and resource factors in the use of acute psychiatric in-patient care in the Atlantic provinces of Canada. *Psychological Medicine* 14, 175–182.

Sainsbury P. (1955) *Suicide in London.* Institute of Psychiatry, London.

Shepherd M. (1957) *A Study of Major Psychosis in an English County. Maudsley Monograph No. 3.* Chapman Hall, London.

Thornicroft G. (1989) Predicting District Health Authority Psychiatric Service Utilisation Ratio in the South East Thames Region using Socio-Demographic Variables. MSc Thesis in Epidemiology, University of London.

Thornicroft G. (1991a) Social deprivation and rates of treated mental disorder: developing statistical models to predict psychiatric service utilization. *British Journal of Psychiatry* 158, 475–484.

Thornicroft G. (1991b) The TAPS Project. 6: New long stay psychiatric patients in relation to social deprivation. *British Journal of Psychiatry* (in press).

Townsend P., Phillimore P. & Beattie A. (1986) *Inequalities in Health in the Northern Region, An Interim Report.* Northern Regional Health Authority and the University of Bristol.

# Chapter 32
# Evaluation of the Transfer of Care from Psychiatric Hospitals to the Community

JULIAN LEFF

## Introduction

A decline in the population of psychiatric hospitals began in the late 1940s and early 1950s in the USA, England and Wales, and some European countries. Over the next 40 years many psychiatric hospitals in these countries were reduced to one-third of their peak bed numbers. At least half a million long-stay psychiatric patients were discharged during this period, and yet this revolutionary policy was not subjected to satisfactory evaluation. There have been a few follow-up studies involving small groups of patients, but no attempt to study comprehensively the closure of a large psychiatric institution. This is not surprising when the scope of such an undertaking is considered. It is necessary to address the effects of relocation in the community on the various types of patients – acute admissions, long-stay non-demented and psychogeriatric. The relatives should be asked their views on the new type of service provided. Comparisons need to be made of the roles of staff in hospital and in the community, and training for the transition should be evaluated. Services in hospital and in the community have to be costed carefully by health economists. The political process of decision making and implementation needs to be monitored so that lessons can be learned for other hospitals attempting the same transition. The respective roles of the public, private and voluntary sectors in providing new facilities should be delineated, and the ways in which they may be integrated. Finally, the views of the public should be sought on the introduction of ex-long-stay patients into local neighbourhoods. These are the main issues, but many subsidiary questions arise in the course of closing a psychiatric hospital which merit investigation in their own right.

In 1983 the North East Thames Regional Health Authority (NETRHA) took the decision to close two of the six psychiatric hospitals in its region over a ten-year period. This provided the opportunity for a comprehensive evaluation of the process of closure, and in 1985 the Team for the Assessment of Psychiatric Services (TAPS) was established with this aim. It is mainly funded by NETRHA but also receives a contribution from the Department of Health, in recognition of the relevance of the research for national policy. In this paper, the research projects undertaken by TAPS will be used to illustrate the issues which need to be faced in evaluating the transfer of care from large psychiatric hospitals to the community.

## Who is left in the hospital?

The drastic reduction in bed numbers in psychiatric hospitals in England and Wales has been achieved by discharging large numbers of long-stay patients. Naturally, the least disabled were discharged first, so that over the course of time the patients remaining in hospital appear an increasingly disabled group. It is necessary to assess the disabilities of the remaining long-stay patients both for the purpose of planning appropriate services and to evaluate how well they cater to the patients' needs.

### The relationship between evaluation and planning

The overlap of requirements for data between evaluators and planners has both advantages and disadvantages. The advantages are that the researchers are likely to collect much more detailed data on patients than is normally available to planners. Furthermore, the sharing of these data with planners improves relationships between the two groups of professionals and helps to ensure continuing cooperation. Researchers are always dependent on the goodwill of planners for their evaluative studies to run smoothly. The disadvantages mainly stem from the need of the evaluators to remain independent of the planning process. The provision of detailed data on individual patients is bound to influence planning, but requests from planners for such data are hard to resist. TAPS has dealt with this problem by supplying all data which have been obtained from professional staff, but only giving data provided by patients if they would not be considered confidential. Thus we give data on the patients' psychiatric state, but not individual patients' opinions about the service they are receiving, nor information about their social networks.

Requests from planners are not confined to the supply of data, but also include invitations to the researchers to contribute to planning. This is because the researchers over time are seen as developing a unique grasp of the effect of re-providing services on the patients. Such requests have been particularly targeted on the social scientists studying decision making and implementation. In our view they have to be politely refused or the ability of the researchers to be critical of the services provided is imperilled. In a long-term research programme, like that of TAPS, the problem cannot be avoided since at some stage during the research preliminary findings need to be disseminated. Inevitably these will influence the planning of future services, indeed it would be regrettable if that were not the case. Thus the researchers cannot avoid altering the process they are evaluating, but at least attention needs to be focused on any changes in planning that follow the dissemination of research findings.

### The residual population of psychiatric hospitals

It is important to recognize that there may be several distinct populations of patients remaining in a psychiatric hospital, each of which requires a different strategy for evaluation. The nature of the populations depends on the functions retained in the hospital. The two hospitals being evaluated by TAPS are Friern and Claybury, both situated in the northern suburbs of London. Friern Hospital serves four different health districts, three of which have established psychiatric admission units in general hospitals. However, at the time of the closure decision, all four districts had admission wards in Friern. Clearly a distinction has to be made between patients being admitted for a short stay, on average six weeks, and the long-stay patients. This division is not entirely absolute since we have found that as long as admission wards remain open, a proportion of acute patients stay more than one year and then technically become part of the long-stay population.

Early on in our research we became aware that the accumulation of new long-stay patients was occurring much more rapidly at Friern Hospital than at Claybury, although their catchment populations were of similar size. We discovered that there was a strong association between the accumulation rate and an index of socioeconomic deprivation of the catchment area (Thornicroft 1990). This problem is not resolved by closing the psychiatric hospitals. Patients will continue to remain for long periods of time on admission wards in district general hospitals, and part of the remit of an evaluation team is to monitor what happens to them when there is no psychiatric hospital to which they can be transferred.

The third type of patient to be found in many psychiatric hospitals is the demented elderly person who has been admitted to spend the last few years of their life there. Demented patients who can no longer look after themselves or be cared for by relatives have traditionally become the responsibility of psychiatric hospitals. Both Friern and Claybury Hospitals have a large population of patients on wards designated as psychogeriatric. When TAPS began to investigate the psychogeriatric population we were quite surprised to find that it comprised a mixture of patients. In addition to the demented patients, most of whom had been admitted less than 5 years previously, there were patients who had been in the hospital for 30 or 40 years. Although admitted initially with a functional psychosis, usually schizophrenia, the staff considered that they had become demented and had transferred them to psychogeriatric wards. TAPS personnel assessed the cognitive abilities and social behaviour of all the patients aged over 70 years at Claybury Hospital to throw some light on this problem (Anderson & Trieman 1990). The cognitive assessment used was the Mini Mental State, while problems with social behaviour were recorded by interviewing staff with the Modified Crichton Royal Behavioural Rating Scale. It was found that the long-stay patients on psychogeriatric wards, termed the 'graduates', were clearly distinguishable from the dements by scoring much higher on the cognitive tests. However, the problems of social behaviour they exhibited were similar to those of the dements. Thus it appeared that their transfer to psychogeriatric wards was determined by issues of management of difficult behaviour and was not on account of a dementing process. This discovery has important implications for the evaluation of reprovision of the psychogeriatric service, which will be discussed below.

Each of the patient populations will be considered in turn with regard to the evaluations required. We will start with the long-stay non-demented patients for two reasons. First they were given the highest priority by NETRHA for reprovision, and second they have been the subject of most concern on the part of the media, the public, and a section of psychiatric professionals who deplore the closure of psychiatric hospitals. Fears have often been expressed that when discharged they will commit suicide, be imprisoned or end up homeless, living on the streets.

## Evaluation of reprovision for the long-stay non-demented

This group of patients, many of whom have lived in a psychiatric hospital for decades, are being resettled in communities which they may not have visited since they were first admitted. This dramatic change in their surroundings and living conditions can be viewed as a natural experiment. The main question to be answered is whether their lives are better in the new circumstances. This deceptively simple question raises a number of methodological issues.

### Designing a study

There is a difficulty in interpreting any changes which are observed following the discharge of long-stay patients into the community. It would not be surprising to find an immediate worsening of their mental state, since patients with functional psychoses are known to be susceptible to life events. However, changes subsequent to the first few months after discharge, either positive or negative, could be due to the change in their environment or might merely reflect the natural history of their condition. It is well documented that manic-depressive and schizophrenic illnesses fluctuate in severity over time. In particular, the handful of long-term follow-up studies of schizophrenia that have been conducted suggest a gradual improvement with the passage of many years. The ideal design to accommodate the natural history of these illnesses would be a randomized controlled trial. In this case it would mean randomly assigning the long-stay patients to a group which would move into the community or a group which would remain in hospital, and comparing the progress of the two groups over time. This design was not feasible for TAPS on two counts. First, NETRHA had announced that for humane reasons patients should be transferred to the community together with their friends, and randomization would inevitably separate friends in many instances. Secondly, the decisions as to which patients should move first were being made by teams in the community who were strongly committed to the ideology of community care and would not accept randomization. As it turned out the mode of selection of patients had a profound influence on the process of reprovision and thereby on the evaluation as well, which will be explained below.

Failing randomization, the next best design is a matched case-control study, and this was the one TAPS utilized. Each long-stay patient selected for discharge is matched with a patient likely to remain in hospital for a further year. Matching ought to be conducted on variables which are associated with a good outcome for discharged patients. However, we cannot be sure which variables should be chosen until we have analysed the outcome of a substantial group of discharged patients. Initially we can do no more than make a guess at the matching variables based on previous research into prognostic factors in schizophrenia. In the event we chose age, sex, length of hospitalization, number of problems of social behaviour, and whether the patient was in Friern or Claybury Hospital. At the beginning of the study it was not difficult to find close matches for the discharged patients. However, as the study proceeded, the pool of remaining patients progressively diminished and it became increasingly difficult to find matches. This problem can be accommodated by appropriate statistical techniques: analysis of variance for parametric data and log linear analysis for non-parametric data.

This design requires the assessment of movers and their matches at baseline and then repeat assessments at various follow-up points. The next issue to be considered is the nature of the assessments.

### Whose quality of life?

The main purpose of transferring long-stay inpatients to the community is to improve their quality of life. However, this nebulous term is difficult to define and even more difficult to measure. There is a tendency for professionals involved in patient care to apply their set of values to the patients. If asked what they value in life, professionals are likely to answer: a fulfilling relationship with another person, being able to take a holiday abroad, having a car, good education for their children, and so on. These kind of values are irrelevant to long-stay patients, whose top priorities are privacy, reasonable meals, and a guaranteed supply of cigarettes.

In considering this problem, we decided to measure those aspects of the patients' lives which might be expected to improve or deteriorate after transfer to the community. It was obvious that an assessment of the patients' psychiatric state needed to be made. We chose to use the Present State Examination (PSE) (Wing *et al.* 1974) as it is well established and accepted internationally.

However, we found that one-third of the patients at Friern and one-quarter at Claybury were unable to complete the interview. This was because they were either mute or incomprehensible or walked away from the interviewer after a few seconds. This is not a result of the nature of the PSE but would occur with any psychiatric interview. The consequence is a large amount of missing data, but this can be compensated for to some extent by accounts from the care staff of the patients' problems. The Social Behaviour Schedule (SBS) (Wykes & Sturt 1986) is used for this purpose. It includes 20 areas of behaviour likely to cause social problems, and the ratings on each record the severity of the problem. The commonest severe problem was found to be neglect of hygiene, which affected over half of the patients in both hospitals. Physical violence and sexually inappropriate behaviour, which are salient features in the public stereotype of the mentally ill, were uncommon problems.

The modal age of the long-stay population is 60 years. In an elderly group like this problems with physical health begin to appear; heart disease, chronic bronchitis, diabetes, and other diseases of later life. It is a reasonable expectation that the patients' physical health will be carefully monitored and any disease detected will be adequately dealt with. In fact, in hospital this is the case since the junior psychiatrists act as GPs to the patients and the nurses are able to give physical as well as psychiatric care. The situation is quite different in the community since many patients are not in frequent contact with psychiatrists and may be in homes in which the staff are not qualified as nurses. Schizophrenic patients are relatively tolerant of discomfort and it is conceivable that they may not readily bring physical symptoms to the attention of staff. Therefore it is important to record any physical illnesses present while they are in hospital and the level of nursing and medical care required. These need to be checked on at follow-up in the community. The instrument TAPS developed for this purpose is the Physical Health Index (PHI) which is used to record the relevant information from case notes and from information obtained from carers. Use of the PHI revealed the surprising fact that nearly a quarter of the Friern patients were incontinent of urine, faeces or both.

Since the patients are the clients of the new community services it is essential to ask them their opinion of what they receive. TAPS designed a new schedule, the Patient Attitude Questionnaire (PAQ), to elicit patients' opinions. There has been some reluctance to ask long-stay patients what they think of services, possibly because of a belief that their answers will be distorted by delusions or will be subject to random variation. In order to check on this possibility, TAPS personnel gave the PAQ to the same 40 patients on two occasions six months apart. It emerged that for most questions there was a high test-retest reliability, and in fact two-thirds of the responses were identical on both occasions. The most reliable responses were to the questions asking whether the patients wanted to leave the hospital or to make their home there permanently (Thornicroft *et al.* 1992). These findings stress that there is no excuse to ignore the opinions of long-stay patients about the care they receive.

One of the main criticisms of psychiatric hospitals has been that they create a very restrictive environment for patients, which is dehumanizing and undermines initiative. To check on whether community life was any less institutional than life in the hospital, TAPS adapted an existing schedule to produce the Environmental Index (EI) which gives a measure of restrictive practices in the patients' living situation.

Finally TAPS addressed the issue of patients' social networks. Existing schedules could not be used or adapted since they had been developed for healthy respondents or neurotic subjects, whose social activity is on a different plane from that of long-stay patients. TAPS developed a new instrument, the Social Network Schedule (SNS), which is used to interview the patient. The respondent is first asked to supply the names of all the people he knows with whom he has had contact in the past month. If he cannot remember a name, he is allowed to identify an individual by some other feature, for example, 'the man I sit next to at mealtimes'. Social networks defined in this way were quite small, with a modal number

of six individuals at Friern and nine at Claybury. For each individual in the network, the patient is then asked whether he would miss them if they were parted, whether they are a friend or an acquaintance, whether he would confide in them, and the quality of their interaction – simply greetings, non-verbal exchange of goods and services, or conversations. Analysis of data gathered with the SNS and naturalistic observations of patients in a social club revealed that the quality of interaction was the most significant indicator of meaningful social bonds between long-stay patients (Dunn *et al.* 1990, Leff *et al.* 1990).

We believe that this range of schedules when taken together gives a good indication of patients' quality of life. It takes about half a day to complete all the schedules on one patient, and it took several researchers 2 years to collect baseline data on all 770 patients who were long-stay in the 2 hospitals.

Before giving a brief summary of the follow-up findings to date, it is necessary to consider the effect of the selection process on the annual cohorts of patients discharged into the community.

### The best first

For administrative reasons the discharged patients are divided up into cohorts, each extending over one year. TAPS began its assessments on 1 September 1985, so that the first year cohort of patients was discharged between that date and 31 August 1986. To date we have information about the first three cohorts of patients, and this shows clearly that each successive cohort has a higher mean age, mean duration in hospital, and median problem score on the SBS. This finding demonstrates that the least disadvantaged and disabled patients are being selected for discharge first. As time goes on the discharged patients are increasingly disabled, but even the third year cohort was substantially better off on each of these measures than the patients still left in hospital.

The process of 'creaming off' the better patients has a number of important implications for the research (Jones 1992). It means that findings from the first few cohorts cannot be generalized to the whole long-stay population, since the remaining patients are likely to have a poorer outlook. The same argument applies to the costing of reprovision for the early cohorts of discharges, since the more disabled patients will undoubtedly be more costly. There is also an implication for staff morale since the remaining patients will include an ever-increasing proportion with difficult behaviour. As far as the findings from the first three cohorts are concerned, which we present next, caution must be exercised in drawing any general conclusions about community reprovision.

### One-year follow-up findings

The data obtained with the batch of TAPS schedules were used to examine any changes in the first 3 cohorts of 278 leavers between baseline assessment and 1-year follow-up in the community. These were compared with data at the same two time points for the matched patients who remained in hospital, using an analysis of variance focused on group-by-time effects. Both groups of patients were found to be remarkably stable over time on the vast majority of data collected. This is perhaps not surprising considering that nearly half the patients had been in hospital for over 20 years and that their modal age was 60–65 years. Only three of the schedules revealed any significant alterations in the leavers compared with their matches, the EI, the SNS and the PAQ. The leavers were found to be living in much less restrictive environments in the community than they had been in hospital. In that sense, the community homes successfully provided a much less institutional way of life. Furthermore, the great majority of patients much preferred their life in the community compared with what they had experienced in hospital.

These changes represent a substantial and meaningful improvement in the discharged patients' quality of life. In terms of cost, care for these patients in the community turned out to be somewhat less expensive than hospital care (Knapp *et al.* 1990). An encouraging finding was that although no expansion occurred in the social networks of discharged patients, they made friends with ordinary members of the public. This suggests that some progress had been made in socially integrating these patients into the community.

TAPS is continuing with a one-year follow-up of all discharged long-stay patients, has conducted two-year follow-ups on a selected group, and has initiated a five-year follow-up on all patients.

### Patients on psychogeriatric wards

The reprovision of community facilities for psychogeriatric patients in Friern and Claybury Hospitals has begun only recently. We have no data for this group as yet, but it is worth outlining the research strategies since they are very different from those used with the long-stay, non-demented patients. First, it is not possible to ask the patients their opinion of the service because of their cognitive impairment. On the other hand, most of them have relatives who can be approached, unlike the long-stay patients. Consequently it is important to ask the relatives for their opinions, since in many instances they would be looking after the patients if they were not in professional care. The second point is that the principal aim is not to follow individual patients from hospital into the community, since one can anticipate that any changes in the cognitive or behavioural deficits due to change in the caring environment would be overshadowed by deterioration caused by the natural history of the organic brain condition. Instead the strategy is to compare one group of patients in the hospital with another similar group in a community setting.

The patients' cognitive state precludes their own assessment of the quality of life, therefore it is necessary for the researcher to make a subjective judgement about this, knowing that it will be supplemented by relatives' opinions. Staff also need to be asked about their satisfaction with working conditions, since the care of psychogeriatric patients places a heavy burden on them. As a more objective measure of this area, staff turnover and absenteeism should be monitored.

The nature of interaction between staff and patients is an important aspect of the quality of the caring environment, but cannot be assessed by interview techniques. It is necessary to make direct observations, which is a very time-consuming but worthwhile approach. Consequently TAPS personnel are conducting observations of staff–patient interaction in the hospital wards and in community settings.

The stated policy of NETRHA is that psychogeriatric reprovision should be in domestic-style facilities with no more than 24 beds. A number of such facilities have been established in the various health districts, but some patients have been moved to more hospital-like settings. Our aim is to compare the two kinds of reprovision to determine whether the domestic-style facilities do in fact provide a better quality of life.

We have introduced the issue of the graduates above, and it has become apparent that some elderly graduates are being moved into psychogeriatric facilities in the community in company with truly demented patients. This raises the question of whether their care will be better or worse in the new settings. The survey of all patients over 70 years old at Claybury Hospital (Anderson & Trieman, 1990) provides a baseline with which to compare the progress of graduates discharged to community psychogeriatric facilities. Consequently a limited follow-up study has been mounted of graduates and true dements from Claybury Hospital discharged to the same community settings. After one year in the new facilities the Mini Mental State and the Crichton Royal Scale are reapplied to assess any changes in cognitive state and social behaviour.

### Reprovision of acute admission wards

The third population of a psychiatric hospital consists of patients admitted for relatively brief periods of about six weeks. As with the demented patients, it is not appropriate to follow them individually through the change in facilities. Again, it is a matter of comparing one group of patients in the psychiatric hospital with another group in the community facilities. In this case, the plans are to close the admission wards in the psychiatric hospitals and open extra beds in the admission units that already exist in district general hospitals. However, in some health districts there will be an overall reduction in the number of acute beds. This situation requires careful evaluation and TAPS is currently engaged in this exercise. TAPS personnel are interviewing patients and relatives to obtain their opinions about the old and new services. In addition they are monitoring difficulties in getting patients admitted to hospital, the occurrence of violent incidents on the wards, and the frequency with which the wards are locked. The latter two kinds of events are considered to be indications of difficulty in running acute admission wards in general hospitals without the advantage of the open spaces in the buildings and grounds of a psychiatric hospital.

### What do the public think?

From the beginning of deinstitutionalization, concern has been voiced that dispersing the institution does not necessarily lead to integration of patients into the community. Since the problem may lie in the attitudes of the public to ex-mental hospital patients, we thought it important to assess these in a separate study. The study forms part of a PhD Thesis (Reda 1992) and is designed to detect the effect of contact with discharged long-stay patients on public attitudes. A survey of attitudes to psychiatric illness and to psychiatric services, including the closure of hospitals, was conducted in two parallel streets. One street contained a new facility for 20 long-stay patients, 10 of whom were resident, while the other 10 commuted daily from Claybury Hospital. Residents in the street were likely to see the patients frequently, while residents in the parallel street would probably have no contact with them. The survey was conducted just before the facility was opened and six months after the patients moved in.

Analysis of the responses to the questionnaire showed that, as expected, individuals in the two streets did not differ in their attitudes before the patients moved in. While there was considerable stigma attached to mental illness, it was interesting to note that many respondents were unable to distinguish between mental illness and mental handicap. More encouraging was the request from a number of respondents for more information about patients moving out of psychiatric hospitals so that they could help. The second survey showed no change in attitudes compared to the first in either street. Thus the presence of patients had no effect on public attitudes, either positive or negative. On the one hand these findings show that fears that patients, whose appearance is often dishevelled, will increase negative attitudes are unfounded. On the other, they suggest that educational campaigns could well tap a reserve of goodwill that might be used to aid integration of patients into the social milieu of the neighbourhood.

## Conclusions

We have presented here the major studies that TAPS is undertaking in evaluating the policy of community reprovision of the services provided by psychiatric hospitals. There are others but lack of space prohibits their inclusion. However, we have attempted to convey the variety of approaches that are necessary to complete even some of the tasks involved in a comprehensive evaluation. The research needs to be both broad and deep, and has a long time-scale. It can be difficult to sustain researchers in the arduous work required with little feedback in the first few years. Nevertheless, once results begin to appear from data analysis, there are substantial rewards, not least the possibility of influencing national policy and improving the quality of life for many thousands of patients.

## References

Anderson J. & Trieman N. (1990) Assessing elderly psychiatric patients: a whole-hospital survey. In *Better Out Than In? Report from the 5th Annual Conference of the Team for the Assessment of Psychiatric Services*. NETRHA, London.

Dunn M., O'Driscoll C., Dayson D., Wills W. & Leff J. (1990) The TAPS Project 4: an observational study of the social life of long-stay patients. *British Journal of Psychiatry* 157, 842–848.

Jones D. (1992) The selection of patients for reprovision. In: The TAPS Project: evaluation of community placement of long-stay psychiatric patients. *British Journal of Psychiatry* Supplement (in press).

Knapp M., Beecham J., Anderson J. *et al.* (1990) The TAPS Project III: predicting the community costs of closing psychiatric hospitals. *British Journal of Psychiatry* 157, 661–670.

Leff J., O'Driscoll C., Dayson D., Wills W. & Anderson J. (1990) The TAPS Project 5: the structure of social network data obtained from long-stay patients. *British Journal of Psychiatry* 157, 848–852.

Reda S. (1992) The discharge of long-stay psychiatric patients into the community: a study of the patients, the staff and the public. PhD thesis, London University.

Thornicroft G. (1990) Accumulating evidence: the new long-stay patients. In *Better Out Than In? Report from the 5th Annual Conference of the Team for the Assessment of Psychiatric Services*. NETRHA, London.

Thornicroft G., Gooch C., O'Driscoll C. & Reda S. (1992) The reliability of the Patient Attitude Questionnaire. In: The TAPS Project: evaluation of community placement of long-stay psychiatric patients. *British Journal of Psychiatry* Supplement (in press).

Wing J.K., Cooper J.E. & Sartorius N. (1974) *Measurement and Classification of Psychiatric Symptoms*. Cambridge University Press, London.

Wykes T. & Sturt E. (1986) The measurement of social behaviour in psychiatric patients: an assessment of the reliability and validity of the SBS schedule. *British Journal of Psychiatry* 148, 1–11.

# Chapter 33
# American Experience in Social Psychiatry

LEONA L. BACHRACH

In American psychiatric circles the definition of social psychiatry has met with little consensus. Schwab & Schwab (1978b) provide a learned analysis of the various ways in which the concept is used and conclude that understandings 'range from its being limited to psychiatrists' research activities in the social area to its emergence as . . . [a major branch] of psychiatry with [a] distinctive conceptual basis, research endeavors, and pluralistic therapeutic approaches'. Indeed, the concepts of social psychiatry and community psychiatry are sometimes used interchangeably in the American psychiatric literature (Schwartz 1972), a situation that is further complicated by the frequent substitution of another vaguely defined concept, community mental health (Schwartz 1972, Group for the Advancement of Psychiatry 1983, Bachrach 1988a).

Such confusion notwithstanding, it is probably fair to conclude that American social psychiatry constitutes a viewpoint more nearly than it does a discrete discipline or subdiscipline. More precisely, social psychiatry in the USA is the conceptual approach that informs the practice of community psychiatry. Community psychiatry, in turn, may be defined as the 'application of the theory and practice of psychiatry in noninstitutional and relatively nontraditional settings' (Group for the Advancement of Psychiatry 1983).

Social psychiatry thus forms a natural meeting ground for academic sociology and clinical psychiatry. The combination of psychiatric illness and social vulnerability – of clinical concerns and societal definitions of, and responses to, those concerns – lends itself readily to such an interdisciplinary focus (Bachrach 1987d). The late H. Warren Dunham, a renowned medical sociologist, gave voice to this common ground when he stated in 1964 that 'sociologists can garner some small satisfaction that the psychiatrist finally has discovered the community' (Dunham 1976a).

Community mental health ideology, on the other hand, has a broader scope than community psychiatry (Thomas & Garrison 1975a) and may be understood as the supportive framework for a 'population-based, prevention-oriented, primarily publicly funded mental health system' characterizing the 1960s and 1970s (Borus 1978) – a definition that suggests clear links with the field of public health. As we shall see, the field of community mental health in the USA is largely identified with a short-lived federal effort to endorse and fund comprehensive mental health services.

Both the practice of community psychiatry and the viewpoint or conceptual framework of social psychiatry have undergone substantial evolution in recent years. During the 1960s, community psychiatry sought not only to improve the life circumstances of individual patients; it was also preoccupied with concepts like primary prevention and community activism. In Kety's (1974) words, community psychiatry 'branched out well beyond mental illness into problems that it . . . [was] not especially qualified to handle – community, national, and international affairs; poverty; politics, and criminality'. Kety added, 'In each of these areas, we have responsibilities as citizens and human beings, [but] we have yet to demonstrate any special competence as psychiatrists'.

Kety was not the only psychiatrist to be concerned with the broad focus of community psychiatry. Zusman (1975) wrote, 'community psychiatrists are bound to be amateurs working in complex areas where it would seem professional skills are very much needed'. Sociologists also expressed some concern. Dinitz & Beran's (1971) observation that community mental health had 'set for itself a boundaryless goal: the improvement of the whole man and every man, in his total environment' applied also to community psychiatry. Dunham (1976b) wrote in typically succinct fashion, that 'community psychiatry must directly face the issue of whether it possesses adequate knowledge of organization functioning for intervention to have significant consequences'.

These kinds of criticisms were in many ways prophetic, for the philosophy of social psychiatry and the practice of community psychiatry have, in more recent years, turned increasingly toward the treatment of illness and away from efforts to change the social structure. More specifically, primary prevention has been brought into sharper focus as having only limited applicability for the full range of psychiatric illnesses, and activism has largely left the social realm and shifted to concerns that are more nearly within the expertise of psychiatrically trained physicians (Lamb 1988). Community psychiatry is also rediscovering some old priorities, most particularly the treatment and long-term care of chronically mentally ill individuals. All of this is occurring within a framework that gives credence to a biopsychosocial emphasis in programme development (Liberman 1988).

In the discussion that follows some of the circumstances leading up to these events will be examined.

## Historical antecedents

The early historical roots of American social psychiatry, which date back to the eighteenth and nineteenth centuries, have been explored and documented in a variety of excellent sources (e.g. see Yolles 1969, Dunham 1976, Schwab & Schwab 1978a, Langsley 1980b, Group for the Advancement of Psychiatry 1983). This chapter focuses on the influence of some more recent events, particularly those underscoring the close relationship between social psychiatry and community mental health which endured for virtually the entire third quarter of this century.

### Pre-1960s influences

Prior to the 1960s the care and treatment of mentally ill individuals in the USA had largely been the responsibility of the individual states. Although there had been some earlier attempts to involve the federal government in such efforts, the precedent for decentralized responsibility was clearly documented. Thus, in 1854, on the premise that he could find no constitutional authority for the federal government to become the 'great almoner of public charity', President Franklin Pierce vetoed legislation to make federal land grants available for the development of public mental hospitals (Task Panel on Community Mental Health Centers Assessment 1978a: hereinafter cited as Task Panel A).

However, as the 1960s approached, several circumstances converged and signalled significant new directions and trends in service planning and service delivery for mentally ill individuals. For one thing, increasing pressure on the federal government to become involved in issues of social concern, which had started during the 1930s, was becoming even stronger, and this, together with the availability of funding for social programmes at the end of World War II, provided a supportive environment for new initiatives.

In addition, mental health causes during the 1960s were heavily influenced by the interaction of several other factors. These included apparent earlier successes in the practice of military psychiatry, the appearance of new psychoactive medications, the increasing popularity of public health concepts, the emergence of civil rights ideology, and a general climate of optimism throughout the country.

MILITARY PSYCHIATRY

The role of military psychiatry, with its emphasis on brief consultation and treatment, is of particular importance (Smith & Hart 1975, Langsley 1980b, Lamb 1988), although it is often overlooked. Certain principles that had been found productive in the treatment of psychiatric casualties during World War II – principles that had proven effective both in returning many members of the armed forces to active military duty and in facilitating their eventual recovery – emerged as focal points for service planning. First, there was the principle of proximity, which was based on the idea that treatment should take place as close as possible to the location where symptoms were exhibited. This was coupled with a second principle, that of immediacy, which held that the early identification and treatment of psychiatric disorders could lead to more favourable outcomes. A third principle, simplicity, held that a major part of psychiatric intervention should consist of rest, nourishment and social support; and a fourth, expectancy, supported the idea that a patient's prompt return to former functioning was both feasible and therapeutic (Lamb 1988).

It was tacitly assumed that these principles could be directly and profitably transferred to the civilian domain and translated into broader goals guiding the development of civilian psychiatric practice. Social psychiatry's endorsement of such concepts as early diagnosis and intervention in order to effect the prompt remission of symptoms, and treatment in environments as close as possible to patients' homes, held a clear relationship to the military principles.

## PUBLIC HEALTH, CIVIL RIGHTS AND MEDICATIONS

These concepts were in fact reinforced by several other forces. Following World War II there was a growing interest in such public health strategies as primary preventive interventions and rehabilitative treatments (Bellak 1969, Bloom 1986, Breakey 1986, Lamb 1988). There was increasing confidence that psychiatric illness could largely be eliminated if early symptoms could be treated promptly. In those cases where illness could not be prevented, rehabilitative interventions could arrest its course and could even restore mentally ill individuals to premorbid levels of functioning.

These assumptions fit readily into the prevailing social climate. This was an era during which a can-do attitude dominated American thought (Freedman 1967, Menninger 1989). It was also a time when the civil rights of various disfranchised populations were being championed. In the field

of mental health, specifically, growing concern about inhumane conditions and violations of the rights of patients in state mental hospitals were capturing the attention of the public, and mental health professionals were beginning to acknowledge a need for basic change.

The positive can-do spirit in the USA was additionally reinforced by the appearance of new psychoactive medications which could markedly reduce the symptomatology of hospitalized mental patients. It had become increasingly easy to conclude that institutionalized mentally ill individuals, who were already perceived as living in inhumane and restrictive environments inappropriate for their needs, should be transferred to community settings where they would be able to function effectively with the help of medications.

In short, it was time for hope and change in American social policy (Dunham 1976a), and this progressive climate was legitimized for mentally ill individuals by the creation of a National Institute of Mental Health in 1949. From the beginning, the fledgling agency stressed both the inalienable rights of mentally ill persons and their legitimate claims on society; and it devoted primary effort to the search for community-based alternatives to the institutionalization of mentally ill individuals. These goals were quickly adopted by social psychiatry.

### The 1960s and later

In 1955 the federal Mental Health Study Act, which authorized the formation of the Joint Commission on Mental Illness and Health, was passed. The formal report of this Commission, published in 1961, contained a number of recommendations including the following: that immediate care be made available to mental patients in community settings; that the major mental illnesses be recognized as the core responsibility of mental health service systems; that fully staffed full-time mental health clinics be accessible to all people living in the USA; that large and remote state mental hospitals be replaced by smaller regional facilities; and that community-based aftercare and rehabilitation services for mentally individuals be greatly expanded.

In 1963 two significant federally inspired developments occurred, and they profoundly affected the course of social psychiatry in the USA. First, categorical Aid to the Disabled (ATD) became available to mentally ill individuals so that, for the first time, they were eligible for federal financial support in the community (Bachrach & Lamb 1989). Patients now had access to federal grants-in-aid, which were in some instances supplemented by state funds, and this enabled them to support themselves or to be supported in the community at comparatively little cost to the state. Although the amount of money made available to patients under ATD was quite modest, it was at least sufficient for them to maintain a minimal standard of living in the community. Additionally, many private individuals discovered that they could earn additional income by taking mental patients into their homes, and this provided needed alternative residences for mental patients.

ATD is known today as Supplemental Security Income (SSI) and is administered by the federal Social Security Administration. However, its distribution has been markedly curtailed during the past decade (Okpaku 1988), and mentally ill individuals have often had great difficulty in accessing its benefits. SSI is not an automatic entitlement, since disabled individuals must undergo stringent eligibility tests to qualify for it.

The second significant federal development of 1963 was the passage of the Community Mental Health Centers Act, a response to President John F. Kennedy's (1963) now famous message calling for a 'bold new approach' in service delivery to mentally ill individuals. With enactment of this legislation and certain supplemental amendments passed during the late 1960s and 1970s, the federal government took on unprecedented responsibility for persons disabled by mental illness. The community mental health initiative, which eventually resulted in the appropriation of $2.9 billion in federal monies (Comptroller General of the United States 1984), finally emerged as a fully legitimated federal endeavour that paralleled, and supported, the ideals, hopes and viewpoints of social psychiatry.

Indeed, community mental health philosophy

and social psychiatry were in some ways indistinguishable in the 1960s. Even the text of President Kennedy's 1963 message held promise for a new kind of psychiatry:

> Private physicians, including general practitioners, psychiatrists, and other medical specialists . . . [will] all be able to participate directly and cooperatively in the work of the [community mental health] center. For the first time, a large proportion of our private practitioners will have the opportunity to treat their patients in a mental health facility served by an auxiliary professional staff that is directly and quickly available for outpatient and inpatient care.

Thus, the 1960s were largely years of encouragement for the twin ideologies: social psychiatry, which served as the foundation for the practice of community psychiatry; and community mental health, which supported the building and operation of federally funded community mental health centres.

As we shall presently see, the optimism of these years was not altogether sufficient to withstand the challenges that the community mental health movement eventually encountered, and by the 1970s some serious problems were recognized. President Jimmy Carter's Commission on Mental Health, established in 1977, tried to breathe new life into federal support for mental health services (President's Commission on Mental Health 1978); and, in fact, a new and stronger commitment followed with passage of the Mental Health Systems Act of 1980. Funding for carrying out this legislation was, however, never appropriated, for the Act was repealed shortly after President Ronald Reagan took office in January 1981 (Bachrach 1991).

The federal involvement in direct mental health service provision in the USA was thus short lived. It came to an abrupt end 18 years after it began, and there has been no substitute since. Although the federal government today does provide some general health and human service block grants to the states, the level of federal funding has decreased drastically, and the mandated focus on mental health service delivery has been severely compromised (Bachrach 1991).

## Principles and problems

It is important to examine more closely the ideological underpinnings of social psychiatry during the 1960s because they formed, in Hegelian manner, a new synthesis which was even in its heyday, moving inexorably toward further change. Social psychiatry embraced a series of complex interrelated principles which defined its viewpoint and goals. These principles included, but were not limited to, the notions of geographical responsibility, humanization of services and equal access to care, comprehensive services and continuity of care, primary prevention and rehabilitation, and clinical egalitarianism. As noted previously, these principles not only formed the ideological basis for social psychaitry, they also epitomized the philosophy of the short-lived federal community mental health movement.

### Geographical responsibility and equal access

As originally conceived, the federal community mental health initiative sought to divide the USA into a series of precisely defined service areas so that all Americans might have equal and ready access to mental health services. There were to have been 1500 such 'catchment areas', each serving a base population of 75 000–200 000 local residents. Each was to contain a community mental health centre as the core mental health service agency and, through the centre, was to identify residents' service needs, formulate plans to meet those needs, and provide relevant programmes.

Geographical responsibility was, in fact, a concept that was intended to operationalize the fundamental goal of substituting community-based for state hospital care in a rational and humane manner. By dividing the country into segments with manageable populations, communities would be able to organize services in such a way that all Americans would have equal access to care. The egalitarian and civil rights antecedents of this goal were apparent: prior to the 1960s there had been a two-class system of mental health care, a situation in which individuals with sufficient resources to do so received primarily private outpatient services, while those who were economically disadvantaged either received custodial state mental hospital inpatient services, or else went totally unserved (Mollica 1983). Moreover, embedded in this differential was a serious imbalance in the availability of services according to race and ethnic origin. It was thought that, with catchmenting, class distinctions could be abolished by what Mollica (1983) has since termed 'unlimited access and universal entitlement'.

Did catchmenting work? With the advent of new facilities and sufficient federal funding to support them, many communities were in fact able to offer mental health care to their residents for the first time. Other communities could, and did, stretch existing offerings appreciably and broadened their target populations. Thus, there is little question that the volume of services did expand in many parts of the country.

At the same time, however, not all communities, and certainly not all Americans, shared in those apparent benefits. Several problems arose with catchmenting almost immediately (President's Commission on Mental Health 1978), not the least of which was the increasing geographical mobility of the American population. Mentally ill individuals who were no longer institutionalized could now, like other Americans, move around a great deal (Bachrach 1982, 1987b), and it became easy for service providers to question whether they should be treating people who had 'just dropped into' their communities.

In their most extreme form, the problems of catchmenting are manifested today in service inequities for homeless mentally ill individuals (Bachrach 1984b, Lamb 1988). People who have no fixed addresses are technically not 'of' any community and so are not the responsibility of any community in the USA. Catchmenting thus, in effect, gives agencies permission to exclude individuals needing mental health services on the grounds that they belong someplace else; and it has given rise to a practice ironically called 'Greyhound therapy', in which people needing psychiatric services are provided with one-way bus tickets out of town (van Winkle 1980, Cordes 1984).

Another problem with catchmenting was its creation of artificial service area boundaries. Catchment areas generally followed the boundary lines previously established for political districts and so did not necessarily represent the natural communities of their residents. In urban places this sometimes meant that people were to receive care not in neighbourhood treatment agencies but rather in facilities to which they were assigned. Very often the two were separate and distinct.

However, it was in smaller and more remote rural communities that some particularly difficult pragmatic issues came to the fore. In order to fulfil the requirements of a 75 000-person population minimum, some catchment areas found it necessary to cover huge geographical expanses (Bachrach 1983, Task Panel on Rural Mental Health 1978b: hereinafter cited as Task Panel B). Thus, most rural catchment areas exceeded 5000 square miles in land area. And a single catchment area in northern Arizona consisted of more than 60 000 square miles – an area roughly the size of all six New England states combined – and was bisected by the Grand Canyon.

In short, there was a growing realization that 'catchment area' and 'community' are not synonymous concepts and that a community mental health system cannot be created merely by drawing boundaries and calling the space within them a mental health catchment area.

Success in eliminating class distinctions in service provision was also mixed. In some places the new programmes did in fact reach racial, ethnic and other minority populations that had previously gone unserved, except perhaps in state hospital settings. However, other kinds of barriers often arose. For example, professional personnel employed in high-income catchment areas tended to have more intensive training and better academic preparation than those employed in low-income catchment areas (National Institute of Mental Health 1978). Once again, the situation in many rural communities reflected some of the more subtle issues encountered in the attempt to eliminate class distinctions in mental health service delivery. Perhaps because they often lacked expertise in 'grantsmanship' (Task Panel B 1978b), rural catchment areas were relatively unsuccessful in competing for federal funding (Task Panel A 1978a), and a disproportionate number of them were still totally unfunded when the federal community mental health initative came to an end in 1981.

Mollica (1983) has argued persuasively that a two-class system of mental health care prevails in the USA to this day despite the federal community mental health effort. The state hospital, in spite of its apparent decline over the past several decades, 'continues to be the principal facility for the acute inpatient care of the lower-class patient'; and, in fact, there has been a 'pooling of the poorest patients at state facilities as middle-class and working-class patients have achieved financial access to private institutions'.

### Humanizing services

With the federal community mental health initiative came great hope – and confidence – that state mental hospitals, widely viewed as custodial warehouses, could be eliminated and replaced by community-based alternatives that would provide more humane care, and during the 1960s reductions in state hospital censuses were both rapid and marked. After 1955, deinstitutionalization proceeded apace, both through the discharge of resident patients from state mental hospitals and the diversion of new admissions (Bachrach 1986). Thus, in 1962, immediately before passage of the federal Community Mental Health Centers Act, there had been some 515 000 patients residing in state hospitals. Twenty years later, in 1982, the count was down to 121 000, a drop of about three-quarters (unpublished data from the National Institute of Mental Health).

However, during the same 20-year period, admissions to state hospitals had risen by over one-fifth. State mental hospitals had thus become busy places where, instead of a relatively few patients' being admitted for long stays, the same individuals were admitted frequently for brief stays – a situation that gave rise to the picture of mental health facilities as having uncontrollably revolving doors. Whether state hospital utilization had truly decreased depended on what criterion one chose to use.

Moreover, there were some real questions about the extent to which the increasing utilization of community-based mental health services and the decreasing state hospital populations were truly paired events. Despite coordinated efforts in some communities, there was little evidence that, on a nationwide basis, the individuals no longer being served in state hospitals were the same ones who were enrolling in community programmes. To the contrary, there was good reason to believe that the two were serving entirely different patient populations and, moreover, that the most severely disabled individuals – those who were chronically mentally ill – were widely underserved or even totally unserved (Windle & Scully 1976, Comptroller General of the United States 1977, Gronfein 1985). Langsley (1980a) has described this situation as one in which community mental health had 'drifted away' from its 'original purpose as defined by Kennedy, the treatment of the mentally ill'.

In retrospect, it now appears that part of the difficulty in reaching chronically mentally ill individuals may be explained by the increasing complexity of their service needs. Prior to the advent of community mental health, service planning for the members of this population had been a relatively simple and uniform affair: most people showing signs of severe mental illness were admitted to state mental hospitals where their stays were generally of long duration, and often for life. Although critics objected (and rightly so) to the direction and quality of care that patients often received in those facilities, there was a simplicity and predictability to programme design that got lost with the community mental health focus.

With the advent of community mental health, by contrast, service planning itself became infinitely more complex. Chronic mental patients now had widely disparate residential and treatment histories, and they were presenting multiple challenges to the planners of community-based mental health service systems. A major obstacle to their care was a frequent failure on the part of those planners to recognize that there were many types of long-term patients, that they varied greatly in their capacity to adjust to life in the community, and that an extensive array of programmes would be essential to meet their complex and diverse needs.

Community-based service systems were, in short, finding it difficult to garner the resources, both material and conceptual, to respond to this diversity. Hence, 'gatekeeping' soon became a serious issue in the delivery of mental health services. Many programmes that were ostensibly designed as initiatives for the most severely disabled ill patients – the chronically mentally ill – in fact resisted admitting, or treating, these individuals and instead focused on providing services to people who were less severely impaired (Langsley 1980a,b Bachrach & Lamb 1989). Therefore, instead of finding more humanized care in the community, chronic patients often discovered that they had no place to go. Caught between emasculated state hospitals that had been forced by public outcry and diminished funding to reduce their services, and community agencies that often acknowledged little responsiblity to them, chronic mental patients frequently became the casualties, not the beneficiaries, of community mental health (Zusman & Lamb 1977).

The situation of homeless mentally ill persons in the USA today provides testimony that the goal of humanizing services has still not been fulfilled (Lamb 1984, 1988). Although not all homeless individuals suffer from mental illnesses, those who do have frequently suffered a unique kind of eviction. The state hospitals that once might have served them are often no longer available to them, and the community alternatives that were to have been created for their care often have not materialized.

### Comprehensive services and continuity of care

Community mental health ideology was largely based on an assumption that all the mental health needs of all community residents could – and indeed should – be met. In fact, the coordination of multiplex service efforts into a comprehensive system of care (Glascote *et al.* 1964) was one of the most fundamental concepts of the federal initiative. 'No longer', proclaimed a federal document, 'will a patient face the choice between hospitalization and no treatment at all'. Instead, the patient in a comprehensive community-based system of care would now 'be able to enter or leave the [community mental health] center from any service component or be able to move from any service to any other service within the center' without interrupting the flow of his or her care (Person 1969).

Such a goal obviously presupposed mechanisms for ensuring continuity of care. With services no longer being provided in a single centralized location, many different providers and agencies would be involved in patient care. There was confidence that techniques for facilitating interagency communication, coordination and linkages would quickly be developed. However, as Hansell (1978) noted, community-based mental health services were too often patterned after programmes developed for the single-episode user of services and thus exhibited 'a deficiency of interest in people with lifelong disorders'.

Thus, community-based service systems regularly and continually encountered major difficulties as they strove to provide comprehensive services within catchment areas and to afford patients with continuity in their care. With a prevailing emphasis on outpatient treatment and short-term interventions, community systems often relied on the patients themselves to be sufficiently motivated and mobile to present for treatment (Lamb 1988). Community mental health programmes often responded to the concerns of an essentially ambulatory and compliant population, even though many severely disabled patients – particularly those suffering from chronic mental illnesses – could not negotiate the overwhelming physical and psychological barriers that kept them from receiving care.

It seems, with hindsight, that the complex nature of providing comprehensive services to chronic mental patients was not fully understood in the early days of community mental health. For these individuals comprehensiveness generally entails the provision of a wide array of psychiatric, medical, residential, social, rehabilitative, vocational and quasi-vocational services. It further requires that agencies ensure the availability of the elusive function of asylum for those persons who need it, for either a limited or an extended period of time (Bachrach 1984a). Unlike the relative ease with which these varied functions could be fulfilled in state hospital settings, community-based systems of care had to contend with fragmentation in services and authority, and sometimes with relentless turf problems that arose among agencies in competition for legitimation and funding.

Concern with these kinds of issues eventually led to a recognition of the importance of case management in community-based mental health services (Harris & Bachrach 1988). Case management, clearly a concept that is meant to redress the difficulties that have accompanied the provision of comprehensive services and continuity of care in community-focused systems of care, is an affirmation of previously underestimated complexities, although it has often brought with it a new set of bureaucratic complications.

### Primary prevention and rehabilitation

It is helpful in discussing the community mental health effort to distinguish among concepts of primary, secondary and tertiary prevention – something that the early proponents of community mental health frequently failed to do. Primary prevention is concerned with actually avoiding or eliminating cases of illness. By contrast, secondary prevention, or treatment, focuses on helping people to control the symptoms of their illnesses to the extent possible and on preventing the development of further illness once it has occurred. Tertiary prevention is concerned with reversing or minimizing the disabilities that are associated with illness (Bloom 1986, Lamb 1988).

In the early years of community mental health it was frequently assumed (and sometimes promised) that primary prevention strategies such as consultation and mental health education would result in a significant reduction of the major mental illnesses and would eventually drastically limit the demand for conventional treatments (Lamb 1988, Zusman & Lamb 1977). The federal community mental health effort thus began with a strong belief in the basic preventability of mental illness, probably as the result of a prevailing view that social conditions, which were subject to change, were independent primary aetiological agents (Scheff 1967). This position was advanced even though the theoretical foundation for such a rationale was, and is, shaky (Zusman & Lamb 1977, Langsley 1980a,b). Certainly, environmental manipulation may be expected to better the life circumstances of mentally ill individuals and even to eliminate some varieties of personal unhappiness and stress, but it cannot be expected to alter the biology and chemistry of mental illness.

Thus, it is not surprising that the answers to preventing schizophrenia and other major mental disorders eluded community mental health (Group for the Advancement of Psychiatry 1983), even though some patients who, short of being cured, benefited greatly from rehabilitative or tertiary prevention initiatives that reduced their illness-related functional disabilities. Even here, however, there was an excess of optimism in the early days of community mental health. Many proponents of rehabilitation believed that, in those instances where illness could not itself be prevented, virtually all patients could still be restored to full societal functioning if they could be afforded appropriate vocational and social opportunities in the community.

For a sizeable number of mental patients, however, high levels of social functioning, competitive employment, and a return to society's mainstream proved to be unrealistic goals. Even today, given the current state of our technology, there are some individuals whose rehabiliation, if that is even an appropriate term, is so slow that it must be conceptualized and measured incrementally (Bachrach 1987c). In fact, our continued insistence on 'rehabilitating' some very seriously disabled mentally ill individuals sometimes does more harm than good, for there may be risks inherent in promoting rehabilitation beyond its logical limits (Lamb 1988). Some programmes that claim to allow patients to proceed incrementally at their own pace actually place such great emphasis on skill achievement and task completion that patients lose the freedom that other citizens have to be temporarily indisposed or disabled. Lamb (1988) has attributed our 'overselling' of rehabili-

tation in community mental health at least in part to a widespread impatience with the concept of dependency in the USA.

## Clinical egalitarianism

It is hardly surprising that a movement born during an era of civil rights and social activism, and nurtured by its values and concepts, subscribed to egalitarian goals. Egalitarianism in fact had several manifestations in the community mental health movement, including efforts to eliminate class distinctions in access to care, involving local communities and their elected or appointed representatives in the administration and delivery of mental health services, involving patients themselves in the treatment process, and equalizing professional roles by creating multidisciplinary treatment teams. Since the first of these has been previously discussed in this chapter, and the next two have received considerable attention elsewhere (e.g. see Bachrach 1991, Lamb 1988), the discussion here focuses only on the last.

If there was a point at which the ideologies of social psychiatry and community mental health parted company to any considerable degree, it was with the question of who specifically should be 'in charge' of the new service delivery efforts. Non-psychiatric service providers perceived President Kennedy's call for multidisciplinary treatment teams as a clear mandate to eradicate line authority in the treatment of mental patients.

Thus, even though Kennedy had actually specified that physicians working in community mental health would be assisted by 'auxiliary treatment staff', multidisciplinary teamwork took on connotations of professional equality and role interchangeability. Professional identities blurred as workers representing different disciplines resisted 'medical model' leadership (Clark 1987a) – a situation supported by the popular notion that mental illness is largely an artefact of undesirable social circumstances that are awaiting amelioration. Indeed, authority in treatment settings was sometimes so diffused that it seemed as if no one at all was in charge of clinical matters (Doyle 1977).

It should, however, be noted that there is an inherent inconsistency in the notions of teamwork and role interchangeability. Teamwork is actually more compatible with concepts of hierarchy and complementarity (Bachrach 1988b), in that its execution is dependent on functional differentiation and leadership. In this sense, an interdisciplinary mental health treatment team may be compared with an American football team which requires a quarterback to call the plays and unify the efforts of the players who perform various functions. In neither team may it be said that one job is more important than the others, for all are equally essential to the functioning of the team. However, the team nevertheless requires a leader who will potentiate the performance of all the necessary team functions.

The community mental health effort largely failed to insist upon a hierarchical concept of teamwork (Langsley & Barter 1983, Jabitsky 1988), and this eventually had several deleterious effects. First, it became increasingly difficult to attract psychiatrists to work in community mental health centres and to persuade those already there to stay (Reinstein 1978, Winslow 1979, Pardes *et al.* 1985, Clark 1987a). Secondly, psychiatric leadership in those centres declined significantly (Clark 1987a). In 1971, 55% of all community mental health centres had been headed by psychiatrists, but by 1980 that representation decreased to 16% (Boyts 1985). Thirdly, territorial conflicts arose among professional groups vying for power (Ribner 1980) – a situation that led many students of the community mental health scene to conclude that mental health professionals were far more interested in their own prestige than in providing patient care.

In summary, then, social psychiatry shared with the federal community mental health initiative in the USA a belief in, and a dedication to, implementing such noble principles as geographical responsibility for patient care, humanization of services, equal access to care, comprehensive treatment, continuity in service provision, primary prevention of illness, rehabilitation of mentally ill individuals, and, to a lesser extent, clinical egalitarianism. If social psychiatry did not entirely approve of the last of these principles, it at least

acquiesced and largely failed to put psychiatrists forth as essential clinical leaders in the provision of community-based mental health services.

In fact, a growing sense that psychiatry was too passive was a primary factor in a rift that was eventually to divide social psychiatry and community mental health. However, it was not the sole factor. Community psychiatrists, those physicians who did the actual work of implementing the principles espoused in social psychiatry's ideology, were beginning to find more generally that the conceptual framework within which the federal effort had been launched had a downside (Thomas & Garrison 1975a).

Thus, the forces that had generated a bold new approach in service planning and service delivery were not destined to dominate social psychiatry for long. Instead, they proved to be incentives for applying, testing, and modifying some new ideas that would be woven into a new synthesis.

## A new synthesis

Should the principles of community mental health, then, be declared invalid for social psychiatry? That seems neither a warranted nor a practicable conclusion. Although these principles have had limitations, they may be regarded as essential elements in the continuing evolution of social psychiatry in the USA. Thus, these principles are not so much to be perceived as wrong or invalid as they are to be regarded as tentative and temporary. As such, they have undergone, and they continue to undergo, considerable rethinking and modification.

In point of fact, social psychiatry in the USA today may be viewed as an ideology that is seeking a new equilibrium. Some of its historically held tenets are being discarded, while others are being retained, and still others are being updated.

What has survived is in itself impressive as a legacy and as a foundation for future direction. More specifically, psychiatrists are generally far more responsive today to the individuality and the unique programme needs of mental patients than they were before social psychiatry 'bought into' the thinking of community mental health, and this is a major and lasting contribution. It is no longer fashionable to plan mental health services for patients as if they are a homogeneous lot of individuals to be warehoused, and even state mental hospitals have become less isolated and altered their programme formats to become more responsive and more humane (Bachrach 1989).

Another positive effect is to be found in our understanding of the importance of cultural phenomena in service planning (Vaccaro 1988). Social psychiatry's close alliance with public health since mid-century has led to mental health professionals' developing a sensitivity, largely lacking in the past, to patients' varying identities and to the social and economic realities that often divide service provider and service recipient (Mollica 1983).

Moreover, there is value not only in what has been retained but also in what has been discarded and what is being modified. The area of prevention provides an excellent example of changing perspectives. Social psychiatry today is clearly adopting a more realistic view of the potential of primary prevention, particularly with reference to the major mental illnesses, since there is at present no evidence that the incidence of these illnesses can be reduced through preventive interventions (Musto 1975, Comptroller General of the United States 1977, Zusman & Lamb 1977, American Medical Association Council on Scientific Affairs 1979, Group for the Advancement of Psychiatry 1983). Thus, social psychiatry is becoming increasingly attuned to the possibilities of secondary and tertiary prevention, particularly for chronically mentally ill individuals, for it is these kinds of approaches that can assist patients in accepting the limitations imposed by their illnesses and enable them to achieve their functional potential (Bloom 1986).

Indeed, rehabilitation itself is being conceptualized in a more realistic manner (Lamb 1988, Bachrach & Lamb 1989). Clinicians have begun to promote an array of rehabilitative interventions ranging from modest incremental goals for lower functioning patients, to stepwise skills training strategies for those patients who are able to tolerate them (Liberman 1988). There is, in general, more comfort with the notion that even high-functioning patients may at times need breathing space from pressures that are sometimes placed upon them always to 'move forward' along some imaginary continuum.

Social psychiatry's determination to place mental patients in the mainstream of American life and to restore their civil rights has also promoted a more realistic understanding of the role that disability plays in the lives of patients with chronic mental illnesses (Meyerson & Fine 1987). There is today a more generalized appreciation of the unique needs of these most severely and persistently disabled individuals (Breakey 1986, Vaccaro 1986, Menninger 1989, Winston 1989), and this is one of the most encouraging outcomes of social psychiatry's efforts of the past three decades.

In fact, a mounting concern for the treatment needs of chronic patients is evident in the literature since the late 1970s. One particularly eloquent contribution by Stern & Minkoff (1979) calls for psychiatrists in training to reorder their priorities and redefine their roles as physicians so that they may more appropriately care for chronically mentally ill individuals. This priority has also been underscored in the writings of several past presidents of the American Psychiatric Association. For example, Donald Langsley (1980a) has written that chronic patients 'are, and must remain, the first responsibility' of community mental health. John Talbott (1985) has asserted that 'the primary problem we face in the area of patient care is our inability to translate into action what we know works best' for these patients.

In short, it would probably not be stretching a point to suggest that social psychiatry has been chastened by its earlier unbridled optimism – or, as some might view it, its grandiosity. This is apparent with respect to one of the early byproducts of social psychiatry's close alliance with community mental health: a general deprofessionalization of mental health service provision. Early efforts in community mental health helped create a milieu in which the importance of professional judgement was often minimized – an atmosphere in which greater value was placed on intuitive interpersonal skills in patient care than on professional training and expertise (Hopkin 1985). Thus, a number of community mental health centres had administrators or boards that adopted frankly antiprofessional attitudes (Clark 1987a, Bachrach 1988a, Clark 1989). In these instances psychiatrists not only had to protect their specific professional turf; they also, more generally, had to justify the very need for professional expertise in caring for mentally ill individuals. It is little wonder that community mental health facilities had become unattractive places for psychiatrists to work (Berlin *et al.* 1981, Peterson 1981, Donovan 1982).

Indeed, the 'boundaryless' nature of the entire community mental health movement played a significant part in psychiatrists' increasing disaffection with community practice (Fink & Weinstein 1979, Clark 1987a, 1989). Mounting resentment over being reduced to 'prescription signers' (Langsley 1980a) finally led to the emergence of a new breed of community psychiatrists who questioned the ideology, emphases, and directions of the community mental health philosophy, even as they retained some of its more positive contributions.

## Future directions

Thus, despite the existence of severe problems and scepticism on the part of many community psychiatrists, portions of the community mental ideology continue to hold appeal, and much of the enthusiasm that characterized social psychiatry during the early years of the community mental health movement has survived to the 1990s. Even though community psychiatry has had to acknowledge earlier errors, and even though the diminution of federal interest in mental health has curtailed programme development (Bachrach 1988c, 1991), there is still widespread hope that services for mentally ill individuals will become more accessible, more equably distributed, and more humane.

There is little doubt that a large part of this optimism should be attributed to the vitality of the new generation of community psychiatrists. Community psychiatry in the 1990s is attracting growing numbers of younger, socially conscious physicians (Breakey 1986, Vaccaro 1986) who believe that psychiatry can, and must, respond to

the treatment needs of psychiatrically underserved populations (President's Commission on Mental Health 1978). They are attuned to concrete circumstances affecting psychiatric service demand, such as homelessness (Lamb 1984), demographic trends (Bachrach 1982) and family burden (Group for the Advancement of Psychiatry 1986).

In 1984 Dr Gordon Clark (1987b) founded and became the first president of an organization now known as the American Association of Community Psychiatrists, a group intended to 'provide mutual support' and develop 'cohesive and politically effective' policies to 'stem the tide of psychiatrists leaving community mental health centers' (Problems 1985). Largely as the result of continuing efforts on the part of Dr Clark and Dr Jerome Vaccaro, editor of the Association's quarterly newsletter, *Community Psychiatrist*, the American Psychiatric Association in 1988 approved a series of guidelines for psychiatric practice in community mental health centres. These include model job descriptions for medical directors and staff psychiatrists, as well as guidelines for patient assessment, emergency intervention, and interdisciplinary clinical collaboration. It is clear that community psychiatrists are no longer passive and that they are today adopting a firm stance toward the issues that affect the practice of their profession.

It is interesting to note as well that *Community Psychiatrist* has an eclectic focus that distinguishes it from publications in the early days of community mental health. It now features regular contributions on psychotropic medications, psychobiology, medical issues, residency training, and concerns that affect the care of chronic mental patients and their families. The newsletter also routinely contains contributions from community psychiatrists located in all the regions of the USA, and its general tone suggests that something very like a grass roots movement is attracting them to the practice of community psychiatry.

One of the most promising prospects for the future lies in community psychiatrists' current efforts to build bridges with other branches of psychiatry, so that social psychiatry's concepts may be extended to the mainstream of psychiatric thought. Several years ago, for example, the

American Psychiatric Association featured a symposium on the relationships between community mental health centres and general hospital psychiatric units, an event to be marked for its unusual interdisciplinary focus. Instead of concentrating on differences within psychiatry, that symposium attempted to promote pluralism and reduce fragmentation of services through mutual understanding and support (Bachrach 1987a).

With such profound changes occurring in rapid succession, it is difficult to offer a summary judgement of the accomplishments of social psychiatry to date: it is probable that better historical perspective is needed. However, the very search for new directions is encouraging. Whatever else it is, social psychiatry in the USA today is not stagnant (Schwab & Schwab 1978a, Fleck 1990). Its new leaders appear to be dedicated physicians who increasingly combine their understanding of the biological aspects of mental illness with a critical appraisal of social psychiatry's history and a continuing devotion to the humanistic ideals that have survived the past four decades.

Thomas & Garrison wrote in 1975 that the community mental health centre 'is clearly a structure in transition between a mental hospital and something else, the outlines of which are only emerging' (Thomas & Garrison 1975b). Similar conclusions may be drawn regarding community mental health in general, community psychiatry, and social psychiatry, all of whose goals and experiences have been exquisitely intertwined. More than one criterion may be used to assess the success of social psychiatry. If we choose to dwell not on the movement's problems but rather on its support of new and innovative thought – on its continuing efforts to humanize services through the application of progressive concepts – we shall probably be inclined to give it fairly high marks. It is, in any case, encouraging to be able to say of a conceptual approach guiding the care of psychiatric patients that it is 'not finished yet'.

## References

American Medical Association Council on Scientific Affairs (1979) *Evaluation of Community Mental Health Centers.* Association, Chicago.

American Psychiatric Association (1988) *Guidelines for Psychiatric Practice in Community Mental Health Centers.* Association, Washington.

Bachrach L.L. (1982) Young adult chronic patients: an analytical review of the literature. *Hospital and Community Psychiatry* 33, 189–197.

Bachrach L.L. (1983) Psychiatric services in rural areas: a sociological overview. *Hospital and Community Psychiatry* 34, 215–226.

Bachrach L.L. (1984a) Asylum and chronic psychiatric patients. *American Journal of Psychiatry* 141, 975–983.

Bachrach L.L. (1984b) The homeless mentally ill and mental health services: an analytical review of the literature. In Lamb H.R. (ed.) *The Homeless Mentally Ill,* pp. 11–53. American Psychiatric Association, Washington.

Bachrach L.L. (1986) Deinstitutionalization: what do the numbers mean? *Hospital and Community Psychiatry* 37, 118–121.

Bachrach L.L. (1987a) General hospitals and CMHCs: a commentary. In *Leona Bachrach Speaks. New Directions for Mental Health Services* no. 35, pp. 91–97. Jossey-Bass, San Francisco.

Bachrach L.L. (1987b) Geographic mobility among the homeless mentally ill. *Hospital and Community Psychiatry* 38, 27–28.

Bachrach L.L. (1987c) Measuring program outcomes in Tucson. *Hospital and Community Psychiatry* 38, 1151–1152.

Bachrach L.L. (1987d) Sociological thought in psychiatric care. *Hospital and Community Psychiatry* 38, 819–820.

Bachrach L.L. (1988a) Community mental health centers and other semantic concerns. *Hospital and Community Psychiatry* 39, 605–606.

Bachrach L.L. (1988b) Egalitarianism and the CMHC treatment team. *Community Psychiatrist* June, 10–12.

Bachrach L.L. (1988c) Progress in community mental health. *Community Mental Health Journal* 24, 3–6.

Bachrach L.L. (1989) The state mental hospital and public psychiatry. In Beels C.C. & Bachrach L.L. (eds) *Survival Strategies for Public Psychiatry. New Directions for Mental Health Services* no. 42, pp. 41–50. Jossey-Bass, San Francisco.

Bachrach L.L. (1991) Community mental health centers in the USA. In Bennett D. & Freeman H.L. (ed.) *Community Psychiatry: The Principles,* pp. 543–569. Churchill Livingstone, London.

Bachrach L.L. & Lamb H.R. (1989) What have we learned from deinstitutionalization? *Psychiatric Annals* 19, 12–21.

Bellak L. (1969) Community mental health as a branch of public health. In Bellak L. & Barten H.H. (eds) *Progress in Community Mental Health* vol. 1, pp. 22–26. Grune & Stratton, New York.

Berlin R.M., Kales J.D., Humphrey F.J. & Kales A. (1981) The patient care crisis in community mental health centers: a need for more psychiatric involvement.

*American Journal of Psychiatry* 138, 450–454.

Bloom B.L. (1986) Primary prevention: an overview. In Barter J.T. & Talbott S.W. (eds) *Primary Prevention in Psychiatry: State of the Art*, pp. 3–12. American Psychiatric Press, Washington.

Borus J.F. (1978) Issues critical to the survival of community mental health. *American Journal of Psychiatry* 135, 1029–1035.

Boyts H. (1985) Overview: recruiting and retaining psychiatrists to work in community mental health centers: overcoming the obstacles. In *Community Mental Health Centers and Psychiatrists*, pp. 7–21. Joint Steering Committee of the American Psychiatric Association and the National Council of Community Mental Health Centers, Washington.

Breakey W.B. (1986) Community psychiatry in residency training. *Community Psychiatrist* April, 8.

Clark G.H. (1987a) *Community Psychiatry: Problems and Possibilities*. McNeil Pharmaceuticals, Spring House, Pennsylvania.

Clark G.H. (1987b) Psychiatrists and community mental health centers. *Hospital and Community Psychiatry* 38, 113.

Clark G.H. (1989) Guidelines for psychiatric practice in community mental health settings. *Psychiatric Annals* 19, 22–26.

Comptroller General of the United States (1977) *Returning the Mentally Disabled to the Community: Government Needs to Do More*. General Accounting Office, Washington.

Comptroller General of the United States (1984) *States Have Made Few Changes in Implementing the Alcohol, Drug Abuse, and Mental Health Services Block Grant*. General Accounting Office, Washington.

Cordes C. (1984) The plight of the homeless mentally ill. *APA Monitor* February, 1, 13.

Dinitz S. & Beran N. (1971) Community mental health as a boundaryless and boundary-busting system. *Journal of Health and Social Behavior* 12, 99–108.

Donovan C.M. (1982) Problems of psychiatric practice in community mental health centers. *American Journal of Psychiatry* 139, 456–460.

Doyle M.C. (1977) Egalitarianism in a mental health center: an experiment that failed. *Hospital and Community Psychiatry* 28, 521–525.

Dunham H.W. (1976) *Social Realities and Community Psychiatry*. Human Sciences Press, New York.

Fink P.J. & Weinstein S.P. (1979) Whatever happened to psychiatry: the deprofessionalization of community mental health centers. *American Journal of Psychiatry* 136, 406–409.

Fleck S. (1990) Social psychiatry – an overview. *Social Psychiatry and Epidemiology* 25, 48–55.

Freedman A.M. (1967) Historical and political roots of the Community Mental Health Centers Act. *American Journal of Orthopsychiatry* 37, 487–494.

Glascote R.M., Sanders D.S., Forstenzer H.M. & Foley A.R. (1964) *The Community Mental Health Center: An Analysis of Existing Models*. American Psychiatric Association, Washington.

Gronfein W. (1985) Incentives and intentions in mental health policy: a comparison of the Medicaid and Community Mental Health Programs. *Journal of Health and Social Behavior* 26, 192–206.

Group for the Advancement of Psychiatry (1983) *Community Psychiatry: A Reappraisal*. Mental Health Materials Center, New York.

Group for the Advancement of Psychiatry (1986) *A Family Affair: Helping Families Cope with Mental Illness: A Guide for the Professions*. Brunner/Mazel, New York.

Hansell N. (1978) Services for schizophrenics: a lifelong approach to treatment. *Hospital and Community Psychiatry* 29, 105–109.

Harris M. & Bachrach L.L. (eds) (1988) *Clinical Case Management. New Directions for Mental Health Services* no. 40. Jossey-Bass, San Francisco.

Hopkin J.T. (1985) Psychiatry and medicine in the emergency room. In Lipton F.R. & Goldfinger S. (eds) *Emergency Psychiatry at the Crossroads. New Directions for Mental Health Services*. Jossey-Bass, San Francisco.

Jabitsky I.M. (1988) Psychiatric teams and the psychiatrist's authority in the New York State mental health system. *New York State Journal of Medicine* 88, 577–581.

Joint Commission on Mental Illness and Health (1961) *Action for Mental Health*. Basic Books, New York.

Kennedy J.F. (1963) Message from the President of the United States Relative to Mental Illness and Mental Retardation. 88th Congress, First Session. House of Representatives Document no. 58, 5 February. Washington.

Kety S.S. (1974) From rationalization to reason. *American Journal of Psychiatry* 131, 957–963.

Lamb H.R. (ed.) (1984) *The Homeless Mentally Ill*. American Psychiatric Association, Washington DC.

Lamb H.R. (1988) Community psychiatry and prevention. In Talbott J.A., Hales R.E. & Yudofsky S.C. (eds) *The American Psychiatric Press Textbook of Psychiatry*. American Psychiatric Press, Washington DC.

Langsley D.G. (1980a) The community mental health center: does it treat patients? *Hospital and Community Psychiatry* 31, 815–819.

Langsley D.G. (1980b) Community psychiatry. In Kaplan H.I. & Freedman A.M. (eds) *Comprehensive Textook of Psychiatry* vol. 3. Williams & Wilkins, Baltimore.

Langsley D.G. & Barter J.T. (1983) Psychiatric roles in the community mental health center. *Hospital and Community Psychiatry* 34, 729–733.

Liberman R.P. (ed.) (1988) *Psychiatric Rehabilitation of Chronic Mental Patients*. American Psychiatric Press, Washington.

Menninger R.W. (1989) Trends in American psychiatry: implications for psychiatry in Japan. *Psychiatria et Neurologia Japonica* 91, 556–565.

Meyerson A.T. & Fine T. (eds) (1987) *Psychiatric Disability: Clinical, Administrative, and Legal Aspects.* American Psychiatric Press, Washington.

Mollica R.E. (1983) From asylum to community. *New England Journal of Medicine* 308, 367–373.

Musto D.A. (1975) Whatever happened to 'community mental health'? *Public Interest* 39, 52–79.

National Institute of Mental Health (1978) *Staffing Differences Between Federally Funded CMHCs Located in Low Income and High Income Catchment Areas.* Division of Biometry and Epidemiology Memorandum no. 30, 27 January. Rockville, Maryland.

Okpaku S.O. (1988) The Psychiatrist and the Social Security Disability Insurance and Supplemental Security Income Programs. *Hospital and Community Psychiatry* 39, 879–883.

Pardes H., Pincus H. & Pomeranz R. (1985) Foreword. In *Joint Steering Committee of the American Psychiatric Association and the National Council of Community Mental Health Centers: Community Mental Health Centers and Psychiatrists*, pp. 1–6. Association, Washington.

Person P.H. (1969) *A Statistical Information System for Community Mental Health Centers*, p. 2. National Institute of Mental Health, Rockville, Maryland.

Peterson L.G. (1981) On being a necessary evil at a mental health center. *Hospital and Community Psychiatry* 32, 644.

President's Commission on Mental Health (1978) Report to the President. The White House, Washington.

Problems in CMHCs spur formation of support group (1985) *Psychiatric News*, March, 1, 16.

Reinstein M.J. (1978) Community mental health centers and the dissatisfied psychiatrist: results of an informal survey. *Hospital and Community Psychiatry* 29, 261–262.

Ribner D.S. (1980) Psychiatrists and community mental health: current issues and trends. *Hospital and Community Psychiatry* 31, 338–341.

Scheff T.J. (1967) Introduction. In Scheff T.J. (ed.) *Mental Illness and Social Processes.* Harper & Row, New York.

Schwab J.J. & Schwab M.E. (1978a) *Sociocultural Roots of Mental Illness: An Epidemiological Survey.* Plenum, New York.

Schwab J.J. & Schwab M.E. (1978b) *Sociocultural Roots of Mental Illness: An Epidemiological Survey*, p. 15. Plenum, New York.

Schwartz D.A. (1972) Community mental health in 1972 – an assessment. In Barten H.H. & Bellak L. (eds) *Progress in Community Mental Health* vol. 2. Grune & Stratton, New York.

Smith W.G. & Hart D.W. (1975) Community mental health: a noble failure? *Hospital and Community Psychiatry* 26, 581–583.

Stern R. & Minkoff K. (1979) Paradoxes in programming for chronic patients in a community clinic. *Hospital and Community Psychiatry* 30, 613–617.

Talbott J.A. (1985) The fate of the public psychiatric system. *Hospital and Community Psychiatry* 36, 46–50.

Task Panel on Community Mental Health Centers Assessment (Task Panel A) (1978a) Reports Submitted to the President's Commission on Mental Health vol. 2. The White House, Washington.

Task Panel on Rural Mental Health (Task Panel B) (1978b) Reports Submitted to the President's Commission on Mental Health vol. 3. The White House, Washington.

Thomas C.S. & Garrison V. (1975a) A general systems view of community mental health. In Bellak L. & Barten H.H. (eds) *Progress in Community Mental Health* vol. 3. Brunner/Mazel, New York.

Thomas C.S. & Garrison V. (1975b) A general systems view of community mental health. In Bellak L. & Barten H.H. (eds) *Progress in Community Mental Health* vol. 3, p. 265. Brunner Mazel, New York.

Vaccaro J.V. (1986) Residents' forum. *Psychiatric News* May, 16, 31.

Vaccaro J.V. (1988) Culture and psychiatry. *Community Psychiatrist* June, 3.

van Winkle W.A. (1980) Bedlam by the bay. *New West* December, 1.

Windle C. & Scully D. (1976) Community mental health centers and the decreasing use of state mental hospitals. *Community Mental Health Journal* 12, 239–243.

Winslow W.W. (1979) The changing role of psychiatrists in community mental health centers. *American Journal of Psychiatry* 136, 24–27.

Winston L.M. (1989) The community psychiatrist's leadership in psychosocial intervention. *Community Psychiatrist* May, 9.

Yolles S.F. (1969) Past, present and 1980: trend projections. In Bellak L. & Barten H.H. (eds) *Progress in Community Mental Health* vol. 1, pp. 3–23. Grune & Stratton, New York.

Zusman J. (1975) The philosophic basis for community and social psychiatry. In Barton W.E. & Sanborn C.J. (eds) *An Assessment of the Community Mental 1975 Health Movement*, p. 26. Heath, Lexington, Massachusetts.

Zusman J. & Lamb H.R. (1977) In defense of community mental health. *American Journal of Psychiatry* 134, 887–890.

# Chapter 34
# Health Economics and Psychiatry:
# The Pursuit of Efficiency

## MARTIN KNAPP & JENI BEECHAM

### Better services, lower costs

Developments in social psychiatry as practised obviously do not stem *solely* from changes in the skills or preferences of psychiatrists. Indeed, in their gloomier moments, psychiatrists may believe that most of their actions and reactions are influenced more by the exigencies of social, economic, demographic, ideological or political imperatives than by the medical needs of patients and accepted medical best practices. Many – perhaps *too* many – factors and forces combine to influence the organization and delivery of mental health services. These forces do not always act in concert, though during the 1980s there was a common theme running through many of them. This was the pressure on all mental health service providers and professionals to deliver better services and/or to cut costs. This pressure to improve value for money, efficiency or cost-effectiveness was one of the more dominant of exogenous influences during the 1980s. It is unlikely to disappear from policy agendas during the 1990s.

The consequences of this emphasis on efficiency are not all welcome, but it would be foolish (and futile) for social psychiatry to reject this particular emphasis or policy theme without further examination of what it can offer. It must be admitted that efficiency is a controversial topic:

> "Efficiency" is a term with unfortunate connotations. Although it appears to some to be self-evidently a good thing, like "sincerity" or "honesty", just as with the pursuit of these latter virtues, there can be unattractive consequences . . . People do not like [efficiency] carried to the extreme where it dominates all other considerations, and especially . . . where the main purposes are

the humane and just treatment of people, and often of people who are having a hard time of it anyway. (Williams & Anderson 1975, p. 1)

What, then, is meant by efficiency? How can it be studied? What can health economics contribute to the discussion of efficiency in social psychiatry, or in mental health care more generally? What, indeed, is the justification for the efficiency imperative?

These four questions concern one of the central topics in health economics and will be used to structure this chapter. However, examination of some recent literature (Knapp & Beecham 1991) shows much variation in the use of economic approaches to issues in psychiatry so we first briefly introduce the broader relevance of a health economics perspective. The chapter continues by outlining a theoretical framework that will facilitate understanding of the economic perspective. The framework is borrowed from economics, though its relevance for the evaluation of mental health services will be demonstrated.

### The contribution of health economics

Economics shares with many of the social sciences (and in common with some of the medical sciences) two interrelated features: it has its own seemingly impenetrable jargon which confuses the outsider, but it also has a certain intuitive appeal and an apparent simplicity which is attractive. It is the tension between the attraction of economics and the confusion it generates which has probably been at the heart of the denigration and over-optimistic misrepresentation of the subject. One does not need a formal qualification in economics to be able to talk with a fair amount of sense about cost-effectiveness or efficiency, but a little knowledge is dangerous.

Readers of this book will most often come into contact with economics via media reports of the state of the national economy or via purchases of goods and services in the high street. In these ways they are exposed to economics the *topic*. This must be distinguished from economics the *discipline* (Culyer 1980). The discipline need not be confined in application to the topic. A general dissatisfaction with the direction or philosophy of macroeconomic policy is not sufficient justification for criticizing the principles of microeconomic theory or their application in practical analysis. One does not have to agree with the economic policies of the government of the day to advocate the sensible pursuit of efficiency in psychiatry; nor does one need to be a free-marketeer to study economics; nor does one have to subscribe to a programme of privatization in order to apply economic techniques to the question of public–private efficiency differences. Health economists are concerned partly with the economic *topics* of health care – expenditure limits, costs, the supply of qualified labour, market forces, contracting-out, and so on – but more often with the application of the *discipline* of economics to practice and policy issues concerning health and health care. To adopt an economic perspective is therefore not necessarily to focus only on what is immediately quantifiable or reducible to monetary magnitudes.

Health economics tackles a wide range of criteria and topics and by concentrating on efficiency in this chapter we do not mean to divert attention away from other areas and applications of the discipline. Health economics textbooks, such as the useful (and accessible) volume by McGuire *et al.* (1988), illustrate the breadth of the subject. Among the social or public policy questions which economic research has successfully addressed, often in collaboration with other disciplines, are the following:

- What is the true cost of care?
- What are the outcomes of care services and how do we measure them?
- What is the relationship between resources and outcomes?
- What are the staffing requirements of a particular service model?

- What are the relative costs and benefits of alternative courses of action?
- What is the relationship between capital and current expenditure?
- Why do the costs of ostensibly similar services or patients vary so markedly?
- Do internal markets raise efficiency? Do they enhance consumer choice?
- What do we mean by an 'optimal balance of care'?
- To what extent can we recoup the costs of care from charges to clients?
- Is 'allocation according to need' substantially different from 'allocation according to willingness to pay'?
- How can we sensibly allocate resources between different areas of the country?
- What do we mean by 'value for money'?
- Can privatization benefit care services?
- Is the private sector cheaper than the public? Is it more efficient?

Few of these questions, however, have been examined for *mental* health or for services delivered to treat it. The shortage of empirical research is particularly acute in the UK. For example, current policy to replace hospital services has generated a huge amount of interest but, to date, has brought forth only a small number of studies which examine the effects of this policy. The cost imperative behind local – if not national – policies is often important and the need to incorporate an economic component should be clear. Despite this policy emphasis, there is only now a UK study which will provide parallel information to the significant work of Weisbrod *et al.* (1980) and Hoult *et al.* (1983) in evaluating the Training in Community Living programmes. The UK replication and evaluation are introduced by Marks *et al.* (1988). To take other examples, despite numerous investigations in the USA, Canada and Germany (and, to a lesser extent, Italy) of the cost consequences of closing mental hospitals, there has been little UK work. Our own work in the North East Thames Region, alongside the Team for the Assessment of Psychiatric Services research (TAPS 1992), which looks at the costs and cost-effectiveness of community care as an alternative to long-stay hospital residence (Knapp *et al.* 1990,

Beecham *et al.* 1991), has disappointingly few parallels in this country. In a recent US paper, Frank & Jackson (1989) examine the impact of payment mechanisms on mental health care provision and utilization of hospital services; only an editorial by Marks & Thornicroft (1990) appears to have raised comparable questions here. Studies of the broad social cost of mental illness *per se* are also not particularly numerous in Britain, though Davies & Drummond (1990) and Croft-Jeffreys & Wilkinson (1989) look at schizophrenia and neurotic disorder, respectively.

Thus, although the efficiency imperative is making itself felt at the policy and practice levels, few economic evaluations have been conducted and the impact of economic research has been substantially less obvious than might have been expected. (The impact of economics as frugality and budget cutting has, however, been all too obvious in some areas.) The libraries of UK literature on the effects of mental health compare with a couple of file boxes on efficiency. This is probably due to several factors: a lack of economic expertise and interest among professionals and managers in psychiatry, a lack of interest among economists, a dearth of suitable data, and a lack of incentives to pursue efficiency. When there is an 'economic component' it is usually reduced to a description of some of the costs and rarely means full integration of all cost and other data.

Economics is arguably more art than science, more a way of organizing thought than of mechanistically allocating resources. It should seek to uncover value judgements, and not unthinkingly impose those of the analyst or the politician. It cannot replace the judgements of decision makers but it can supplement and inform them. It can help the decision maker formulate the practice or policy questions sensibly and logically and then (generally) provides a *range* of answers from which to choose. If the decision maker misinterprets these answers it is the economist's responsibility to point this out, but it is *not* the economist's responsibility to determine policies. Exploitation of the interplay of economic appraisal, political priorities and clinical expertise is the most sensible way to proceed.

This chapter will focus rather more on health economics than social psychiatry. This focus is hardly a surprising choice given the qualifications of the authors, but it is also important to have a chapter with this kind of focus so that policy makers, managers and clinicians can be aware of what health economics can *and* cannot contribute to discussions on mental health care and delivery of services. The need for a sensible balance of interests, expertise, and empirical evidence must not be overlooked when taking concepts from a textbook to the real world. We do not mean to suggest that economics (the discipline) should have the upper hand in evaluations, policy discussions or practice. The chapter also focuses in particular on the concept and evaluation of efficiency, and we have already noted that economists have a wide frame of reference.

## Defining efficiency

The pursuit of efficiency is predicated on the assumption that resources are scarce relative to the demands placed upon them. There will never be enough resources to meet all of society's needs or wants, not because members of society are greedy, prodigal or selfish, but because need is relative and not absolute. In provision of care it seems that almost every time service boundaries are pushed forward to reach more clients or to better serve existing clients, so more needs are revealed and more demands stimulated. Scarcity suggests that it would be prudent to make careful use of available resources, and economics has developed as the study of allocation under conditions of scarcity. Efficiency is simply one criterion for guiding or operationalizing the careful use of resources in the face of scarcity.

*Efficiency*, therefore, refers to a situation in which the allocation of a given level of resources maximizes the outcomes of a system of care (or component parts thereof), or minimizes the resource requirements to achieve specified ends. (We will define terms like outcomes and resource requirements below.) Absolute efficiency is hard to conceptualize for activities with such varied objectives as mental health care. However, whilst it may be impossible to say what is the *most* efficient utilization of resources, it ought to be possible to say whether a policy or practice change results in a *more* efficient utilization. Relative efficiency is an accessible concept in principle and practice. Defined in even these rather vague terms, a change in clinical practice or resource allocation which results in greater efficiency, without damaging clinical or other objectives, is undeniably a good thing. The crucial qualifier here is that efficiency is not, of course, the only criterion for good resource allocation. *Equity* (fairness or justice) is also fundamentally important, concerned as it is with the distribution of resources in accordance with an individual's or society's value judgements on the equal or unequal treatment of equal wants or needs. Thus, the scarcity of resources necessitates a choice which should be based at least on the twin criteria of efficiency and equity, and decision makers may also want to introduce additional criteria such as autonomy, liberty and diversity. Health economists, particularly those working within the mental health field, have tended to concentrate more on the efficiency criterion than on equity.

The concept of efficiency in broadest terms is thus straightforward, although there are alternative definitions and concepts for practical applications. Although common parlance might use the word efficiency as a euphemism for cheap, it should really be reserved for a criterion which looks at both achievements and resources, outputs and inputs, benefits and costs, ends and means. We will offer some alternative definitions below, but we first consider the theoretical basis for efficiency examinations.

### A theoretical framework

Most applied research in psychiatry includes an examination of effectiveness or outcomes, based upon a description of the objectives of mental health care intervention. These objectives are of two types. *Final* objectives are ends in themselves, even though there will be causal connections between them, whilst *intermediate* objectives are couched in terms of means to those ends. Providing mental health services where they are needed is really an intermediate objective, and so too is offering a supportive, high quality environment in a residential facility, for these are means to achieve various desired changes in, for example, the mental and physical health of individual patients or clients. The latter are final objectives in so far as they are desired for their own sake. Others might include improving individual competence and independence in the activities of daily living, promoting the well-being of relatives or informal carers, and protecting the rights of other members of society. Deficiencies in respect of these objectives are generally taken to be *needs*, and improvements along the dimensions spanned by these objectives are usually defined as *outcomes* (equivalent to reductions in need). This suggests a distinction between intermediate and final outcomes, depending on the objectives under discussion or study. Other chapters in this book describe in more detail the different meanings to be attached to the terms needs and outcomes, and also provide illustrations of their measurement and use in practice.

The objectives of mental health services are usually discussed by reference to hypothesized influences on outcome. Much applied research in psychiatry is designed to test the impact on users of one or more service, drug or social situation, frequently using an experimental or carefully executed quasi-experimental design to control for extraneous influences. The range of factors with a potential influence on outcomes is broad. The personal characteristics, experiences and circumstances of patients or clients will be of particular importance, but there are also the various social characteristics such as the quality of a care environment and the availability of support and stimulation. Characteristics of the physical setting – such as the fabric of a facility, and the level of support from income maintenance programmes – would also need to be included in a list of possible determinants of needs and outcomes.

We can introduce a more specific terminology here. *Resource inputs* are defined as the tangible resources such as staff, physical capital (including buildings and vehicles), provisions and other consumable items which go to create service packages and help achieve the desirable outcomes. Associated with each of them is a *cost*, this being a shorthand term and summary measure for all these resource inputs. *Non-resource inputs*, by contrast, are those determinants of final and intermediate outcomes which are neither physical nor tangible: they are embodied in the personalities, activities, attitudes and experiences of the principal actors in the mental health care system or process. For the non-resource inputs it is impossible to sensibly define a cost. (Because these non-resource inputs do not have a cost but exert an influence on outcomes, the discussion or study of efficiency needs to include them. Some of the non-resource inputs are correlated with, and perhaps determined by, the resource inputs or costs, but some are determined outside the care system, and these need either to be comprehensively purged from an evaluation by rigorous design, or built into the analyses.)

The basic assumption we are making here, and this is the basic premise of the *production of welfare theory* or approach, is that final and intermediate outcomes are determined by the level and modes of combination of the many and various resource and non-resource inputs.

This is not the place to attempt either a comprehensive description of the processes of care and support for people with mental health problems or a summary of previous research. The terms introduced here, and the framework in which they have been discussed, suggest that analogies can be drawn between, on the one hand, the practice of psychiatry and the delivery of mental health services, and, on the other, the terms, concepts and theories of economics. What we have described is what the economist would recognize as a model of production, with patient or client health and welfare being the product or output. This production of welfare perspective is not suggesting that the support and treatment of people with mental health problems is a production line or is mechanistic, nor does it seek to reduce the myriad interrelationships between outcomes and treatment characteristics to simple summary formulae. The influence and relevance of any one factor upon client or other outcomes depends on a combination of factors, the sequence in which they appear or are experienced, and the marginality of the stimulus which they bring

to the care setting. The production of welfare approach allows us to organize or locate efficiency research within both a theoretical framework and a clinical or service delivery context. We have described it in more detail elsewhere for other social and health care services (e.g. Knapp 1980, 1984, Davies & Knapp 1981, 1988). The point we wish to stress is that the framework requires no leap of faith, no departure from the implicit 'models' of service delivery underpinning psychiatric practice and research.

With this theoretical framework we can now define efficiency with more precision.

### Definitions of efficiency

*Effectiveness*, as the term is conventionally employed, refers to a simple increase in outcome following the introduction of an additional unit of input. An effective production process is simply a process which produces or achieves something desirable. A necessary but not sufficient condition for efficiency is effectiveness. A mental health service or activity cannot be efficient if it is not effective, and the effectiveness of some forms of treatment such as ECT, has sometimes been doubted. A closely related concept is *productivity*, the capacity to produce, which can be simply defined as the ratio of outcome to input. As we move from effectiveness and productivity to efficiency we need to distinguish a number of component definitions. The terms employed for them are not unique, even though the concepts are widely employed. (For example, the previously cited textbook by McGuire *et al.* (1988) employs a different terminology to the one we favour.) A process is *technically efficient* when it produces maximum outcomes from given inputs. *Price efficiency* is attained when the various inputs are employed in such proportions as to produce a given level of outcome at minimum cost. A technically efficient production process which is also price efficient can be called *cost-effective*.

A cost-effective technique might not be 'socially efficient'. Cost-effectiveness indicates only the most sensible among alternative ways of doing something; it does not tell us whether we should be doing that thing in the first place. It does not, for example, tell us whether we are better allocating money to ballistic missiles or community mental health services, nor must it ever pretend that it can. Full *social efficiency* is achieved when net social benefits (social benefits less social costs) are maximized. By considering social benefits and costs we immediately concentrate attention on the *full* ramifications of the options under consideration. The social benefits, preferably measured in units commensurate with the units of social costs, cover each and every output or outcome of a policy change or practice innovation.

The move from effectiveness through to social efficiency thus proceeds logically: effectiveness is a necessary prerequisite for technical efficiency; cost-effectiveness is defined with reference to the set of all technically efficient and price-efficient activities or techniques; and social efficiency builds on top of these lower level concepts.

One further concept has attracted attention. *Target efficiency* is the efficiency with which resources are allocated to and among those for whom receipt has been judged the most cost-effective method of intervention (Bebbington & Davies 1983). It measures the extent to which a particular principle of equity (embodied in allocation according to need or allocation according to some individually based measure of cost-effectiveness) is met in practice. Thus equity and efficiency are of equal importance in defining target efficiency. There are two dimensions to target efficiency: *horizontal target efficiency*, which indicates the extent to which those deemed to be in need of a particular service actually receive it; and *vertical target efficiency*, which is the extent to which the available resources are received by those deemed to be in need.

Efficiency in whatever form is a statement about, or measure of, the achievements of a service or policy and the resources and other factors which combine to secure them. Some of those influential factors are difficult to measure or impossible to cost – these are the *non-resouce inputs* introduced earlier – and they should not be overlooked. This means that they must either be tackled head on or controlled in a discussion or evaluation. For example, an evaluation of hospital and community locations as alternative places of

treatment for a particular group of patients would either need to measure patient preferences, the social milieu of different settings, staff attitudes and so on, or would need to employ a research design, such as an appropriately timed randomized control trial, which neutralized their influences. We will not say much more in this chapter about these non-resource inputs, but this should not be interpreted as implying that they are unimportant. They are crucial intervening variables between the resource inputs or costs and the outcomes or effects of mental health services.

We now turn our attention to these costs and outcomes by considering the study of efficiency in practice. This will take us to the most common of the 'efficiency analyses' to be found in the health economics literature: cost-benefit, cost-effectiveness, cost-utility and cost-function analyses. (These techniques are not restricted to answering questions about efficiency, for increasingly evaluations have sought to examine *distributional* implications, though we shall maintain our efficiency focus.) These analyses can provide information needed for a variety of decisions:

- *What* care service (treatment, drug, programme of support, . . . ) is more or most appropriate in given circumstances?
- *When* should care be provided?
- *Where* should care be provided?
- *To whom* should care be provided?
- *How* should care be provided?

### Efficiency in practice: measures and analyses

Efficiency analyses do not seek to replace the sound or educated judgement of the decision maker, whether clinician, manager or politician. Final decisions will be made by these people in the light of the information made available to them. It is the principal aim of all evaluative research, and efficiency analyses are certainly no exception, to provide a more considered and sound information base for policy decisions. Weisbrod (1979), an early and widely respected exponent of the art of cost-benefit analysis in psychiatry, made the point that these techniques will never 'make decisions', but if vigorously pursued they will 'make decisions better informed'.

In the study of efficiency in practice there are numerous techniques which can be used. None is simple or uncontroversial. Each is simply 'an effort to bridge the gap between a conceptual model – theoretic welfare economics – and actual social policy' (Weisbrod & Helming 1980). Welfare economics is that branch of the discipline of economics concerned with the relationship between an economic system and the well-being of individuals. It has developed the techniques of cost-benefit, cost-effectiveness, cost-utility and cost-function analyses as alternative means of appraising efficiency in contexts where markets either do not exist or cannot be relied upon automatically to generate efficiency. (This is not the place to delve into basic economic theory. There are circumstances in which an efficient allocation of society's resources will result automatically from market forces – 'the invisible hand of the market' as Adam Smith described it two centuries ago. The prerequisites for such an outcome are demanding, and are most unlikely to obtain in a market for mental health services.)

In principle, these techniques of efficiency evaluation are simple. The costs of a project are compared with the benefits or outcomes; if the latter exceed the former the policy or service is worth undertaking. If two or more projects are vying for selection, the one with the greatest excess of benefits over costs should be selected. Benefits and costs which fall to or upon any member of society are to be included. Unfortunately, it is this simplicity which has been the cause of much difficulty. In application these are complex tools, harbouring a host of practical problems.

Common to each of these techniques of efficiency analysis is the measurement of outcomes and costs. What are these two central components of the production of welfare approach?

## Outcomes

As noted earlier, outcomes can be conceptualized and measured at two levels: final outcomes reflect the changes in client welfare along various dimensions, together with the impacts upon clients' relatives and other significant actors; intermediate outcomes are defined and measured in terms of the volume and quality of care. It would be inappropriate to go into the measurement of outcomes for psychiatric services in tremendous detail in this chapter, given that some other contributors to this volume are better positioned than we are to describe the principles. However, it is useful to rehearse briefly the approach favoured by some health economists.

Outcome measurement proceeds through two obligatory and two optional stages. Having agreed the dimensions along which outcomes are to be explored, the first stage is to develop scales of client characteristics ('well-being') for each. At the second stage the task is to assess the impact of intervention along each dimension over a period of time. By reference to the objectives of mental health care it is usually possible to identify the dimensions of well-being over which the outcome measures should range, and judicious use of well-validated instrumentation provides empirical indicators.

Thus far, outcome measurement will be familiar territory for non-economists. The two further stages may be less familiar, and are generally to be found only when economists are involved. They are optional. One of these further stages is to place monetary values on the outcomes, the other is to combine the scale scores (or monetary values) into a unidimensional outcome measure. Clearly neither is without complexity or controversy, for the information needed for monetary valuation and dimension weighting is difficult and costly to obtain, and laden with even more value judgements and subjectivities than other facets of evaluation. (We must not overplay these difficulties, for a thorough evaluation which is any good is almost inevitably complex, and value judgements are made at *every* stage of a social psychiatric evaluation, even if it is not fashionable to make them explicit.)

The advantages of moving through these two optional stages should be clear. First, outcomes measured in monetary terms can be directly compared with costs. (Does treatment X generate more benefits than it costs? Is service innovation Y worth doing?) Second, the multidimensional changes that result from a treatment or innovation are reduced to a single indicator. Simplicity and manageability are the common characteristics, but they are also the principal drawbacks, for conflation to a single dimension and reduction to monetary measures wastes information, and may also unwittingly disguise the value judgements and methodological assumptions that have been made. The Quality Adjusted Life Year (QALY) measure is an example of a conflated, unidimensional measure of (physical) health status which is now being extended to mental health applications (Kind 1990, Kind *et al.* 1990, Loomes & McKenzie 1990, Wilkinson *et al.* 1990; and see ongoing work by Rachel Rosser). The QALY does not put monetary values on health status changes. It is fashionable to cavil at the QALY, and there are undoubtedly methodological weaknesses in the original instrument that have long been recognized but are only now being rectified, but the technique has the considerable signal virtue of highlighting the stages that *any* outcome evaluation must go through. Far too many outcome studies in psychiatry, and in medicine more generally, fail to make clear their underlying assumptions, fail to explicate their implicit weightings, and fail to make the distinction between categorical, ordinal and cardinal measures. The considerable contributions of the QALY approach are to bring these all-too-often-neglected methodological issues to the fore.

Outcomes measure the movement towards objectives. They need to be *net* measures, and it is thus necessary to make comparisons between individuals or between time-periods using a before-after design. Single observations at one point in time are not enough except in very special circumstances. We must also introduce a dynamic component: a measure of 'flow' or trending. Many mental health care interventions are not occasioned by transient needs but by longstanding problems. Well-being thus has both *intensity* (measured, for example, by points on a set of scales of disability or symptoms) and *duration*. Outcome is the differential effect of care – the 'additional well-being' that it generates. Four practical decisions have to be taken. What kind of comparison is needed in order to measure the differential or net effect of care on patients? How

often should this differential effect be measured? For how long is it necessary to monitor these effects? How are errors and distortions associated with measurement to be minimized? These are all standard (if tricky) questions of research design which are considered at length in the evaluation and social statistics literatures. Outcome evaluation by economists is no different in intent, methodological design or constraint from outcome evaluation by social psychiatrists.

## Costs

On the opposite side of the production of welfare relationship to outcomes are the resource and non-resource inputs and the costs. These have known or hypothesized influences on the achievement of the intermediate and final outcomes of psychiatric interventions. Although the resource inputs are usually measured as costs, and the non-resource inputs taken into account by statistical standardization or evaluative design, it is frequently desirable to work with disaggregated concepts and measures, such as in the examination of the impact of staff skills or professional backgrounds on patient welfare. However, we concentrate on summary resource measures (costs) in what follows.

Elsewhere we have discussed and illustrated a recommended set of rules for costing mental health services and it is unnecessary to repeat the detail in this chapter (Knapp & Beecham 1990). There are four rules. First, costs should be measured comprehensively to range over all relevant service components of a service, treatment or care 'package'. Second, the cost variations that will be revealed between patients, facilities, or areas of the country when undertaking such a comprehensive costing, should be examined for their policy and practice insights. Third, like-with-like comparisons should be attempted, taking out or statistically standardizing for the influences of extraneous factors, and ensuring that comparable samples of patients or facilities are being studied. Fourth, cost information should be integrated where possible with information on patient outcomes: sole reliance on cost findings is scientifically acceptable only under special circumstances, even if it has political acceptability. Equally, neglecting costs when making policy decisions, or when undertaking the evaluations which inform them, should also prompt questions about scientific validity and generalizability.

We can illustrate the application of these costing rules from some of our own recent work. As noted earlier, we have been examining the costs and cost-effectiveness of the reprovision of services for residents at Friern and Claybury Hospitals. By September 1988, comprehensive cost data had been collected for 216 people who had been discharged from the hospitals and had been living in the community for 12 months. The comprehensive approach to costing made comparison with the cost of hospital care valid, but also ensured that policy requirements were met as the reprovision programme under which most of the clients left hospital is supported by a 'dowry' mechanism which transfers an amount equal to the average cost of hospital to the community mental health care budget. A 15-fold variation in the costs of care packages required to support the client in the community was revealed. In this evaluation we are fortunate to be working in collaboration with the TAPS researchers, and so have access to a rich data-set relating to the effects of reprovision on individual clients. This offers the facility for examining the costs of community care alongside the *final* outcomes (Beecham *et al.* 1991).

Costs are utilized outside evaluations of efficiency, for example in the costing of diseases, the pricing of services for contract, the description of expenditure flows and the examination of the 'burden of care', though we do not discuss these uses here (see Knapp & Beecham 1991, for a review of recent uses of cost information).

With these outcome and cost measures, we can now describe the primary tools of efficiency analysis within health economics. We start with cost-effectiveness analysis, setting out the stages through which an actual study would proceed.

## Cost-effectiveness analysis

There are essentially six stages in a cost-effectiveness analysis (CEA):

1 Define the alternatives to be examined in the analysis.
2 List the costs and effects (the outcomes).
3 Quantify and value the costs and effects.
4 Compare them.
5 Qualify or revise the comparison in the light of risk, uncertainty, and sensitivity.
6 Examine the distributional implications.

At the first stage the exact nature of the range of policy or treatment options needs to be made explicit so that the research question is clear. This is neither trite nor trivial, for once selected, the nature of the whole study is determined, and some policy or practice issues do not lend themselves to a straightforward evaluative design. The second stage is the listing of all likely costs and outcomes to draw attention to those which might prove beyond the technology or politics of measurement: it is important to be aware of all factors necessary to the implementation of, or likely to result from, the policy, practice or treatment regime options being examined within the CEA, even if they do not later figure in the empirical evaluation. The next stage, the first of the empirical activities, is to quantify and value (in monetary magnitudes) the costs and outcomes. These activities proceed along the lines set out above. The technique of cost-*effectiveness* analysis does not, in fact, attempt to place monetary values on the outputs; cost-*benefit* analysis does attempt it.

With a CEA, the efficiency rule would be to compare the costs of obtaining levels of outcome, and to conclude that the option with lowest cost per given level of outcome is the more efficient. This is obviously not always an easy rule to apply in practice, particularly with multidimensional outcome measures which do not move in concert. In the case of the cost-effectiveness evaluation of the rundown of Friern and Claybury Hospitals, and the earlier evaluation of the Care in the Community demonstration programme (Knapp *et al.* 1992), community care costs were lower than inpatient hospital residence for people with chronic mental health problems (excluding dementia). In both cases, the outcome results suggested that community care was no worse than inpatient residence and, along one or two dimensions, significantly better (TAPS 1990). If some outcome dimensions register improvements and others indicate deterioration, or if the cost and outcome comparisons point to different preferred solutions, it is not the task of the CEA researcher to advocate a particular policy or treatment option. It is the task of the researcher to point to the various consequences and to leave decisions to the politician, clinical manager, or care-giver.

The costs and effects calculated for the various options are likely to be subject to some error, and a good CEA would include sensitivity analyses, examining the implications of different assumptions regarding the estimation of costs, effects, and so on. To give an example, McGuire (1991) suggests that the conclusions from the seminal work of Weisbrod *et al.* (1980) are sensitive to the assumption made about the costing of capital. Dramatic turnarounds in the results from a CEA are not common, but the assumptions should nevertheless be checked.

Finally, the distributional consequences of the different options should be addressed. For example, as many people have pointed out, community care may be less costly overall than inpatient residence, but more costly for informal carers, which would suggest that a policy of dehospitalization should be accompanied by some redistribution to assist or compensate the latter. There is a danger that the distributional findings, and equity more generally, might get subsumed under and dominated by efficiency, and there is also the danger that CEA becomes a vehicle for the analyst's or sponsor's own prejudices. Thus, whilst it would be wrong for the analyst not to make clear the implications of alternative projects for individuals in different socioeconomic groups, in different areas of the country, or with different needs, it would be equally wrong to give the treatment of the distributional consequences any scientific, value-free veneer.

### Cost-benefit analysis

The CEA is designed to examine the technical and price efficiency of one or more mental health procedures; in contrast, a cost-benefit analysis examines social efficiency. The stages of a cost-benefit analysis (CBA) exactly mirror those of a CEA, except that the former places monetary values on the outcomes and the latter does not. The CEA technique aims to show how a given level of outcome can be achieved at minimum cost (or maximum outcome at given cost); the CBA can compute cost-benefit ratios or differences. Many economists would agree with Sugden & Williams that CEA is of most value when 'choosing between mutually exclusive ways of achieving a particular, very clearly defined benefit' (1978, p. 19). It cannot, however, be used to say whether or not the benefits of a project or procedure actually outweigh the costs, which is the prerogative of the CBA. This should not make one too dissatisfied with a CEA, for it can ensure that a full range of costs is estimated and that measures are sought for all relevant dimensions of outcome, and it does so without introducing all of the difficulties and additional value judgements associated with the attachment of monetary values to outcomes. The information thus gathered can then be presented so as to make plain the efficiency and distributional implications of the alternatives under consideration and allow policy makers to make the necessary trade-offs.

The only studies labelled as CBAs in the psychiatric field have employed rather narrow outcome or benefit measures. For example, it has been common to define benefit as expenditure or cost saved, which is not only misleading, but also makes the strong assumption of identical outcome implications of the alternatives under consideration.

### Cost-utility analysis

Cost-utility analysis (CUA) is the label attached to a particular data configuration; it is a cost-effectiveness analysis conducted with outcomes measured in terms of QALYs. With a CUA it is possible to calculate the *cost per QALY* for different procedures or even different health problems, comparing kidney transplants with treatment of cystic fibrosis with cetfazidime, for example (Gudex 1990). This opens up a whole new area, for it provides the clinical, managerial or financial decision maker with a set of precise looking statistics. The dangers of these measures must not be overlooked, although many of the criticisms to date have focused on the technical construction of the QALY rather than the broader strategic difficulties. Our primary concern would be the loss of information if the many outcome dimensions generally deemed to be relevant in the evaluation of mental health services were squeezed into a unidimensional straitjacket.

We are not aware of any CUAs conducted for psychiatric procedures.

## Cost functions

In economics it is rarely possible to set up a controlled study: it is hard to persuade companies to allow themselves to be randomly allocated to different market regimes, and national economies are unique. Thus, applied economics research has developed around some fairly complex multivariate statistical techniques in order to get around the problems of less-than-ideal samples. If data allow, cost differences between units (companies, public authorities, years, and so on) can be examined with the help of 'statistical cost functions'. The cost function is the estimated relationship between the cost of providing a service, the outcomes, the prices of resource inputs, and other factors with a hypothesized influence on cost (such as product mix, the arrangements and organization of care, and the characteristics of users). The aim of the technique is to estimate the relationship between cost and these hypothesized influences, using multiple regression analysis, in an attempt to 'explain' observed cost variations. The form of the function is determined by the interaction of *a priori* theoretical considerations and statistical findings. The simple production of welfare framework set out above provides the theoretical context within which to suggest specific forms for cost functions. This is, however, a data-hungry tool, which limits its application.

The cost function takes a rather different approach from CEA, CBA and CUA. It is partly a statistical technique, and is most commonly estimated for a cross-section sample of 'production units' which are known or assumed to have reasonably similar objectives and to employ reasonably similar production techniques. In service applications there is no engineer's blueprint to guide the study of costs, and 'production' is certainly not routinized or standardized, but 'behavioural cost functions' have been estimated to good effect, either for facilities or for individual clients. (We are not aware of any mental health service examples of the use of cost functions at the facility level; our own work in the North East Thames study is an example of an application of the technique at the individual client level. See Beecham *et al.* 1991.)

## The pursuit of efficiency

Efficiency is not a new objective, though its high profile during the 1980s and 1990s has sometimes fooled disgruntled professionals into thinking that it was part of a Thatcherite plot to control the medical profession or float the NHS off into the private sector. In the early years of the NHS, and indeed until the oil crises of the early 1970s, there were periodic funding problems and reorganization traumas which forced decision-makers to look more carefully at how resources were being allocated and utilized. Efficiency was always an objective, but it generally had a low profile, and it was anyway designated as a responsibility of managers and accountants. Clinicians were encouraged to concentrate on clinical matters, and efficiency remained a largely administrative concern.

There were at least three problems with such an approach. First, efficiency often remained a hidden objective – hidden from clinicians, patients, tax payers and opposition politicians – or was dressed up as some other aim, such as regional redistribution, managerial reform or 'good practice'. There was no public debate about efficiency. Second, a consequence of clinicians being excluded from this level of decision making was that efficiency came to be narrowly defined. Indeed, the policy historian would be hard pressed to find examples of efficiency-inspired policies or changes which adequately dealt with the clinical dimension. A 'more efficient' health care system or practice was invariably taken to mean one that treated more patients at lower cost. The health status of patients and their views about the service were not part of the efficiency discussion. The third problem, again stemming from the exclusion of clinicians and other mental health practitioners and service providers from the discussion, was that the resource or cost side of the efficiency criterion came to be interpreted as of no relevance in clinical practice. Indeed, clinicians and others fought to keep costs at arm's length, and many denigrated any attempt to introduce a financial dimension to their work.

Thus, for many years efficiency was a hidden and poorly understood aim of policy, a narrowly operationalized criterion, and one widely criticized by those providing services. Efficiency was imposed upon – or 'done to' – psychiatrists by managers remote from the realities of day-to-day mental health care delivery.

The contrast with the situation today is not total, for efficiency is still often regarded as an externally imposed objective, and cost information is still regarded with some suspicion, but there has nevertheless been a sea change. It would be nice to think that the proselytizing skills of health economists have succeeded in re-educating a sceptical medical profession, but any such influence has probably been marginal. The main reasons for this change have been a shift in the locus of responsibility for efficiency and the sheer cumulative weight of shrinking budgets and political pressure. Efficiency is no longer to be done *to* psychiatrists but done *by* them, and after a dozen years of performance reviews, value for money audits and efficiency scrutinies (in various guises), few are now likely to argue that efficiency is not here to stay.

Successive reforms and directives during the 1980s brought the clinical and the resource or cost sides of mental health provision closer together. Joint finance, dowry transfers, budget-holding case or care managers, clinical budgeting experiments, contracting out, and the care programme and the specific grant were among the contributory influences. The NHS and community care reforms introduced from April 1991 will go even further. Far from ignoring questions of efficiency or relegating them to an appendix, central government and other policy documents on mental health care sometimes *lead* with financial ques-

tions, and certainly always remind providers that efficiency must be one of the component objectives of service initiatives. With the Audit Commission extending its responsibilities from local authorities to the NHS, regular monitoring of health service activities will include value for money auditing. Even this chapter is an example of how far we have come, for there can have been few if any previous social psychiatry source books which have included a chapter on economics.

As we have suggested in this chapter, we do not find the trend to greater efficiency emphasis or awareness regrettable. On the whole, the trend is to be applauded, though the implementation of efficiency-inspired reforms, and the very examination of efficiency in research and planning exercises, often leave a lot to be desired. Indeed, as clinical and financial considerations meet under the same policy umbrella, so a number of inadequacies and misconceptions come to light. The integration of cost and effectiveness information within performance reviews has revealed the inadequacies of the costs data lovingly tended by local and health authority treasurers over the years, and the limitations of the so-called effectiveness data. Rightly, though belatedly, extant information systems have been strongly criticized and new systems devised. Nevertheless, we must still strive to get away from a situation in which overworked psychiatrists with no economic training are grappling with policy and practice decisions which have huge financial ramifications, and in which treasurers and auditors with no clinical training are trying to incorporate perspectives on psychiatric practice so as to adjudge efficiency. The continued application of health economics to psychiatry is essential.

## References

Bebbington A.C. & Davies B.P. (1983) Equity and efficiency in the allocation of the personal social services. *Journal of Social Policy* 12, 309–330.

Beecham J., Knapp M.R.J. & Fenyo A. (1991) Costs, needs and outcomes: community care for people with long-term mental health problems. *Schizophrenia Bulletin* 17, 427–439.

Croft-Jeffreys C. & Wilkinson G. (1989) Estimated cost of neurotic disorder in UK general practice. *Psychological Medicine* 19, 549–558.

Culyer A.J. (1980) *The Political Economy of Social Policy.* Martin Robertson, Oxford.

Davies B.P. & Knapp M.R.J. (1981) *Old People's Homes and the Production of Welfare.* Routledge and Kegan Paul, London.

Davies B.P. & Knapp M.R.J. (eds) (1988) The production of welfare approach: evidence and argument from the PSSRU. *British Journal of Social Work* 18, supplement.

Davies L.M. & Drummond M.F. (1990) The economic burden of schizophrenia. *Psychological Bulletin* 14, 522–525.

Frank R.G. & Jackson C.A. (1989) The impact of prospectively set hospital budgets on psychiatric admissions. *Social Science and Medicine* 28, 861–867.

Gudex C. (1990) The QALY: how can it be used? In Baldwin S., Godfrey C. & Propper C. (eds) *Quality of Life: Perspectives and Policies*, pp. 218–230. Routledge, London.

Hoult J., Reynolds I., Charbonneau-Powis M., Weekes P. & Briggs J. (1983) Psychiatric hospital versus community treatment: the results of a randomised trial. *Australian and New Zealand Journal of Psychiatry* 17, 160–167.

Kind P. (1990) Issues in the design and construction of a quality of life measure. In Baldwin S., Godfrey C. & Propper C. (eds) *Quality of Life: Perspectives and Policies*, pp. 63–71. Routledge, London.

Kind P., Gudex C. & Godfrey C. (1990) Introduction: what are QALYs? In Baldwin S., Godfrey C. & Propper C. (eds) *Quality of Life: Perspectives and Policies*, pp. 57–62. Routledge, London.

Knapp M.R.J. (1980) Production Relations for Old People's Homes. Unpublished PhD thesis, University of Kent, Canterbury.

Knapp M.R.J. (1984) *The Economics of Social Care.* Macmillan, London.

Knapp M.R.J. & Beecham J. (1990) Costing mental health services. *Psychological Medicine* 20, 893–908.

Knapp M.R.J. & Beecham J. (1991) Mental health service costs. *Current Opinion in Psychiatry* 4, 275–282.

Knapp M.R.J., Beecham J., Anderson J. *et al.* (1990) Predicting the community costs of closing psychiatric hospitals. *British Journal of Psychiatry* 157, 661–670.

Knapp M.R.J., Cambridge P., Thomason C., Beecham J., Allen C. & Darton R.A. (1992) *Care in the Community: Challenges and Demonstration.* Ashgate, Aldershot.

Loomes G. & Mckenzie L. (1990) The scope and limitations of QALY measures. In Baldwin S., Godfrey C. & Propper C. (eds) *Quality of Life: Perspectives and Policies*. Routledge, London.

McGuire A., Henderson J. & Mooney G. (1988) *The Economics of Health Care.* Routledge and Kegan Paul, London.

McGuire T. (1991) Measuring the economic cost of schizophrenia. *Schizophrenia Bulletin* 17, 375–388.

Marks I., Connolly J. & Muijen M. (1988) The Maudsley Daily Living Programme: a controlled cost effectiveness study of community-based versus standard in-patient care of serious mental illness. *Bulletin of the Royal College of Psychiatrists* 12, 22–24.

Marks I. & Thornicroft G. (1990) Private inpatient psychiatric care. *British Medical Journal* 300, 892.

Sugden R. & Williams A. (1978) *The Principles of Practical Cost Benefit Analysis*, p. 191. Oxford University Press, Oxford.

TAPS (1992) The TAPS Project: evaluation of community placement of long-stay psychiatric patients. *British Journal of Psychiatry* Supplement (in press).

Weisbrod B.A. (1979) *A Guide to Benefit–Costs Analysis as Seen Through a Controlled Experiment in Treating the Mentally Ill.* (Discussion Paper 559–79.) Institute for Research on Poverty, University of Wisconsin, Madison.

Weisbrod B.A. & Helming M. (1980) What benefit cost analysis can and cannot do: the case of treating the mentally ill. In Stromsdorfer E.W. & Farkas G. (eds) *Evaluation Studies Review Annual*. Sage, Beverly Hills.

Weisbrod B.A., Test M.A. & Stein L.I. (1980) Alternative to mental hospital treatment: economic benefit–cost analysis. *Archives of General Psychiatry* 37, 400–405.

Wilkinson G., Croft-Jeffreys C., KreRorian H., McLees S. & Falloon I. (1990) QALYs in psychiatric care? *Psychiatric Bulletin* 14, 586–589.

Williams A. & Anderson R. (1975) *Efficiency in the Social Services*, p. 1. Basil Blackwell, Oxford.

# Chapter 35
# The Role of Facilitated Relatives' Groups and Voluntary Self-Help Groups

## LIZ KUIPERS & JERRY WESTALL

## Introduction

The management of mental illness has to include dealing with the family network of the patient wherever possible. As the popular sector of health care, i.e. individual, family and social network, is reportedly responsible for dealing with 70–90% of all illness episodes in the USA (see Chapter 5), it is of paramount importance that relatives are involved in management. Often relatives need help in their own right. The two contributors to this chapter look at the role of voluntary self-help and facilitated relatives' groups. The first half of the chapter is devoted to a facilitated group and the second half to voluntary self-help groups taking the National Schizophrenia Fellowship (NSF) as its model.

## A. Running a Facilitated Group for Relatives of the Long-term Adult Mentally Ill

### LIZ KUIPERS

Groups which include a professional are different from self-help or voluntary groups, although it seems likely that many of their functions overlap. There is an argument that a professional who facilitates a group cannot, by definition, be an integral member, and may even lessen the ability of group members to help each other (Avebury 1986). There is certainly a danger of this if a professional is seen only as the 'expert' and/or if the professional 'takes over' the group. However, the use of the word facilitator is meant to suggest that it is possible for a professional to use skills

that may not be available to other group members, and that these skills should enable the group to help each other in specific ways that might not otherwise occur. There is now quite clear research evidence that such facilitated groups can improve coping skills, reduce emotional upset and help share the burden of care. In addition, they also help to bring about changes in attitudes and behaviour that improve outcome in patients (Leff *et al.* 1982, 1989, MacCarthy *et al.* 1989, Berkowitz *et al.* 1990, personal communication).

However, this is not to suggest that such groups are preferable to self-help or voluntary groups, nor that such changes can only take place in facilitated groups. It seems clear that different groups serve important but different needs and that a variety of support should be on offer to relatives and clients with long-term psychiatric problems.

As an example, I would like to use the facilitated relatives' groups run as part of two research projects over the last decade. These were multiple family groups which did not include patients. Those set up for the initial study were run fortnightly (Leff *et al.* 1982); relatives of more long-term patients had groups offered once a month, and this is the model discussed in detail here (MacCarthy *et al.* 1989).

The aims of such a group are based on research findings concerning the social environment (Leff & Vaughn 1985). For relatives of adults with long-term mental illness who may continue to be high users of care over many years, obvious aims are to offer reassurance, support and structure in order to counteract the very common feelings of resignation and pessimism that carers may exhibit (MacCarthy 1988). Carers typically find the 'communality' – the feelings that they share experiences and burdens with others and that they 'are not alone' – is an important part of the support that a group can offer.

### Aims

*1 Facilitate social interaction.* We know that once relatives have been carers for some time they begin to share the stigma, isolation and reduced social networks that patients with long-term illnesses such as schizophrenia often face (Anderson *et al.* 1984, MacCarthy 1988). One of the clear aims of a relatives' group should be to counteract these feelings and facilitate social interaction. This can help to share the emotional burden of care; the relief of being able to talk freely to others who know your situation can often be dramatic.

*2 Answer questions.* There are now a number of written information packages (e.g. Smith & Birchwood 1985, Leff *et al.* 1988) which can be an important part of a pregroup or initial group meetings. However, for long-term carers information about diagnosis is usually well established and the information that tends to be required is a more thorough understanding of the facts that other professionals have imparted. A relatives' group can be an important forum for the detailed discussion and repetition of issues that arise, for example, the use of medication, the cause of mental illness, are relatives to blame? An important aim is to offer to answer all questions that arise either from the facilitator's own knowledge or from the group's considerable experience. Such information is not 'learnt' by the group but the process of understanding and continuing to absorb the emotional and practical impact of long-term mental illness can be enhanced in this setting.

*3 To offer specific help with problem solving,* using the group's own experiences and a behavioural skills perspective.

*4 To help relatives increase their tolerance* particularly of the negative symptoms and poor role performance of patients that are commonly misinterpreted or attributed as the patient's 'fault' and thus can increase levels of frustration and tension in carers.

*5 To help carers develop a sense of perspective about problems,* and for them to adjust their expectations of the patient to more realistic levels.

*6 To help both carers and patients achieve* an appropriate level of adult independence despite a patient's residual disabilities and perceived vulnerability.

It can be seen that these aims are based on the research literature which shows that high Expressed Emotion (EE) in carers makes it difficult for them to cope with the very difficult and intractable problems that they may be facing (Kuipers & Bebbington 1990).

### Structure

The long-term group met once a month for one and a half hours in a comfortable setting based in the hospital site. Tea and biscuits accompanied the meeting and a sociable and relaxed atmosphere was encouraged. Sessions were tape recorded, with the permission of relatives, for purposes of analysis; this did not seem to impede the flow of discussion. Even for the purposes of noting what was discussed, a tape recorder is helpful, as with a large group information is easily missed or recorded partially from memory alone.

The same two facilitators ran the group whenever possible. Although this is not necessary, continuity and trust are important components of a group and can be jeopardized by staff changes. The long-term group ran for 18 months. Previous groups have run for several years but always with a final end because of research requirements. Other facilitated groups run continuously.

The group was open rather than closed. The latter is often difficult to organize because of limitations on numbers. Although it takes longer to establish trust in an open group, it has the advantage of novelty, because new members introduce new issues, and they help avoid a feeling of repetition.

At the beginning of the group, and every time there is a new member, it is important to allow carers to get to know each other. A useful strategy is to ask for the carer's story. This allows a carer to control the information they give and also gives a chance for others to hear similarities in another's situation. Allowing carers this control reduces anxiety and automatically brings out the common issues and burdens that are shared by members.

While running an open group it is useful to have some ideas about optimum numbers. These have ranged from 2 to 11 over the years and there is no predetermined preferred number. However, with as few as 2 relatives there are limited possibilities for group support and the session begins to have a more individual feel. Eleven relatives may not be a maximum, but it is harder to ensure that all the concerns that 11 people have brought to a group have been heard, let alone discussed in any detail. A pool of about 12 relatives of whom 6–10 attend regularly allows for adequate time for individuals, with the variety and adequacy of group support also available.

### Strategies

The model described here has aims based on the research evidence and uses strategies with elements from three main approaches. These are:
1 The research-derived ideas – based on the EE work.
2 Group counselling techniques.
3 Behavioural skills training, e.g. problem solving.

There was a deliberate policy of not using psychodynamic interpretations of either group or individual processes. These have not been found to be useful (Kottgen *et al.* 1984).

### Leadership style

A non-confrontational but directive style is one that has been found to be the most appropriate for facilitators of this kind of group. It is necessary for the facilitators to be able to focus the group on one topic at a time and also to follow a theme through to a constructive conclusion. Unless channelled in this way, it is easy for a group,

particularly one with more than five or so members, to disintegrate into concurrent conversations in which no one can hear all the topics discussed. It is also important to foster a positive and non-judgmental atmosphere, where difficult and negative issues can be discussed frankly but where the relatives' assets of humour, sociability and tolerance can be maximized.

### Engaging relatives

It is known that it is not easy or even possible to engage all relatives in a group (e.g. Leff *et al.* 1989). High levels of motivation are required plus reassurance that the group will not expose individuals to increased anxiety and distress. It has been found to be helpful to meet relatives at home first before a group starts. Subsequently, if the people who make the home visits are also the facilitators everyone who attends will know at least one person and can be welcomed personally. It can be useful to use these pregroup home visits as an opportunity to offer education to relatives, i.e. to answer questions about schizophrenia and give information. It is helpful to do this in the more relaxed setting of the relatives' home and also demonstrates that the facilitator has made an effort and offered the relatives a service. The group meeting can then be described as an opportunity to meet others in the same situation and also to continue the process of asking and answering questions. It is also true that relatives will be able to offer help to each other from their experiences, and this aspect can be emphasized. We know from the literature that offering education in a pregroup or group setting increases relative optimism and rates of engagement in later interventions (Berkowitz *et al.* 1984, Smith & Birchwood 1987). It seems likely that making an effort to meet all relatives before a group, answer queries and provide reassurance fulfils several of these functions even if a specific education package is not provided.

### Facilitating communication

Helping relatives' communication skills may not only enhance the effective functioning of the group but also improve interactions with the patient at home. Experimental work shows that high EE relatives are poor listeners (Kuipers *et al.* 1983), and either escalate or produce largely negative interaction patterns with patients (Hooley & Hahlweg 1986, Hubschmidt & Zemp 1989). Thus listening, turn taking, not interrupting and not talking in parallel with other relatives are skills that may need to be fostered. It can be necessary to state these as rules early on in group meetings. Alternatively, the rules can be modelled consistently by the facilitators and this can set the scene, particularly if it becomes obvious that a group becomes chaotic if everyone talks at once.

Sometimes a facilitator must be directive because of a monologue that is inappropriately dominating the group. This may have to be interrupted and channelled into a more general concern that the group as a whole can contribute to. Alternatively some group member may need to be asked directly for their views and encouraged to participate if they find that the process is too daunting unaided.

### Problem solving

Relatives often have a wide range of expertise and one of the advantages of meeting together is the way in which the group can be canvassed to provide ideas on how to solve the problems of individuals. There will usually be somebody else who has met and coped with a problem, however bizarre, difficult, frightening or mundane, and the fact that others have faced and survived similar difficulties is reassuring in itself. Often a current problem for one member will be in the past of another, and the fact that problems can change and that others have been there before helps members in crisis to gain a sense of perspective.

One of a facilitator's chief roles in the group is to help members actually get round to the important job not just of discussing problems but of trying to help them to effect some change. This can be seen as risky and will often be resisted. However, a professional may be able to focus a group on one issue and prevent either diversion or a feeling of being overwhelmed by trying to cope

with more than one problem at a time. The most useful techniques for problem solving are those drawn from behavioural skills training and involve breaking down a problem into small components, separating the individual from the behaviour (thereby reducing feelings of blame and resentment), asking for a range of solutions from the group, valuing each contribution, and then trying to help the group reach a consensus.

In order to solve a problem, solutions must be negotiated, not imposed, so that some degree of compromise has to be modelled in the group in order for it to be modelled at home. One of the advantages of using the group process to look at problems is that a wide variety of novel and creative solutions can be proposed – usually ones that a professional would not have thought of. The fact that in this setting the professional is not an expert is worth emphasizing. Once a small and manageable solution has been decided upon, a task is suggested as a trial run which can be reported back on the next time. Feedback of this task is important regardless of the success or otherwise of the venture. Any small change can be positively discussed and noted as an important and difficult achievement by carers. This helps to counteract the conviction that nothing ever changes and may begin to suggest the feeling of hope that is so essential to foster in long-term care.

If the task was not successful, unpacking the further difficulties it reveals can be equally useful. If it can be accepted by the facilitators that this task was too difficult and another should be negotiated then relatives can feel supported and not blamed. Feedback is also important, both because it suggests that attempts to change things are valued and worth the effort, even if unsuccessful, and because it stresses continuity – that issues are not dropped by the group even if solutions are difficult to find. This mirrors the burden of the care itself.

Overall, it is helpful for group members to aim at a consistent and predictable home environment for patients that is also flexible and responsive to changing circumstances.

*Emotional processing*

One of the most important and successful functions a relatives' group can fulfil is to be able to share and help process the emotional burden of care and the wide range of feelings, many of them negative, that it can provoke. As cohesion and trust develop in a group it will become easier for members to share these negative emotions, which need to be expressed, normalized and allowed. It is vital for facilitators to adopt an accepting and non-blaming stance (Ferris & Marshall 1987) when faced with these negative feelings and to re-emphasize how understandable this response is to the abnormal and stressful situations that many carers find themselves having to cope with. Anger, rage, rejection of the patient, hostility, grief, guilt, sadness, blame, bitterness and frustration are all commonly found. It may be helpful for facilitators, too, to acknowledge that it is not just carers who feel these things and that staff may share in the helplessness, frustration and anger that carers experience.

The fact that all carers will have felt these emotions at some stage is deeply reassuring and supportive and enables relatives to allow and share their impact. Finding that others have identical feelings can also help to ease the guilt and blame that relatives assume must be their sole responsibility – how can just *they* have caused the patients' problems if others have to cope with the same difficulties?

Another aspect of this processing is to look at relatives' expectations and perspectives on the problems. Having unrealistically high expectations of a patient's abilities after their illness, and of how long the process of recovery may take, will frequently lead to dashed hopes and a sense of failure, both for patient and relatives. If the aim is to get back to work when a patient is still coping with impaired concentration and a range of negative symptoms then this will not be successful. However, by reframing a behaviour so that a small overall change is seen as progress, for example, doing one independent task at home, such as shopping or cooking a meal, enables relatives to build on these behavioural gains. Sometimes the expectations are based on a denial

of reality – 'the patient is well now, we don't have to think about preventing relapses in the future'. Particularly at the beginning of the illness relatives may prefer to think in this way. However, meeting other carers who have coped for longer and have also managed continued crises is often a specific way of helping relatives accept that the illness may return, and that this can be dealt with positively, for instance by maximizing prevention and early treatment strategies. Similarly the length of time that recovery takes, the slow pace of change but also the likelihood that persistent and consistent measures will improve the situation, can be emphasized by the fact of the variety of the group's experiences.

A final facet of emotional processing is to look with the group at how difficult limit setting can be for some members. Many carers are very aware of how sensitive patients can be to the social setting and try to avoid arguments and criticism at all costs. However, the price of this 'calm' environment is often a feeling of intense resentment by relatives of the 'power' of patients to be demanding and to get away with things because they are unwell. Attempts to change this are either stifled by relatives, when frustration increases in line with the patient's often increasingly unhelpful behaviour, or lead to bitter conflicts and sometimes even violence. Being able to negotiate, set limits and keep to them consistently with the patient, is a skill that is not available to everybody without help but may be a very vital aspect of change. Again, helping relatives to face the problem and then apply the problem-solving methods discussed earlier is a way of beginning to break down these conflicts. However, it is often necessary to help relatives deal with their fear of escalating the problem and their worries about totally losing control of a fragile situation, that may need to be confronted and shared before any solutions can be tried.

*Themes*

The groups that I have been involved with have had a variety of themes but there is usually some consistency. These can be grouped into issues that commonly arise. With carers of the long-term mentally ill there is a tendency at the beginning of a group to focus on relatively external issues, such as the need for information, the role of medication, current intractable problems. There is normally a focus on the stigma of mental illness in the family and how difficult it can be to explain convincingly to neighbours and friends why a healthy-looking son, daughter or spouse stays at home and does not participate in ordinary community activities. The burden of the caring process, particularly as it continues over many years, and the bad experiences often found in the early days of the illness are compared. Later on, as a group develops, the more internal and negative emotional themes begin to surface. These include the guilt, grief, the necessity of changing expectations and having to come to terms with the reality of 'another person in his body'.

There are particular worries about the vulnerability of patients to exploitation by more competent friends or strangers. Sexual exploitation is a worry for some, together with a general concern as to how to handle the fact of the sexual activity of adult sons and daughters. Other kinds of exploitation are also a concern, that patients will be robbed or conned or be otherwise unable to handle a variety of social situations. These worries can be the central reason why carers are not able to allow patients to act as autonomous adults, sometimes even to the extent of not allowing a patient on the bus or to cross a road alone. Often the patients' confidence in their abilities will have receded and the group can discuss how to change these ideas and how to maximize patient functioning despite continuing, accurately perceived, levels of disability.

Other themes tend to include the long-term impact of schizophrenia on the patient and relatives' lifestyle, the loss of hope and the loss of 'quiet retirement'. Finally there is always a worry about what the future will hold and who will continue to provide high levels of care for a patient when relatives no longer can. Given that facilities for care in the community continue to be very piecemeal and dependent upon local initiatives, these worries are often all too reasonable.

### Ending a group

Not all groups will have an ending but it may be worth discussing options with members about the sort of contact they may prefer in the future. Some groups will have a life of their own and may continue without a facilitator. To some this might be a preferred option or even an aim – that a facilitator's role is to enable a group not to need one. The group discussed above did not want meetings to continue after about 18 months. However, relatives did want to feel that they could contact staff easily at *non*-crisis times and said that continued family sessions which included the patient, every six weeks or so, would be useful.

Some continuity, even if only the offer of a telephone number, is an essential aspect of intervening with relatives in this way and is not abused. Such a lifeline is a reassurance that help can be activated easily and that the continuing burden of care that relatives face will not be left to them alone.

### Conclusions

Running a facilitated group requires commitment, continuity and an ability to let the group build up trust, cohesion and social links, while helping members to try out constructive efforts for change. This latter I would see as the most important function and the main justification for a facilitator's presence. Whilst other groups may also manage these functions, the actual process of change may be harder to achieve without the possibility of an objective view which is a facilitator's asset. In running a group it has been found that the easier it is to establish the common ground between members the easier it is to enable the group to function optimally, engage all members and offer help. Where there are large differences, for example, different diagnoses, disparity in relationships (e.g. only one spouse in a group full of parents), it will be harder to offer anything constructive to these 'outsiders' (Kuipers *et al.* 1989). Groups of any kind also assume a basic level of cognitive and social skills, together with motivation and ability to get out of the house to a central meeting place. Not all relatives will have these advantages and although if they attend such groups can be of considerable benefit to members, it has to be borne in mind that there will always be people who cannot or will not engage and who will need other channels of intervention.

## References

Anderson C.M., Hogarty G., Bayer T. *et al.* (1984) EE & Social Networks in parents of schizophrenic patients. *British Journal of Psychiatry* 144, 247–255.

Avebury K. (1986) *Volunteers in Mental Health.* The Volunteer Centre, in association with the Mental Health Foundation, London.

Berkowitz R., Eberlein-Fries R., Kuipers L. & Leff J. (1984) Educating relatives about schizophrenia. *Schizophrenia Bulletin* 10, 418–429.

Ferris P.A. & Marshall C.A. (1987) A model project for families of the chronically mentally ill. *Social Work* 32, 110–114.

Hooley J. & Hahlweg K. (1986) The marriages & interaction patterns of depressed patients and their spouses: comparison of high and low EE dyads. In Goldstein M.J., Hand L. & Hahlweg K. (eds) *Treatment of Schizophrenia: Family Assessment & Intervention.* Springer, Berlin.

Hubschmidt T. & Zemp M. (1989) Interactions in high and low EE families. *Social Psychiatry and Psychiatric Epidemiology* 24, 113–119.

Kottgen C., Sonnichsen I., Mollenhasser K. *et al.* (1984) Group therapy with the families of schizophrenic patients: results of the Hamberg Camberwell Family Interview Study III. *International Journal of Family Psychiatry* 5, 84–94.

Kuipers L. & Bebbington P. (1990) *Working in Partnership: Clinician and Carers in the Management of Longstanding Mental Illness.* Heinemann Medical Books, Oxford.

Kuipers L., MacCarthy B., Hurry J. & Harper R. (1989) Counselling the relatives of the long-term adult mentally ill II: A low cost supportive model. *British Journal of Psychiatry* 154, 775–782.

Kuipers L., Sturgeon D., Berkowitz R. & Leff J.P. (1983) Characteristics of expressed emotion; its relationship to speech and looking in schizophrenic patients and their relatives. *British Journal of Clinical Psychology* 22, 257–264.

Leff J.P., Berkowitz R., Eberlein-Fries R. *et al.* (1988) *Schizophrenia Notes for Relatives and Friends.* Surbiton National Schizophrenic Fellowship, Surbiton, Surrey.

Leff J.P., Berkowitz R., Shavit N. *et al.* (1989) A trial of family therapy v. a relatives' group for schizophrenia. *British Journal of Psychiatry* 154, 58–66.

Leff J.P., Kuipers L., Berkowitz R. *et al.* (1982) A controlled trial of social intervention in the families of schizophrenic patients. *British Journal of Psychiatry* 144, 121–134.

Leff J. & Vaughn C. (1985) *Expressed Emotion in Families.* Guilford Press, London.

MacCarthy B. (1988) The role of relatives. In Lavender A. & Holloway F. (eds) *Community Care in Practice.* John Wiley, Chichester.

MacCarthy B., Kuipers L., Hurry J., Harper R. & Le Sage A. (1989) Counselling the relatives of the long-term adult mentally ill I: Evaluation of the impact on relatives and patients. *British Journal of Psychiatry* 154, 768–775.

Smith J.V. & Birchwood M.J. (1985) *Understanding Schizophrenia.* Health Promotion Unit, West Birmingham Health Authority Mental Health Series.

Smith J.V. & Birchwood M.J. (1987) Specific and non-specific effects of educational interventions with families of schizophrenic patients. *British Journal of Psychiatry* 150, 643–652.

# B. Voluntary Self-Help Groups

## JERRY WESTALL

In considering the perceptions of relatives and patients as regards voluntary and self-help groups, one needs to bear in mind the assembly of people, of whom I am representative, who work for self-help groups, yet do not have the illness/problem which is the *raison d'être* of the organization we are working for. In the main, we are not sufferers, relatives or carers.

The bulk of the staff of the National Schizophrenia Fellowship (NSF) are in this category. We are the intermediaries, possibly more detached than the members, but, in a sense, suspect to everyone. From one angle we are viewed as people who could not possibly know about something we have never experienced ourselves. We do not feel where the shoe pinches. From another point of view we are not quite acceptable to the statutory services as being the equivalent of other professions. I have heard the 'intermediaries' being referred to as 'fourth class professionals' coming after doctors (first), nurses (second), social workers (third).

Two observations one could make on this situation are that reliance on empathy is important for an intermediary who has the advantage of being acquainted with a wide variety of experiences (some dissimilar) conveyed by those 'at the receiving end'. The other factor is that the expertise in a particular area built up by intermediaries gradually over the years can become a formidable source of information and knowledge.

A friend of mine observed some years ago that voluntary organizations are becoming a significant area of 'opposition' in this country. It is apparent that recognition of the definite power that resides within the voluntary sector is not always welcomed by the administration. However, if the power is based on membership, respect for that source of influence is also evident.

With the NSF the constituency is mainly one of carers although the organization is keen to develop self help among those who have experienced schizophrenia and are now stabilized and living in the community. The organization started some 20 years ago with a parents' plea for the gathering together of those who had been through the trauma of seeing a relative develop schizophrenia and had witnessed the lack of help in coping with the experience.

The value of self-help groups to relatives (very often mothers of the afflicted person with the illness) is that there is a source of established information and support which is not controlled by the authorities. Not only is there a sympathetic shoulder to cry on provided by a person who understands what you are going through, simply because they have known similar trauma to your own; but with schizophrenia, there is a means of combating the mythology – still sadly present to this day – of the supposed parental (usually maternal) responsibility for the illness.

To add to this support comes the regional and/or national organization run full time by intermediaries (the staff) who assist with empowerment. Staff can improve the situation both as regards individual problems and for the wider constituency of schizophrenia sufferers and their relatives. The position for those who have experienced schizophrenia is influenced by the National Association for Mental Health (MIND) who have for a number of years presented users as the group needing empowerment. For those who have experienced schizophrenia, the knowledge of the effect of the illness and the medication prescribed to deal with symptoms is very varied. It is mistaken to believe that only sentiments encompassing antipsychiatry and opposition to medication are apparent among users. The NSF has encouraged the emergence of a valuable semiautonomous grouping – the Voices forum – which is establishing groups around the country to present a balanced approach to self help for users.

One member of Voices gave me an account of how he views the support provided:

> I come to the socials every two weeks. It helps. I attend the forums ever two months, as well. That's a business meeting with an outside speaker . . . I think there's biological, psychological, mental, spiritual ways in which schizophrenia affects different people, different ways of getting schizophrenia. I see so many people claiming this, that and the other but they cannot seem to relate that its that for them but something else for someone else. They seem to think that what they have is what everyone else has, but I can see it's different things for different people.

This particular individual's approach to schizophrenia in fact included the view that his family was partly responsible. It is inevitable that among those with schizophrenia some have experienced poor parenting which has not helped. From the carers' point of view, the word user can mean that their own role as 'user of services' is disregarded.

However, alternative words have their drawbacks. The description 'sufferer' can be regarded as reducing the status of an individual for all time to that of supplicant; even 'patient' and 'client' may denote a relationship to medical or social authority portraying the recipient as a passive and powerless individual. So often words such as these do not have prejudicial overtones in the mind of this author but may be seen in such a light by others. Perhaps the interests of users and carers cannot be represented by one organization but clearly a measure of cooperation between users and carers over the issue of schizophrenia is important for all concerned.

When asked how best the NSF could help with the training of community psychiatric nurses, social workers or psychiatrists, the immediate response is drawn from my own experience. It is advice that has been given and taken with declared gratitude by senior civil servants and a Minister at the Department of Health: it is to attend meetings of the self-help groups, as many varied meetings as possible. Certainly it is worth seeing how a successful group operates on several levels of self help in fund raising, innovative projects and local and national publicity, but also illuminating is the experience of a struggling group, people trying to get themselves together after the shock of destroyed dreams for a loved one where suffering of great intensity leaves little strength for organization. Any organization has clashes of personality and approach but few people are more vulnerable than the exhausted carers of those who can be a trial at times for the saintliest person. Although self-help groups are not for everyone it is helpful to know that they are available if needed. They can be an important means of coping and learning to cope. It seems that for those with a relative suffering severe illness they can be particularly important.

In this respect it is interesting to note that the membership of the Association to Combat Huntington's Chorea is about the same numerically as the NSF, whereas the incidence of Huntington's chorea is about a tenth that of schizophrenia. Huntington's chorea is a serious long-term progressive illness. Because it is an autosomal dominant genetic disease (50/50 chance of inheritance from male or female parent), this makes it more of a family problem than even schizophrenia.

Both the Association and NSF have clear constitutional regulations ensuring that control of the organization remains with relatives. The advantage of this is that management is with the elected members of the organization and although intermediaries have a certain leeway within agreed policy outlines, there is not a danger of a professional take-over – which is how some carers view the organization of MIND. Over the last 25 years there has been a huge increase in the number of self-help groups in this country; estimates of local branches exceed 25 000. In health fields particularly, where emotional support for families is provided, professionals have gradually recognized their value.

In the 1960s only a few academics and pro-

fessionals saw self-help groups as part of the solution to problems. Nowadays, it is common to find, at a minimum, lip service being given to the value of such groups. Possibly Sir Roy Griffiths and the Department of Health are mainly responsible for this. Griffiths gave authoritative backing to the voluntary sector and the Department of Health has been a major funder of many self-help initiatives.

Griffiths (1988) made it clear in *Community Care: Agenda for Action* that:

> A failure to give proper levels of support to informal carers not only reduces their own quality of life and that of the relative or friend they care for, but it is also potentially inefficient as it can lead to less personally appropriate care being offered. Positive action is therefore needed to encourage the delivery of more flexible support, which takes account of how best to support and maintain the role of the informal carer.

He also outlined the variety of roles the voluntary sector has in addition to the direct provision of services. These were:

1 Self-help support group.
2 Information source/source of expertise.
3 Befriending agency.
4 Advocate for individuals.
5 Constructive critic of service providers.
6 Public educator.
7 Campaigns.

Several other references in the Griffiths report are significant and Griffiths draws from the evidence of the Department of Health and Social Security to the House of Commons Social Services Committee (HC 13 1984–85) in locating an 'official statement of principles and objectives of community care' as including the wish 'to give support and relief to informal carers (family, friends, and neighbours) coping with the stress of caring for a dependent person'.

This element of the caring process was taken up in the Community Care White Paper and become formalized into the National Health Service and Community Care Act. The Minister for Health, Virginia Bottomley, in the debate in which the then Secretary of State, Kenneth Clarke, announced the phasing of the community care policies, emphasized the particular reference to 'the importance of carers. We are funding caring organisations to the tune of about £100 000 this year. They are deeply involved in our consultation on guidance and the implementation of the important work' (Hansard 18 July 1990 Col 1052). Clarke had previously reiterated the position that 'beyond anything provided by the statutory bodies, it is the families and the friends who carry the main burden of coping with the problems of the elderly and the disabled' (Col 1008).

The self-help groups themselves are varied, although overall there is an increased capacity to deal with relevant issues. The mainstream groups who in the health field usually accept the conventional wisdom of the acknowledged authorities on the matter in question are part of the accepted model of health. Collaboration between professionals (especially younger ones) and self-help groups has been increasing. A clear majority of professionals now favour self-help groups and have followed pioneers like John Wing in the area of schizophrenia with their own support and encouragement.

Alternative health groupings have also come into the frame. With schizophrenia, the Schizophrenia Association of Great Britain tends in this direction. Where people are desperate for a cure for a severe illness there is a tendency for sometimes sincere exponents of diets or psychotherapies to acquire the adherence of vulnerable people. Among the sincere and honest if sometimes misguided proponents may be charlatans or quack remedies exploiting the suffering of the distressed. Such areas of 'self-help' need fair attention; for voluntary organizations the risk of being viewed as an unreliable or 'crank' outfit if they should get heavily involved in suspect remedies is something that needs to be carefully borne in mind.

Credibility for voluntary organizations is very important. It can fluctuate quite rapidly when certain people leave or join a group, but 'street knowledge' of the standing of varying groups is fairly accessible to professionals who take a reasonable interest.

A drawback in the organization of self-help groups is that they tend to give the field to those with the time and inclination to establish a presence. This means that a white, middle-class bias in membership can be widely evident. It is always important to try and involve all sections of society in any self-help group, but with schizophrenia it is even more crucial since the high representation of people from the black community with a diagnosis of schizophrenia in the population is such a troubling finding of recent research. It could be that this is an area for self-help groups where a specific push from the intermediaries is called for in attempting to promote the value of the voluntary organization among ethnic minority groups. The NSF has made a small start in this direction but a great deal more needs to be done.

A value of an organized self-help group is to provide a constituency for research. This can lead to work of value to the collectivity. Social research is aided greatly by having this public assembly of interested people. The weakness of this research, however, is that an unrepresentative sample is being utilized and thus ethnic and class bias may be incorporated into research findings.

Schizophrenia, described by Marjorie Wallace (1985) as the 'forgotten illness', has by means of fairly shrill whistle blowing made sure it is not now ignored. In the circumstances legitimate tactics, in the main, were used to achieve this end result. The media assisted in increasing a general awareness of the illness. None the less, the translation of a complex medical and social matter such as schizophrenia into a form which has impact and interest to a reasonably informed public is difficult and can cause unintended problems.

The NSF and SANE (Schizophrenia: A National Emergency), together with the grouping of professionals chaired by Malcolm Weller named Concern, have together built a high public profile for schizophrenia. Sometimes the impression conveyed can be disadvantageous to those with a diagnosis of schizophrenia when trying to find a job, accommodation or a friend. There is a responsibility in constantly emphasizing the small number of people with schizophrenia who are suicidal or violent, and a variety of symptoms in those who suffer from it. Clearly the opinion that mental hospitals need to be maintained for long-term mentally ill people is worthy of serious consideration, together with the requirement that one should only close hospitals when alternative provision is established. It is a line of argument that has struck a chord of concurrence with a wide public. The Mental Health Foundation in a survey of 100 representative members of Parliament (reflecting political parties, urban/rural, age range, etc.) found that 56% of the sample favoured halting the closure of mental hospitals (Mental Health Foundation 1990).

The reality of the media is that factors such as 'watchability' cannot be overlooked if the object is to obtain television attention. The main enemy of the media is a yawn. The role of the media is further discussed in Chapter 22.

The emphasis on the failures of community care for those with mental health problems was valid in the main; it was as relevant as exposing the scandals within hospitals which shocked many people a few years ago. There is evidence which suggests media coverage can induce authorities to provide much needed resources; pressure of public opinion can when stimulated exert particular weight in areas such as the mentally ill homeless population or for those in prison. The end result of media coverage is visibility. You are known about and in some respects obtain more clout and credibility. Mental illness, we are told, has moved up the political agenda. From this position we need to emphasize that more adequate resources need to follow, otherwise community care for those with psychiatric problems will be discredited in the public mind. Voluntary organizations can be seen as part of the strategy to induce sufficient funding from the Treasury.

On balance, self-help groups benefit their members by being more visible. They are then in a position to give more people support in coping with problems since there is greater knowledge of one's existence. There is a great fund of information within self-help groups and they can become a primary source of knowledge on specific subjects. The best of the self-help groups are highly respected by informed professionals.

The findings of an opinion poll carried out by ICM of 1478 adults aged 15+ in 103 randomly selected constituencies, interviewed between 22 and 23 June 1990, are highly significant. The poll was carried out for *The Guardian*, the NSF and SANE (see *The Guardian* 23 July 1990 and *NSF News* August 1990) and indicated that 79% of respondents thought mental health was a specific health issue that required increased government spending (compare this with 77% wanting increased expenditure on heart disease and 63% on AIDS). Whilst 55% of respondents felt that people with mental illnesses should live in the community and be treated as outpatients if treatment is required, 81% thought the government was not providing enough care and support for the mentally ill in the community.

Ideally, at some future date, self-help groups should be able to persuade a body such as the Health Education Council to mount a campaign with the same strength as the one on AIDS for the area of mental health. That mental health is an area of controversy and dispute is no excuse for not having done so already. Since community care involves the public in its exercise, public education bodies should have the responsibility to inform and advise the general public of the nature of mental illness.

### References

Griffiths R. (1988) *Community Care: Agenda for Action* Sec 4.3. HMSO, London.

MHF (1990) *Political Perceptions of Mental Health*. MHF, London.

Wallace M. (1985) *The Forgotten Illness*. Reprinted by Times Newspapers Ltd 1987, London.

# Chapter 36
# Looking Forwards

## J.P. LEFF

We work in an era in which biological psychiatry is in the ascendant. New imaging techniques offer fascinating glimpses into the structure and function of the living brain. The number of known receptors in cortical neurones is increasing exponentially and we are beginning to grasp the complexity of their interrelationships. The sense of excitement and impending discovery generated by these advances is epitomized in the declaration by the National Institute of Mental Health in the USA that this is the Decade of the Brain. At the same time, research in molecular genetics has been rewarded by several Nobel prizes in medicine. There have been two recent claims to have identified a gene linked with schizophrenia and although these have not been substantiated, a Nobel prize in psychiatry is not a remote possibility.

Social psychiatry is not invested with the glamour of glittering new machinery or breakthroughs in basic science. Rather there has been slow but steady progress on its central theme: the study of relationships between patients and their social environment. The salient problem in this endeavour is the understanding of relationships between people and the ways in which they can influence psychiatric conditions. This does not preclude an acceptance of a biological basis to some of the conditions studied. It is very unfortunate that there has been a tendency to polarization in psychiatry, with people occupying the extreme positions denying any validity to the concepts of those they see as their opponents. A rapprochement can be found between social and biological psychiatry, but it requires open-mindedness on the part of the adherents of both schools, as they must work together to find a common language. This is not, solely, a matter of communication: concepts need to be developed that link phenomena at a biological level with phenomena at a social level. The term 'arousal' has been pressed into service for this function in the past, but neither psychophysiologists nor social psychiatrists have been satisfied with it. A wider range of terms needs to be developed that refers to processes linking the biochemical and physiological with the psychological.

Within social psychiatry, measurement techniques have been increasingly refined. Areas which began somewhat simplistically, such as life events, have now reached a high level of sophistication. Approaches have been made to delineating the interrelationships between measures of different aspects of the social environment, for example life events and relatives' Expressed Emotion. It is by no means easy to gain an understanding of the complex social systems which surround an individual. The direction and strength of some of the social vectors operating in these systems are being explored by studies which employ social interventions, such as Newpin for depression and work with the families of schizophrenic patients. These studies have not only furthered our theoretical understanding of the social forces that play on the individual, but have led to the development of new psychosocial treatments. This is evidently a most promising area of social psychiatry which is likely to produce more clinical benefits in the future.

This century has been characterized by unprecedented mass movements of peoples. The remarkable changes occurring in both Eastern and Western Europe will undoubtedly increase these migratory moments. The upsurge in psychiatric morbidity which appears to be an inevitable accompaniment of such migrations remains unexplained. Biological psychiatrists are seeking an answer in the physical environment, but there is vast scope here for social psychiatrists using epidemiological and individual interviewing techniques and drawing on the insights provided by transcultural psychiatry. Benefits that might be gained are reduction in morbidity, improvement of services, and possibly even clues to the aetiology of schizophrenia.

The combination of epidemiological surveys and in-depth interviewing has yielded valuable results in the past, as evidenced by much of the work presented in this book. They will continue to be the technical mainstay of social psychiatry, although further refinements in the design of trials of psychosocial treatments can be expected.

It is ironic that as families get smaller and smaller to the point of extinction in the west, there is a growing awareness of the importance of social support for the maintenance of mental health. The global concept of social support is not particularly useful: research in this area has already revealed extensive differences between the needs for and nature of support of healthy people and those of long-stay schizophrenic patients in institutions. Detailed analyses are needed of the transactions between people that maintain mental health and prevent psychiatric illness. These will draw social psychiatry into the ambit of individual psychology and the dynamics of interpersonal relationships. At the beginning of the book we traced the development of social psychiatry in the UK and showed that its origins were closely intertwined with the therapeutic community movement and psychotherapy. This link, though varying in intensity over the years, remains intact. In the future it could provide the basis for fruitful collaboration, leading to a deeper understanding of what happens between people in the process of healing the sick mind.

# Index

*Index*